Biochips and Medical Imaging

Biochips and Medical Imaging

Adam de la Zerda and Shan Xiang Wang

Stanford University, CA
USA

WILEY

This edition first published 2022

Registered Office
John Wiley & Sons, Inc., 111 River Street, Hoboken, NJ 07030, USA

Editorial Office
111 River Street, Hoboken, NJ 07030, USA

For details of our global editorial offices, customer services, and more information about Wiley products visit us at www.wiley.com.

Wiley also publishes its books in a variety of electronic formats and by print-on-demand. Some content that appears in standard print versions of this book may not be available in other formats.

Library of Congress Cataloging-in-Publication Data

Names: De la Zerda, Adam, author. | Wang, Shan X., author.
Title: Biochips and medical imaging / Adam de la Zerda, Shan Xiang Wang, Stanford University, California, United States.
Description: First edition. | Hoboken, NJ, USA : John Wiley & Sons, Inc., 2021. | Includes bibliographical references and index.
Identifiers: LCCN 2021003996 (print) | LCCN 2021003997 (ebook) | ISBN 9781118910504 (hardback) | ISBN 9781118910634 (adobe pdf) | ISBN 9781118910481 (epub)
Subjects: LCSH: Biochips. | Diagnostic imaging.
Classification: LCC R857.B5 D4 2021 (print) | LCC R857.B5 (ebook) | DDC 616.07/54–dc23
LC record available at https://lccn.loc.gov/2021003996
LC ebook record available at https://lccn.loc.gov/2021003997

Cover Design: Wiley
Cover Image: © luchschen/Getty Images

Set in 9.5/12.5pt STIXTwoText by Straive, Pondicherry, India

In Loving Memory of
Professor Sanjiv Sam Gambhir, MD, PhD
23 November 1962–18 July 2020

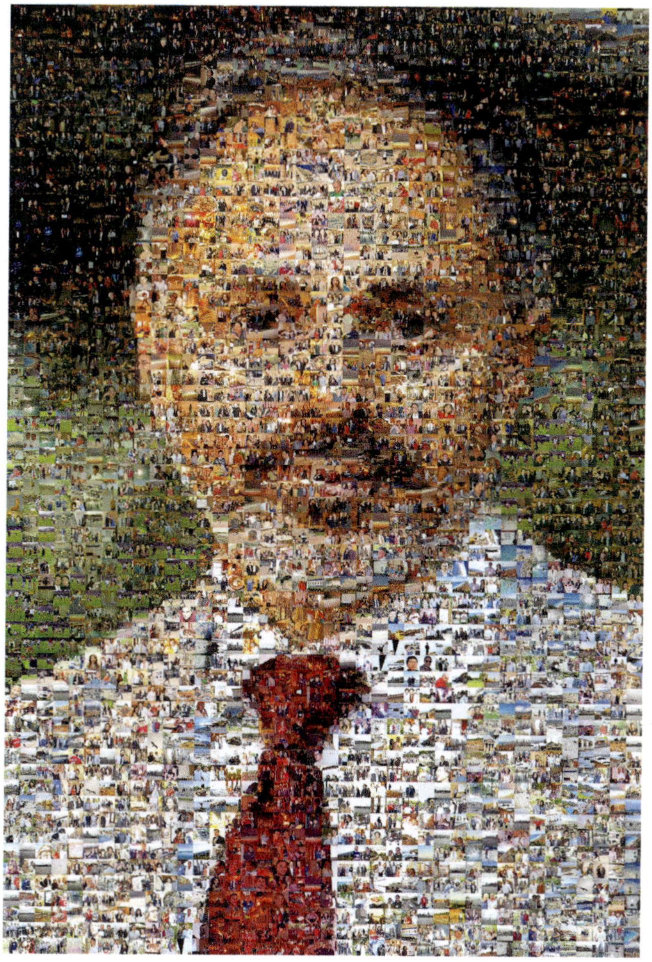

Image Courtesy of Drs. Sandip Biswal and Edward Graves, First Appeared in https://web.stanford.edu/group/radweb/cgi-bin/ssg/

Contents

Foreword

Dr. Sanjiv Sam Gambhir was a pioneer in the field of molecular imaging and early cancer detection and an outstanding mentor and advisor to hundreds. His legacy lives on with the mark he made in precision medicine and molecular imaging, his hundreds of manuscripts and many patents, and in those who benefited from his passion, dedication, and hard work as his mentees. As one of his mentees (PhD 2000–2004), I continue to be influenced by his approach to science in my own work at the forefront of developing iPSC biology as a platform for improving cardiovascular health.

Sam's dedication to the field, ability to bring together different scientific disciplines, and emphasis on collaboration among departments and schools paved the way to innovative and decisive advancements. We remember him for his impact in the field as the "Father of Molecular Imaging."

Sam was known for his revolutionary work in developing positron emission tomography (PET) reporter genes to enable early cancer detection and disease characterization. In this way, he hoped we would one day achieve precisely tailored cancer treatments. He also developed microbubbles for cancer detection and was a visionary who revolutionized the field of immunodiagnostics. His work always pointed toward precision medicine as the ultimate goal post, with a push toward early disease (cancer) detection beyond the conventional focus on late-stage disease. Beyond trailblazing the fields of molecular imaging, Sam's work also led to a paradigm shift in how to consider disease research and treatment by redirecting our focus toward early cancer detection that may save the lives of millions in the years to come with our growing ability to tailor optimal treatment for individual patients.

Sam's dedication to his work was infectious. He convinced us that early detection of disease like cancer was the best approach, and inspired us to strive for making that a scientific and clinical possibility. The hundreds of trainees, mentees, and collaborators across disciplines and institutions are carrying on his vision to create a world in which cancer can be detected before any classic symptoms or deterioration in health manifest themselves, at a time when intervention and treatment will prove to be the most crucial not only in timing but also in outcome. Not only will far fewer patients die, but many fewer patients and families will suffer long-term health and other consequences because they are treated in time, thanks to Sam's vision.

This book allows you, the student, to learn about a different discipline. It will provide you with knowledge and new ways of thinking that will inform and improve your own work. It is intended to lead you to innovate new ideas on your own. We hope that you will help carry on the tradition of interdisciplinary, big picture thinking that Dr. Sanjiv Sam Gambhir was known for and has continued to inspire in us.

Sincerely,
Joseph C. Wu, MD, PhD
Director, Stanford Cardiovascular Institute
Simon H. Stertzer, MD, Professor of Medicine & Radiology

Preface

This textbook covers state-of-the-art biosensors, biochips, and imaging modalities that are either extensively practiced as standard care or widely disseminated in scientific literature. These subjects will be studied systematically and holistically in the context of human biology and physiology, biomarkers, disease diagnostics, and disease management. The students and other readers will gain comprehensive and foundational knowledge in the broad areas of bio-diagnostics and medical imaging.

The book is organized into three sections by and large. It begins with a biology section consisting of five chapters: cell biology, biological lab techniques, human physiology (the nervous system, the circulatory system, the endocrine system, the lymphatic system, and the immune system), cancer, and cardiovascular diseases. These topics are particularly useful to the students who are less familiar with biology and physiology but want to delve into biochips and medical imaging as part of their majors or research interests. The contents on the lymphatic system and the immune system are conducive to studying infectious diseases. The biology section serves as a compelling steppingstone for the readers to explore the biochip and medical imaging sections in great depth and convenience.

The biochip section consists of seven chapters and covers a wide spectrum of bioassays with analytes ranging from nucleic acids (e.g. DNA and RNA), proteins (e.g. antigens and antibodies), to cells. Many of these assays manifest in the form of biosensors and biochips. The three chapters on DNA chips and sequencing, next-generation sequencing (NGS) and FET-based biochips, and protein assays and chips, respectively, form the "bread and butter" of the modern-day methods and tool sets in biotechnology and diagnostics industries. The next three chapters on label-free affinity-based biosensors, magneto-nanosensor biochips, and microfluidic chips for capturing circulating tumor cells (CTCs), respectively, represent quintessential examples of emerging biochip development, which eventually lead to nascent and/or burgeoning products. The section culminates with a chapter on molecular diagnostics where the fundamental concepts of diagnostic sensitivity, diagnostic specificity, positive predictive value, negative predictive value, receiver operating characteristics (ROC), among others, are presented. These are essential to the practice of clinical diagnostics, medical imaging, and disease treatment.

The medical imaging section consists of six chapters, focusing on both conventional in vivo medical imaging and molecular imaging modalities. The two chapters on magnetic resonance imaging (MRI) and radionuclide imaging expand on some of the most widely used imaging modalities in today's hospitals. The next two chapters, fluorescence and Raman imaging and optical coherence tomography, belong to the domain of optical imaging. These optical imaging modalities have gained increased prominence and wider applications over recent years. The next chapter covers photoacoustic imaging that marries optics with acoustics. This imaging mechanism can be traced back to A. G. Bell's 1880 patent on photophone, although its commercialization is still in its infancy. The last chapter on imaging controls and concepts put the imaging section altogether by espousing the indispensable control experiments when formulating biological hypothesis and study design in any medical imaging modality. Such considerations are even more critical in multimodality imaging. The considerations of signal to noise ratio, sensitivity, and specificity are critical to medical imaging, with interesting parallels in molecular diagnostics of the biochip section.

Importantly, each chapter of this textbook ends with relevant problems for practicing or examination, which the instructors and teaching assistants at Stanford have composed for their own classes. They should be quite helpful and illustrative to the instructors and students at other institutions.

Each section in the biochips and imaging portions of the book emphasizes the physical basis of the technology as well as its medical applications in real world. No prerequisites are required for most readers. Of course, basic knowledge of electromagnetism, optics, chemistry, thermodynamics, or human biology will be complementary.

The textbook is written primarily for the graduate students fulfilling their breadth/depth requirements in Physical Science and Technology; the upper-level undergraduate students in Electrical Engineering, Bioengineering, Materials Science, Applied Physics, Mechanical Engineering, Chemical Engineering, Premed Majors, etc.; and anyone with an interest in diagnostic and therapeutic technologies. The book will also be useful to scientists and engineers in the industry who desire to review or learn more about medical diagnostic technologies.

Although great efforts have been made to write and edit the book, there are inevitably some errors, typos, and even misconceptions undetected by the authors and editors. If you notice any shortcomings, or simply have a comment, please contact the authors at sxwang@ee.stanford.edu and adlz@stanford.edu, who will be very grateful.

This book is suitable as a textbook for a one-semester or one-quarter course on biochips and medical imaging, together or separately. It has worked quite well at Stanford. Obviously, an instructor may choose to use some chapters and add their own supplemental materials. The authors do have solutions to the problem sets that can be shared on an informal basis.

COVID-19 pandemic is still looming large as we are putting the finishing touches to this book. It has challenged all of us in numerous ways and taught us many valuable lessons. One takeaway message is that "chance favors the prepared mind." We sincerely hope that this book will also facilitate interested readers to appreciate an explosive body of literature on the diagnostics of COVID-19 (e.g. Weissleder et al., *Science Translational Medicine* 12, eabc1931, 2020; Ravi et al., *Biosensors and Bioelectronics* 165, 112454, 2020) and the world will be better prepared for the next pandemic.

Adam de la Zerda, PhD
Associate Professor of Structural Biology, and by courtesy, Electrical Engineering

Shan Xiang Wang, PhD
Leland T. Edwards Professor in the School of Engineering
Professor of Materials Science and Engineering, Electrical Engineering, and by courtesy, Radiology

Acknowledgments

The writing of this book is a substantial endeavor, which would not have been possible without the help and support of many individuals. We wish to thank Nuvia Pacheco and Lily Friebel at Stanford University, who have ably and tirelessly gathered all the copyright permissions for the numerous figures and illustrations contained in this textbook. Identifying and chasing down the leads to some dormant copyright owners to obtain use consents seemed like the mission impossible, but they were able to persist and persevere. They also fielded long lists of inquiries from the publisher and kept the authors organized. We also wish to thank Dr. Gennifer (Genna) Smith, who proofread most chapters, located many alternative figures, or recreated a large number of figures when necessary. "A picture is worth a thousand words" – the numerous and polished figures and illustrations throughout this book have made it more pleasing to the eyes and more straightforward to teach and learn. Of course, the original creators of these figures and illustrations are gratefully acknowledged, and their copyrights are credited individually where they appear in the book.

The chapters in this book evolved from the lecture notes and problem sets developed for a graduate course on biochips and medical imaging at Stanford University, California. We are deeply grateful to the significant contributions from our teaching assistants, particularly Dawson Wong, Umit Yoruk, Gennifer (Genna) Smith, Elliott SoRelle, Adi Gani, Edwin Yuan, Sarah Divel, Jung-Rok Lee, and Bryce Yao, among others. Each chapter is generally self-contained and allows the readers to follow its content without undue interruptions. Some technical papers (and web pages) are listed at the end of each chapter, which are cited for relatively specialized topics and should be studied optionally. We try to be fair in citing the right papers for original contributions, but sometimes we cite references just for convenience and easy access to students.

The authors are indebted to Stanford University that has provided an atmosphere conducive to productive work and scholarship. In particular, the late Professor Sanjiv Sam Gambhir, MD, PhD, was the doctorate advisor and mentor to Adam de la Zerda, and he was a pivotal collaborator to Shan Wang for over 15 years including the vital and successive leaderships of the Center for Cancer Nanotechnology Excellence Focused on Therapy Responses (CCNE-TR), the Center for Cancer Nanotechnology Excellence and Translation (CCNE-T), and the Center for Cancer Nanotechnology Excellence for Translational Diagnostics (CCNE-TD). Both authors have benefited tremendously from Sam's extraordinary vision, insights, energy, network, and working style and are forever grateful for everything he stood for. We thank Professor Joseph C. Wu, MD, PhD, for his support over many years and for providing a very moving foreword as a tribute to Sam. We are also grateful to our research group members and alumni who have contributed significantly to our scholarship over the years, some of which are reflected in this book.

Both authors wish to thank Daniela Bez and Devi Ignasi from Wiley for their professionalism and assistance during the production of this book and for pushing us past the finish line.

Last but not the least, we wish to thank our spouses and families for their inspiration and unwavering support through the ups and downs in our academic careers. It has been an awesome journey.

Adam de la Zerda, PhD
Associate Professor of Structural Biology, and by courtesy, Electrical Engineering

Shan Xiang Wang, PhD
Leland T. Edwards Professor in the School of Engineering
Professor of Materials Science and Engineering, Electrical Engineering, and by courtesy, Radiology

1

Cell Biology

1.1 Cell Biology Introduction

A study of the human body can be approached from many different levels. At a broad level, the human body consists of several systems (e.g. digestive, nervous, and endocrine). Each one of these systems is composed of functional units called organs (e.g. heart, brain, and liver). Similarly, each organ is composed of different tissues that perform different tasks. Tissues are then composed of cells that perform different functions (e.g. myocytes, neurons, and stem cells). The **cell** is the smallest unit of life in the human body. Cells are composed of smaller functional units called organelles (e.g. nucleus and mitochondria). These organelles perform various tasks to keep the cell alive and functional. On an even smaller scale, cells and organelles contain biomolecules (e.g. proteins and DNA).

The cell is the basic structural and functional unit of all organisms. The human body is composed of about 10 trillion cells. Cell biology focuses on the study of cells, including their structure and function, organelles, interaction with other cells, and life cycle (including division and death). There are many types of cells that are typically named according to their functioning, e.g. nerve cells, muscle cells, bone cells, gland cells, reproductive cells (sperm and ovum), and blood cells (including red blood cells, lymphocytes, and neutrophils).

1.2 Cell Structure

Human cells range in size from 7.5 to 150 μm. Human cells are eukaryotic, meaning they have a nucleus. Although the structure of eukaryotic cells can be very complex, their three basic components are the membrane, cytoplasm, and nucleus. A typical eukaryotic cell structure is seen in Figure 1.1. The membrane is an envelope that surrounds the cell and serves as a protective barrier (blue in Figure 1.1a). The cytoplasm (yellow in Figure 1.1a) is the interior of the cell and contains the cell organelles. The nucleus (violet in Figure 1.1a) contains the genetic information of the cell. Figure 1.1b is a microscopic image of human epithelial cells. The distinction between the membrane, cytoplasm, and nucleus is clear in this image.

Biochips and Medical Imaging, First Edition. Adam de la Zerda and Shan Xiang Wang.

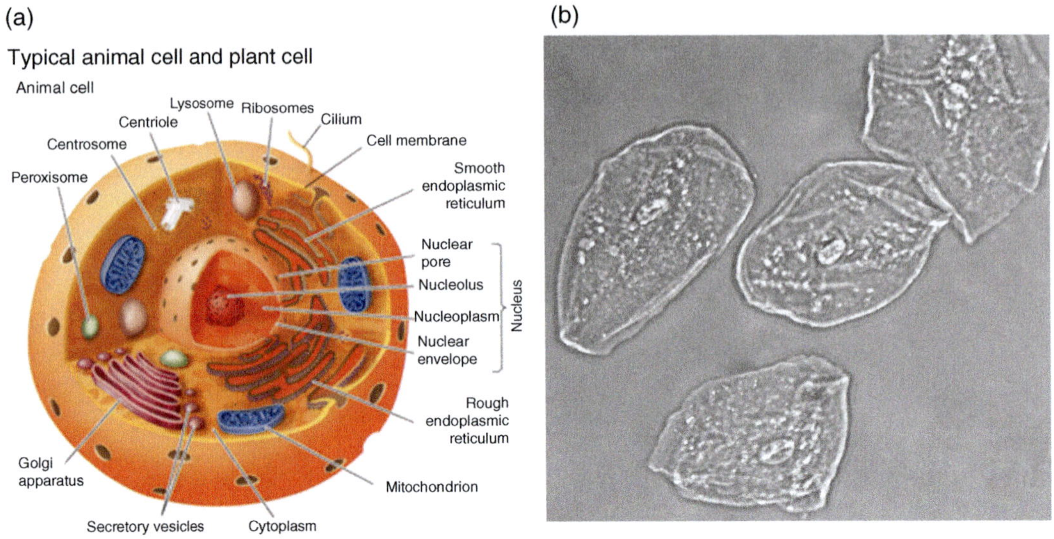

Figure 1.1 (a) Eukaryotic cell schematic. (*Source:* Reprinted with permission from Encyclopedia Britannica, © 2018 by Encyclopedia Britannica, Inc.), (b) human epithelial cells.

1.3 Cell Membrane

The **cell membrane** is approximately 4–7 nm thick and forms a semipermeable boundary between the intracellular space (inside the cell) and the extracellular space (outside the cell). It mainly consists of phospholipids, proteins, and cholesterol. **Phospholipid** molecules (Figure 1.2a) have a hydrophilic ("water-loving") head and hydrophobic ("water-hating") tails. In the cell membrane, two phospholipids face each other, with the hydrophobic tails in the interior of the membrane, to form a **phospholipid bilayer** (Figure 1.2b). **Cholesterol** molecules are embedded within the phospholipid bilayer, and they provide stability and rigidity to the cell membrane (Figure 1.2c). There are two main classifications of **membrane proteins**: **receptors** and **transporters**. Receptors help send information to and from the cell. Transporters help selectively transport molecules into and out of the cell. Remember that the bilayer has hydrophilic surfaces on both sides and a nonpolar hydrophobic layer in the center. This nonpolar layer prevents the transportation of polar molecules through the membrane. Only small nonpolar molecules can pass through this structure because they can squeeze through the spacing between polar heads and pass the nonpolar barrier by dissolving in it. Large nonpolar molecules, polar molecules, and ions cannot pass through the membrane. However, the cell needs these molecules in order to survive (e.g. glucose). Thus, the role of transport proteins is to selectively transport vital proteins across the membrane. Various carbohydrate chains (sugars) are attached to membrane proteins and lipids as a tagging mechanism. These carbohydrates are involved in cell recognition and immunity.

1.4 Proteins

Membrane proteins, although important, are not the only types of proteins used by the cell. **Receptors**, which bind to other molecules to transmit signals, exist in abundance both inside and outside of the cell. **Enzymes** are an important subcategory of proteins that catalyze biological reactions. Their names typically end in "-ase" (e.g. endonuclease and ligase). **Structural** proteins

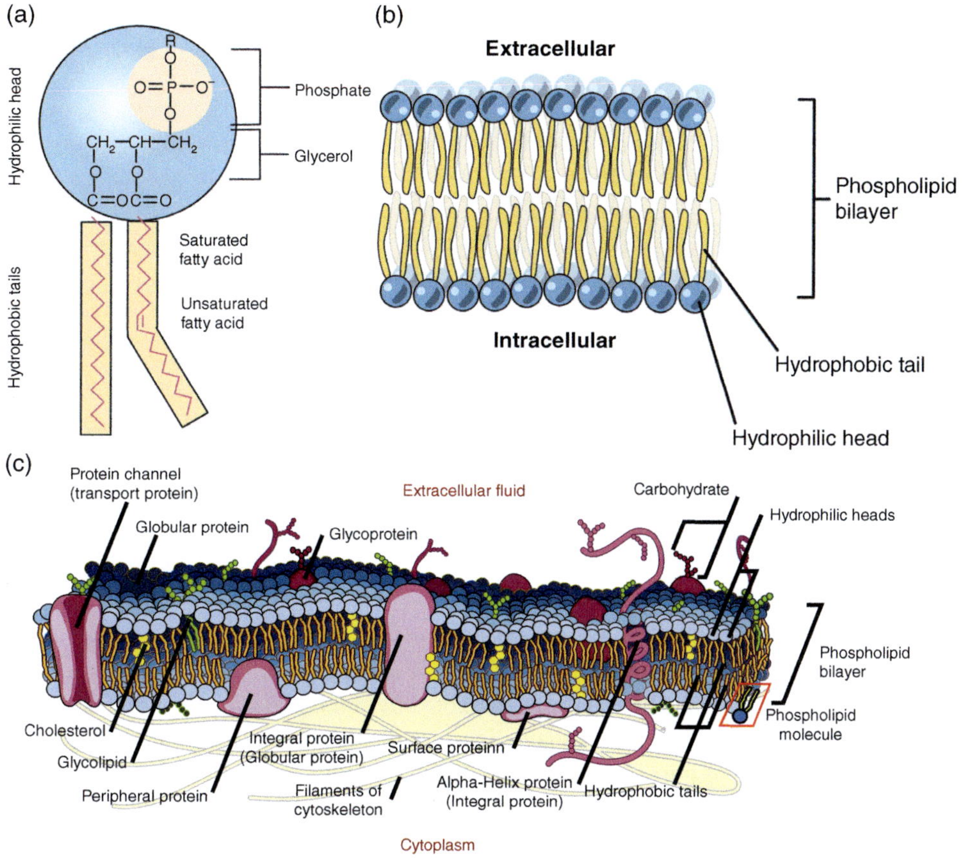

Figure 1.2 (a) Phospholipid (*Source:* OpenStax [1], used under CC BY- SA 4.0 https://creativecommons.org/licenses/by-sa/4.0/), (b) phospholipid bilayer (*Source:* OpenStax [2] used under CC BY-SA 4.0 https://creativecommons.org/licenses/by-sa/4.0/), (c) cell membrane.

give shape and structure to cells and organelles (e.g. collagen, actin, and myosin). There exist many other protein types that serve specific functions (e.g. antibodies).

1.5 Cytoplasm and Organelles

The **cytoplasm** is a gel-like substance inside the cell membrane that holds all the cell's organelles. Many cell activities occur inside the cytoplasm, including glycolysis (the enzymatic process that converts glucose to energy) and protein synthesis. **Organelles** are smaller sub-cell structures with specific functions. Some important organelles are ribosomes, endoplasmic reticulum (ER), Golgi, mitochondria, lysosomes, centrioles, cilia, and flagella.

Did You Know?

A bilayer is not the only possible stable arrangement of phospholipids. Phospholipids can also form single-layered structures called micelles. If the hydrophobic tails are short enough (or if the molecules have single tails), then the tails can pack together to form a nonpolar sphere surrounded by a shell of polar phospholipid heads. A micelle structure is shown in Figure 1.3.

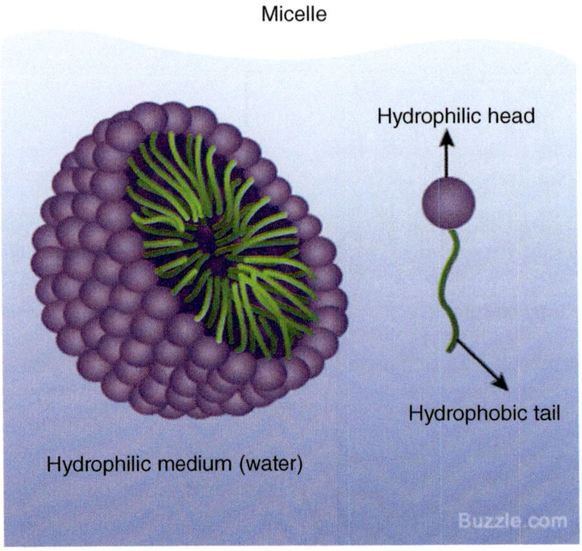

Figure 1.3 Micelle structure. *Source:* buzzle.com.

What is special about this structure? It is better known as soap. Have you ever wondered why water and soap remove greasiness from your hands but water alone cannot? When you scrub your hands with soap, you break soap micelles on the surface of your hands exposing the nonpolar tails to the dirt. Because grease is nonpolar, it normally does not dissolve in water. However, it easily dissolves in the nonpolar tails of phospholipids. Then, phospholipids form the micelle structure again (because they are still in a water environment) and trap the dirt in the core as seen in Figure 1.3. The outside of the sphere is hydrophilic and the whole structure can dissolve in water. Now with the help of the micelle, the nonpolar dirt can dissolve in water and get washed away.

The **nucleus** contains the cell's genetic material (DNA). **Ribosomes** are responsible for synthesizing proteins. They are approximately 25–30 nm in size and consist of ribosomal RNA (rRNA) and ribosomal proteins. Ribosomes play a significant role in the translation of mRNA into proteins (discussed later).

There are two types of **endoplasmic reticulum** (ER): the rough ER and the smooth ER (Figure 1.4). The **rough ER** receives newly made proteins, chemically modifies them, and then

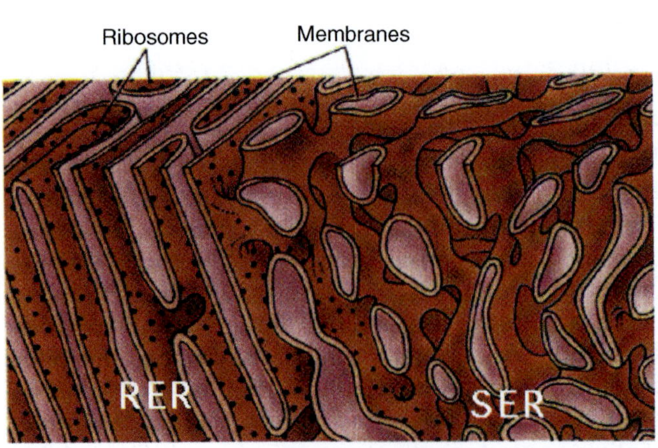

Figure 1.4 Rough ER (RER) vs. smooth ER (SER). *Source:* Sadava et al. [3], figure 4.19 on p. 78, By permission of Oxford University Press.

transports them to the Golgi. The surface of the rough ER is covered with ribosomes that give the ER a rough appearance. The **smooth ER** makes new membrane components (e.g. fats and carbohydrates) and stores calcium ions. Unlike the rough ER, the smooth ER does not have ribosomes attached to its membrane, so it has a smooth appearance under a microscope.

The **Golgi** apparatus receives proteins from the rough ER, chemically modifies them, and transports them to their final destination (e.g. nucleus, cytoplasm, cell membrane, and cell exterior).

Mitochondria (singular: mitochondrion) are the powerhouses of the cell. They provide energy (in the form of ATP) to the cell through a process called oxidative phosphorylation. In this process, the mitochondria uses molecules produced during glucose metabolism to make ATP. Mitochondria range from 500 to 1000 nm in diameter (Figure 1.5a). The mitochondrion consists of two membranes: the outer membrane and the inner membrane. The inner membrane surface contains

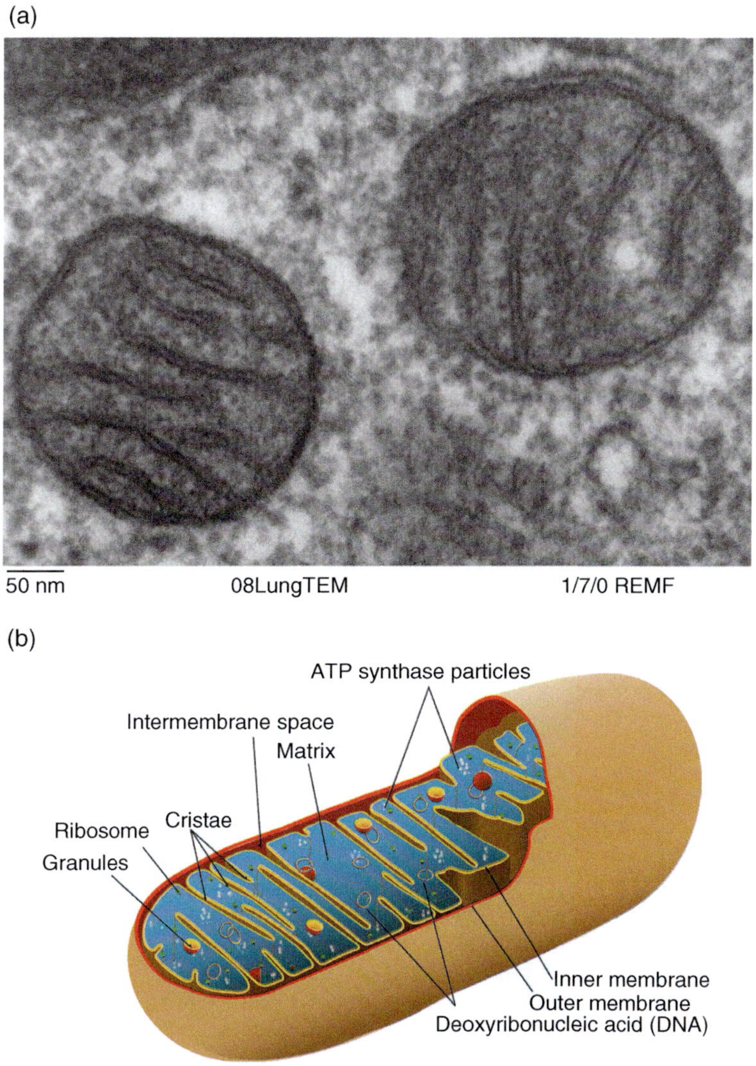

Figure 1.5 (a) Mitochondria from mammalian lung tissue (*Source:* courtesy of Dartmouth Electron Microscope Facility.), (b) structure of mitochondrion.

proteins and peptides required for converting glucose metabolites into energy. In order to maximize surface area for energy production, the inner membrane forms a labyrinth-like structure called cristae, depicted in Figure 1.5b. Interestingly, mitochondria have structural similarities to bacteria, and they even possess their own circular DNA. This is because mitochondria originated as endosymbiotic prokaryotes. In other words, at some point during evolution, eukaryotic cells incorporated a bacterium (ancestor of mitochondrion) into their own cell structure and then transformed it into an organelle. The mitochondria and the eukaryotic cell formed a symbiotic relationship because without the mitochondria, the cell would have been able to extract only a fraction of the potential energy present in a glucose molecule.

The cell also contains **lysosomes** which are digestive "bags" that digest and destroy microbes. Lysosomes are formed in the Golgi apparatus and are released into the cytoplasm. They contain very destructive enzymes such as lipases (digest lipids), amylases (digest complex sugars like starch), proteases (digest proteins), and nucleases (digest nucleic acids). Since these digestive enzymes work best under acidic conditions, the lysosome creates an acidic internal environment (pH = 4.8) by pumping protons H+ into the organelle. The cytoplasm itself is slightly alkaline (pH = 7.2), so if these digestive enzymes get released into the cell accidentally, their functions slow down significantly and the cell survives. However, if multiple lysosomes burst in a short period of time, the cumulative effect of the digestive enzymes can cause cell death (called autolysis). Hence, lysosomes play some role in programmed cell death (apoptosis).

Centrioles assist in cell division by organizing mitotic spindles. Mitotic spindles play a role in the arrangement and distribution of chromosomes during cell division. **Cilia** are tiny extensions from the cell that can propel material upward over the cell (e.g. mucus). **Flagella** are a single large extension responsible for propelling male sperm cells toward the female ovum.

1.6 Nucleus

The **nucleus** contains the genetic information of the cell. The anatomy of the nucleus is seen in Figure 1.6. The nucleus is covered by the nuclear envelope – a porous layer that allows certain molecules to pass in and out. Inside the nucleus, we can find the **nucleolus** (where ribosomes are

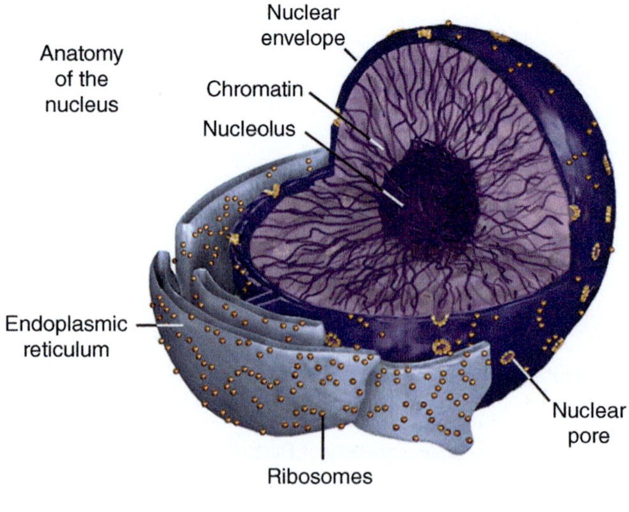

Figure 1.6 Anatomy of the nucleus. *Source:* "Molecular Expressions" at Florida State University.

manufactured) and **chromatin** (a packed form of DNA). DNA must utilize a very efficient packing mechanism for storing genetic material as chromatin inside the nucleus. If the DNA from a single human cell were uncoiled, its average length would be about 2 m. In eukaryotic cells, this 2 m of DNA needs to be stored inside a 6-μm-diameter nucleus. Stuffing this material into the nucleus like a ball of string is not very efficient because a certain portion of the genetic material needs to be accessible for cells to function properly. This is why DNA packing into chromatin is highly organized.

A human's DNA is assorted into 46 chromosomes that are 23 pairs of chromosomes. One chromosome in each of these 23 pairs is inherited from the individual's mother and the other chromosome in each of the 23 pairs is inherited from the father. Microscopic images of the 23 human chromosome pairs are called **karyograms** (Figure 1.7). In this karyogram, each chromosome pair is labeled with a number. The 23rd chromosome is the **sex chromosome** where the gender is determined by the chromosome from the father. An XX pair is female, while an XY pair is male, and since females can only give an X chromosome, the gender is determined by whether the father gave an X or Y chromosome. **Each chromosome** consists of a double-helix strand of DNA, which is wrapped around **histones.** Histones are then wrapped around themselves to form **chromatin** structures (Figure 1.8). This tight packing allows a large amount of genetic information to be stored on a micron scale. When the cell is not dividing, the chromosomes are stored inside the nucleus as chromatin. In preparation for mitosis (cell division), chromosomes replicate and then condense into a more tightly packed structure called **condensed chromosomes** (X-shape on the

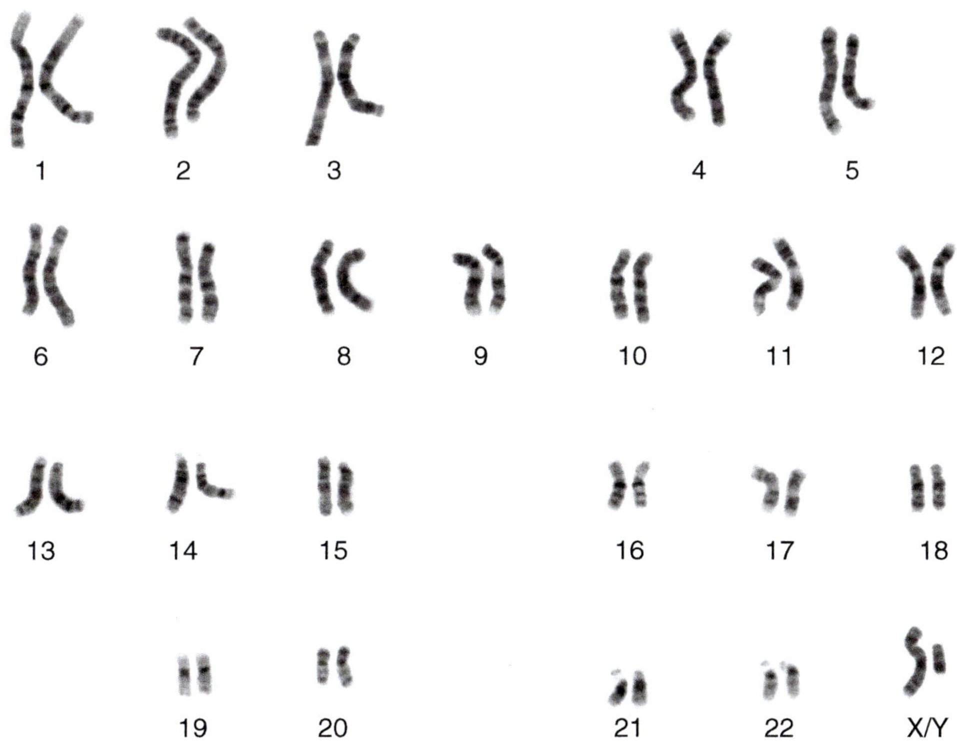

Figure 1.7 Human karyogram. *Source:* Earthsound [4]. Courtesy of National Human Genome Research Institute.

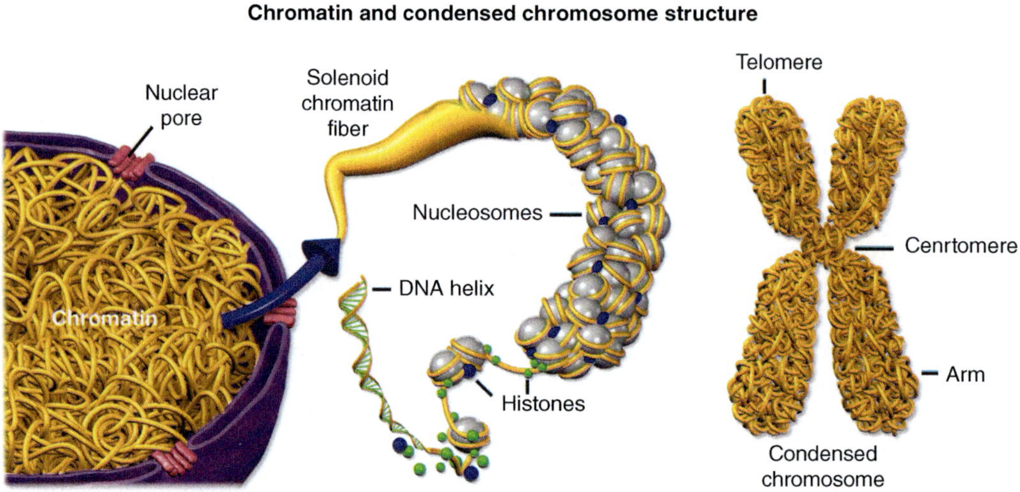

Figure 1.8 Efficient packing of genetic material. *Source:* "Molecular Expressions" at Florida State University.

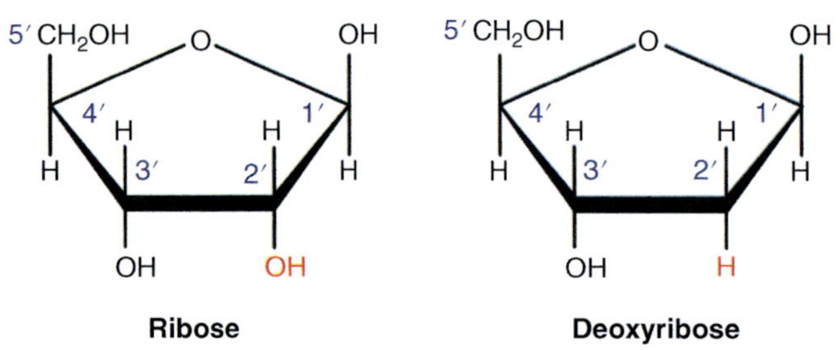

Figure 1.9 Ribose and deoxyribose sugars.

right side of Figure 1.8). The right-hand side of the condensed chromosome is identical to the left side of the condensed chromosome. Each one of these halves is called a **chromatid**.

1.7 Nucleic Acids (DNA and RNA)

1.7.1 DNA

DNA stands for deoxyribonucleic acid. The name comes from the deoxygenated ribose sugar, which forms the backbone of the molecule along with phosphate. The difference between ribose and deoxyribose is the missing oxygen on the 2′ carbon of deoxyribose (Figure 1.9).

The building block of DNA is called a nucleotide. Each **nucleotide** contains a 5-carbon sugar (deoxyribose), a phosphate group, and a nucleobase (A = Adenine, T = Thymine, G = Guanine, and C = Cytosine). The nucleotides create a chain (or strand) by forming ester bonds between the 5-carbon sugar and the phosphate group, and two such chains intertwine to form a **double-helix structure** (Figure **1.10**). The two DNA strands are attracted together by weak hydrogen bonds between complementary nucleotide pairs, which are (A, T) and (G, C). The **hydrogen bond** is a weak interaction that can be broken at high temperatures.

The sequence of nucleotides in DNA encodes genetic information. This sequence depends on which direction you read the signal. So, it is important to clarify the directionality of the strands.

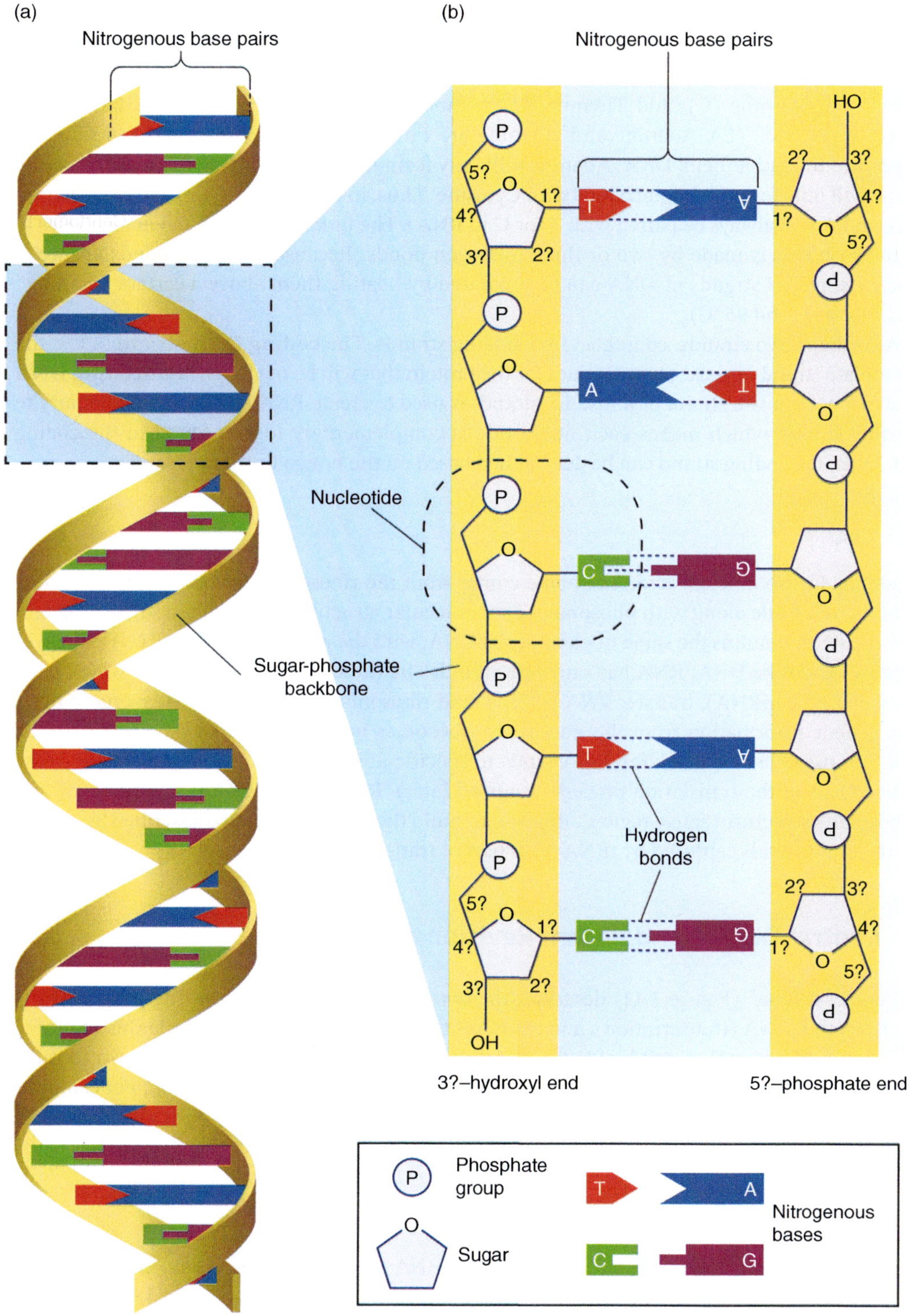

Figure 1.10 (a) DNA double-helix structure and (b) base-pair interactions. *Source:* Reprinted with permission from Encyclopedia Britannica, © 2018 by Encyclopedia Britannica, Inc.

DNA strands are read from 5′ to 3′ direction. The 5′ end of the DNA terminates with a phosphate group and the 3′ end of the DNA terminates with an OH group.

The nucleobases encode the genetic information. There are four nucleobases, Adenine (A), Guanine (G), Cytosine (C), and Thymine (T), although in RNA (discussed later) Thymine is replaced with Uracil (U). Adenine and Guanine are Purines, while Thymine and Cytosine are Pyrimidines. In double-helix DNA, Adenine will only form hydrogen bonds with Thymine, while Guanine will only form hydrogen bonds with Cytosine. Thus, in a base pair, C will always be paired with G, and A will always be paired with T (or U in RNA). The linkage between the nucleobases to form the base pair is made by two or three hydrogen bonds. Because hydrogen bonds are weak interactions, paired strands of DNA can be separated by heating them above a certain "melting" temperature (around 95 °C).

DNA contains two strands: coding and noncoding strands. The **coding DNA strand** (a.k.a. the non-template strand or sense strand) codes for the protein that will be made. The **noncoding DNA strand** (a.k.a. template strand or antisense strand) is used to create RNA and is complementary to the coding strand, which means each nucleotide is complementary to that found in the coding strand. Thus, the coding strand can be determined based on the noncoding strand, and vice versa.

1.7.2 RNA

RNA stands for ribonucleic acid. The name comes from the ribose sugar which forms the backbone of the molecule along with phosphate. The molecular structure of the ribose sugar is seen in Figure 1.9. RNA contains the same nucleotides as DNA, with the exception of Uracil (U) instead of Thymine (T). Unlike DNA, RNA has only one strand. The three most common types of RNA are messenger RNA (mRNA), transfer RNA (tRNA), and ribosomal RNA (rRNA). **Messenger RNA** carries genetic information from the nucleus to ribosomes in the cell (part of the transcription process discussed later). **Transfer RNA** binds to specific amino acids and transfers them to the ribosome (part of the translation process discussed later). **Ribosomal RNA** is incorporated into the ribosome's structure (active region). Ribosomes build the protein sequence described by mRNA using the amino acids captured by tRNA (also part of translation, discussed later).

1.8 Central Dogma and Recent Revisions

The "central dogma" (Figure 1.11) describes the two-step process of synthesizing proteins from DNA: DNA to mRNA (transcription), and mRNA into proteins (translation). While this sequence of events is fundamental to cell biology, research from the past two decades has shown that the central dogma only provides a partial picture of the diverse roles of RNA in the cell. For example, some RNA structures are capable of performing enzyme-like activities without the aid of proteins. Other RNA structures play significant roles in regulating gene expression.

1.8.1 Transcription (DNA → mRNA)

Transcription is the process of creating messenger RNA (mRNA) that is a complementary copy of a DNA sequence. The mRNA carries the actual code that specifies the amino acid sequence in a polypeptide (protein). Genes are organized in DNA by segments located in between a promoter DNA sequence and a terminator DNA sequence. Transcription consists of three steps: initiation, elongation, and termination (Figure 1.12).

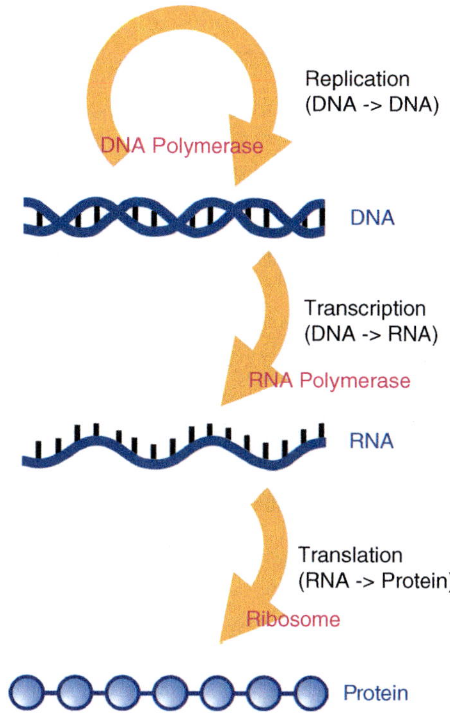

Figure 1.11 Central Dogma (DNA -> mRNA -> Protein). *Source:* Dhorspool [5], used under CC-BY-SA 3.0 https://creativecommons.org/licenses/by-sa/4.0/.

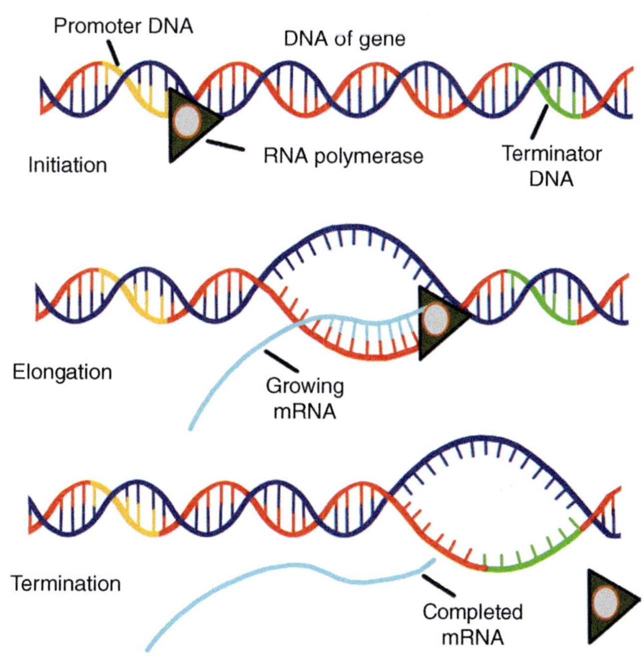

Figure 1.12 Steps of transcription.

During the **initiation step**, RNA polymerase binds to a **promoter**, a region of bases in the DNA that signals the beginning of a gene in the noncoding DNA strand (template strand). Transcription factors aid in bringing and anchoring the RNA polymerase to the promoter. The DNA's double

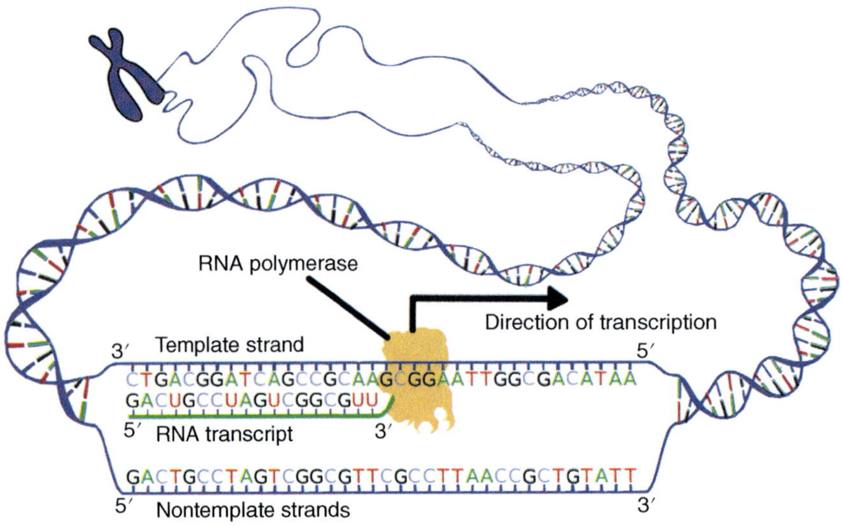

Figure 1.13 Elongation step of transcription.

helix unwinds slightly at the promoter, and the gene downstream of that promoter is ready to be transcribed into a complementary mRNA strand.

During the **elongation step**, the RNA polymerase moves along the DNA strand, adding new RNA nucleotides (A, C, G, and U) in the 5′ to 3′ direction, complementary to the DNA template strand (Figure 1.13). This process occurs very rapidly, at up to 60 nucleotides per second. Once a region is finished with elongation, the template and non-template strands will reform the double-helix structure. Notice that the coding DNA strand (a.k.a. non-template strand) is read in 5′ to 3′ direction. The resulting RNA sequence is also built from 5′ to 3′ and is identical to the coding strand except T bases are replaced by U bases in the RNA strand.

During the **termination step**, the RNA polymerase reaches the terminator region of the protein-encoding gene. This causes all the enzymes and factors to release from the DNA along with the product RNA strand, called pre-mRNA. Sections in this pre-mRNA are called introns and exons. The introns are taken out ("spliced") in a process called *splicing*, leaving only exon sections in the final mRNA strand. When there are multiple exons in a gene, some of them may be skipped in the splicing process creating a different protein. This allows one gene to code for multiple proteins.

In summary, the determination of which part of the DNA is transcribed into mRNA is highly regulated. When a certain protein is needed by the cell, the cell produces transcription factors specific to that protein's gene. These transcription factors help the enzyme RNA polymerase assemble at the promoter and start the transcription process. Transcription by RNA polymerase produces an mRNA strand that encodes the needed protein. The transcription process ends when the RNA polymerase reaches the terminator sequence in the DNA, causing the release of RNA polymerase and the pre-mRNA transcript.

1.8.2 Translation (mRNA → Protein)

After transcription is completed, the mRNA strand leaves the nucleus and goes to the cytoplasm where proteins are made. The mRNA is composed of codons (sequences of three nucleic acids) and each codon codes for a specific amino acid. The reading frame of the mRNA, which is translated into a polypeptide (protein), begins with a start codon and ends with a stop codon (Figure 1.14).

The mRNA also contains leader and trailer sequences that are not translated. Even though the leader sequence is not translated into a polypeptide chain, it is still very important for the translation process because it contains a ribosome-binding site. The 64 possible codons determine one of 20 different amino acids, which form a chain with peptide bonds (polypeptide) to make a protein. The list of all codons and their corresponding amino acids is shown in Figure 1.15. Each amino acid has the same basic structure, including an amino group (H_2N), a carboxylic acid group (COOH), and an organic group (R_1, R_2, etc.) that determines the amino acid identity. They are linked with peptide bonds to form chains (polypeptides) which fold into proteins.

The transcribed mRNA travels to a ribosome that binds to the mRNA at a specific location called the ribosome-binding site located on the leader sequence of the mRNA. The ribosome reads the base sequence one by one until it detects the start codon "AUG" (see Figure 1.14). Once the start codon is detected, translation begins and the following bases are read in groups of 3 (i.e. a codon). For each codon, the ribosome finds a transfer RNA (tRNA) with the complementary codon and attaches the amino acid transferred by this tRNA to the growing chain of amino acids (Figure 1.16). For example, when the ribosome sees an AAA codon in the mRNA, it looks for its complementary tRNA, which is UUU. The tRNA with the UUU sequence carries with it the amino acid lysine to the ribosome (see mRNA AAA codon in Figure 1.15). The amino acid (e.g. lysine) is attached to the

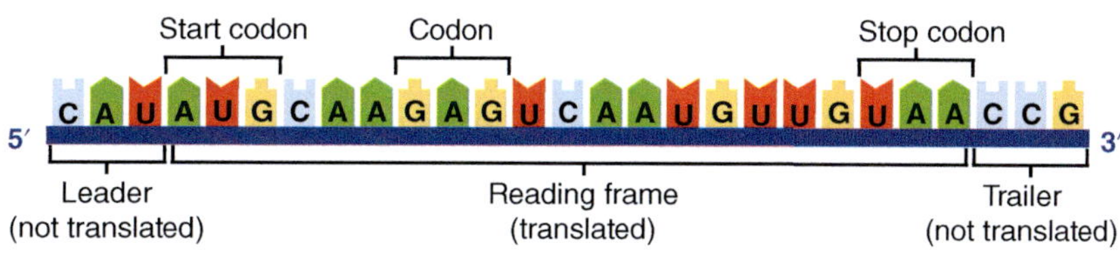

Figure 1.14 Reading frame of mRNA.

Second letter

First letter	U	C	A	G	Third letter
U	UUU Phe	UCU Ser	UAU Tyr	UGU Cys	U
U	UUC Phe	UCC Ser	UAC Tyr	UGC Cys	C
U	UUA Leu	UCA Ser	UAA Stop	UGA Stop	A
U	UUG Leu	UCG Ser	UAG Stop	UGG Trp	G
C	CUU Leu	CCU Pro	CAU His	CGU Arg	U
C	CUC Leu	CCC Pro	CAC His	CGC Arg	C
C	CUA Leu	CCA Pro	CAA Gln	CGA Arg	A
C	CUG Leu	CCG Pro	CAG Gln	CGG Arg	G
A	AUU Ile	ACU Thr	AAU Asn	AGU Ser	U
A	AUC Ile	ACC Thr	AAC Asn	AGC Ser	C
A	AUA Ile	ACA Thr	AAA Lys	AGA Arg	A
A	AUG Met	ACG Thr	AAG Lys	AGG Arg	G
G	GUU Val	GCU Ala	GAU Asp	GGU Gly	U
G	GUC Val	GCC Ala	GAC Asp	GGC Gly	C
G	GUA Val	GCA Ala	GAA Glu	GGA Gly	A
G	GUG Val	GCG Ala	GAG Glu	GGG Gly	G

Figure 1.15 Codons for amino acids.

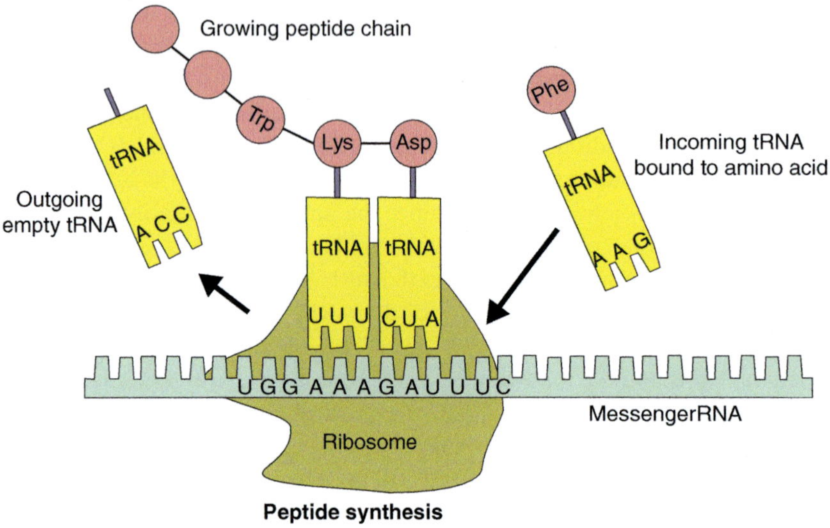

Figure 1.16 Role of tRNA in peptide synthesis. *Source:* Boumphreyfr, [6], used under CC-BY-SA 3.0 https://creativecommons.org/licenses/by-sa/3.0/.

existing peptide chain. When a stop codon (UAA, UAG, or UGA) is reached, the polypeptide chain is released from the ribosome. Upon release, this polypeptide chain can fold in on itself to produce the final functional protein.

Note that the start codon "AUG" also encodes the amino acid methionine (Met). Since all mRNA sequences begin with a start codon, all polypeptide chains produced in the ribosomes start with methionine. Depending on the protein being produced, this first Methionine may be removed later in the post-processing stage of the protein. Therefore, not every protein begins with methionine.

1.9 Mutations

DNA mutations often cause harmful outcomes to the gene expression process. For example, sickle cell anemia is a trait in which a person's DNA for hemoglobin (which carries oxygen in red blood cells) differs by a single nucleotide. This single DNA nucleotide difference means that mRNA transcribed from the hemoglobin gene also contains a single different nucleotide. Therefore, when the ribosome translates the mRNA, the final polypeptide sequence has a single amino acid substitution: individuals with sickle cell anemia have the amino acid valine at a position that has a glutamic acid in healthy individuals (Table 1.1).

This mutation has a severe effect on the function of the resulting hemoglobin that causes the red blood cells of the individual that carry the mutation to look sickle-shaped rather than the normal round disk-shaped (Figure 1.17).

1.10 Cell Cycle

Every cell that undergoes division is found in one of four possible phases (Figure 1.18): G_1 is the growth phase where growth and normal metabolic processes occur, S is the synthesis phase where DNA is replicated, G_2 is the second growth phase where growth and preparation for mitosis occur, and M is the mitosis phase where actual cell division occurs.

Table 1.1 Template DNA, translated mRNA, and resulting amino acid (AA) for normal hemoglobin and sickle cell hemoglobin.

	Normal hemoglobin			Sickle cell hemoglobin		
Template DNA	**GCA**	**CTT**	**GCA**	**GGA**	**CAT**	**GCA**
mRNA	CCU	GAA	CGU	CCU	GUA	CGU
AA	PRO	GEU	ARG	PRO	VAL	ARG

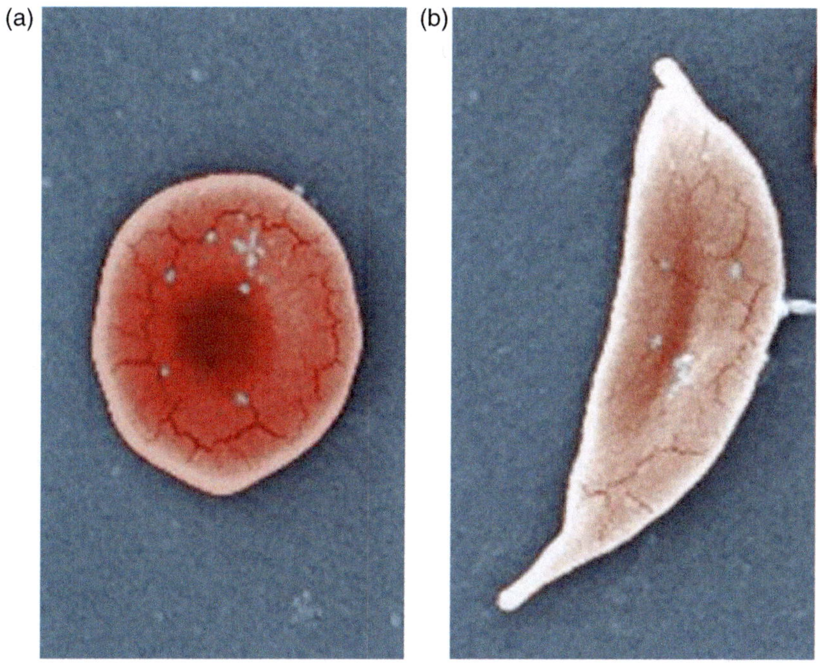

Figure 1.17 (a) Healthy red blood cell, and (b) sickle-shaped red blood cell. *Source:* OpenStax College [7], used under CC BY 3.0 http://creativecommons.org/licenses/by/3.0.

During the S phase, DNA is replicated. The key enzyme responsible for this replication is DNA polymerase, which was discovered in 1956 by Arthur Kornberg (who won the Nobel Prize in 1959). Another enzyme, helicase, first opens up the DNA double helix into two strands, after which the DNA polymerase adds nucleotides to each strand to form two DNA copies (Figure 1.19). This process contains a proofreading mechanism that guarantees minimal errors, on the order of 1 error in 10^9 bases in humans.

1.10.1 Cell Division – Mitosis

Mitosis is the process by which cells divide. In order to create two identical daughter cells, the genetic material needs to be replicated. As humans, we have 46 chromosomes. Each chromosome is a long double-helix DNA polymer. When a cell is not replicating, the chromosomes are stored in the nucleus as chromatin. During the S phase, an identical copy of each chromosome is created. However, since both copies are attached to each other (using a centromere), they are still considered one chromosome and each of the copies is named a chromatid. There are a few key definitions needed to

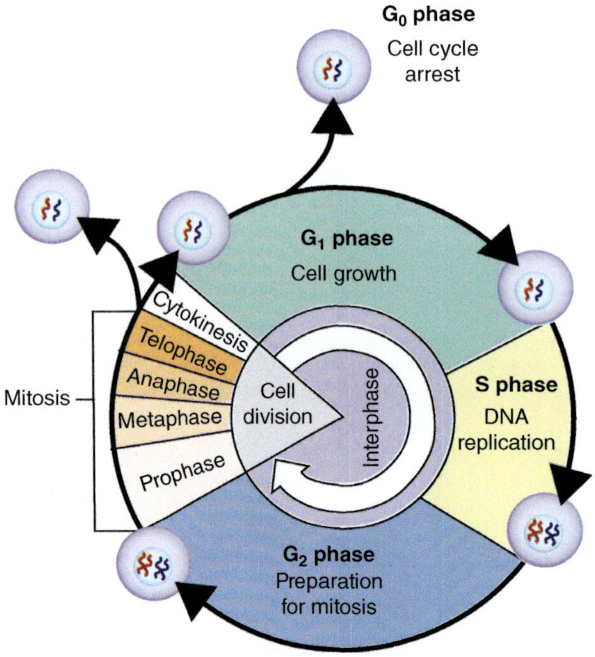

Figure 1.18 The cell cycle.

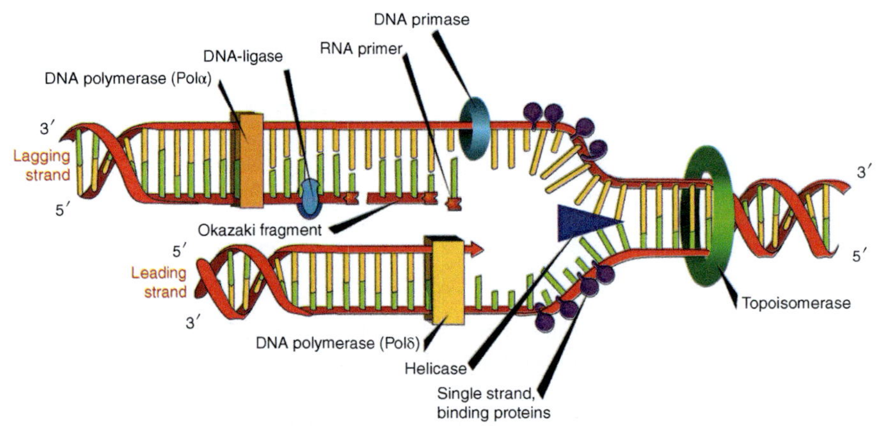

Figure 1.19 DNA replication.

understand mitosis. **Chromatin** is dense DNA content in the nucleus. **Chromosomes** are long double-helix DNA strands. Note that only in the context of mitosis, a chromosome is referred to as the construct of two identical DNA strands connected at their center by a centromere. **Chromatids** are one of the two identical copies of double-helix strands (during mitosis). **Centromeres** are constructs used to connect two sister chromatids together at their center. **Centrioles** are protein structures that construct spreading spindle fibers to pull each sister chromatid to one side of the cell during anaphase. **Spindle fibers** are a net of tubules spread by centrioles.

1.10.1.1 Stages of Mitosis

Mitosis consists of four stages: prophase, metaphase, anaphase, and telophase (Figure 1.20).

Prophase: The chromatin condenses into visible condensed chromosomes. The spindle fibers (a net of tubules spread by centrioles) appear, and the nuclear envelope disappears.

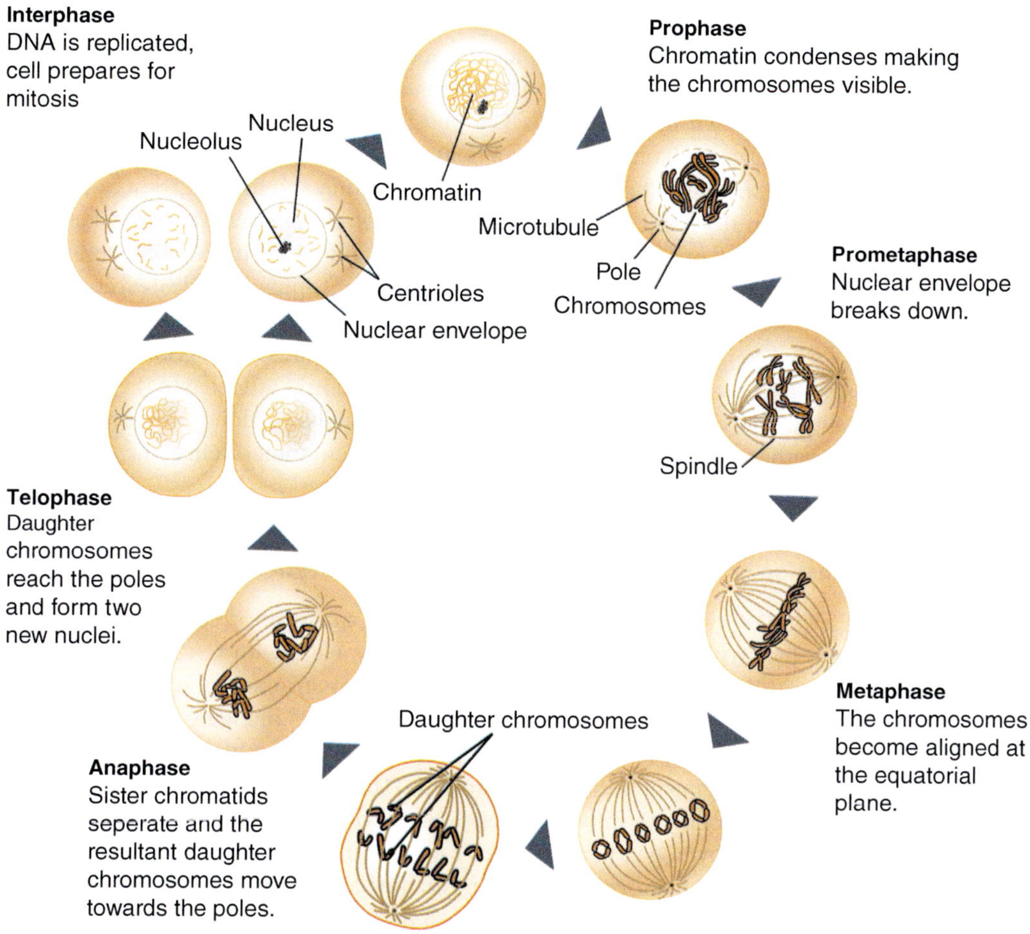

Figure 1.20 Stages of mitosis. *Source:* Jpablo [8], used under CC BY- SA 3.0 https://creativecommons.org/licenses/bv-sa/3.0.

Metaphase: The spindle fibers attach to each chromatid, and chromosomes align across the center of the cell. At the end of this stage, there are 46 chromosomes (each with two chromatids).

Anaphase: The centromeres break apart and spindle fibers pull the chromosomes away from the center of the cell. A cleavage (named cleavage furrow) on the cell membrane begins to appear. At this point, two sister chromatids detach from each other and now each of them is called a daughter chromosome. At the end of this stage, there are 92 chromosomes.

Telophase: The nuclear envelope and both nuclei appear, the cytoplasm and organelles divide equally, and the process of cell division is completed. At the end of this stage, there are 46 chromosomes per daughter cell. Hence, the number of chromosomes is conserved.

1.11 Additional Information

1.11.1 More Information on Lipids and Lipid Bilayers

Lipids have a polar head and a nonpolar tail. Polar molecules generally dissolve in polar solvents. Since water is a polar solvent, the polar phospholipid head likes water. Similarly, nonpolar molecules dissolve better in nonpolar solvents, hence, the hydrophobic phospholipid tails attract each other tail-to-tail. When you add phospholipids into the water, the polar heads want to dissolve in water, but the tails want to stay away from it. One simple formation to guarantee this is the **bilayer** formation, with the resulting structure shown in Figure 1.21. The phospholipid heads on both surfaces face water and the nonpolar tails face each other to create a nonpolar environment for themselves.

However, the lipid bilayer structure shown in Figure 1.21 is too fluid and fragile to be a cell membrane. It has a consistency similar to oil. The phospholipids stay on the surface (therefore, keeping the same lipid bilayer structure), but they can move around and change their positions, similar to a sea of phospholipids. The cell membrane needs some structural integrity. **Cholesterol**, like phospholipid but much smaller, is an amphipathic molecule. **Amphipathic** molecules have both a hydrophilic part and a hydrophobic part. The hydrophilic portion of cholesterol is attracted to the polar head of a phospholipid molecule, while the hydrophobic portion is attracted to the nonpolar tails of this phospholipid and the tails of neighboring phospholipids. By doing this, cholesterol binds phospholipids together and reduces the fluidity of the cell membrane. Hence, the structural integrity of the cell membrane increases.

1.11.2 More Information on DNA Bases, Base Pairing, and Applications

Why is it that the bases in DNA form in pairs rather than triples, quadruples, etc.? And why does Adenine almost always pair with Thymine (A–T) while Guanine pairs with Cytosine (G–C)? To better understand these DNA "rules," we can look at the molecular structure of each nucleobase (Figure 1.22). Each base is connected to a deoxyribose sugar (labeled "R" in Figure 1.22) within the DNA helix backbone. The bases interact with each other through hydrogen bonds.

Note that because of their differing molecular structures, G–C base pairs can form three hydrogen bonds while A–T base pairs can only form two hydrogen bonds. Depending on the other bonding atoms (e.g. O, N, etc.), a single hydrogen bond releases roughly 10–30 $kJ\,mol^{-1}$ of energy. Because Guanine and Cytosine share more hydrogen bonds than Adenine and Thymine, G–C base pairs are slightly more energetically stable than A–T pairs. Because of these differences in hydrogen-bonding capabilities, A–T and G–C base pairs (also called Watson–Crick base pairs, after James Watson and Francis Crick, the discoverers of the DNA double-helix structure) form most commonly.

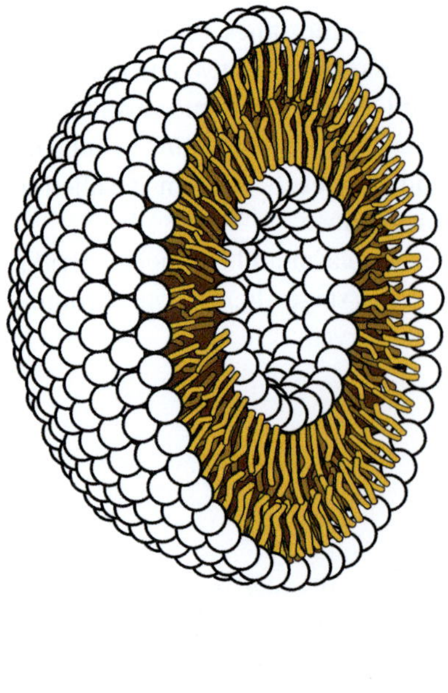

Figure 1.21 Lipid bilayer forming liposome.

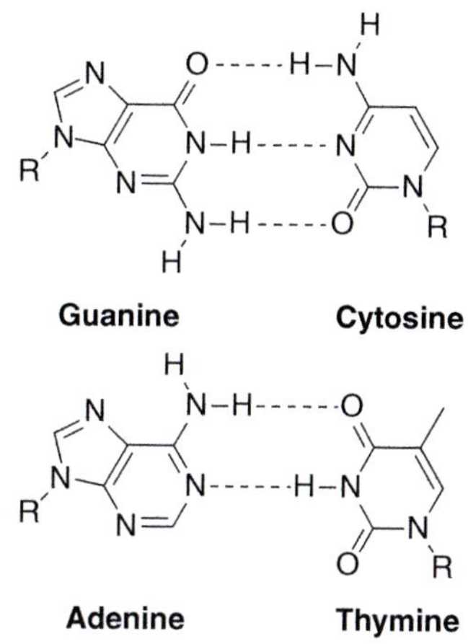

Figure 1.22 Hydrogen bonds in Watson–Crick base pairs.

In addition to the hydrogen bonding, there is also another factor that causes A–T and G–C base pairs. Note that A and G (the purines) are both made up of two "rings," while C and T (the pyrimidines) have only a single ring. In other words, A–T pairs are three rings wide and G–C pairs are also three rings wide. What if a G was paired with an A at one point within the double helix? Not only would the A–G pair not be able to form the proper hydrogen bonds, but that base pair would also be four rings wide. The DNA backbone at this location would be "pushed out" by the extra ring. Using the same logic, a C–T pair would only be two rings wide. The DNA backbone at a C–T pair would be narrower at this location. In either case, the base pair mismatch would actually deform the DNA backbone into an energetically unfavorable structure. It is important to note that thermodynamic principles govern the way molecules like DNA assemble. Knowing these principles can help explain why DNA exhibits its famous properties (double-helix) and why because of its single-stranded structure, RNA can (and does) occasionally form non-Watson–Crick base pairs.

On a different note, the molecular properties of the different nucleobases can be exploited in a number of practical engineering applications. Because of their different atomic compositions, each base has different electronic properties. For example, bases with more oxygen and nitrogen tend to have more free electrons. It turns out that the tiny electronic differences between the four bases can be used to distinguish them from each other. Technologies have been developed to pull strands of DNA through microscale sensors that can detect pico-amp (pA) currents. As the DNA is pulled through the detector, each base generates a slightly different current due to its specific electronic properties. Although very preliminary, this kind of approach could provide improvements to DNA-sequencing technologies.

1.11.3 More Information on Amino Acids, Proteins Folding, and Applications

The proteins formed by translation are composed of amino acids that are linked in sequence by peptide bonds. These peptide bonds (formed by the NH_2 group of one amino acid and the COOH group of the adjacent amino acid) make up the backbone of the folded protein. While the importance of this protein backbone cannot be understated, the sidechains of each amino acid are also crucial for determining protein structure and function. Each amino acid has a different sidechain (sometimes called an "R-group"), as shown in Figure 1.23. These different sidechains impart different properties; they can be ionic, polar, nonpolar, acidic, basic, some can form hydrogen bonds while others cannot, etc. Because of these properties, side chains can influence protein folding and functional properties. Thus, the proper sequence of amino acids is of critical importance to functional proteins.

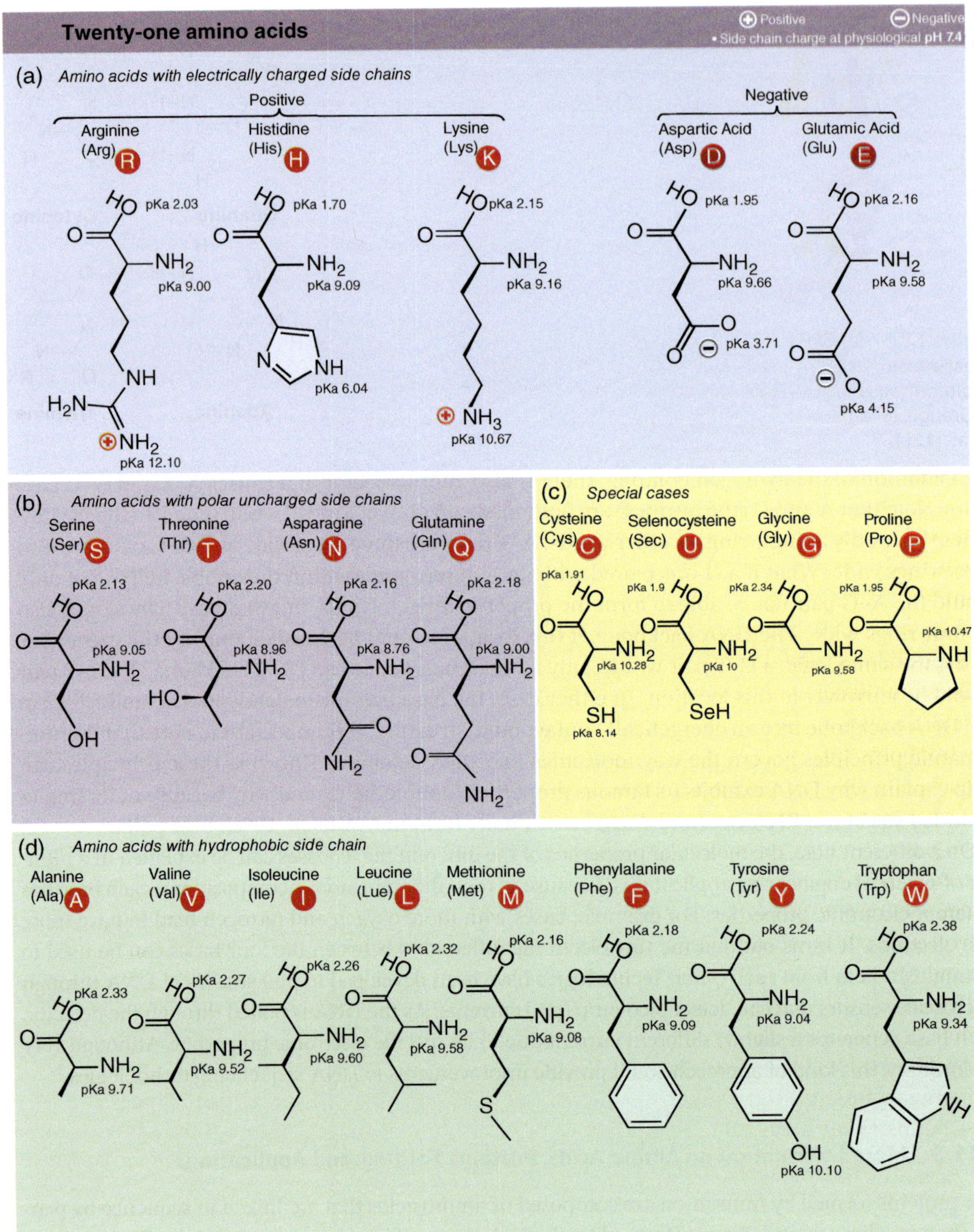

Figure 1.23 Amino acids (20 natural and 1 natural derivative, selenocysteine). *Source:* Fred the Oyster [9], used under CC-BY-SA 3.0 https://creativecommons.org/licenses/bv-sa/3.0/.

Recall that we briefly discussed how a single genetic mutation in hemoglobin can lead to sickle cell anemia. We discussed this example from the standpoint of the genetic code but now let us consider it from the standpoint of the protein that is produced by that genetic mutation. That single amino acid substitution of valine rather than Glutamic Acid can actually explain the morphology of sickle-shaped red blood cells.

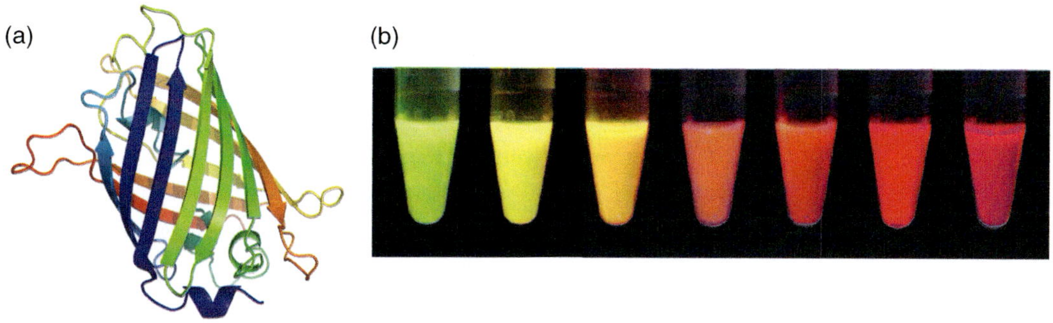

Figure 1.24 (a) GFP protein structure. (*Source:* Zephyris [10], used under CC-BY-SA 3.0 https://creativecommons.org/licenses/by-sa/3.0/. Courtesy of Jawahar Swaminathan and MSD staff at the European Bioinformatics Institute) (b) Engineered fluorescent proteins (from left to right: mHoneydew, mBanana, mOrange, tdTomato, mTangerine, mStrawberry, and mCherry). (*Source:* Reprinted by permission from Shaner et al. [11].).

Glutamic acid is a polar, hydrophilic amino acid that is expressed on the outer surface of hemoglobin. On the other hand, valine is a nonpolar, hydrophobic residue that is usually not found on parts of the protein that are exposed to water. In sickle cell hemoglobin, hydrophobic valine at this position is exposed to water, which is energetically unfavorable. This energetic instability causes multiple hemoglobin proteins to aggregate to try to "bury" the exposed valine residues and shield them from water molecules (this aggregation is caused by the phenomenon called the Hydrophobic Effect). Long rod-like aggregates of hemoglobin form and actually deform the red blood cells in which they are carried.

There are also many practical applications of proteins with unique structures and functions. Using genetic approaches, proteins with interesting properties can be engineered for optimized or altered functions. A now-classic example is Roger Tsien's discovery and work with green fluorescent protein (GFP), which is naturally found in a species of jellyfish. GFP has a barrel-shaped structure called a beta-barrel (Figure 1.24a). Inside this structure is a cluster of amino acids that produce a fluorescent "chromophore." Along with others, Tsien substituted different amino acids in place of the native GFP chromophore to produce a wide range of proteins with different fluorescent wavelengths (Figure 1.24b). Because of their distinct optical properties, these engineered proteins have many applications for biological research and imaging techniques (more on this in future chapters). Tsien was awarded the 2008 Nobel Prize in Chemistry for this work.

Problems

1.1 Match each function in Column B with the proper cell structure in Column A.

Column A	Column B
1. ___ Ribosome	A. A long cell projection used to propel sperm cells
2. ___ Endoplasmic reticulum	B. Bags of digestive enzymes in the cell
3. ___ Golgi apparatus	C. Tube-like passages that carry substances through the cytoplasm
4. ___ Mitochondria	D. Short hair-like structures on the free surface of some cells

Column A	Column B
5. ___ Lysosomes	E. Chemically process and package substances from the endoplasmic reticulum
6. ___ Flagella	F. Directs protein synthesis; the brain of the cell
7. ___ Cilia	G. "Protein factories" in the cell, made of RNA
8. ___ Nucleus	H. "Powerhouse" of the cell; most of the cell's ATP (energy) is formed here

1.2 An organism has DNA with 60 000 kbp (kilobase pairs). It is known that 21% of the base pairs contain T residues. Calculate the number of A, C, G, and T residues in the DNA of each cell in this organism. If RNA is transcribed from this DNA, calculate the number of residues that would be present in the RNA.
Assume transcription of entire 60 000 kbp DNA and even distribution of nucleotides in coding and noncoding strands of DNA.

1.3 Given a DNA coding strand of TTATGACACATAAACATTAAT, write the sequence of the following:

A Noncoding DNA strand
B mRNA strand that is transcribed
C Amino acid sequence that is translated

1.4

A Examine the following nucleotide sequence from the coding strand of DNA. What is the mRNA strand that will be transcribed from this DNA and the amino acid sequence of the encoded protein?
5′ G T A A T T C A A A A T G C C T T A C G C C C C T G G A G A C G A A A A G A A G G G T G C T A T T A C G T A T T T G A A G A A G G C C A C C T C T G A G T A A A T G T G A C 3′

B After translation, it is observed that the amino acid sequence contains Ala-Pro-Arg. Explain why and how this can occur.

1.5 Given a DNA-coding strand of 5′GAATGCCTACCTCAAAATAGG 3′, write the sequence of the following:

A Noncoding DNA strand
B mRNA strand that is transcribed
C Amino acid sequence that is translated
D A scientist tried to express this DNA sequence and received the following amino acid sequence: Met-Pro-Thr. Assuming only a single mutation has occurred, help the scientist find the position of the mutation and what the mutation was (if you believe there are more than one possible answer, list them all).
E If the mutation had occurred in the noncoding (template) strand only, but not in the coding (non-template) strand, would the same amino acid sequence (Met-Pro-Thr) still result? Explain.

1.6 As shown in Figure 1.25, antibodies are composed of two identical heavy chains attached to two identical light chains. The diversity of antibodies can be explained by the fact that each heavy chain is composed of Variable (V), Diversity (D), and Joining (J) regions, while each light chain is composed of Variable (V) and Joining (J) regions. The recombination process joins together various VDJ regions for a heavy chain and various VJ regions for a light chain. Suppose the following is the DNA-coding strand of a heavy chain joining sequence (J_H):
5′ TTAT GT AT CAT GGCAAT GGTT AAGC 3′

A What is the noncoding DNA sequence?

B What would be the transcribed mRNA sequence?

C What would be the translated amino acid sequence? An amino acid reference table is available on the last page of the exam.

D Now let's assume that the genome contains various permutations in the bases underlined in the joining sequence: TTATGT<u>AT</u>CATGGCAATGGTTAAGC.
How many different amino acid sequences are possible, assuming that all valid joining sequences must have five different amino acids?

E Now assuming the following number of VDJ regions for Heavy Chains and VJ regions for Light Chains (Table 1.2), what is the total number of different combinations of antibodies that can be made?

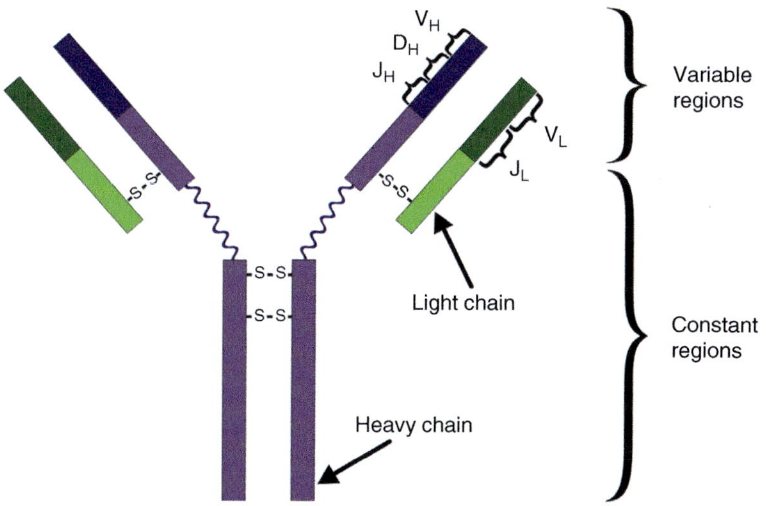

Figure 1.25 Structure of antibodies, including the composition of the heavy and light chains.

Table 1.2 Number of possible variations for the components of the heavy and light chains.

	Number of possible gene segments	
Segment	**Light chains**	**Heavy chains**
Variable (V)	70	65
Diversity (D)	0	27
Joining (J)	5	6

References

1 OpenStax (2016). A level notes: Biological membranes. https://commons.wikimedia.org/wiki/File:0301_Phospholipid_Structure.jpg.
2 OpenStax (2016). A level notes: Biological membranes. https://commons.wikimedia.org/wiki/File:0302_Phospholipid_Bilayer.jpg.
3 Sadava, D.E., Hillis, D.M., Heller, H.C., and Berenbaum, M. (2013). *Life: The Science of Biology* by Sadava et al. Fig. 4.19 on, 78. **Oxford University Press**.
4 Earthsound (2012). NHGRI human male karyotype. https://en.wikipedia.org/wiki/File:NHGRI_human_male_karvotvpe.png.
5 Dhorspool (2008). Central dogma of molecular biochemistry with enzymes. https://commons.wikimedia.org/wiki/File:Central_Dogma_of_Molecular_Biochemistry_with_Enzymes.jpg.
6 Boumphreyfr (2009). http://en.wikipedia.org/wiki/File:Peptide_syn.png.
7 OpenStax College (2013). https://commons.wikimedia.org/wiki/File:1911_Sickle_Cells.jpg.
8 Jpablo (2011). Mitosis schematic diagram. https://commons.wikimedia.org/wiki/File:Mitosis_schematic_diagram-en.svg.
9 Fred the Oyster (2010). Amino acids. https://commons.wikimedia.org/wiki/File:Amino_Acids.svg.
10 Zephyris (2007). https://commons.wikimedia.org/wiki/File:GFP_structure.png.
11 *Nature Biotechnology*, Improved monomeric, red, orange and yellow fluorescent proteins derived from Discosoma sp. Red fluorescent protein, Nathan C Shaner, Robert E Campbell, Paul A Steinbach, Ben N G Giepmans, Amy E Palmer et al., (2004) Volume: 22, Pgs: 1567–1572. https://www.nature.com/articles/nbt1037.

Further Reading

Adam-Day, S. A level notes-biological membranes. http://alevelnotes.com/Biological-Membratnes/128.

Boumphreyfr (2009). http://en.wikipedia.org/wiki/File:Peptide_syn.png.

Courtesy of National Human Genome Research Institute (2012). NHGRI human male karyotype. http://en.wikipedia.org/wiki/File:NHGRI_human_male_karyotype.png.

Davidson, M.W. (2000). Molecular expressions: Cell biology and microscopy structure and function of cells & viruses – the cell nucleus. http://micro.magnet.fsu.edu/cells/nucleus/nucleus.html.

Davidson, M.W. (2005). Molecular expressions: Cell biology and microscopy structure and function of cells & viruses – chromatin and chromosomes. http://micro.magnet.fsu.edu/cells/nucleus/chromatin.html.

http://academic.brooklyn.cuny.edu/biology/bio4fv/page/phosphb.htm

http://academic.brooklyn.cuny.edu/biology/bio4fv/page/rougher.htm

http://cellfunctioning.wikispaces.com/Epithelial+cells

http://chemistrv.gravitywaves.com/CHEMXL153/NucleotidesCompandStruc.htm

http://en.wikipedia.org/wiki/Amino_acids

http://en.wikipedia.org/wiki/Base_pair

http://en.wikipedia.org/wiki/File:Mitochondria._mammalian_lung_-_TEM.jpg

http://www.bio.miami.edu/~cmallery/255/255chem/gk2x20.gif

http://www.cholesterol-and-health.com/Cholesterol-Cell-Membrane.html

http://www.rikenresearch.riken.ip/eng/frontline/5514

Pratt, C.W. and Cornely, K. (2004). *Essential Biochemistry*. Wiley.
Shionyu, M., Yamaguchi, A., Shinoda, K. et al. (2009). AS-ALPS: a database for analyzing the effects of alternative splicing on protein structure, interaction and network in human and mouse. *Nucleic Acids Res.* **37** (Database issue): D305–D309. http://as-alps.nagahama-i-bio.ac.jp/.
Thibodeau, G.A. (2008). *Structure & Function of the Body*, 13e. Mosby.
Villarreal, M.R. (LadyofHats). (2006). Animal mitochondrian diagram. http://en.wikipedia.org/wiki/File:Animal_mitochondrion_diagram_en_(edit).svg
Wheeler, R. (Zephyis) (2005). Ribose structure. http://en.wikipedia.org/wiki/File:Ribose_structure_2.png.
Zimmer, M. *Green Fluorescent Protein: A Molecular Microscope*. Dept. of Chemistry Connecticut College http://www.photobiology.info/Zimmer.html.

2

Biological Lab Techniques

2.1 Overview

A variety of biological lab techniques are covered in this chapter. (i) **Spectrophotometry** uses Beer Lambert's law to measure the concentration of a molecule in a solution. (ii) **Restriction endonucleases** are used to cut DNA in specific locations. (iii) **Recombinant DNA** technology uses restriction enzymes to insert one DNA sequence into another. (iv) **Polymerase Chain Reaction (PCR)** is the most widely used method to replicate DNA in a lab. (v) **Gel Electrophoresis** is used to separate pieces of DNA based on size. Finally, we will discuss how these techniques are applied to make forensic DNA fingerprinting possible.

2.2 Beer Lambert's Law

Beer Lambert's Law defines the relationship between the concentration of a molecule in a solution and how much light the molecule absorbs. To determine a molecule's concentration, the experimental setup requires a light source, a cuvette filled with a solution of the molecule, and a photodetector. A sample setup is illustrated in Figure 2.1, where I_0 is the intensity of the incident light beam and I_2 is the intensity of the attenuated light beam. The incident light and attenuated light are related to each other through the attenuation coefficient (α) and length of the cuvette (l):

$$I_1 = I_0 \times 10^{-\alpha l}.$$

Transmission (T) is the ratio of attenuated intensity to the incident intensity and it is given by the following equation:

$$T = \frac{I_1}{I_0} = 10^{-\alpha l}.$$

Through a series of experiments, Beer and Lambert discovered that there is a direct relationship between the concentration of the molecule in the solution (c) and the attenuation coefficient (α), where the slope of the curve describing the relationship between the two terms is defined as the extinction coefficient (ϵ) of the molecule, such that: $\alpha = \epsilon c$. The extinction coefficient, ϵ, represents the intrinsic ability of the molecule to absorb light and is independent of the molecule's

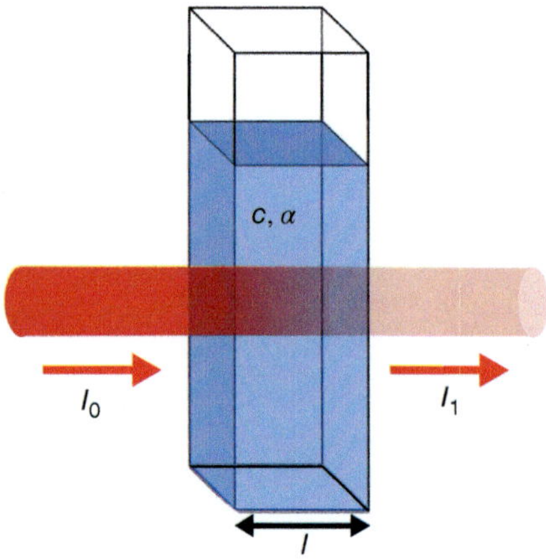

Figure 2.1 Beer Lambert's Law. *Source:* Oscar2 [1]. Used under CC-BY-SA 3.0 https://creativecommons.org/licenses/by-sa/3.0/.

concentration (in most cases). Given a molecule with extinction coefficient ϵ and cuvette of length l, one can compute the molecule concentration in the solution by measuring the light transmission through the cuvette using the following equation:

$$T = \frac{I_1}{I_0} = 10^{-\epsilon lc}.$$

Finally, the absorbance, A, is defined as the negative $\log_{10}$ of the ratio of intensities. Hence, the absorbance is expressed as:

$$A = \epsilon lc,$$

where ϵ is the extinction coefficient ($M^{-1}\ cm^{-1}$), l is s the length of the cuvette (cm), and c is the concentration of the solution ($M = mol\ L^{-}$). Note that absorbance is defined on a logarithmic scale with respect to light intensity. An absorbance of 1 means that 1 out of every 10^1 source photons makes it to the detector. Likewise, an absorbance of 2 means that 1 out of every 10^2 source photons makes it to the detector.

Each molecule has its own constant ϵ, which gives the ability of the molecule to absorb light. Given an absorbance measurement, Beer Lambert's Law can be used to measure the concentration of a known molecule. Note that ε is actually a function of wavelength. Hence, it is conventional to refer to ϵ at the peak of the extinction–wavelength curve.

2.3 DNA Lab Techniques

Four lab techniques will be discussed in this chapter: restriction enzymes (cut DNA in specific locations), recombinant DNA (insert one DNA into another), PCR (replicate DNA), and gel electrophoresis (separate DNA based on size).

2.3.1 Restriction Endonucleases

Restriction endonucleases (a.k.a. restriction enzymes) are "molecular scissors" that can cut DNA at certain locations. In 1978, Smith and Nathans won the Nobel Prize for discovering EcoR1, a bacterial enzyme that cuts double-stranded DNA at the sequence GAATTC. This discovery was the pillar for creating the field of biotechnology. Different bacterial strains contain different restriction enzymes that cut precise sequences of 4–8 base pairs in length and hundreds of restriction enzymes have been discovered to date. Restriction enzymes can be used to shorten DNA into fragments for analysis. While different restriction enzymes cut different DNA sequences, nearly all these DNA sequences have the property of being (semi-) **palindromic** sequences. This means that both DNA strands (the coding and noncoding) read the same from their respective 5′ ends. For example, the sequence recognized by EcoR1 is:

5′	GAATTC	3′
3′	CTTAAG	5′

There are some restriction enzymes that are not palindromic (e.g. AciI targets the 5′ CCGC 3′ sequence).

Figure 2.2 shows five different restriction endonucleases and their target sequences. The frequency of occurrence for each sequence depends on the sequence length. For example, HaeIII targets a four-base-pair-long sequence. The probability of getting these four bases in the same order (GGCC) is given by $(G = 1/4 \times G = 1/4 \times C = 1/4 \times C = 1/4) = 1/(4^4)$. Similarly, NotI targets an eight-base-long sequence and there is $1/(4^8)$ chance to see this particular sequence (probabilities assume random bases).

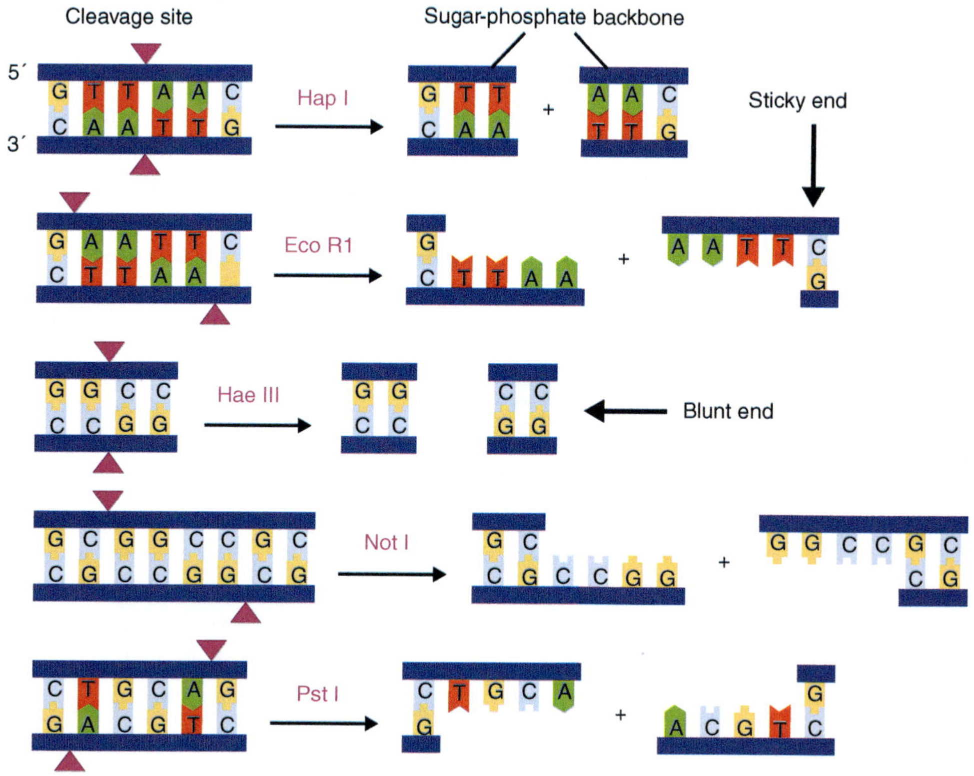

Figure 2.2 Restriction endonucleases and their targets.

Restriction enzymes make cuts on the sequence at specific locations called **cleavage sites**. Restriction endonucleases can create "sticky ends" or "blunt ends" after cutting DNA, depending on the location of cleavage sites. For example, EcoR1 creates **"sticky ends"** with exposed nucleotides, which can easily attract neighboring nucleotides (Figure 2.2). In contrast, AluI creates **"blunt ends,"** so that the resulting two DNA strands will not attract each other as much. Once DNA is cut, different ends can be joined together to create a new DNA sequence, which is the process of genetic engineering (Figure 2.3). There are several options of joining strands together: either two complementary staggered ("sticky") ends together, or two blunt ends together, or a blunt end with a sticky end, where the sticky end is first complemented by a DNA polymerase.

Restriction enzymes were first discovered in bacteria. Bacteria use these enzymes as a weapon to fight bacteriophages (viruses that infect bacteria), other bacteria, and invaders by cutting their DNA. The bacterial host DNA is not affected by its own restriction enzymes because methyl groups ($-CH_3$) are attached to the restriction site on the host DNA. These methyl groups block the part of the restriction enzymes that are responsible for making cuts in the DNA.

2.3.1.1 Exonucleases

Exonucleases are enzymes that also cut DNA. However, unlike restriction endonucleases, exonucleases cut DNA (and RNA) strands at their 3′ or 5′ ends. They remove nucleotides one by one from the ends of the strands. Exonucleases are important for proofreading by DNA polymerase and RNA polymerase (the enzymes that make DNA and RNA, respectively) by stopping DNA replication or transcription (respectively) if errors occur. Exonucleases are also used for recycling mRNA strands back into nucleotides.

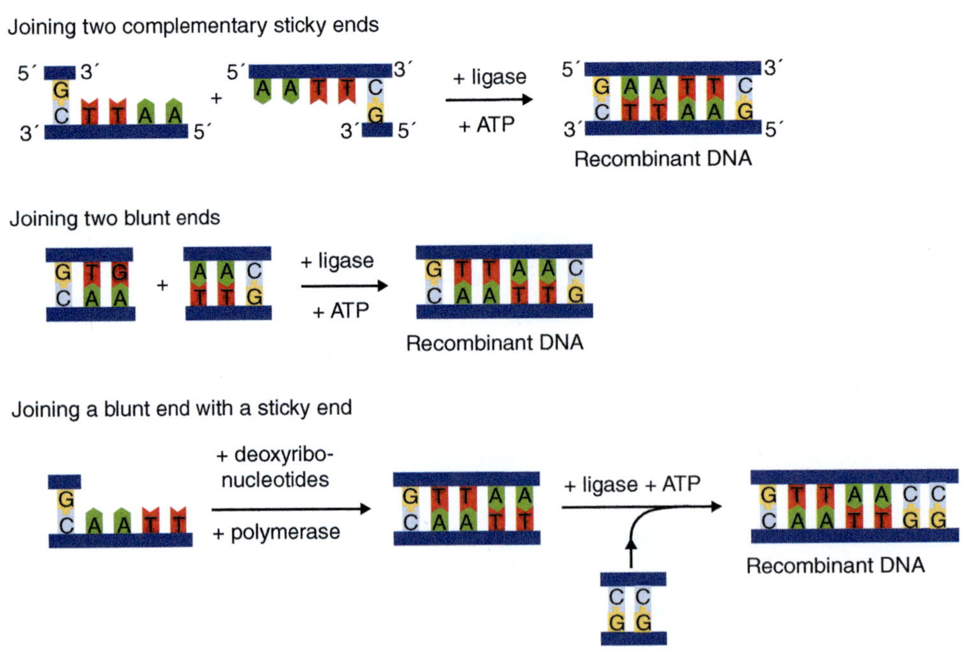

Figure 2.3 Joining DNA fragments.

2.3.2 Recombinant DNA

Recombinant DNA technology is a method to combine DNA from two different sources and transfer DNA from one organism to another. For example, the recombinant DNA technique allows for insertion of DNA that encodes for human insulin into bacteria or yeast, which allows insulin to be made outside of the body. Once the vector transfection is complete, the vector is inserted into the host organism (e.g. bacteria). The organism is then cultured and produces the protein of interest. The protein of interest (e.g. insulin) is then harvested and used (e.g. for medical applications). The primary use of this method is to produce therapeutic proteins on a large and cost-efficient scale.

2.3.2.1 Recombinant DNA Process

The recombinant DNA process involves restriction enzymes and two DNA double-strands. First, a restriction enzyme cuts one of the double-stranded DNA at its recognition sites, producing a DNA fragment with two sticky ends. Then, the same enzyme is used to cut the other DNA to expose similar sticky ends. When two fragments of DNA cut by the same restriction enzyme come together, they can join by base-pairing (A–T and G–C). The joined fragments will usually form either a linear molecule or a circular one (depending on their size). Note that other combinations of fragments can also occur. DNA ligase is then used to unite the backbones of the two DNA fragments, producing a recombinant DNA strand (Figure 2.4).

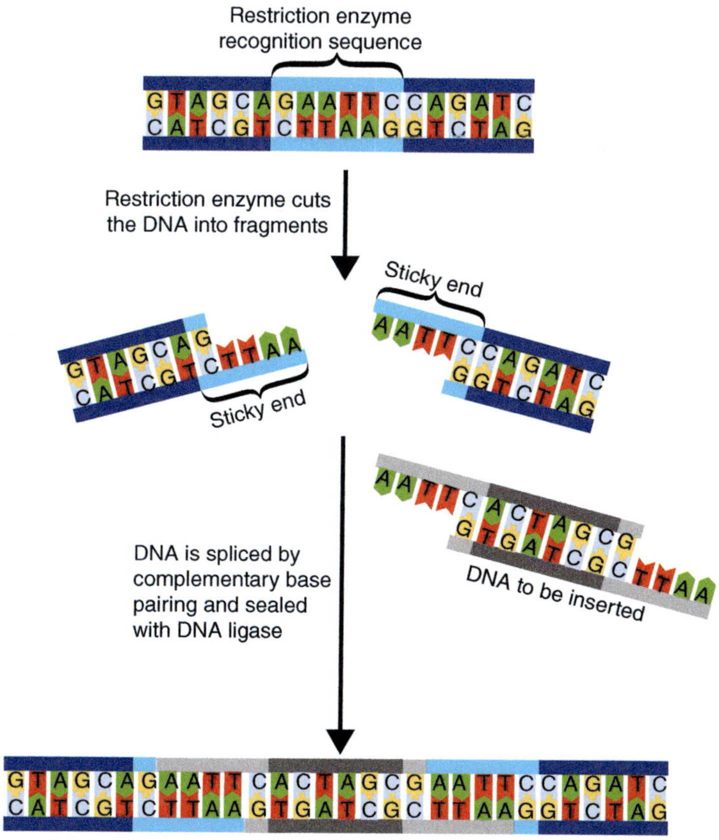

Figure 2.4 Recombinant DNA process.

Using the insulin example, a restriction enzyme is used to cut a human DNA right before and after the gene that encodes for insulin. The resulting DNA fragment will have "sticky ends" specific to the restriction endonuclease used. The same restriction enzyme is applied to bacterium DNA. The bacterial DNA fragments will have the same sticky ends as the human DNA. The human and bacteria DNA are put together and a ligase is added to join the fragments. One of the resulting DNA strands will be a bacterial DNA infused with the human insulin gene (i.e. recombinant DNA).

2.3.2.2 Recombinant DNA – Origin

Bacteria have small, circular, extrachromosomal DNA, called **plasmids** (Figure 2.5). Plasmids often carry genes that help the bacteria resist antibiotic drugs (this mechanism is the basis for bacterial antibiotic resistance). These plasmids are also called "cloning vectors" or "expression vectors" in the context of recombinant DNA technology. Once the recombinant DNA process is performed on the plasmid, it is inserted into a host organism (e.g. bacteria). The organism is left to reproduce by dividing, and produce the protein of interest, that was encoded by the gene inserted into the plasmid. The primary application of recombinant DNA in plasmids is to use bacteria to produce therapeutic proteins (e.g. insulin).

2.3.2.3 Recombinant DNA – Validation

After the DNA recombination process is completed, how can one determine which (bacterial) hosts have a copy of the human gene? One method is to use a **cloning vector** that has a reporter gene (e.g. lacZ, which encodes for the enzyme β-galactosidase) that produces a visible change in the host (e.g. blue color) if the human DNA was not inserted (Figure 2.6a).

Notice the lacZ gene at the top of the vector: within this gene, there are 13 different restriction sites. The plasmid is cut at one of these sites and human DNA is inserted. The bacteria are then grown with X-gal supplement. If the insertion is successful, the original lacZ gene is ruined and the resulting colony turns out to be white. This can be seen in the colonies grown on agar (Figure 2.6b).

The lacZ gene encodes for an enzyme called β-galactosidase. In bacteria, β-galactosidase is used for breaking β-galactosides (a group of complex sugars like lactose) into monosaccharides (simple sugars like glucose). When X-gal (a colorless artificial sugar similar to lactose) is presented to this enzyme, X-gal is broken into smaller units. These smaller units oxidize in the environment and the resulting product is blue in color. Hence, if one takes a bacteria colony with a functioning lacZ gene (i.e. the human DNA insertion did not succeed) and feed them with X-gal, they will turn blue. However, if the insertion was successful, the lacZ gene is broken in the middle. Therefore, the bacteria will not be able to produce β-galactosidase, and the colonies will appear white.

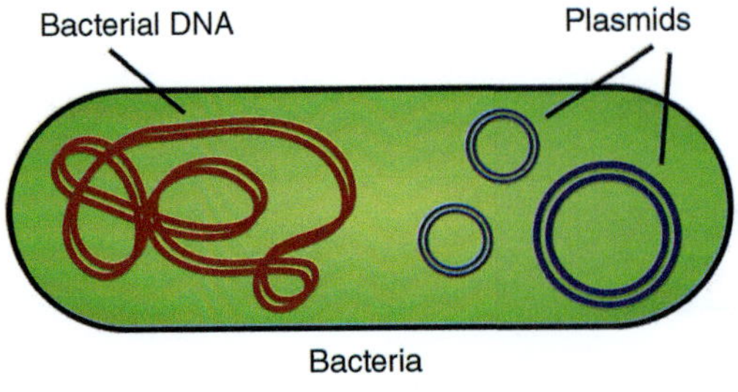

Figure 2.5 Plasmids in bacteria. *Source:* Fibonacci [2]. Used under CC-BY-SA 2.5 https://creativecommons.org/licenses/by-sa/2.5/.

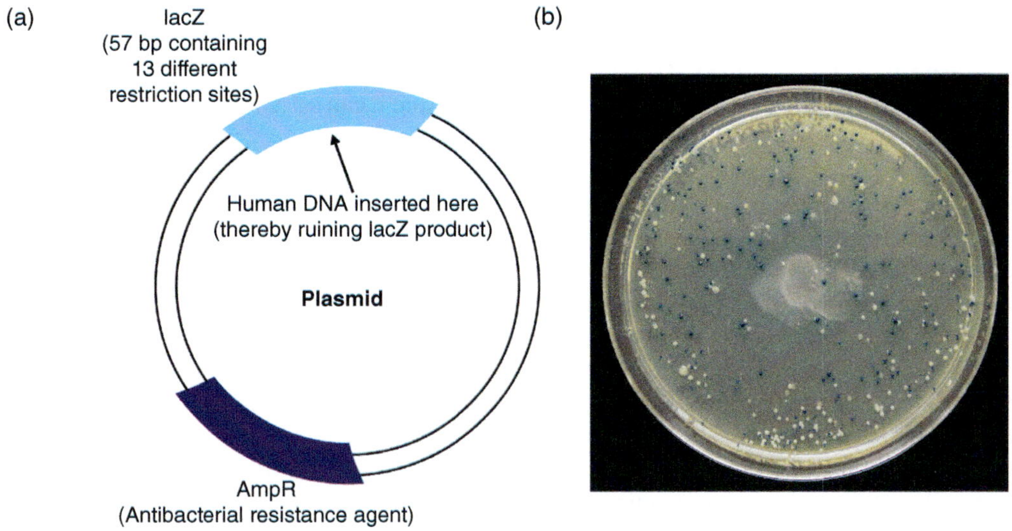

Figure 2.6 (a) Recombinant DNA validation, (b) resulting colonies. *Source:* Navaho [3]. Used under CC-BY-SA 4.0 https://creativecommons.org/licenses/by-sa/4.0/.

Did You Know?

San Diego beach scene on a petri dish – eight different bacteria colonies (expressing fluorescent genes at different colors) were used as a palette to create this artwork in Roger Tsien's lab in 2006: Reporter genes and proteins are not limited to lacZ and β-galactosidase. There are many other reporter genes, such as luciferase (derived from fireflies) and fluorescent proteins (initially derived from jellyfish). Green fluorescent proteins (GFPs) are especially interesting. The GFP gene was discovered by Martin Chalfie, Osamu Shimomura, and Roger Y. Tsien who were awarded the 2008 Nobel Prize in Chemistry. Multiple derivatives (mutants) of GFP gene have been created. Some of these mutants increased the fluorescence quality of the protein while other mutations caused the protein to fluoresce in different colors (Figure 2.7). By including fluorescent reporter genes in a vector with a gene of interest, researchers can identify when that gene is expressed in an organism.

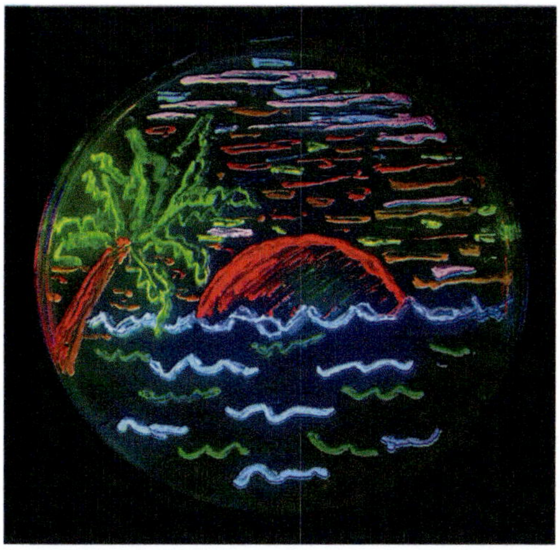

Figure 2.7 San Diego beach scene on a petri dish. *Source:* Nathan Shaner/Paul Steinbach [4]. Used under CC-BY-SA 3.0 https://creativecommons.org/licenses/by-sa/4.0/.

2.3.3 Polymerase Chain Reaction (PCR)

Polymerase Chain Reaction (PCR) is a process that is used to make many copies of a piece of DNA (a.k.a. DNA amplification). One advantage of PCR is that it can selectively amplify a specific target DNA sequence, even in a mixture of many other DNA sequences.

Each cycle of PCR happens in three steps: denaturation, annealing, and elongation.

Denaturation: First, the DNA is heated up to ~95 °C for five minutes, which separates the DNA strands by breaking the weak hydrogen bonds between base pairs.

Add ingredients: Primers, nucleotides, and DNA polymerase are then added to the mixture. To allow amplification of a specific region in the DNA strand, primers, which are DNA strands 18–22 base pairs long, are designed to complement the beginning and ending of the region on the coding and noncoding strands, respectively (Figure 2.8).

Anneal: After cooling the solution to ~60 °C, the primers can anneal (hydrogen bond) to their complementary sequences at the beginning and end of the target strand.

Elongation: Finally, the DNA polymerase finds the primers and synthesizes complementary DNA strands (DNA polymerase requires such primers to "jump-start" the polymerization process).

The PCR process described above repeats itself over many cycles of heating and cooling, at the end of each, the number of DNA strands approximately doubles. These cycles are repeated until the desired DNA amplification is reached. If there is 100% efficiency, one expects to double the amount of DNA in every cycle, resulting in an exponential growth (Figure 2.8). In reality, the growth is indeed exponential; however, the amplification is less than twofold per cycle. PCR has several modifications (such as real-time PCR and reverse transcriptase PCR). Those modifications will be discussed later in the course.

Since DNA polymerase denatures (deactivates) in high temperatures, more DNA polymerase was needed after each denaturing step, resulting in a very expensive and long process. This problem was solved by using a heat-stable DNA polymerase isolated from bacteria (Thermus aquaticus, Taq) that live in the hot springs of Yellowstone. This Taq DNA polymerase has optimal activity at 75–80 °C, and does not denature during PCR. This discovery made Roche over two billion dollars and won Kary Mullis the Nobel Prize in 1993.

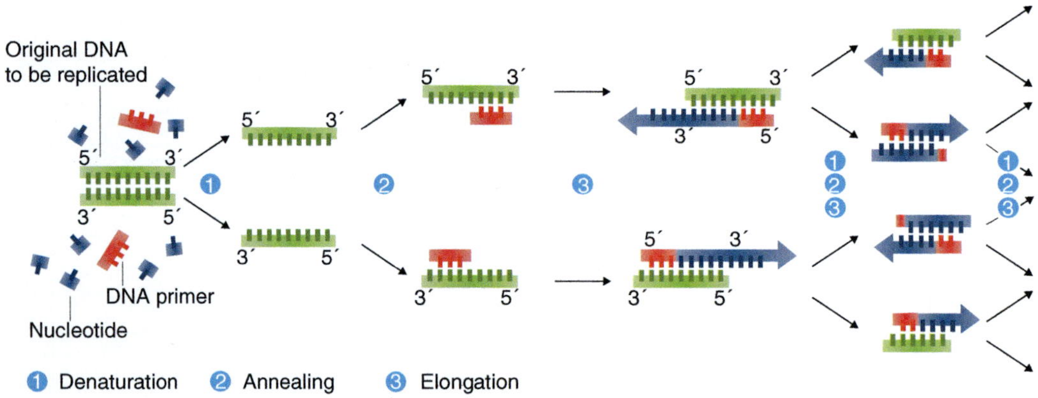

Figure 2.8 Steps of PCR cycle. *Source:* Enzoklop [5]. Used under CC-BY-SA 3.0 https://creativecommons.org/licenses/by-sa/3.0/.

2.3.4 Gel Electrophoresis

Gel Electrophoresis is a method to separate DNA based on its size. Since DNA and RNA have a phosphate backbone with a negative charge, they will experience a force under an applied electric field and move along a gel. This movement, when charged species drift when placed under an electric field, is called electrophoresis. It is governed by the equation:

$$v = -\mu \frac{dV}{dx'}$$

where v is the electrophoretic velocity, μ is the electrophoretic mobility, and dV/dx is the applied electric field. The separation region of the gel electrophoresis setup is filled with a gel matrix with pores, through which the DNA molecules pushed by the electric field can traverse in a snake-like fashion. A sample setup is shown in Figure 2.9.

Mixtures of DNA fragments of different sizes in solution are placed at the top "lanes" in the gel (Figure 2.10). The DNA molecules are then pushed by the electric field and traverse through the gel. The longer the DNA strand, the slower it will travel through the gel. This may be counterintuitive as the longer the DNA strand is, the greater its charge is and hence the greater the Coulomb force that is applied on it. However, in the case of gel electrophoresis, the difficulty of moving through the gel pores dominates the speed of movement through the gel. As a result of the differential motion of the DNA strands, bands are formed in the gel, where each band corresponds to DNA fragments of a different length. To visualize the DNA strands, the gel is later exposed to a fluorescent dye that binds to DNA (e.g. ethidium bromide). A sample of the visualization is seen in Figure 2.10b.

Gel electrophoresis is not quantitative in the sense that it is hard to correlate movement through the gel to a specific DNA length. For this reason, samples are usually run with a DNA ladder. DNA ladders are commercially available samples with several fragments of known sizes. Putting a

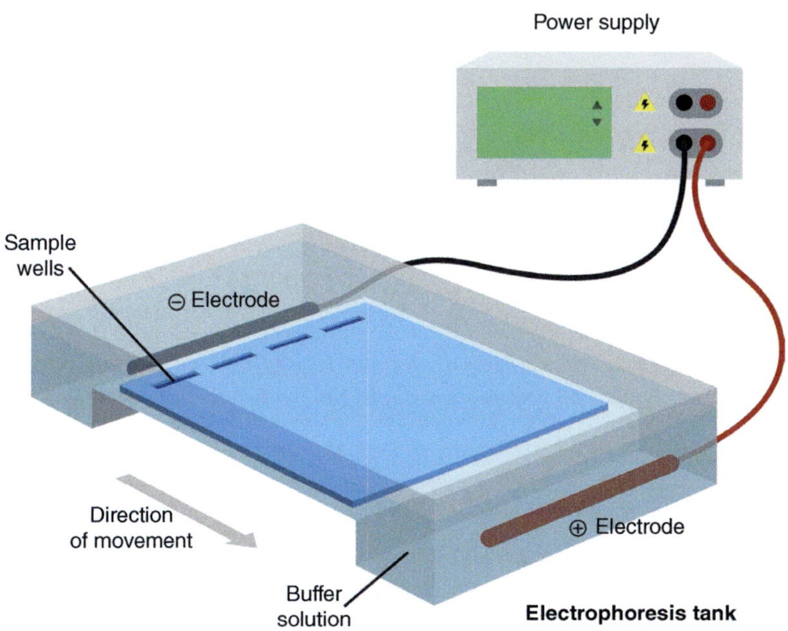

Figure 2.9 Sample gel electrophoresis setup. *Source:* yourgenome [6].

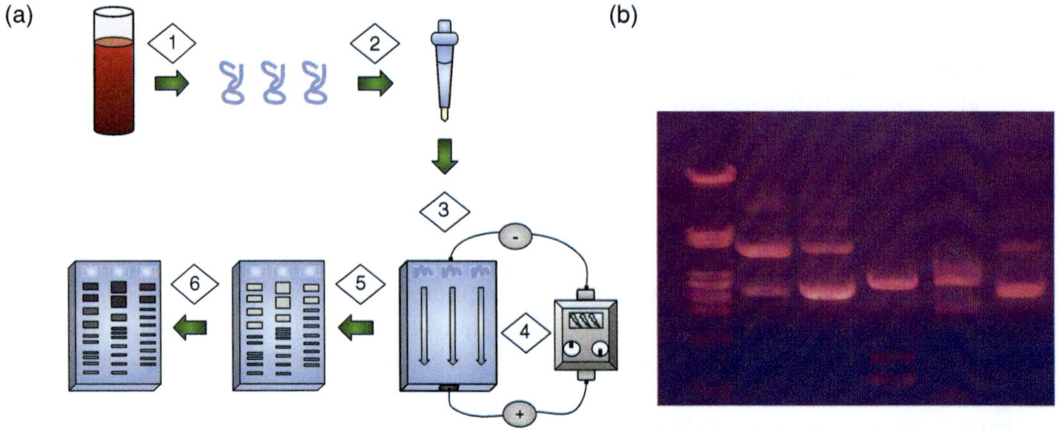

Figure 2.10 (a) Sample electrophoresis run. *Source:* Jennifer0328 [7]. https://commons.wikimedia.org/wiki/File:Gel_Electrophoresis_in_DNA_Fingerprinting.svg Used under CC BY-SA 4.0 https://creativecommons.org/licenses/by-sa/340/. (b) actual electrophoresis result. Under UV light, ethidium bromide glows orange. *Source:* Mnolf [8]. Used under CC-BY-SA 3.0 https://creativecommons.org/licenses/by-sa/3.0/

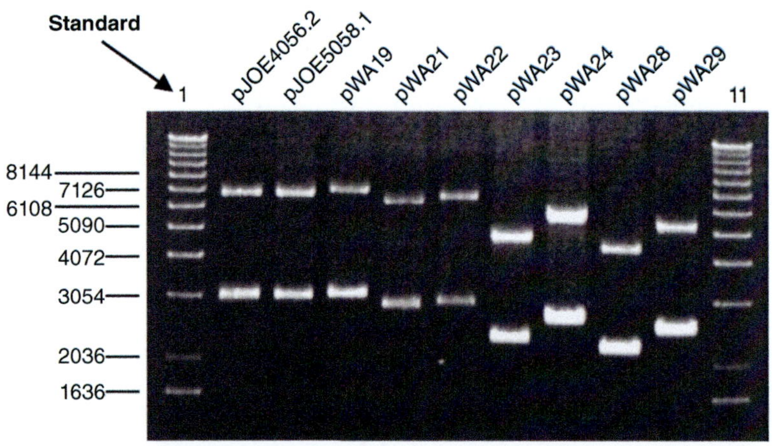

Figure 2.11 Sample electrophoresis run with DNA ladders in lanes 1 and 11. *Source:* Reprinted with permission from Springer (BMC Biotechnology) under CC-BY-SA 2.0 https://creativecommons.org/licenses/by-sa/2.0/.

ladder sample in one of the electrophoresis wells creates a reference result (like a ruler) to compare the lengths of unknown fragments. Figure 2.11 shows a sample run with two ladders placed at wells 1 and 11.

2.3.5 Forensic DNA Fingerprinting

2.3.5.1 Restriction Fragment Length Polymorphism

Forensic DNA fingerprinting uses several biological lab techniques to match a suspect's DNA to a sample of DNA collected from the field (e.g. saliva or blood residue at a crime scene). First, a DNA sample is extracted from a suspect's blood, saliva, or other bodily fluid. This DNA is cleaved by

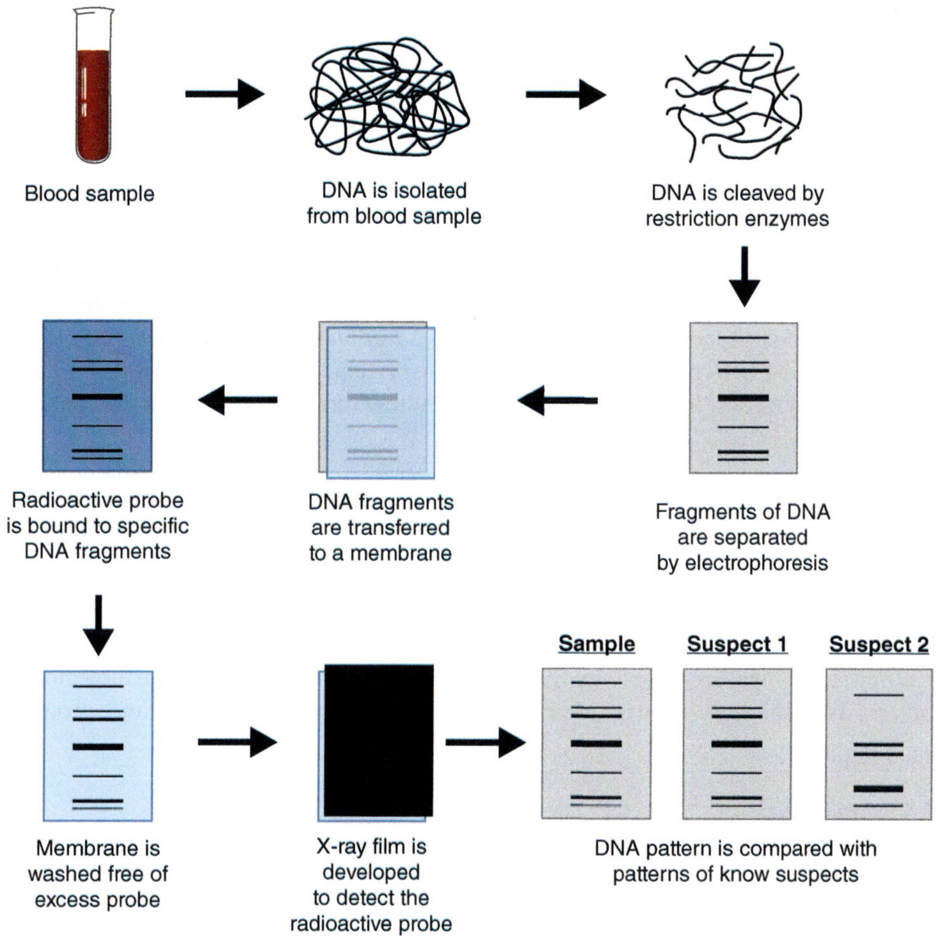

Figure 2.12 Restriction fragment length polymorphism method.

restriction enzymes and separated by gel electrophoresis into different bands corresponding to DNA fragment length. After transferring the DNA fragments to a membrane, radioactive DNA probes are bound to specific DNA fragments. The membrane is then washed free of excess probes and an X-ray film is used to detect a radioactive pattern of bands. Finally, the pattern of DNA bands from the suspect is compared to an unknown DNA sample to determine if they match. See Figure 2.12 for an illustration of this process.

Did You Know?

Short Tandem Repeat Polymorphism

Most of the modern forensic labs today use a different method called Short Tandem Repeat (STR) analysis. As we discussed earlier, not all of the DNA is used in coding proteins. There are regions called introns and exons. While exons are used in the translation process, the introns of the mRNA are cut during splicing. Some of these introns contain repeating sequences of 2–5 base pairs. For example, the CSF1PO locus of DNA contains repeats of $[AGAT]_n$ sequence.

These are called **short tandem repeats (STRs).** The number of repeats changes from person to person. This is called **short tandem repeat polymorphism (STRP).** This forensic analysis technique focuses on detecting STRPs at certain loci.

The process is as follows: first, a DNA sample is acquired from the suspect. Then, the DNA segment with a repeating sequence (for example, CSF1PO locus) is amplified using PCR. These amplified segments are then passed through gel electrophoresis. Depending on the number of repeats (hence the length of the segment), fragments move to a certain position. Using a DNA ladder, it is possible to determine the length of the segment and the number of repeats. The same process is repeated for different STR loci and an STR profile of the suspect is acquired. In the US, the Combined DNA Index System (CODIS) uses 13 different STR locations (CSF1PO is one of them) to create a DNA profile for everyone in the system. The possibility of 2 people having the same configuration in all 13 locations is very low (unless they are monozygotic twins).

2.4 Additional Information

2.4.1 More Information on Biological Spectrophotometry

Now that we know the physical principles of spectrophotometry, let's look at some practical examples of how absorbance measurements can provide information about biological molecules. Spectrophotometry is commonly used to determine the concentration of DNA and protein samples.

2.4.1.1 DNA Spectrophotometry

DNA bases (A, T, G, and C) have molecular structures (called aromatic rings) that absorb ultraviolet (UV) light. Specifically, double helix DNA has a characteristic absorbance peak of light with a wavelength of about 260 nm. In other words, DNA has a higher molar extinction coefficient (ϵ) around 260 nm than it does at other wavelengths.

Because each nucleobase has its own characteristic extinction (ϵ) at 260 nm, you can determine the total extinction expected per DNA molecule at 260 nm. For example, the total extinction from Adenine is the number of Adenines in the DNA molecule (n_{Adenine}) multiplied by the extinction coefficient for Adenine ($\epsilon_{\text{Adenine}}$). Applying this logic to each of the four bases, we find that the total extinction per DNA molecule can be mathematically expressed as:

$$\varepsilon_{260\,\text{nm DNA}} = n_{\text{Adenine}}\varepsilon_{260\,\text{nm Adenine}} + n_{\text{Guanine}}\varepsilon_{260\,\text{nm Guanine}} + n_{\text{Thymine}}\varepsilon_{260\,\text{nm Thymine}} + n_{\text{Cytosine}}\varepsilon_{260\,\text{nm Cytosine}}.$$

We now know the molar extinction, ϵ, of our DNA molecule at 260 nm. Now suppose we have a solution of this DNA, but we don't know the concentration of the molecule in the solution. The first step to find the sample's concentration is to use a spectrophotometer to take an absorbance scan of this sample. This measurement will tell us the total absorbance of the solution at 260 nm. Since we know the sample's absorbance (A), our molecule's extinction (ϵ), and the length of the cuvette in which we prepared our sample, we can use Beer–Lambert's law ($A = \epsilon lc$) to solve for the concentration.

2.4.1.2 Protein Spectrophotometry

The same principles described above can also be applied to protein samples but in a slightly different way. Because proteins do not contain nucleobases, they do not have strong absorbance at

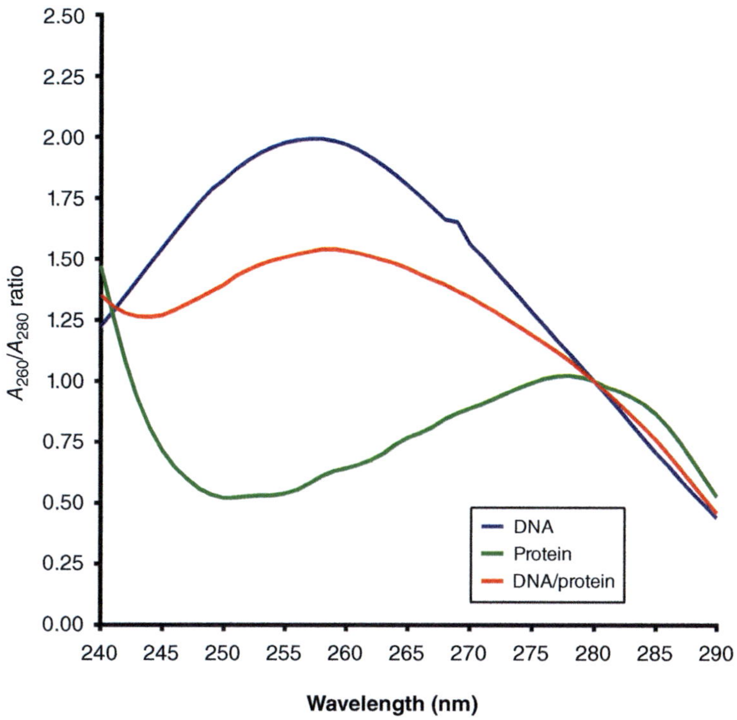

Figure 2.13 Absorbance of DNA and protein samples. *Source:* Figure obtained courtesy of Paul Held, BioTek Instruments.

260 nm like DNA does. However, some of the amino acids that make up proteins have characteristic absorbance properties. These amino acids (tryptophan, tyrosine, and phenylalanine) are also made up of aromatic rings, and they have strong absorbance of light around 280 nm. If you know the sequence of your protein, then you can count up the number of each of these three amino acids and determine the protein's total extinction at 280 nm in the same way we did for DNA at 260 nm:

$$\varepsilon_{280\,\mathrm{nm\,Protein}} = n_{\mathrm{Tryptophan}}\varepsilon_{280\,\mathrm{nm\,Tryptophan}} + n_{\mathrm{Tyrosine}}\varepsilon_{280\,\mathrm{nm\,Tyrosine}} + n_{\mathrm{Phenylalanine}}\varepsilon_{280\,\mathrm{nm\,Phenylalanine}}.$$

Again using a spectrophotometer and Beer–Lambert's law, we can find the concentration of our protein sample. The difference in protein and DNA spectra (Figure 2.13) can be used to help identify unknown biological samples or to determine the concentration of a known sample as described above.

2.4.1.3 Other Applications of Spectrophotometry

There are just a few uses of spectrophotometry. This simple technique can also be used to perform very elegant studies of enzyme activity rates and even to distinguish different forms of the same protein. For example, hemoglobin absorbs different wavelengths of light depending on whether it contains oxygen (O_2) or carbon dioxide (CO_2). By measuring the absorbance of hemoglobin at two different wavelengths (one where hemoglobin-O_2 absorbs strongly and one where hemoglobin-CO_2 absorbs strongly) and taking the ratio of the two measurements, it is possible to determine the relative ratio of each of the two forms. In fact, this is the principle behind a technique called **pulse oximetry**. A pulse oximeter (Figure 2.14) is designed to measure a patient's blood oxygenation

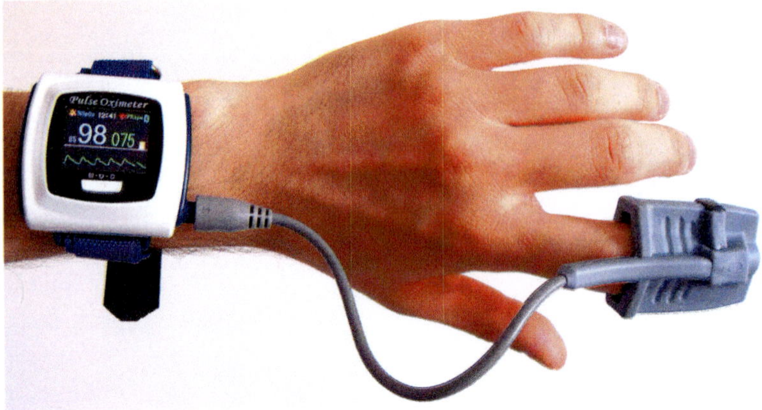

Figure 2.14 A pulse oximeter is used to easily monitor a patient's blood oxygenation level. *Source:* Mysid [9]. CC0-1.0 public domain https://creativecommons.org/publicdomain/zero/1.0/.

level. To do this, the pulse oximeter emits two different wavelengths of light that pass through the patient's fingertip. The amount by which each wavelength is attenuated is dependent on how much hemoglobin-O_2 and hemoglobin-CO_2 are present in their blood. Pulse oximetry is just one example of how Beer–Lambert's Law can be used in practical design applications.

Did You Know?

RNA vs. DNA spectrophotometry

We talked about how to distinguish DNA from protein using spectrophotometry, but what about RNA? RNA and DNA are both made of aromatic nucleobases, so how do we tell them apart? Recall that, in most cases, DNA is double-stranded and RNA is single-stranded. If you look closely at the DNA double helix, adjacent bases in the same strand are arranged so that they "stack" on top of each other. These interactions actually change the electronic resonance properties of each nucleobase, which, in turn, affects the absorbance properties of DNA. On the other hand, single-stranded RNA is more flexible and does not exhibit these stacking interactions. Therefore, RNA actually has a slightly different absorbance than DNA, despite being made up of (mostly) the same nucleobases.

Problems

2.1 A biologist has received an optical dye from a friend in a liquid form. The friend did not indicate the concentration of the dye. However, he did mention that the extinction coefficient of this dye is $\epsilon = 280\,000\,\text{cm}^{-1}\,\text{M}^{-1}$ at the peak absorbance point. The biologist then scanned the sample he received in his lab's spectrophotometer using a 1.5 cm cuvette and received the absorbance spectrum in Figure 2.15. Can you help the biologist calculate the concentration of the dye sample he received?

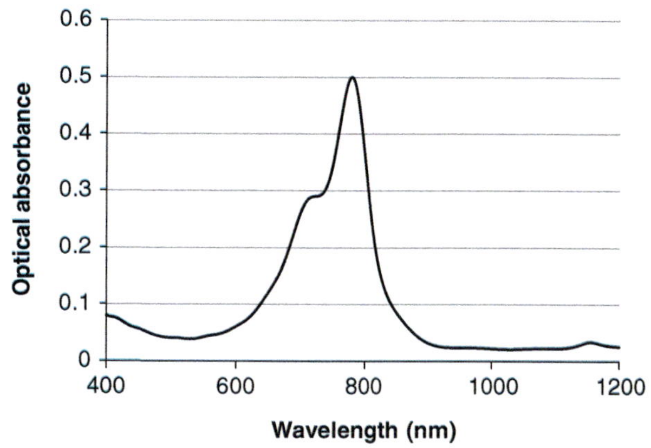

Figure 2.15 Absorption profile of dye with unknown concentration.

2.2 In an experiment, bacteria are transfected with a gene whose product is Protein-X, which exhibits a strong blue color. Protein-X has a known extinction coefficient of $\varepsilon = 30\,000\,\text{cm}^{-1}\,\text{M}^{-1}$. In a volume of 1 ml, a scientist counted 10^6 bacteria. He then poured the bacteria solution to a 1 cm-wide (path length) cuvette and measured absorbance $A = 0.5$ from that solution. Help the scientist determine how many copies of the Protein-X each bacterium has produced?

Assume that the mean amount of the protein expressed by each bacterium is uniform.
For your reference, Avogadro's number is: $N_A = 6\times10^{23}$ molecules mol^{-1}

2.3 Beer Lambert's law indicates that for a cuvette filled with an absorbing dye, $T=10^{-\alpha l}$ where α is *linearly* related to the dye concentration by $\alpha = \varepsilon\, c$.

A A cuvette is filled with 1 ml of dye #1 and out of 1 000 000 photons that hit its surface, 1 000 photons make it through the other side of the cuvette. A different cuvette is then filled with 1 ml of dye #2 and out of 1 000 000 photons, only 160 photons make it through the other side of the cuvette. A new solution is made by mixing 0.5 ml of dye #1 with 0.5 ml of dye #2 and is poured into a new cuvette. How many photons will make it through the other side of the cuvette this time?

B Unlike an absorption event where the absorbed photon disappears, in a scattering event, the photon changes its direction of propagation. Briefly explain:

i) Why a spectrophotometer is not a good instrument for measuring scattering dyes
ii) Under what circumstances could a spectrophotometer instrument be used to measure scattering dyes?

Hint: You may find the drawings in Figure 2.16 helpful in your explanation.

2.4 A cloning vector that has a reporter gene such as lacZ is used to identify bacteria that have insulin. Human DNA that encodes insulin is inserted into lacZ and this combination is introduced into the bacterial colonies in the presence of X-gal. Blue and white colors are observed in the colonies. Explain what do these signify.

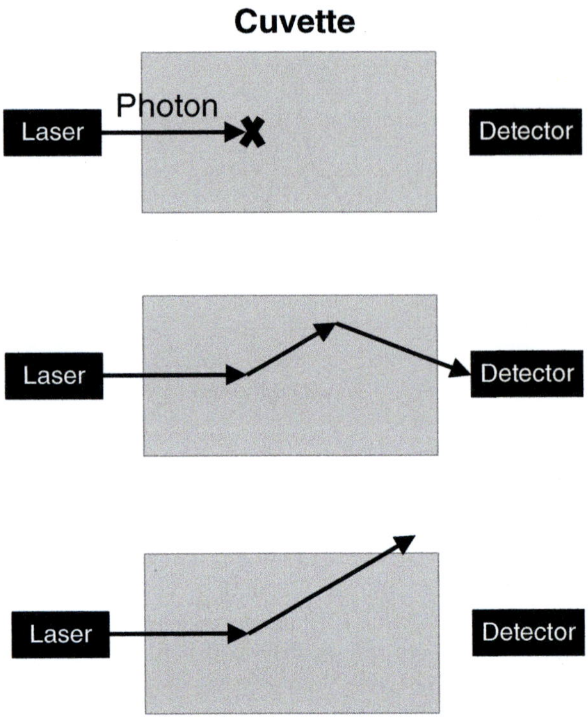

Figure 2.16 Photon interactions.

2.5 PCR is used to generate large quantities of a particular sequence of DNA. The binding sites of interest in the DNA are shown below and the dotted lines indicate the rest of the DNA sequence.

Primer 1 should bind here   Primer 2 should bind here

5′ AATTCGCGCGCGCGAATTCGATCGA------TTAAGCGCGCGCGCGCTTAATACGTACTAG 3′

3′ TTAAGCGCGCGCGCTTAAGCTAGCT------AATTCGCGCGCGCGCGAATTATGCATGATC 5′

Among the following sets of primers, identify those that can amplify this DNA.

i) **Primer 1: 5′ AATTCGCGCGCG 3′ and Primer 2: 5′ TATTCCGCGCCG 3′**
ii) **Primer 1: 5′ GCTTAAGCTAGC 3′ and Primer 2: 5′GATCATGCATAA 3′**
iii) **Primer 1: 5′ GAATTCGATCGA 3′ and Primer 2: 5' CTAGTACGTATT 3′**
iv) **Primer 1: 5′ CGAATTCGATCG 3′ and Primer 2: 5' TTAAGCGCGCGC 3′**

2.6 Restriction enzymes are used to construct restriction maps of DNA. These are diagrams of specific DNA molecules that show the sites where the restriction enzymes cleave the DNA. To construct a restriction map, purified samples of the DNA are treated with one or more restriction enzymes. The reaction products are then separated by agarose gel electrophoresis, a technique that separates the DNA fragments based on size (the smaller fragments travel more quickly and are found near the bottom of the gel, whereas the larger fragments are found near the top of the gel). Use the results of the agarose gel electrophoresis separation (Figure 2.17) to construct a restriction map for the sample of DNA.

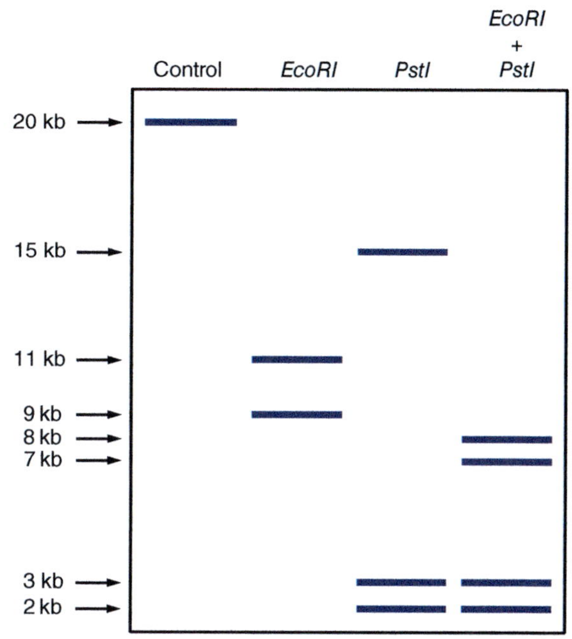

Figure 2.17 Gel electrophoresis used for creating a restriction map.

2.7 A cloning vector v_1 (Figure 2.18) is 90k base-pairs-long (90 kbp); the two specified locations are recognized by EcoR1 (the restriction endonuclease).

We want to use EcoR1 to insert gene g_1 into the vector. g_1 is 20 kbp long. We make three samples (v_1 only, v_1 with EcoR1, and v_1 with EcoR1 and gene g_1) and run them in a gel electrophoresis, results are shown in Figure 2.19.

Five bands are seen in the third column. Explain what each band in the third column represents.

A gene g_1 is defined as: A T G (G A T A T C)$_{500}$ G A A T T C (G A T A T C)$_{500}$ T A A, where (AAA)$_n$ means that the sequence AAA is repeated n times consecutively.

A vector v_1 is 100k base-pairs-long (100 kbp, a circular form) and has two specified locations recognized by two restriction endonucleases: EcoRI (with DNA recognition site of GAATTC) and EcoRV (with DNA recognition site of GATATC), as shown in the restriction map below (Figure 2.20).

We try to insert gene g_1 into the vector v_1. We prepared four samples and ran them in a gel electrophoresis:

1) $v_1 + g_1$
2) $v_1 + g_1$ + EcoRI

Figure 2.18 Restriction map of cloning vector v_1 with cleavage sites indicated.

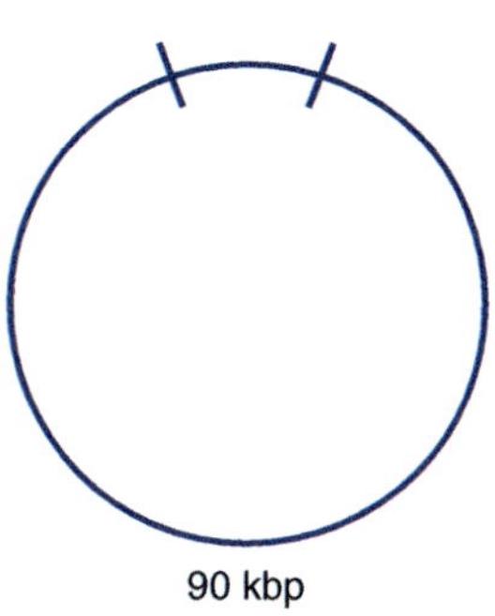

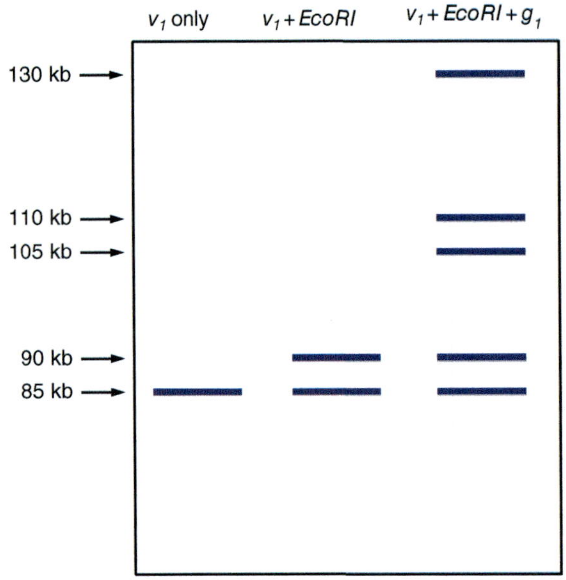

Figure 2.19 Gel electrophoresis results from insertion of gene g_1 into cloning vector v_1.

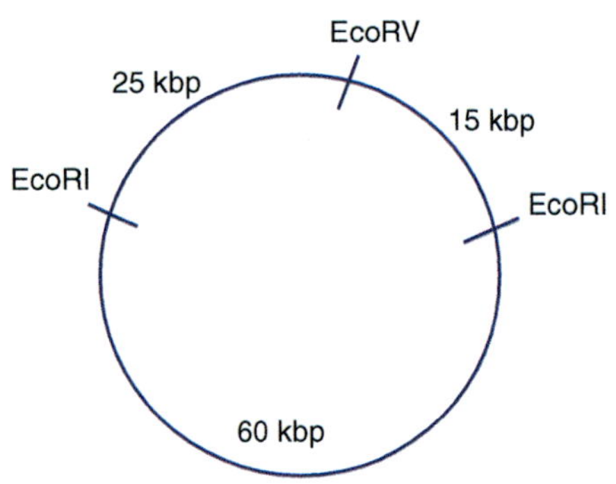

Figure 2.20 Restriction map of vector v_1 with cleavage sites of EcoRI and EcoRV indicated.

3) $v_1 + g_1$ + EcoRV
4) $v_1 + g_1$ + EcoRI + EcoRV
   A What is the length of gene g_1?
   B Describe/draw the output of the completed gel electrophoresis with important bands labeled with lengths.

2.8 Figure 2.21 shows the structure of an antibody molecule. It consists of two light chains and two heavy chains.

The molecular weight of each of the light chains is 25 kDa, and each of the heavy chains is 50 kDa, giving a total molecular weight of 150 kDa for the whole antibody molecule. You run antibody solutions through gel electrophoresis. What would the gel look like in each of the conditions below?

A Intact antibody
B Antibody cleaved with β-mercaptoethanol, a reducing agent that breaks disulfide bonds.
C Antibody cleaved with Pepsin. Pepsin has the ability to cleave the heavy chains near the hinge region, but leaving the disulfide bonds intact (see Figure 2.21).

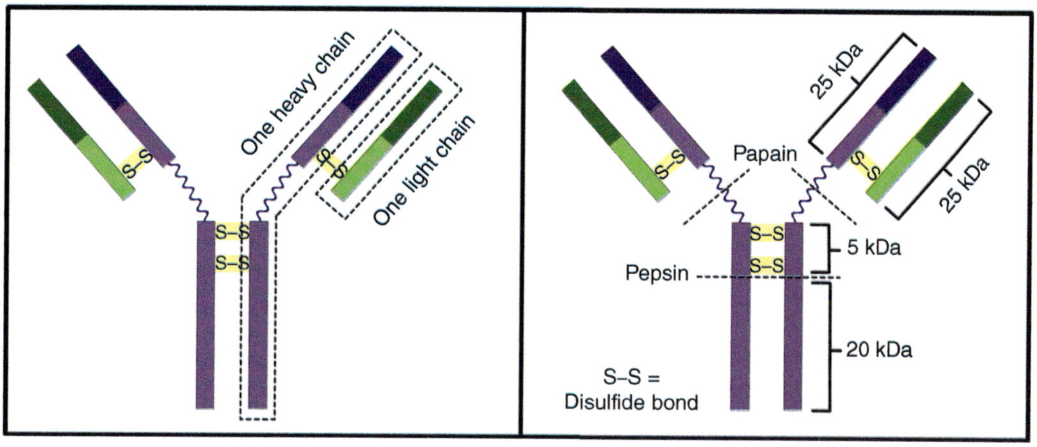

Figure 2.21 Structure of an antibody molecule.

D Antibody cleaved with Papain. Papain has the endopeptidase activity to cleave antibody molecules in the hinge region (see Figure 2.21).
E Antibody cleaved with β-mercaptoethanol, then Pepsin.
F Antibody cleaved with β-mercaptoethanol, then Papain.

References

1. Oscar2, https://commons.wikimedia.org/wiki/File:Cuvet.jpg.
2. Fibonacci, https://commons.wikimedia.org/wiki/File:Plasmid_(english).svg.
3. Walkowski, S. (17 December 2009). Navaho, https://commons.wikimedia.org/wiki/File:Blue-white_test.jpg.
4. Cressey, D. (2016). Roger Tsien's legacy: the creations that lit up biology. *Nature* https://doi.org/10.1038/nature.2016.20532.
5. Enzoklop, https://commons.wikimedia.org/wiki/File:Polymerase_chain_reaction.svg.
6. yourgenome, Genome Research Limited. https://www.yourgenome.org/facts/what-is-gel-electrophoresis.
7. Jennifer0328, https://commons.wikimedia.org/wiki/File:Gel_Electrophoresis_in_DNA_Fingerprinting.svg.
8. Mnolf, https://en.wikipedia.org/wiki/File:Gel_electrophoresis_2.jpg.
9. Mysid, http://en.wikipedia.org/wiki/File:Wrist-oximeter.jpg

Further Reading

Pratt and Cornely (2004). *Essential Biochemistry*. Wiley.

Reporter Genes and Proteins (2002). Malcolm Campbell, Dept. of Biology, Davidson College, Davidson, NC.

Thibodeau, G.A. (2008). *Structure & Function of the Body*, 13ee. Mosby.

Wegerer, A., Sun, T., and Altenbuchner, J. (2008). Optimization of an E. coli L-rhamnose expression vecor: test of various genetic module combinations. *BMC Biotechnol.* 8: 2.

http://www.tsienlab.ucsd.edu/Images.htm

https://openi.nlm.nih.gov/detailedresult?img=PMC2254391_1472-6750-8-2-3&req=4

3

Human Physiology

3.1 Overview

Physiology is the science of the function of living systems the focus of which is the study of the organ systems, organs, and cells that carry out functions in the human body. There are many physiological systems in the human body (e.g. skeletal, muscular). This chapter will cover only a subset of these systems, including the nervous system, the circulatory system, the endocrine system, the lymphatic system, and the immune system. Each system will be discussed in terms of specialized cell types (e.g. neurons as part of the nervous system) and organs (e.g. heart as part of the circulatory system).

3.2 Nervous System

The **nervous system** (Figure 3.1) can be divided into two component systems: the **Central Nervous System (CNS)** and the **Peripheral Nervous System (PNS)**. The CNS consists of the brain and the spinal cord, and the PNS consists of autonomic (involuntary) motor nerves, somatic (voluntary) motor nerves, and sensory nerves. The specific functions and organization of the CNS and PNS will be discussed soon, but let's first take a broader look at the different cells that make up the nervous system.

3.2.1 Cells of the Nervous System: Neurons and Glia

3.2.1.1 Neurons

Neurons are the cells of the nervous system that carry electrical impulses throughout the body. Neurons are made up of three components: **dendrites**, the **cell body**, and **axons** (Figure 3.2). Dendrites collect a signal and transmit it into the neuron cell body. The signal then travels from the cell body to the axon. A single neuron can have many dendrites but only one axon. The axon ends in many terminals that can transmit the signal to the dendrites of many other nerve cells. Note that an impulse only travels in one direction: from dendrites to the cell body to the axon. **Impulses** are action potentials that can originate when neurons experience pressure, temperature, vibrational, or other physical; stimuli.

There are three types of neurons: **sensory (afferent) neurons**, **motor (efferent) neurons**, and **interneurons**. Each of these three types has a different signaling function and direction. Sensory neurons transmit signals from the PNS to the CNS. In other words, they deliver the information that the body senses to the brain and spinal cord. Motor neurons signal in the opposite

Biochips and Medical Imaging, First Edition. Adam de la Zerda and Shan Xiang Wang.

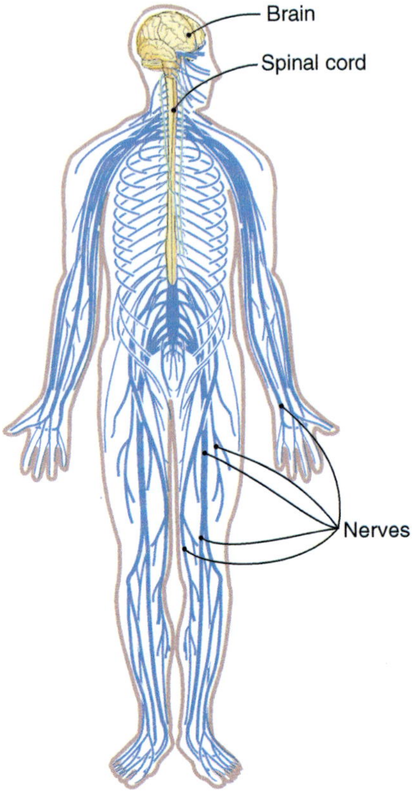

Figure 3.1 Nervous system. *Source:* Jmarchn [1], used under CC-BY-SA 4.0 https://creativecommons.org/licenses/by-sa/4.0/.

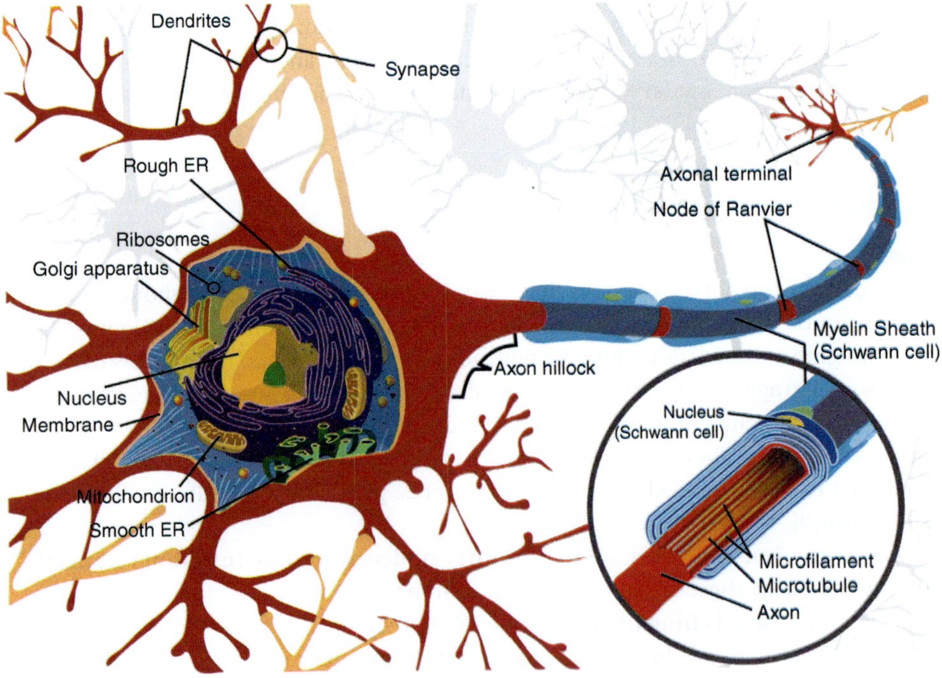

Figure 3.2 Diagram of a neuron, including a close-up of an axon coated in Schwann cells and myelin.

direction: they transmit signals from the CNS out to the nerves of the PNS. Interneurons are cells that are responsible for transmitting signals from sensory neurons to motor neurons.

Recall that the axon is the part of a neuron that carries an impulse away from the neuron toward other neurons. Axons are very thin, and they must be protected in order to preserve their ability to properly transmit nerve impulses. Axons within the CNS are protected by white fatty layers of myelin. These layers produce what is called a **myelin sheath**, which insulates each axon and facilitates the transmission of impulses. Some axons outside of the CNS are coated by a protective layer of cells called **Schwann cells** that produce the myelin sheath (see Figure 3.2).

3.2.1.2 Glia

Unlike neurons, **glia** (e.g. glial cells) do not conduct electrical impulses. However, glia are critically important to the nervous system because they provide structural support and other helpful functions for neurons. The term "glia" is derived from the Greek word for glue, but we will see that glia do more than just glue the nervous system together. Most glial cells reside in the CNS, but some are present in the PNS. There are three types of glia: **astrocytes**, **microglia**, and **oligodendroglia (oligodendrocytes)**.

Astrocytes (Figure 3.3a) are relatively large glia that help attach neurons to small blood vessels. Astrocytes can hold several blood vessels together and they also wrap around blood capillaries. By

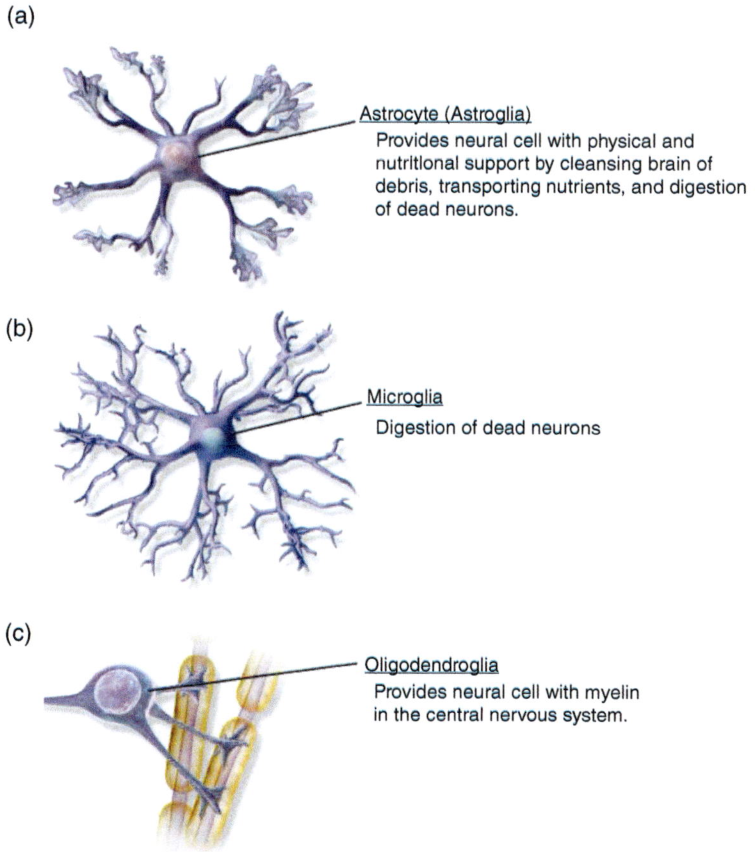

Figure 3.3 (a) Astrocytes, (b) microglia, (c) oligodendroglia (oligodendrocytes). *Source:* BruceBlaus [2], used under CC-BY-SA 4.0 https://creativecommons.org/licenses/by-sa/4.0/.

wrapping around capillaries, astrocytes prevent certain contents in the blood from leaking into the brain. This physical layer of astrocytes is often referred to the **Blood–Brain Barrier (BBB)**, and it provides a lateral coating of capillaries located throughout the brain (for more information on the importance of the BBB, see the "Did you know?" box below).

As we will see in the section on the lymphatic system, the brain is an "immune-privileged" organ (in part because of the BBB). This means that the brain is not protected by the kinds of immune cells that protect the rest of the body from foreign invaders. Instead, the brain contains **microglia** (Figure 3.3b) which are another type of glial cell that actually provide the brain with its own immune system. Microglia are small cells that can recognize foreign microbes and destroy them in a process called **phagocytosis** (this process will be discussed in more detail in the immune system section). Once a microglial cell destroys a pathogen, the cell becomes activated and begins to move around the brain in search of more pathogens to destroy. Because of their immune function, microglia are widely studied to try to understand why the brain does not recognize tumor cells as harmful.

The third type of glial cell is the **oligodendrocyte** (Figure 3.3c). Oligodendrocytes help bundle multiple nerve cells together into a nerve fiber. These cells also form the myelin sheath that envelopes and protects the nerve fibers in the brain and spinal cord.

Did You Know?

Capillaries in most parts of the body are leaky and can easily deliver nutrients (like glucose) from the blood into local tissues through simple diffusion. However, this also means that pathogens (viruses, bacteria, fungi, etc.) can easily travel from the blood to these tissues as well. To fight these pathogens, the lymphatic system (discussed later in the chapter) produces many cells and molecules that act throughout the body. Unlike the rest of the body, the brain is protected from most pathogens by the BBB, which prevents blood from leaking into the brain by coating brain capillaries. The BBB even contains special transport proteins so that glucose can still get out of the blood and into the brain. However, some pathogens can still get into the brain because they are very small and can "squeeze past" the BBB. Because normal immune cells can't get past the BBB, microglia are vital for their ability to neutralize these pathogens. The BBB also poses many challenges for trying to create imaging agents and therapeutics for brain diseases. Some of these challenges will be discussed in more detail in the chapters on *in vivo* imaging methods.

3.2.2 Nerves and Tracts

Neurons are often bundled together into larger nerve fibers. Many such nerve fibers are also bundled together into structures commonly called **nerves** or **tracts**. Nerves are bundles of nerve fibers that are part of the PNS (Figure 3.4). Tracts are bundles of nerve fibers that are part of the CNS. Because nerves and tracts contain many neurons, they contain many long axons that are covered in myelin sheaths. Recall that myelin sheaths are fatty in composition. Fatty tissue appears white in an MRI scan because of its water content (much more on this in Chapter 13). As a result, regions of the brain that are rich in tracts are commonly referred to as "white matter." On the other hand, regions of the brain that have many cell bodies but very few tracts generate MRI signal that appears gray. Such regions are therefore referred to as "gray matter."

3.2.2.1 Reflex Arcs

If you have ever been to the doctor for a physical examination, then you may have had your reflexes tested. Usually, the doctor will hit a certain spot on your knee that makes your leg kick, even

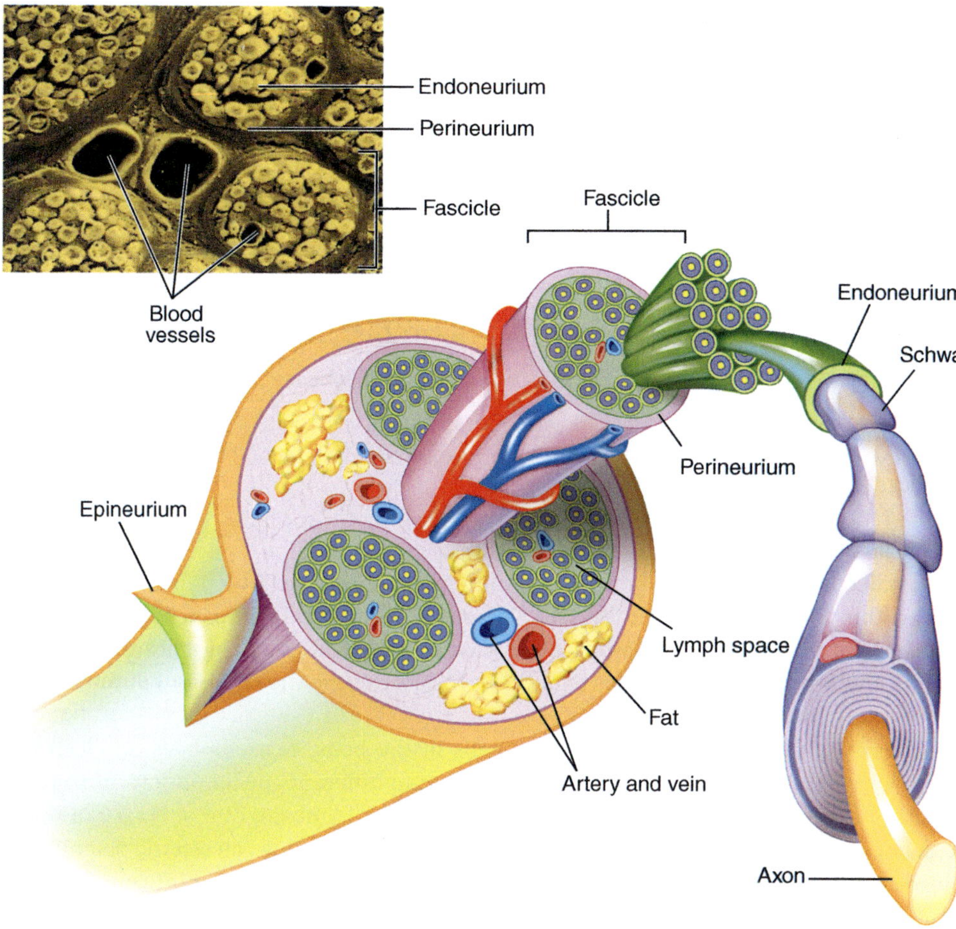

Figure 3.4 Nerve composed of several bundles of neurons. *Source:* Thibodeau and Patton [3]. This article was published in Structure and Function of the Body, Copyright © 2008 Published by Elsevier.

though you don't "think" to move your leg. This "knee-jerk" reaction is a kind of response commonly called a **reflex** or **reflex arc**. "Reflex" refers to an action that your body does without thinking. What makes us react so involuntarily? To answer this question, let's take a look at what is happening at the level of a single neuron.

When the doctor hits your knee (usually with a triangular rubber hammer), the pressure from the hammer acts as a stimulus that initiates an impulse in the dendrites of a nearby sensory neuron. This impulse then travels from the dendrites into the cell body of the neuron (which is grouped with other neuron cell bodies in a structure called a ganglion). From the cell body, the impulse travels through the axon until it reaches the spinal cord. This axon terminates near the dendrites of a motor neuron (although sometimes an interneuron will exist between the sensory neuron axon and the motor neuron dendrites). The result is that the motor neuron will cause the muscles of your leg to move in an almost immediate "knee-jerk" response. Note that the original impulse from the doctor's hammer only has to travel in two neurons before it produces a mechanical movement (see Figure 3.5). Further note that a single axon can be as long as 1 or 2 m and can travel all the way from the knee to the brain (or vice versa).

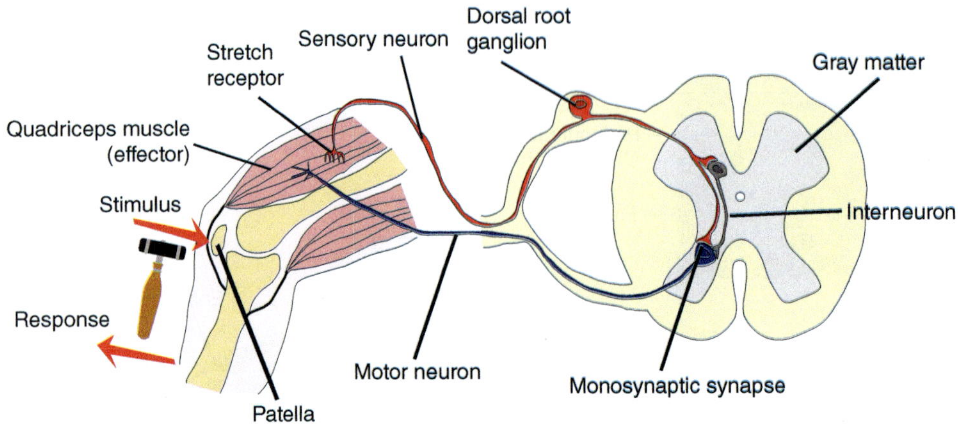

Figure 3.5 Reflex arc taken in a "knee-jerk" reaction. *Source:* Adapted from Юкатан [4], used under CC-BY-SA 3.0 https://creativecommons.org/licenses/by-sa/3.0.

3.2.2.2 Nerve Impulses (Action Potentials)

We can go even deeper to understand how a nerve impulse is transmitted by looking at what actually happens within the neuron. Physically, what is a nerve "impulse?" A **nerve impulse** is also called an **action potential**. It is a self-propagating wave of electrical potential that travels in one direction along a neuron's cell membrane (Figure 3.6a). Let's explore the stages of neuron signaling and the return to the resting state:

Resting (Steady) State Potential: Like other cells in the body, neurons have an electrical potential across their cell membrane. This potential is due to different concentrations of sodium ions (Na^+) and potassium ions (K^+) inside and outside of the cell. Amazingly, it only takes a small difference in the number of ions on either side of the membrane to produce an electric potential of tens of millivolts. The cell uses membrane-bound proteins that pump ions either into or out of the cell to maintain a slightly negative resting potential across the membrane (the inside of the cell is negatively charged and the outside of the cell is positively charged).

Impulse Propagation: The neuron also has membrane proteins called ion channels. When there are pressure, temperature, or chemical changes within a neuron's environment, certain ion channels temporarily activate (open up), allowing positive ions like Na^+ and Ca^{2+} to rush into the cell. This causes a local section of the cell membrane to switch from a negative to a positive potential. This flip in potential causes other nearby ion channels to open up and thus causes the membrane potential to switch in an adjacent region of the neuron. This process repeats along the length of the neuron, resulting in a propagating electric potential.

Return to Resting Electric Potential: Now that we know how a signal propagates, it's important to know how an impulse is "turned off." To turn off the signal, the membrane must return to its original negative polarization. Recall that Na^+ ions rush into the cell to flip the potential to positive during the impulse. In addition to propagating the signal, this flip in potential activates another type of ion channel in the cell membrane, the potassium ion channel. When potassium channels are activated, K^+ ions inside the cell rush out, counterbalancing the Na^+ influx and restoring the original negative electric potential. These potassium channels therefore prevent the same neuron from continuously firing.

Return to Resting Chemical Potential: Now that the electric potential has been restored, we might assume that the neuron is ready to "fire" again. But let's take a closer look at the state of the cell. At this point, the cell has a negative membrane potential that is caused by extracellular K^+ and

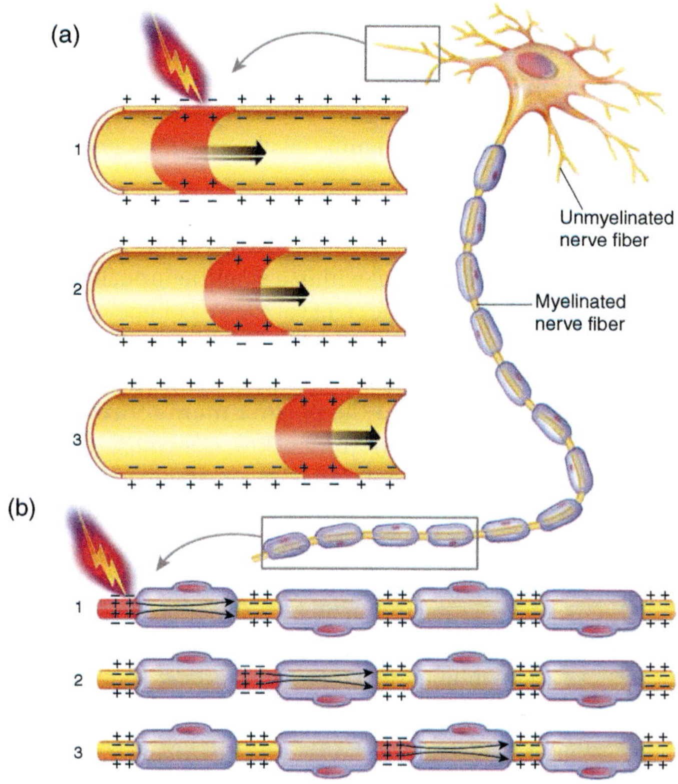

Figure 3.6 (a) Action potential propagation. (b) Saltatory conduction (myelin "jumping") of an action potential. *Source:* Thibodeau and Patton [5]. This article was published in Structure and Function of the Body, Copyright © 2008 Published by Elsevier.

intracellular Na^+. But the cell started with K^+ *inside* and Na^+ *outside* the cell! So, the neuron cannot yet be activated by new stimuli. While the membrane's electric gradient has returned to the resting state, its chemical gradient (Na^+ and K^+ distribution) must also return to the resting state. Luckily, neurons possess yet another membrane protein that can exchange Na^+ and K^+ ions across the membrane. This **Na^+K^+ pump** can transport Na^+ back out of the cell and bring K^+ back into the cell, thereby re-establishing the original electrochemical gradient. Now, the neuron can conduct a new impulse. Note that Na^+ ion channels and K^+ channels allow **passive transport** down a chemical gradient while the Na^+K^+ pump uses **active transport** that requires energy from the cell to exchange the ions.

The fact that both the electric and chemical potentials of the membrane must be re-established helps explain why neuron impulses only travel in one direction. Restoring the membrane potential takes time (even if it only takes a few milliseconds), and the impulse is propagating further and further away by the time the potential in the original part of the neuron is restored.

Saltatory Conduction: The propagation of the impulse is actually sped up even more by the presence of the myelin sheath. Myelin does not provide a continuous coat along the length of the axon (see Figure 3.6b). Rather, there are uncoated junctions between segments of the axon that are myelin-coated. The "bare" regions of the axon are called **nodes of Ranvier** and they have interesting electrical properties. As shown in Figure 3.6b, membrane polarization flipping occurs at these nodes (depicted in yellow when resting and red when active). Parts of the membrane that are coated in myelin actually do not experience this potential flipping because myelin functions as an electrical insulator. Rather, polarization at one node of Ranvier causes a voltage change that can propagate directly through the cytoplasm of a myelin-coated segment and induce potential flipping at the next node of Ranvier. In this way, the myelin sheath actually speeds up the propagation of an electrical impulse. This ability of an action potential to "jump" myelin-coated segments of the axon is called **saltatory conduction**.

3.2.2.3 Nerve Synapses

Action potential propagation explains how nerve impulses travel within a single neuron, but how does that signal get transmitted from one neuron to the next? The signal at the end of one neuron's axon must get conducted into the dendrites of "downstream" neurons. This transmission occurs at junctions called **nerve synapses**, one of which is shown in Figure 3.7. A synapse is composed of three main parts: the **synaptic knob**, the **synaptic cleft**, and the **plasma membrane of the postsynaptic neuron**. Each of these parts of the synapse is described below. Generally, the synapse is the site where an electric signal (action potential) is temporarily converted into a chemical signal and then converted back into an electrical signal in the dendrites of the next neuron. The synapse is also the site that provides the basis for nerve impulse "learning."

Synaptic Knob: This region is made up of the end of one neuron's axon. The cytoplasm of the synaptic knob contains many small vesicles that each contains a small quantity of neurotransmitters. When an action potential reaches this knob, the change in potential triggers a number of biochemical reactions that cause these vesicles to migrate to the far end of the axon. Once at the axon membrane (also called the presynaptic cleft), the vesicles fuse with the membrane and release their neurotransmitter molecules into the synaptic cleft.

Synaptic Cleft: The synaptic cleft is a very narrow (~20 nm-wide) extracellular space between the axon of an upstream neuron and the dendrite of a downstream neuron. Neurotransmitters are released into the synaptic cleft from the presynaptic cleft as described above. Once released, these molecules naturally diffuse along a chemical gradient across the synaptic cleft toward the postsynaptic neuron.

Postsynaptic Cleft: Once the neurotransmitters reach the postsynaptic neuron, they bind to receptors on the dendrite membrane. These neurotransmitter receptors then generate a new action potential in the postsynaptic neuron. At this point, the nerve impulse can continue to propagate as described in the section on action potentials.

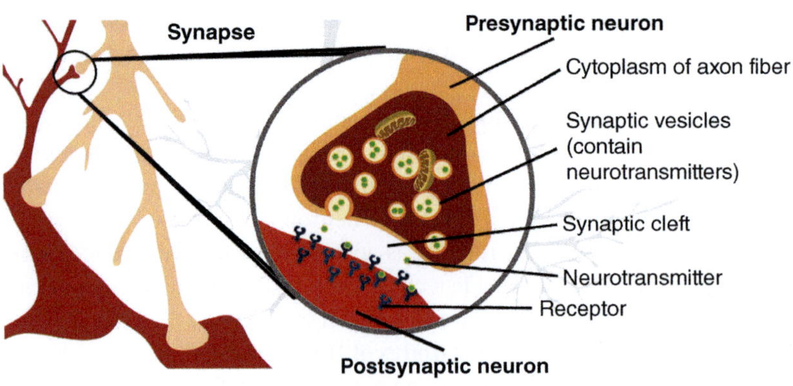

Figure 3.7 Nerve synapse.

Did You Know?

The proper function of neurons seems to depend heavily on the coordinated movement of Na^+ and K^+ ions into and out of the cell. This raises a very fundamental question: how does the cell distinguish an Na^+ ion from a K^+ ion? After all, both of these ions have the same charge.... The answer is that different ion channel proteins have inner regions called ion selectivity filters. The Na^+ and K^+ ion channel proteins are made of different amino acids. Recall that the type and sequence of amino acids are critical for protein structure and function. The middle of the Na^+ ion channel has several amino acids that actually prevent K^+ ions from passing through because K^+ is a few Ångstroms (10^{-10} m) larger in diameter than Na^+! These amino acids function as a "gatekeeper" to make sure that the right ion can pass through. The K^+ ion channel has a slightly different ion selectivity filter that recognizes the hydration shell around a K^+ ion but does not recognize the smaller hydration shell of Na^+. Ion selectivity filters are just a few more examples of the tiny differences that make neuron signaling possible.

3.2.3 Nervous System Organization

Now that we have a basic understanding of how the cells of the nervous system work, let's take a more global view of the parts of the body in which those cells are organized. Recall that the nervous system can be divided into the **CNS** and the **PNS**.

3.2.3.1 Central Nervous System (CNS)

The CNS is composed of the brain and the spinal cord, shown in Figure 3.8. We will briefly discuss the different regions and functions of both of these components of the CNS.

3.2.3.2 The Brain

The brain can be divided into four main regions: the **brainstem**, the **diencephalon**, the **cerebellum**, and the **cerebrum**. Each of these regions can be further subdivided into areas that are

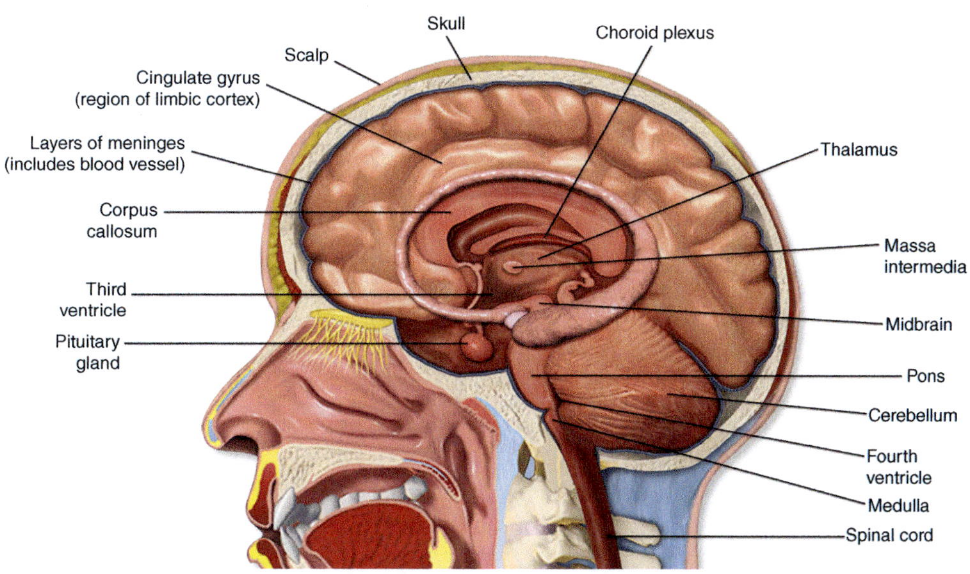

Figure 3.8 Central Nervous System. *Source:* BruceBlaus [6], used under CC-BY-SA 4.0 https://creativecommons.org/licenses/by-sa/3.0.

Table 3.1 Functions of the brainstem.

Brainstem area	Function
Medulla oblongata	Two-way conduction pathway between the spinal cord and higher brain centers; cardiac, respiratory, and vasomotor control center
Pons	Two-way conduction pathway between areas of the brain and other regions of the body; influences respiration
Midbrain	Two-way conduction pathway; relay for visual and auditory impulses

responsible for coordinating specific bodily functions and responses. The functions of each region of the brain have largely been determined through trigger and response experiments in which a certain region is physically stimulated and the living subject's reactions are observed.

The **brainstem** is the region that links the brain to the spinal cord. It is composed of the medulla oblongata, the pons, and the midbrain. The functions of each of these regions are given in Table 3.1 to the right. Each region of the brainstem can receive and transmit nerve signals in order to communicate with the spinal cord. The **diencephalon** is composed of two regions: the hypothalamus and the thalamus. The functions of each of these regions are summarized in Table 3.2. The **cerebellum** is the region of the brain that is responsible for the coordination of muscle movement and several other related functions described in Table 3.3. The **cerebrum** is perhaps the most widely recognized region of the brain. It is also the largest region of the brain. Different lobes of the cerebrum are responsible for controlling sensory perception, emotions, memory, and consciousness (Table 3.3 and Figure 3.9).

3.2.3.3 The Spinal Cord

The spinal cord is responsible for making sure that signals from the brain reach the right part of the body. In this sense, the spinal cord functions like a telephone switchboard that routes signals to different locations. The spinal cord contains very thick bundles that are rich in tracts that go to and from various regions of the body. The spinal cord also contains interneurons and other centers that conduct reflex arcs (described earlier). The spinal cord conducts nerve impulses to the brain through **ascending tracts** and conducts signals from the brain through **descending tracts**. It is interesting to note that the axon bundles within a given spinal tract tend to serve the same general

Table 3.2 Functions of the diencephalon.

Diencephalon area	Function
Hypothalamus	Regulations of body temperature, water balance, sleep-cycle control, appetite, and sexual arousal
Thalamus	Sensory relay station from various body areas to cerebral cortex; emotions and alerting or arousal mechanisms

Table 3.3 Functions of the cerebellum and cerebrum.

Others	Function
Cerebellum	Muscle coordination; maintenance of equilibrium and posture
Cerebrum	Sensory perception, emotions, willed movements, consciousness, and memory

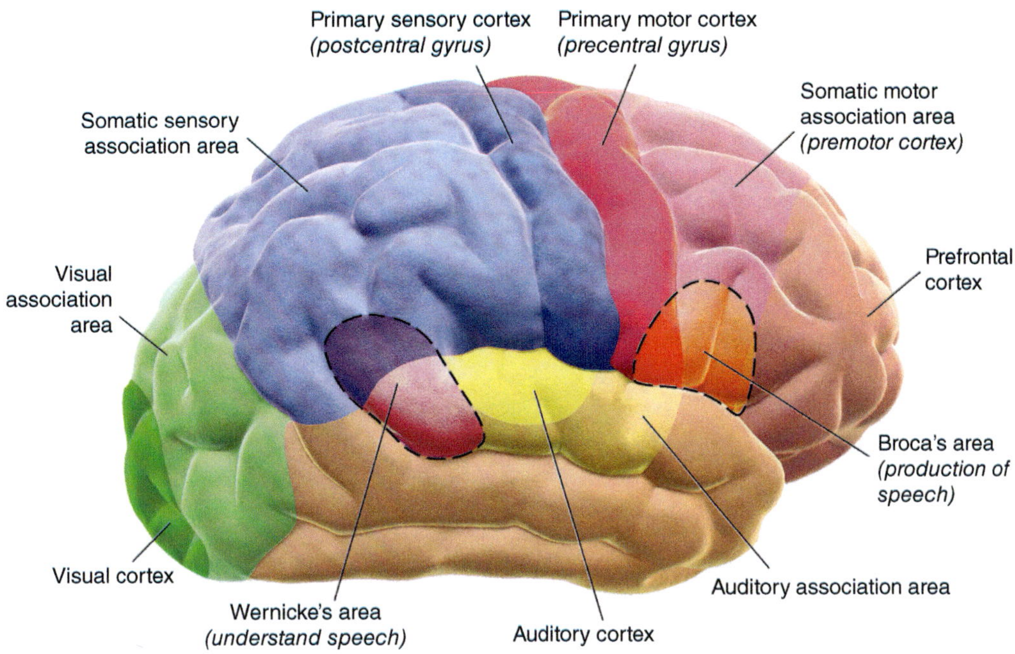

Figure 3.9 Regions and functions of the cerebrum. *Source:* BruceBlaus [7], used under CC-BY 3.0 https://creativecommons.org/licenses/by/3.0/.

signaling function. In other words, regions of the spinal cord are organized by the type of signal they carry. For instance, axons within the spinothalamic tract conduct impulses for sensory functions. The axons in the lateral corticospinal region control voluntary movements. The organization of these tracts within the spine is depicted in Figure 3.10.

3.2.3.4 The Meninges

Neurons are really quite sensitive and delicate cells that can be harmed or killed if exposed to even mild pressure. Therefore, the neurons of the CNS are protected by a tough, continuous membrane called the **meninges** (Figure 3.11). The meninges are composed of three separate layers. The outer layer called the dura mater provides a tough overcoating. The middle layer is a fibrous network called the arachnoid mater. The inner layer, called the pia mater, wraps directly around the spinal cord. Between the arachnoid and pia layers is a particularly important component called **cerebrospinal fluid (CSF)**.

3.2.3.5 Cerebrospinal Fluid (CSF)

CSF is a clear fluid that is derived from the blood by the *choroid plexus*. CSF circulates through the spine and the veins within the brain. This fluid plays many very important functions to protect the CNS. The CSF provides buoyancy to the brain cortex, which serves a cushioning function that helps protect the brain from trauma caused by rapid movements and pressure. Because of the buoyancy provided by the CSF, a normal human brain that weighs about 3 lb has an effective mass of only about 25 g in the skull (Figure 3.12).

The cushion provided by the CSF has consequences for diseases like cancer as well. Note that the skull is rigid and limits the brain's total volume. If a tumor mass begins to grow in the brain, the CSF can flow out and prevent pressure from building up in the brain. Without CSF, the first thing

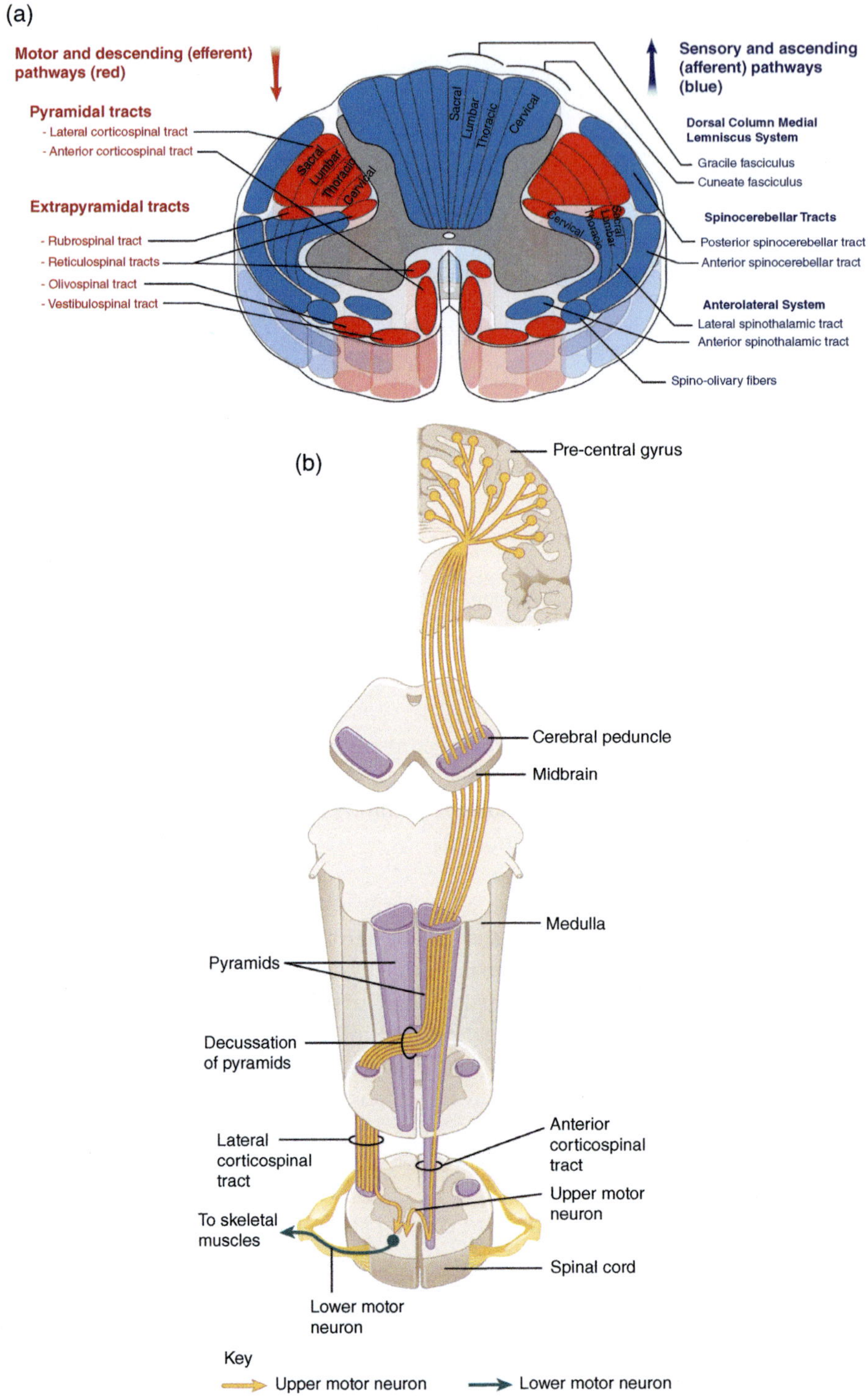

Figure 3.10 (a) Ascending and descending spinal tracts. *Source:* Polarlys and Mikael Häggström [8], used under CC-BY-SA 3.0 https://creativecommons.org/licenses/by-sa/3.0. (b) Organization of spinal tracts. Source: OpenStax College [9], used under CC-BY 3.0 http://creativecommons.org/licenses/by/3.0.

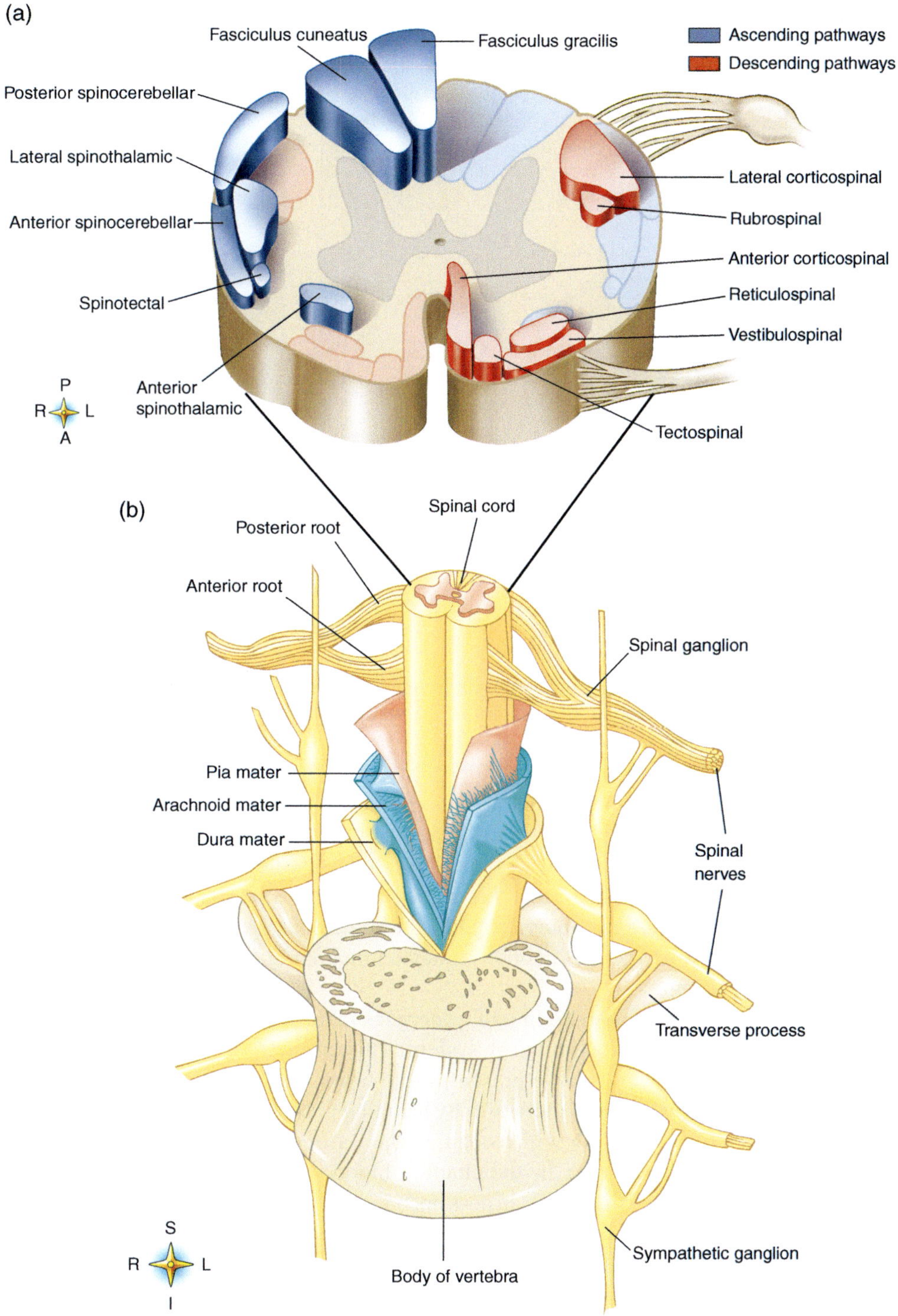

Figure 3.11 (a) Ascending and descending spinal tracts. *Source:* Thibodeau and Patton [10]. This article was published in Structure and Function of the Body, Copyright © 2008 Published by Elsevier. (b) Meninges. Source: Thibodeau and Patton [11]. This article was published in Structure and Function of the Body, Copyright © 2008 Published by Elsevier.

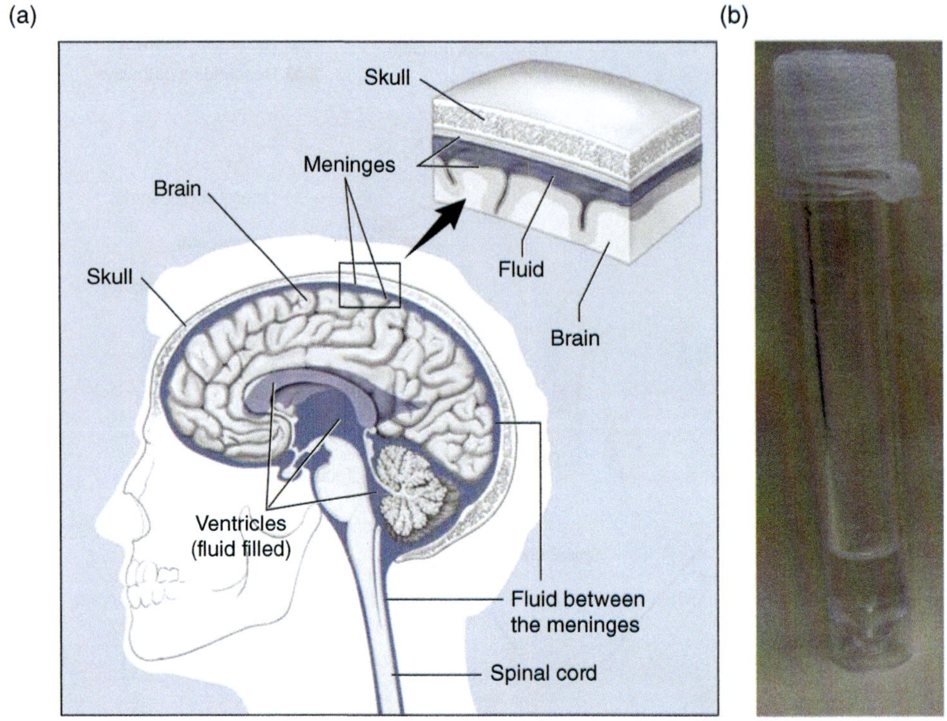

Figure 3.12 (a) Location of Cerebrospinal Fluid (CSF) within the body. *Source:* Courtesy of Alan Hoofring [12]. (b) Vial containing CSF. Source: Doc James [13], used under CC-BY 3.0 https://creativecommons.org/licenses/by/3.0/.

that would happen during tumor growth would be constriction of blood flow to the brain because of the added pressure within the skull. The CSF can flow out of the skull and prevent this constriction from occurring. However, this function of the CSF is a double-edged sword from the standpoint of diagnosing brain tumors. As a result of this cushioning effect, a person with a brain tumor may not develop symptoms from brain pressure until the tumor has grown substantially. Most brain tumors are diagnosed after the person observes some impaired function, so this function of the CSF can hinder early diagnosis.

Importantly, CSF flows through the brain and undergoes turnover. After it flows out of the brain, the CSF returns to the blood circulatory system. This circulation improves the body's ability to recognize pathogens that may be present in the brain. CSF that flows back into the bloodstream may carry pathogens from the brain. By bringing pathogens to the blood, the CSF helps improve the odds that the body will recognize the pathogens and mount the proper immune response (as we will see later in the chapter, blood circulation plays a major role in immune recognition). Remember that the brain does not have full access to the cells of the immune system, so this function of CSF is particularly important. A good example of the immune function of CSF is highlighted by the condition called **meningitis**. Meningitis is an illness caused by bacteria (or, in some cases, viruses) that infiltrate into the layers of the meninges and get dangerously close to the tracts in the spinal cord. Recall that the CSF exists between the middle (arachnoid) and inner (pia) layers of the meninges. CSF can help carry invading pathogens to the blood so that the body can mount an immune response before the infection reaches the spinal cord.

3.2.3.6 Peripheral Nervous System (PNS)

The **PNS** is composed of nerves that connect the brain and the spinal cord to other parts of the body. The nerves of the PNS can be divided based upon two different criteria: (a) by physical location or (b) by the types of signals they carry.

Physically, the PNS is made up of **cranial nerves** which connect the CNS to the eye, tongue, face, and other parts of the head, and **spinal nerves** which connect the CNS to parts of the body outside of the head.

In terms of signaling, the PNS is composed of **somatic nerves** which carry signals from voluntary movements like arm and leg movements and **autonomic nerves** which carry involuntary signals like contractions of the heart and abdominal cavity muscles.

Autonomic nerves can be further divided into the **sympathetic system** nerves and the **parasympathetic system** nerves (Figure 3.13). Nerves in the sympathetic system are responsible for what is known as the "fight-or-flight" response. These nerves carry impulses that make the heart beat faster, cause blood vessel constriction to increase blood pressure, cause skeletal muscles to dilate, and slow down digestion. In other words, the sympathetic nerve system induces physiological changes that favor quick responses to danger. On the other hand, nerves of the parasympathetic

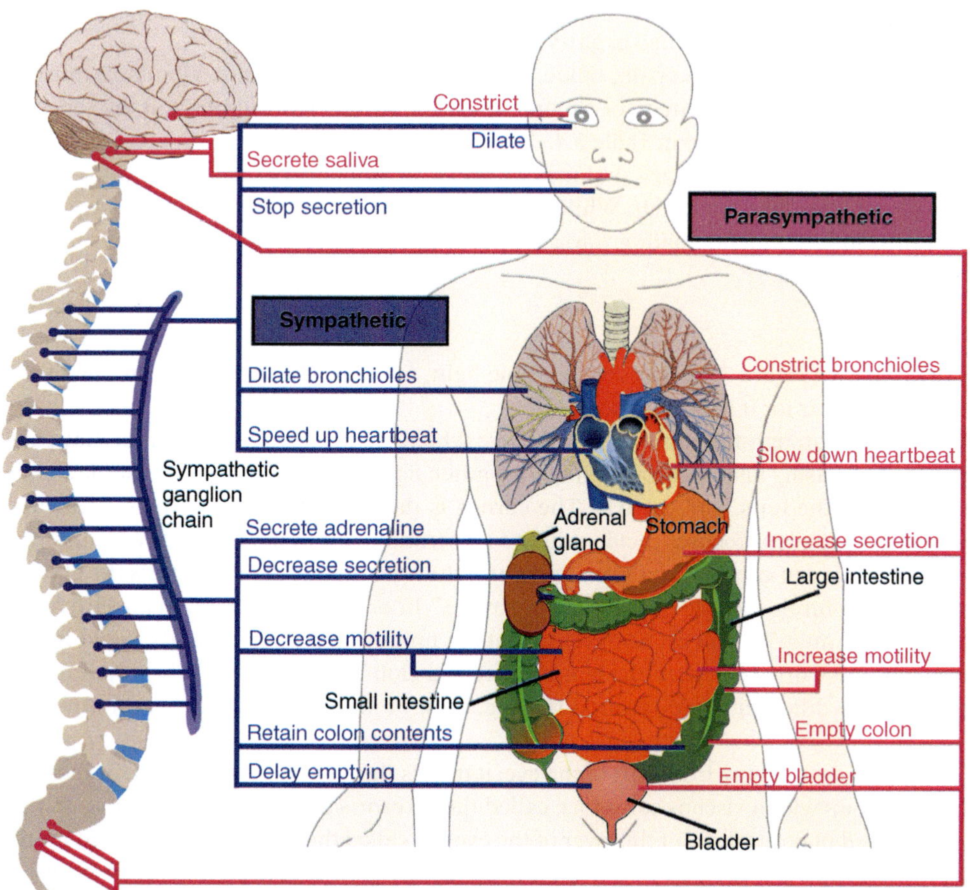

Figure 3.13 Sympathetic and parasympathetic nerve systems. *Source:* Madhero88 [14], used under CC-BY-SA 3.0 https://creativecommons.org/licenses/by/3.0/.

system function in the opposite fashion to control resting levels of breathing, heartbeat, and digestive functions. While these two systems send very different signals to the same organs, they are always both "on." Organs like the heart, stomach, intestines, and many others are constantly receiving signals from both sympathetic and parasympathetic neurons. The ultimate response of each of these organs is therefore determined by which signals are most intense. In other words, whichever system "shouts loudest" is the one whose message gets heard and processed into a response.

3.2.4 The Senses

We have looked briefly at how neurons are organized into different systems that enable communication between the brain and spine with the rest of the body. We have also discussed how neurons can detect a physical stimulus and transmit that stimulus through these systems to generate a response or reaction. But up to this point, we have not detailed the tremendous variety of physical stimuli that the body is capable of converting into electric impulses. The senses of the human body help demonstrate this variety. The body can sense pain, touch, temperature, itch, tickle, vibration, smell, taste, sound, and visible light, just to name a few. Incredibly, the same neurons can be arranged in different architectures that can detect each of these stimuli. Sensory organs can be divided into two groups: **general sense organs** and **special sense organs**.

General sense organs can sense pain, tickle, touch, temperature, pressure, vibration, muscle tension, and muscle length. A summary of general sense organ cell architectures and the sensory information they detect is provided in Table 3.4.

Special sense organs are the organs that may be the most familiar sensory organs to us. They include the eye, ear, nose, and taste buds. While all of these organs are capable of detecting specific sensory stimuli in unique and fascinating ways, we will focus our discussion on two organs in particular: the eye and the ear.

3.2.4.1 The Eye

We know that the eye (Figure 3.14) can detect visible light, but let's see what path a photon takes through the eye in order for it to be detected.

Photons first pass through the front part of the eye which contains several elements that play important roles in focusing light and controlling how much light can enter the eye. These elements include the **cornea**, the **lens**, and the **iris**. The cornea is the window through which light first travels into the eye. The lens focuses incident light to a certain point in the back of the eye (more on this soon). The iris can contract and relax to control the amount of light that enters the eye. In this sense, the iris controls the size of the eye's "aperture." In order to maintain visual clarity, the front part of the eye must be kept moist by tears that are produced in nearby glands called **lacrimal glands**. If the eye dries out, then the lens can become cloudy and vision will be impaired. In fact, there are many different glands around the eye; each produces tears that contain different molecules.

Once light passes through the front part of the eye, it travels through the middle space of the eye. This space is filled up with a viscous substance called the **vitreous gel**. After passing through the vitreous gel, focused photons then hit the layer of the eyeball called the **retina.** The retina contains photoreceptor cells and it is the part of the eye where signals from visible photons get converted into electrical impulses that travel to the brain. The retina is actually one of the three layers that make up the eyeball. The other two layers are the **sclera** and the **choroid**. The sclera gives most of the eye its visible white color. The choroid is a layer of heavily vascularized tissue that helps deliver blood to parts of the eye.

Table 3.4 Nerve architectures of different general sense organs.

Type	Main location	General senses	
Free nerve endings:			
	Skin and mucosa (epithelial layers)	Pain, crude touch, temperature, itch, tickle	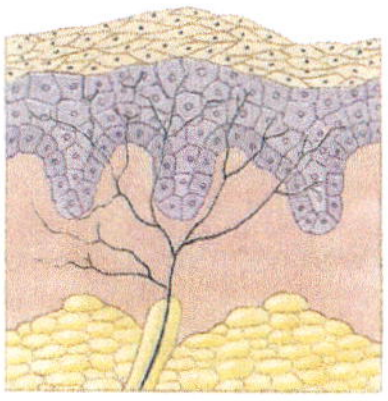
Encapsulated nerve endings:			
Meissner (tactile) corpuscles	Skin (in papillae of dermis) and fingertips and lips (numerous)	Fine touch and low-frequency vibration	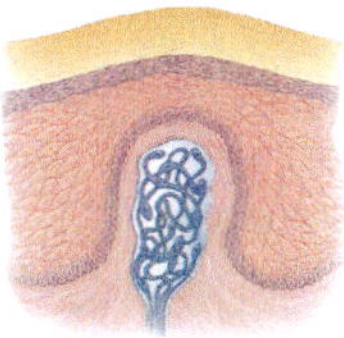
Ruffini (bulbous) corpuscles	Skin (dermal layer) and subcutaneous tissue of fingers	Touch and pressure	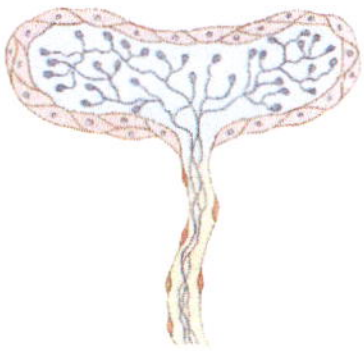
Pacini (lamellar) corpuscles	Subcutaneous, submucous, and subserous tissues; around joints, in mammary glands, and external genitals of both sexes	Pressure and high-frequency vibration	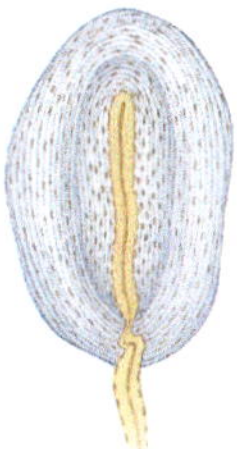
Krause end bulbs (bulboid corpuscles)	Skin (dermal layer), subcutaneous tissue, mucosa of lips and eyelids, and external genitals	Touch	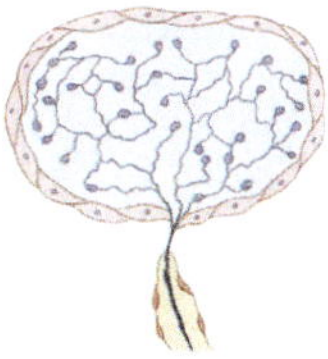
Golgi tendon organs	Near junction of tendons and muscles	Proprioception (sense of muscle tension)	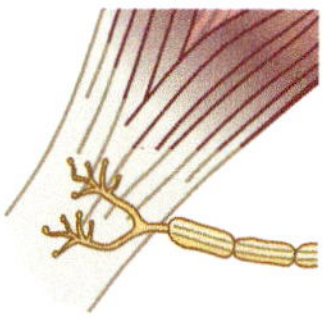
Muscle spindles	Skeletal muscles	Proprioception (sense of muscle length)	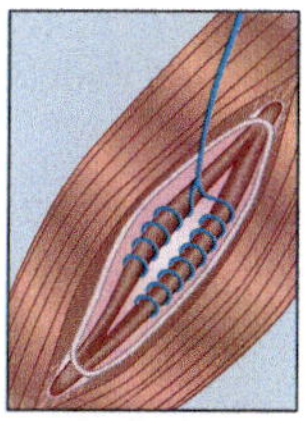

Source: Thibodeau and Patton [5]. This article was published in Structure and Function of the Body, Copyright © 2008 Published by Elsevier.

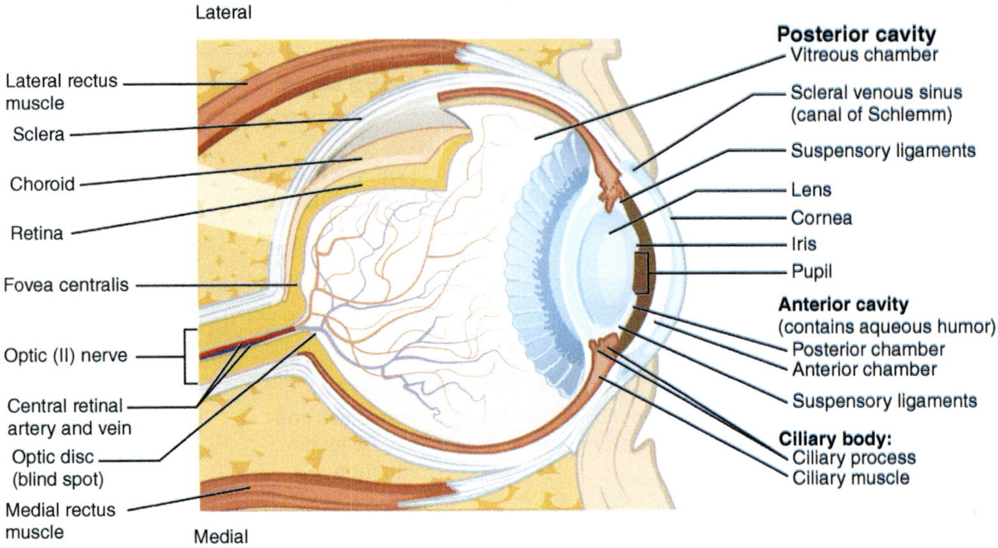

Figure 3.14 The eye. *Source:* OpenStax College [15], used under CC-BY 3.0 http://creativecommons.org/licenses/by/3.0.

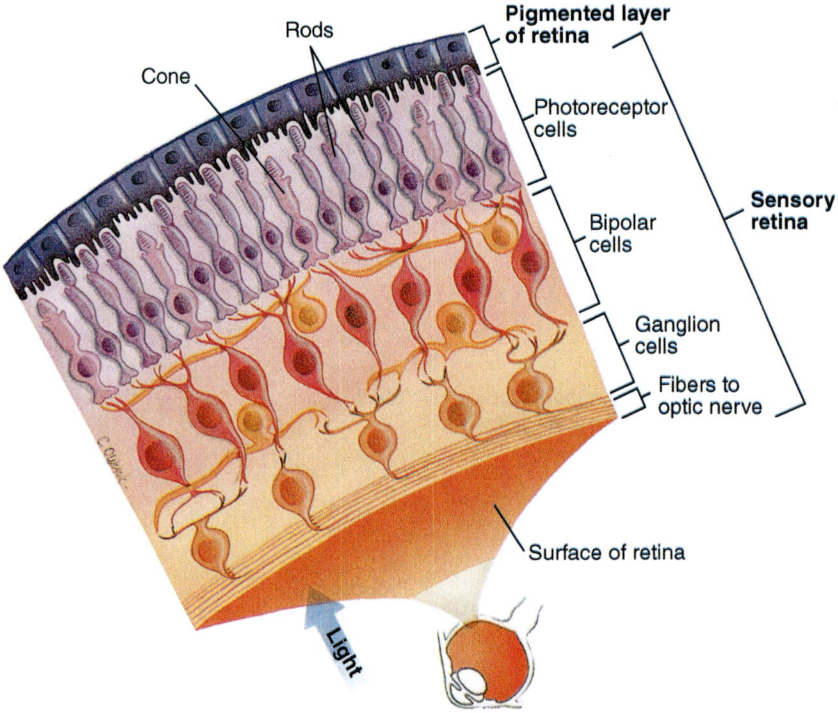

Figure 3.15 The layers of the retina. *Source:* Thibodeau and Patton [16], this article was published in Structure and Function of the Body, Copyright © 2008 Published by Elsevier.

3.2.4.2 The Retina

The retina is very critical for the eye's ability to convert light signals into electric impulses, so let's take a closer look at the different layers of cells within the retina. The retina is only about 200 μm thick and it is made up of 10 different cell layers. We will discuss the main layers of the retina that make our sense of vision possible (Figure 3.15).

Photons travel from the vitreous gel in the middle of the eye into a layer of fibers that lead to the optic nerve. These nerve fibers transmit electrical signals that contain information about the image that the eye perceives.

Once light passes through these fibers, it then travels through a layer of **ganglion cells**. These ganglion cells are neural cells that transmit image-forming and nonimage-forming information to the brain.

The next major layer of the retina includes **bipolar cells** that transmit electrical impulses from a layer of photoreceptors (described next) to the ganglion cells (described previously). The bipolar cell layer is responsible for processing a lot of image information including rapid movements and the recognition of patterns.

After photons pass through the layer of bipolar cells, they encounter a layer of **photoreceptor cells**. There are two types of photoreceptor cells: **rods** and **cones**. **Rods** are very sensitive cells that detect contrast in the form of black and white information. **Cones** are less sensitive to light intensity, but they are capable of distinguishing different colors. The eye has three types of cone cells, each of which can see a different range of wavelengths. For example, one type of cone cell perceives a spectrum of red wavelengths, one perceives a spectrum of green wavelengths, and the third type perceives a range of blue wavelengths. Rods and cones are particularly interesting because they are the cells that are responsible for converting photons into electrical impulses.

Behind the photoreceptor layer is a layer of **pigmented cells** that supplies the retina with nutrients and also helps protect it from excess light. These pigmented cells contain large quantities of melanin and can appear in a number of colors. In fact, the color of a person's eyes is determined by this layer. For example, a person with blue eyes has pigmented cells that reflect blue light out through the front of the eye. Because pigmented cells do not absorb much red light, they are also the source of the "red-eye" effect in photography.

It is important to clarify a potentially confusing point. We have just described the layers of the retina in the order in which photons actually pass through them. However, you may have noticed that this is the *reverse order* from how their signal is transmitted once photons are converted to an electric impulse. In other words, a *photon* will first encounter the layer of fibers that leads to the optic nerve. Next, the photon will pass through the ganglion cell layer, the bipolar cell layer, the photoreceptor layer, and the pigmented cell layer. The cells within the photoreceptor layer convert the photons into electrical impulses, and now the electrical signal travels back through the photoreceptors, bipolar cells, and ganglion cells. The electrical signal is then transmitted to the layer of optic fibers, which transmits the impulses to the **optic nerve**, which, in turn, transmits those signals to the brain (see Figure 3.15 for a visual illustration of these layers).

Did You Know?

The human eye is very complex and capable of perceiving subtle visual information including spatial depth, color, and object movements. However, it is far from being the most complex eye design found in living organisms. For example, the eye of the mantis shrimp (Figure 3.16), a small crustacean that lives in saltwater, contains 16 different types of photoreceptor cells (recall that the human retina contains 3 types of cone cells for color vision and rod cells for detecting black and white). Of the mantis shrimp's 16 photoreceptors, 12 are used to perceive color. Some of these cells may even interpret UV light into color, meaning that the mantis shrimp can perceive "new" colors that are invisible to the human eye. In addition to its enhanced color perception, each of the shrimp's eyes possesses trifocal vision. Moreover, the shrimp is even capable of distinguishing different polarized planes of light and may even be able to distinguish circularly polarized light.

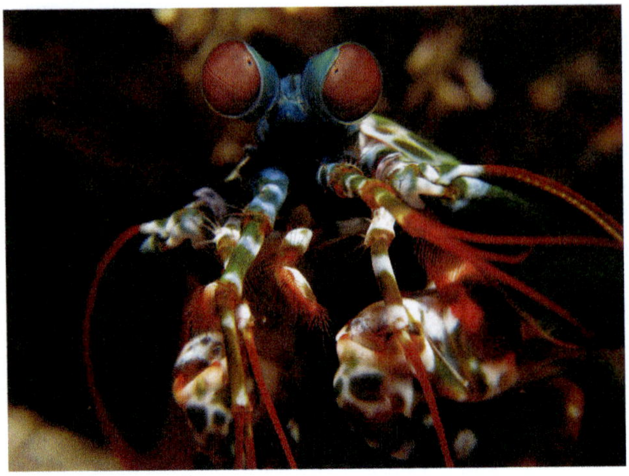

Figure 3.16 Mantis shrimp. *Source:* Jacopo Werther [17], used under CC-BY 2.0 https://creativecommons.org/licenses/by/2.0/.

3.2.4.3 The Ear

The ear is responsible for converting yet another type of stimulus, sound, into nerve impulses. The ear (Figure 3.17) is composed of three basic regions: the **outer ear**, the **middle ear**, and the **inner ear**. Let's track how a sound wave traveling through the air travels through each of these regions and ultimately results in an electrical impulse.

Outer ear: The **outer ear** collects sound waves that travel through the air and channels them through the auditory canal to the **tympanic membrane**, also known as the eardrum. Sound waves hit the eardrum and cause it to vibrate at a given frequency.

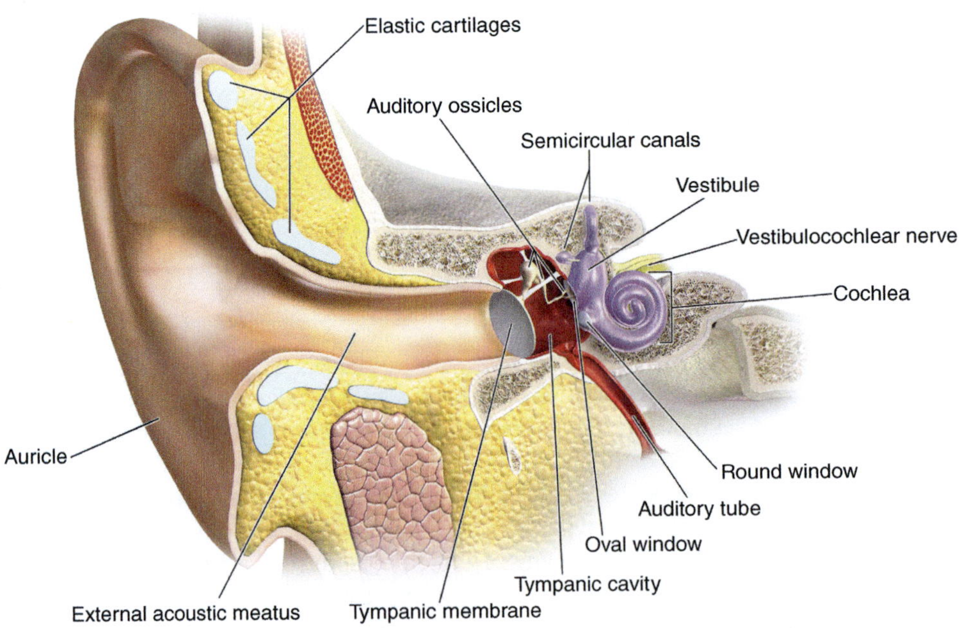

Figure 3.17 The ear. *Source:* BruceBlaus [7], used under CC-BY 3.0 https://creativecommons.org/licenses/by/3.0/.

Middle ear: The eardrum then transfers this vibration to the bones of the **middle ear**. The eardrum transmits the signal to a small bone called the **malleus** (Latin for "hammer," since it is a hammer-shaped bone). The malleus then transmits the vibration to the **incus** (Latin for "anvil," since it is an anvil-shaped bone), and the incus then transmits the vibration to the **stapes** (Latin for "stirrup," since it is a stirrup-shaped bone). The stapes then transmits the vibrational signal to the **cochlea** which is part of the **inner ear**.

Inner ear (Figure 3.18)**:** The cochlea is composed of three different canals that are each filled with thick fluid. The vibrating stapes in the middle ear transmits the sound signal into the fluid of the outermost canal of the cochlea. From here, the vibration travels through the middle canal and into the inner canal of the cochlea. The inner canal of the cochlea contains an organ called the **Organ of Corti** (Figure 3.18a). This organ is composed of **hair cells** that can detect even very tiny movements. These sensory hair cells function as the mechanoreceptors of the ear. In other words, they detect even micron- or nanometer-scale deflections caused by acoustic waves (sound) and convert that signal into a neuronal impulse that goes to the brain. These hair cells can be excited by a range of vibration frequencies, which defines the limits of what pitches we can and cannot hear. Note that the hair cells are present only within the innermost region of the cochlea. This

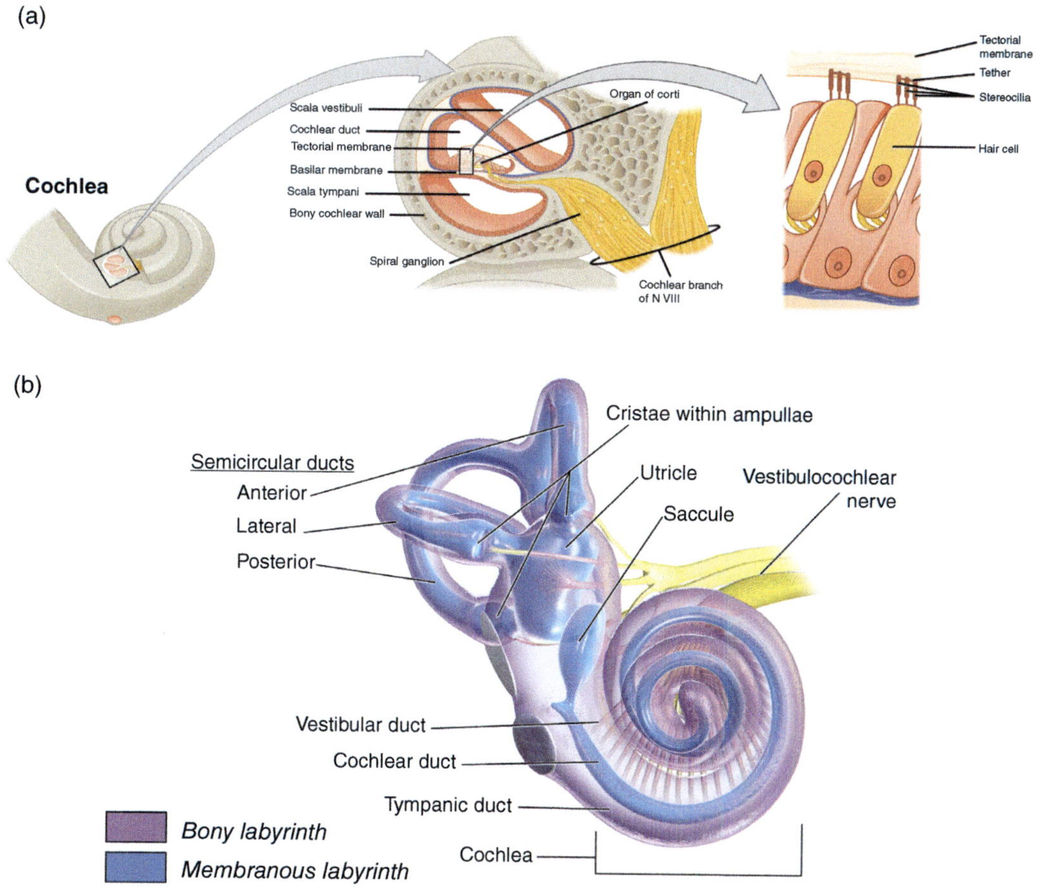

Figure 3.18 (a) Anatomy of the cochlea. *Source:* Adapted from OpenStax [18], used under CC-BY 4.0 http://creativecommons.org/licenses/by/4.0. (b) Anatomy of the inner ear. *Source:* BruceBlaus [7], used under CC-BY 3.0 https://creativecommons.org/licenses/by/3.0/.

should make some intuitive sense because if sound waves encountered hair cells in earlier canals, the cells themselves would alter the signal that could be detected in more interior regions. Another sidenote, as you go deeper into the ear, fewer frequencies can travel. Only lower frequencies (bass sounds) can get deeper into the ear. High-pitched frequencies are mainly detected at points in the ear that are closer to the outer regions.

The inner ear also contains structures that are important for more than just our sense of hearing. In addition to the cochlea, the inner ear contains three **semicircular canals** (Figure 3.18b) that are oriented along three orthogonal axes (approximately *x*, *y*, and *z*). Each of these three canals is about half-filled with fluid. Together, they control our sense of balance. Specifically, the location of the fluid within each canal (caused by gravity) sends information that gets integrated into our sense of our body's spatial orientation.

3.3 Circulatory System

The **circulatory system** consists of three components: blood, the heart, and blood vessels (Figure 3.19). It has several vital body functions, such as transportation, temperature regulation, immunity, and communication. **Transportation:** Blood transports many chemicals to and from tissue cells, including nutrients to the cells (amino acids, glucose, vitamins, minerals, and lipids), oxygen (by red blood cells), and waste from cells (urea and CO_2, mainly as HCO_3 in solution in the

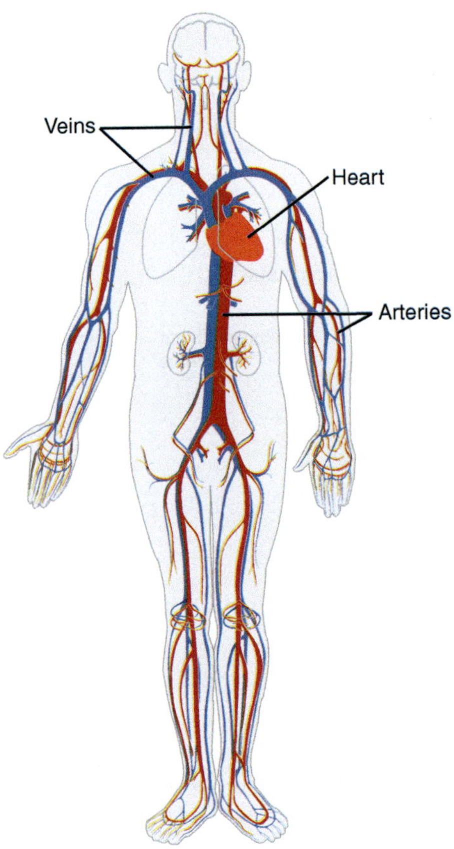

Figure 3.19 Circulatory system.

plasma). **Temperature regulation:** Blood also aids in temperature regulation by altering the blood flow through the skin. **Immunity:** The circulatory system plays an important role in immunity by providing protection against pathogens through blood clotting (following a wound), phagocytes, lymphocytes, and circulating antibodies. **Communication:** Finally, the circulatory system aids in communication through hormones distributed to all parts of the body through the blood.

3.3.1 Blood Content

Blood contains approximately half water by volume, about 45% formed elements (platelets, leukocytes, and erythrocytes), and small amounts of proteins and other solutes, such as nutrients and waste products (Figure 3.20). **Platelets** play a role in homeostasis by leading to the formation of blood clots. **Leukocytes** (a.k.a. **white blood cells**) are used by the immune system to defend the body against infectious disease and foreign materials. **Erythrocytes** (a.k.a. **red blood cells** or **RBC**) carry oxygen to the cells and carbon dioxide from the cells. When formed elements (platelets, white blood cells, and red blood cells) are removed from the blood, the remaining yellowish clear liquid is called **blood plasma**.

3.3.1.1 Red Blood Cells

Red blood cells (RBCs) are shaped like biconcave disks with a diameter of 7–8 μm (Figure 3.21). RBCs are made in the bone marrow of the skull, ribs, vertebrae, and other bones. They contain large quantities of hemoglobin, the protein that is used for oxygen transport. Each hemoglobin molecule can carry up to four oxygen molecules. Unlike most other human cells, red blood cells lack a nucleus and have a life span of 120 days, after which they are dismantled in the liver and spleen. An adult human has

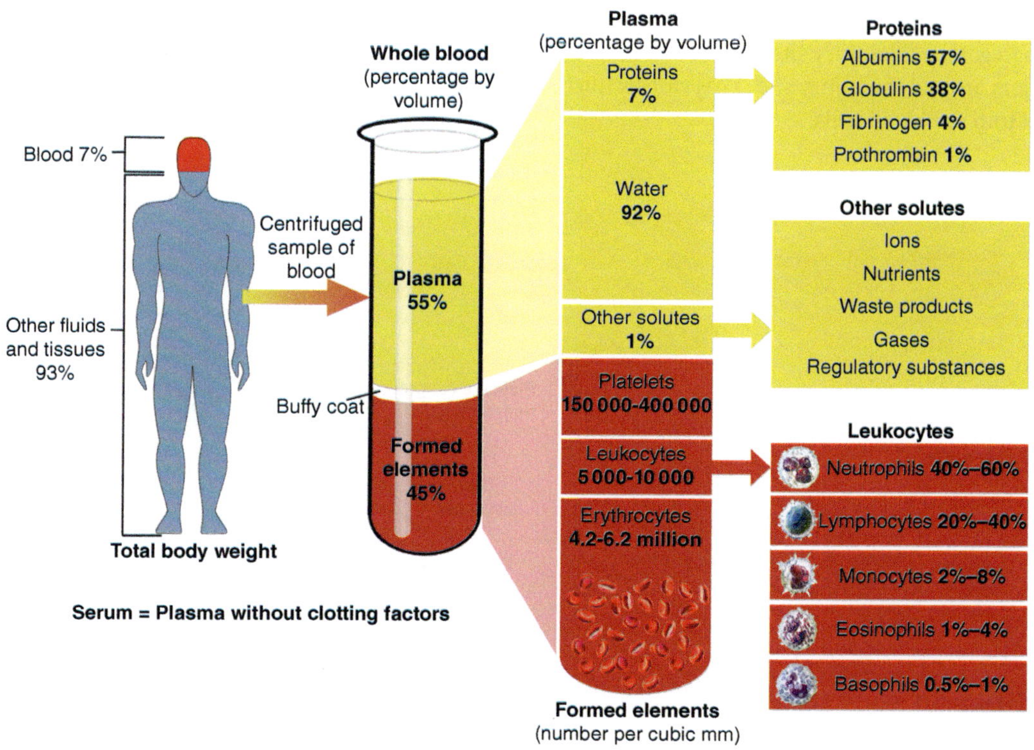

Figure 3.20 Components of blood.

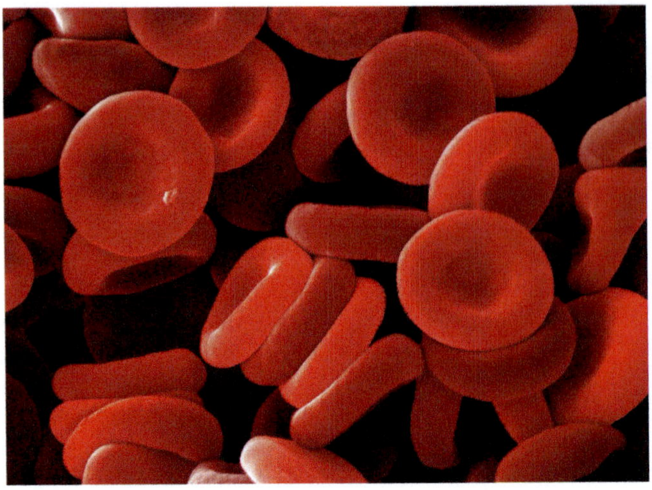

Figure 3.21 Red blood cells (RBCs). *Source:* Red Blood Cells, C003/6575 – Power and Syred/Science Photo Library.

about 25 trillion RBCs at any given time. Hence, to maintain a steady supply of RBCs to the body, the bone marrow creates ~2.5 million RBCs per second. Red blood cells can fold to squeeze into the small capillaries. People who lack a sufficient number of RBCs suffer from a condition called anemia.

3.3.1.2 Platelets

Platelets cause blood clotting at injury sites (Figure 3.22). After a blood vessel is injured, platelets congregate at the injury site and form a plug. Platelets and injured tissue cells both secrete clotting factors around the injury site. This causes fibrin threads to form around the plug to seal the injury and trap red blood cells.

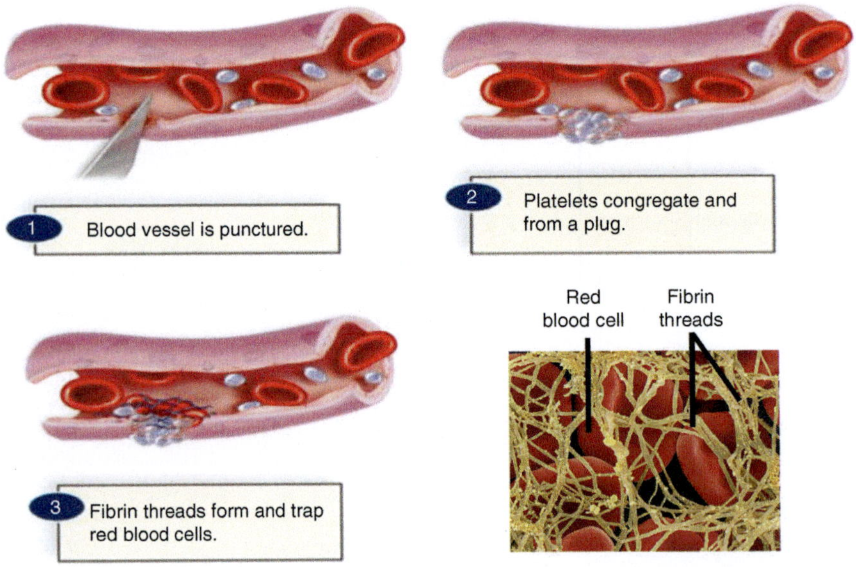

Figure 3.22 Blood clot formation. *Source:* The Blood Clot, C036/9640 – Dennis Kunkel Microscopy/Science Photo Library and Mader and Windelspecht [19].

3.3.2 Heart

The **heart** is a cone-shaped, muscular organ located between the lungs and behind the sternum. The muscular wall of the heart is called the myocardium. The pericardium is the outer membranous sac that is filled with lubricating fluid. The heart has four chambers: two upper, thin-walled atria, and two lower, thick-walled ventricles. A wall called the septum separates the right and left sides of the heart. Valves exist between the atria and ventricles – the tricuspid valve on the right and the bicuspid valve on the left (shown in Figure 3.23a and b).

3.3.2.1 Circulation

Circulation occurs through the pulmonary circuit (to and from the lungs) and the systemic circuit (to and from the rest of the body) (Figure 3.23b). In the **pulmonary circuit**, O_2-poor blood from all regions of the body collects in the right atrium and then passes into the right ventricle, which pumps it into the lungs. As blood passes through the alveolar capillaries in the lungs, CO_2 is released and oxygen is picked up. The O_2-rich blood then returns to the left atrium of the heart through pulmonary veins. In the **systemic circuit**, oxygenated blood goes from the left atrium to the left ventricle, where it is pumped to the aorta (the major artery), which then branches to various tissues in the body. Deoxygenated blood returns from the organs through the veins to the vena cava (the major vein), which enters the right atrium. Systemic capillaries facilitate the exchange of oxygen and nutrients to the cells and waste products from the cells.

3.3.2.2 Blood Pressure

There are three main categories of blood vessels: arteries, capillaries, and veins. **Arteries** carry the blood away from the heart. Arteries split into smaller branches called **arterioles** throughout the body. These arterioles split into even smaller branches called capillaries. **Capillaries** are narrow vessels with very thin walls that facilitate the exchange of substances (e.g. oxygen, CO_2, nutrients, and waste) between blood and the surrounding tissues. Even though they are narrow, capillaries are abundant in number and have a higher total cross-sectional area than the other blood vessels in the body. **Veins** return the blood from capillaries back to the heart. Like arteries, veins also form small branches called **venules**. The blood travels through the blood vessels in the following order: arteries, arterioles, capillaries, venules, and veins (Figure 3.24).

The pumping of the heart sends out blood under pressure to the arteries. Blood pressure is highest in the aorta, the main artery in the systemic circuit. The wall of the left ventricle is thicker (stronger) than that of the right ventricle since it pumps blood to the entire body. Blood pressure then decreases as the total cross-sectional area of the vessels increases (e.g. in the arterioles and capillaries).

3.3.2.3 Capillary Exchange

Capillaries are tiny blood vessels (5–10 μm in diameter) that allow some materials to go in and out of them to the tissue bed. Two forces control the movement of fluid through the capillary wall: blood pressure, which tends to cause water to move out of a capillary and into the tissue fluid, and osmotic pressure, which tends to cause water to move from the tissue fluid into a capillary. Red blood cells and almost all plasma proteins remain in the capillaries and are not exchanged. Osmotic pressure is the pressure that is built by water aiming to cross a semipermeable membrane (e.g. blood vessel membrane) to equate osmolarities across the membrane. The arterial end of the capillary, which carries oxygenated blood from the heart, has a greater blood pressure than osmotic pressure; hence materials such as water, oxygen, amino acids, and glucose leave the capillary and

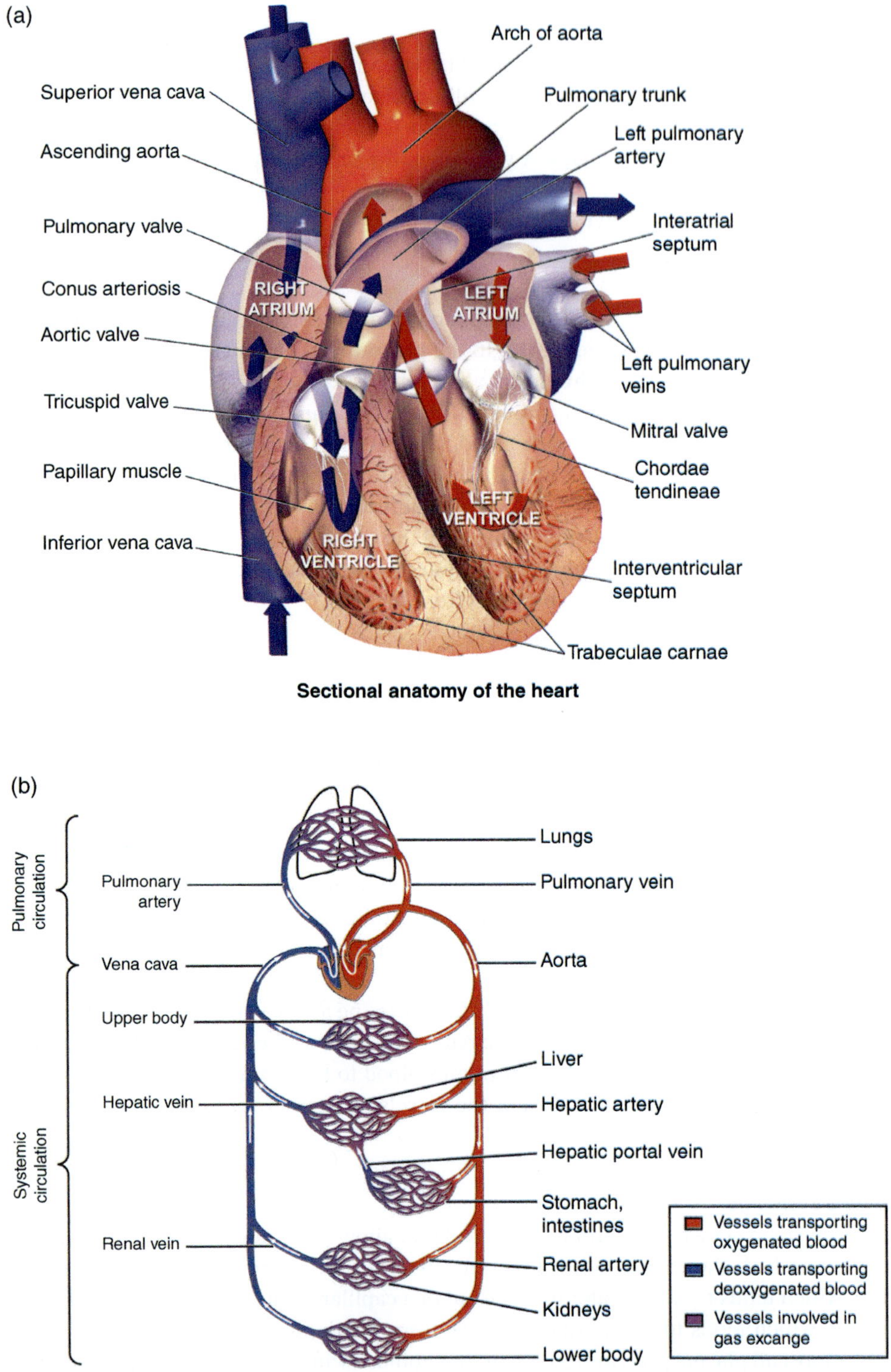

Figure 3.23 (a) A front view of the heart. *Source:* Dcoetzee [20], used under CC-BY 3.0 https://creativecommons.org/licenses/by/3.0/. (b) Pulmonary and systemic units. Source: OpenStax College [21], used under CC-BY 3.0 https://creativecommons.org/licenses/by/3.0/.

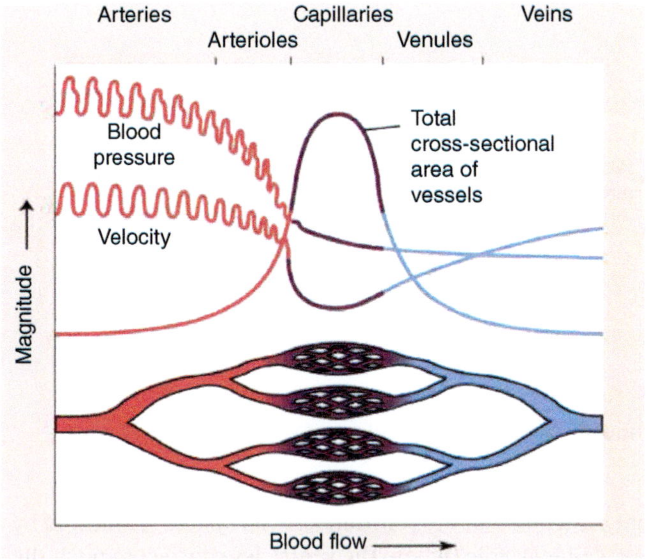

Figure 3.24 Blood pressure and velocity. *Source:* Mader and Windelspecht [22].

enter the tissue fluid. At the venous end of the capillary, blood pressure has fallen below osmotic pressure; hence materials such as water, carbon dioxide, and urea leave the tissue fluid and enter the capillaries (Figure 3.25).

3.3.2.4 Heartbeat

Each heartbeat is called a **cardiac cycle**. During a heartbeat, the two atria contract together, then the two ventricles contract, followed by a relaxation of the whole heart. **Systole** is the contraction of heart chambers, while **diastole** is their relaxation. The cardiac cycle begins with atrial systole.

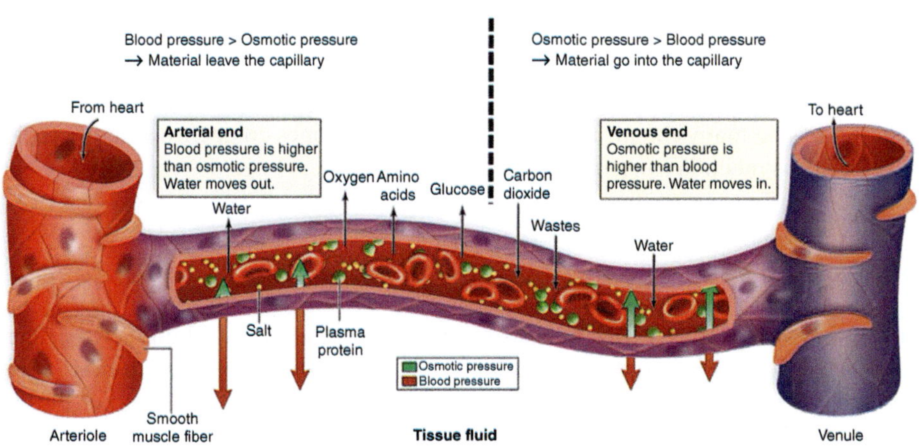

Figure 3.25 Capillary exchange of standards. At the arterial end of the capillary, the blood pressure is greater than the osmotic pressure, which causes material to leave the capillary. At the venous end of the capillary, the osmotic pressure exceeds the blood pressure, which causes material to enter the capillary. *Source:* Mader and Windelspecht [22].

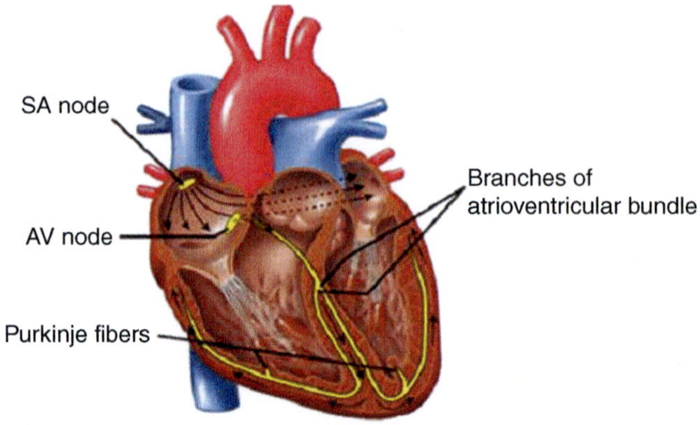

Figure 3.26 Location of the nodes that control heartbeat. *Source:* Mader and Windelspecht [22].

During this phase, both atria contract and push blood to the ventricles. Atrial systole is followed by atrial diastole (when atria relax) and ventricular systole (where the ventricles contract to push the blood into arteries). During ventricular systole, the pressure in the ventricles increases. This pressure closes the atrioventricular valves located between atria and ventricles. Atrioventricular valves prevent the blood from moving back into atria, effectively forcing the blood to the arteries. Ventricular systole is followed by ventricular diastole where ventricles relax. Semilunar valves (between ventricles and arteries) close because of the pressure difference created between arteries and ventricles during this relaxation. The "lub-dup" sound made by the heart is caused by the closing of the atrioventricular valves, followed by the closing of the semilunar valves.

The SA (sinoatrial) and AV (atrioventricular) nodes are responsible for internal control of the heartbeat. The SA node, sometimes called the pacemaker, initiates the heartbeat and causes the atria to contract on average every 0.85 second. The AV node conveys the stimulus and initiates the contraction of the ventricles. The signal for the ventricles to contract travels from the AV node through the atrioventricular bundle to the smaller Purkinje fibers (Figure 3.26).

The heartbeat is also controlled by other body systems that are not part of the circulatory system. The nervous system (particularly, the medulla oblongata in the brain) can speed up or slow down the heart rate in response to many chemical stimuli. Also, the hormones epinephrine and norepinephrine from the adrenal medulla can stimulate a faster heart rate.

3.4 Endocrine System

The glands in the human body are divided into two categories: exocrine and endocrine. The **exocrine glands** (exo = outside) produce chemicals and secrete them into ducts that open into either the lumen (i.e. cavities inside the organs) or outside the body. On the other hand, **endocrine glands** (endo = inside) produce chemicals and secrete them into the blood. The endocrine system is the system of glands that is responsible for secreting specific hormones into the bloodstream to regulate bodily functions. **Hormones** are chemicals that travel in the bloodstream to a target tissue and generate a response. They perform general functions of communication and control that are typically slower and longer-lasting than the type of control provided by nerve impulses. Cells acted on by hormones are called target cells. In order to

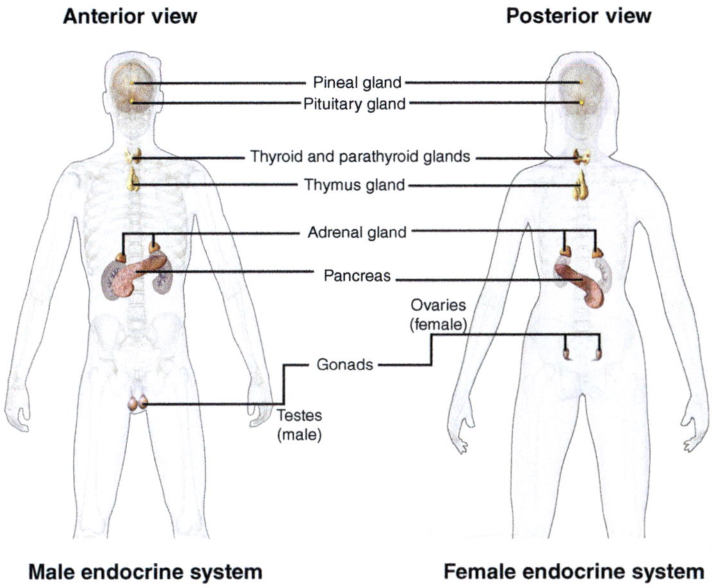

Figure 3.27 Endocrine glands and their location. *Source:* Adapted from BruceBlaus [7], used under CC-BY 3.0 http://creativecommons.org/licenses/by/3.0.

maintain stable conditions in the body, or homeostasis, hormone balance is important. The endocrine glands include hypothalamus, pineal, pituitary, thyroid, parathyroid, thymus, adrenals, pancreas, and ovaries or testes (Figure 3.27).

3.4.1 Types of Hormones

Hormones are divided into two categories based on their solubility: water-soluble (e.g. peptide hormones and protein hormones) and lipid-soluble (e.g. steroid hormones).

Protein hormones are hydrophilic and they travel in the bloodstream as free soluble molecules. These hormones cannot cross the cell membrane (due to their hydrophilic nature), so they must bind to receptors on the target cell membrane. This binding triggers secondary messengers inside the cell to affect the cell's activities through signaling pathways (Figure 3.28). Human growth hormone (HGH) and insulin are two examples of protein hormones.

Steroid hormones are hydrophobic and therefore need a hydrophilic molecule (transport protein) to transport them through the bloodstream. Since they are hydrophobic, they can easily cross the cell and nuclear membranes. Once inside the target cell's nucleus, steroid hormones bind and activate molecules that influence cell activity by acting directly on DNA. All steroid hormones are derived from cholesterol. Some examples of steroid hormones are cortisol, aldosterone, testosterone, and estrogen.

3.4.2 Mechanisms of Action

3.4.2.1 Action of Protein Hormones

Protein hormones can travel in the bloodstream freely, but they cannot easily enter the cell (recall from Chapter 1 that the cell membrane prevents the passage of hydrophilic molecules). Hence, protein hormones rely on interaction with messengers to activate enzymes inside the cell

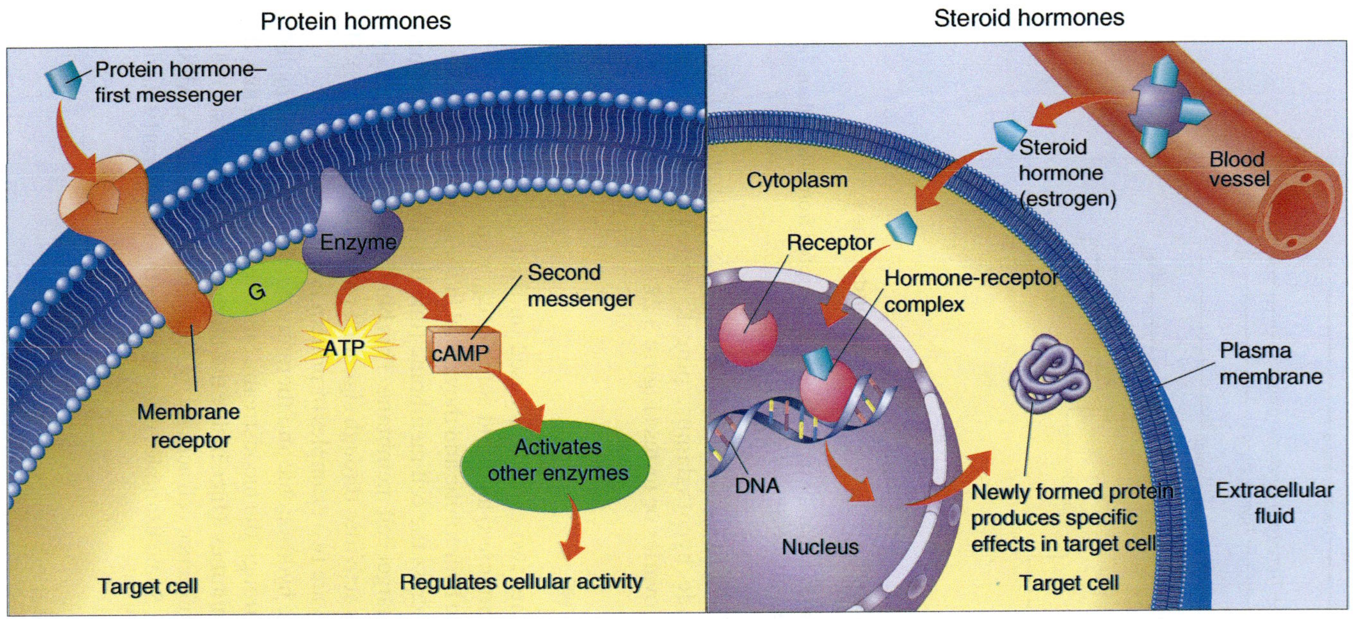

Figure 3.28 Protein vs. steroid hormones. *Source:* Thibodeau and Patton [23]. This article was published in Structure & Function of the Body – The Endocrine System, Copyright © 2008 Published by Elsevier.

membrane. The action mechanism of protein hormones is shown in Figure 3.28. The protein hormone itself is called the **first messenger** (or primary messenger). The first messenger finds its target membrane receptor on the cell membrane and binds to it. This binding causes activation of G protein located inside the membrane. The activated G protein, in turn, activates an enzyme that converts ATP to cyclic AMP (cAMP) in the cytoplasm. In this mechanism, cAMP is called the **second messenger** (or secondary messenger) because it freely moves in the cytoplasm and activates other enzymes that regulate cellular activity. Secondary messengers, in turn, activate protein kinases (enzymes that turn on/off certain proteins). The result is the physiological response of the cell to the hormone. In addition, it is important to note that the conversion of ATP to cAMP (and all other enzyme activities) continues to occur as long as enzymes stay active. This causes amplification of the signal (i.e. one hormone molecule can cause activation of millions of proteins).

3.4.2.2 Action of Steroid Hormones

Steroid hormones are carried in the blood bound to transport proteins. When they are released from these proteins, they leave the blood vessel and diffuse into the cell through the cell membrane (recall from Chapter 1 that small hydrophobic molecules can diffuse through the membrane). Once inside the cell, they bind to their target receptor either in the cytoplasm or in the nucleus. This receptor–hormone complex can turn certain genes in the DNA on or off (recall that promoters and transcription factors attract RNA polymerase to start transcription). When a gene is turned on, the cell starts to produce the protein that is encoded by this gene (through transcription and translation mechanism). The action mechanism of steroid hormones is shown in Figure 3.28.

3.4.3 Pituitary Gland

The **pituitary gland** is an important gland in the endocrine system, secreting many hormones that regulate homeostasis. The pituitary gland has two parts: the anterior pituitary and the posterior pituitary (Figure 3.29). The **anterior pituitary** secretes six major hormones: thyroid-stimulating hormone (TSH), adrenocorticotropic hormone (ACTH), follicle-stimulating hormone (FSH), luteinizing hormone (LH), growth hormone (GH), and prolactin (PRL). The secretion of anterior pituitary hormones is strictly controlled by the hypothalamus. The **posterior pituitary** secretes two major hormones: antidiuretic hormone (ADH) and oxytocin (OT). The posterior pituitary receives its hormones from the hypothalamus; it does not produce hormones itself. The hormones of the anterior and posterior pituitary are summarized in Table 3.5.

3.4.4 Thyroid and Parathyroid Glands

The **thyroid gland** is located in the neck (Figure 3.30), just under the larynx (voice box), and secretes three different hormones: thyroxine (a.k.a. T4 because it has four iodine atoms), triiodothyronine (a.k.a. T3 because it has three iodine atoms), and calcitonin.

T4 and **T3** stimulate the energy metabolism in all cells (i.e. increase the body's metabolic rate). When the energy metabolism increases, cells burn more glucose, and as a side effect, the body temperature rises (calorigenic effect). The **calorigenic effect** plays an important role in survival at low temperatures. Mammals cannot survive freezing temperatures if their thyroids have been removed. **Calcitonin** inhibits the breakdown of bone and causes a decrease in blood calcium concentration.

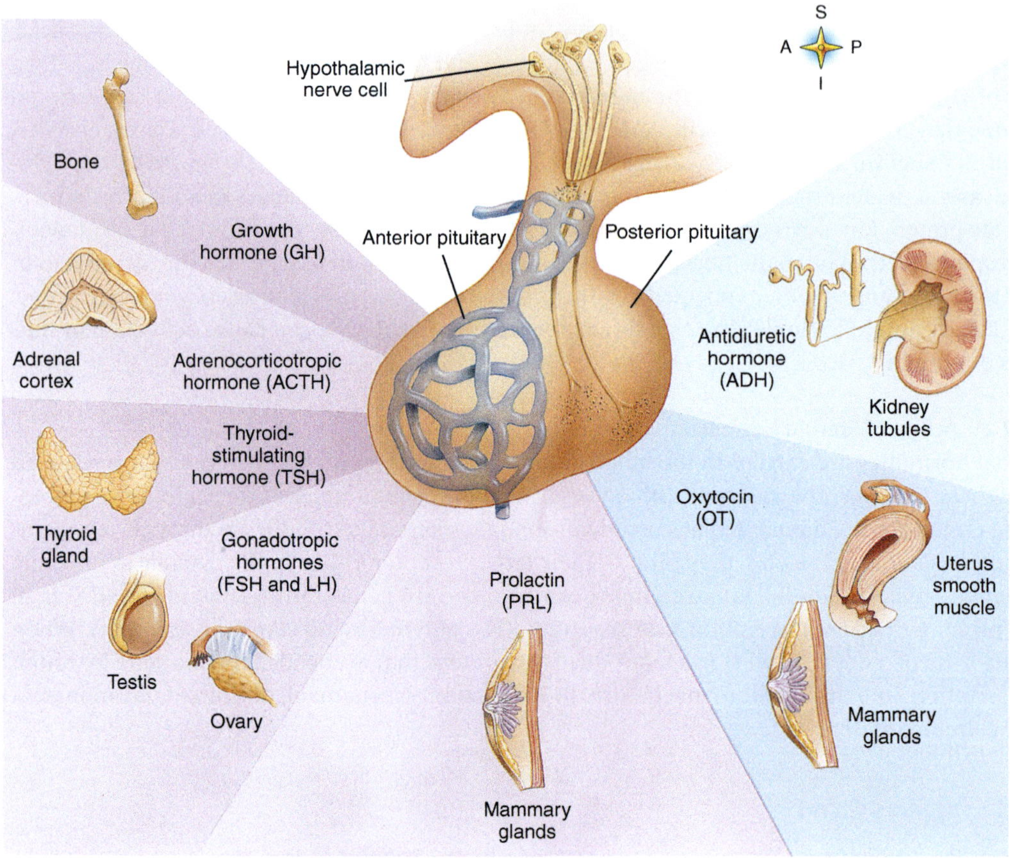

Figure 3.29 Pituitary hormones and their targets [24].

The **parathyroid glands** are embedded on the posterior (back) surface of the thyroid gland. A normal individual has four parathyroid glands. These glands secrete only parathyroid hormone.

Parathyroid hormone (PTH) stimulates the breakdown of bone and causes an increase in blood calcium concentration. The thyroid and parathyroid activity act to balance out the effects of high or low blood calcium levels, respectively (Figure 3.31).

The thyroid and parathyroid glands together regulate the calcium homeostatic balance. If for some reason the blood calcium level drops below normal, parathyroid glands increase PTH secretion. PTH causes an increase in blood calcium level by stimulating the breakdown of the bone matrix. As a result, the blood calcium level returns to normal. If for some reason the blood calcium level increases, the thyroid gland increases the secretion of calcitonin hormone. Calcitonin inhibits bone breakdown and the blood calcium level decreases. PTH and calcitonin hormones stabilize the concentration of calcium in the blood.

3.4.5 Adrenal Glands

The **adrenal glands** are small glands located on top of each kidney (Figure 3.32). Each adrenal gland has two distinct regions: adrenal cortex and adrenal medulla. The **adrenal cortex** secretes mineralocorticoids (e.g. aldosterone), glucocorticoids (e.g. cortisol), and androgens (sex hormones).

Table 3.5 Pituitary hormones and their functions.

Anterior pituitary hormones	
TSH (thyroid-stimulating hormone)	Targets the thyroid gland. Stimulates secretion of thyroid hormones.
ACTH (adrenocorticotropic hormone)	Targets the adrenal cortex. Stimulates the secretion of adrenal cortex hormones.
FSH (follicle-stimulating hormone)	Targets the ovaries in females and testes in males. Stimulates the development of ovarian follicles (which contains the ovum) and the secretion of estrogen in females, and the production of sperm in males.
LH (luteinizing hormone)	Targets the ovaries in females and testes in males. Stimulates the maturation of ovarian follicle and ovum, secretion of estrogen, and beginning of ovulation in females. Stimulates secretion of testosterone from testes in males.
GH (growth hormone)	Targets liver, muscle, cartilage, bone, and other tissues. Stimulates these organs and tissues to secrete insulin-like growth factors (IGFs). IGFs cause growth in all organs.
Prolactin (lactogenic hormone)	Targets mammary glands. Stimulates breast development during pregnancy and milk secretion after pregnancy.
Posterior pituitary hormones	
ADH (antidiuretic hormone)	Targets the kidney. Accelerates water reabsorption from urine into blood, thereby decreasing urine secretion.
OT (oxytocin)	Stimulates the pregnant uterus to contract, may initiate labor, and causes glandular cells of the breast to release milk into the ducts.

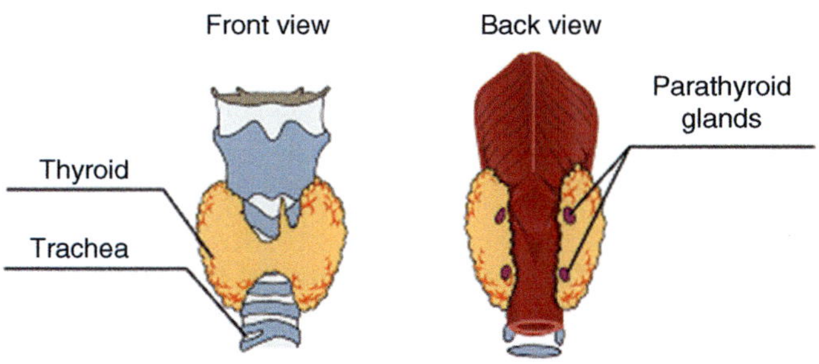

Figure 3.30 Physical location of thyroid and parathyroid glands.

The **adrenal medulla** secretes epinephrine (adrenaline) and norepinephrine which prolong and intensify the sympathetic nervous response (for stress response).

3.4.5.1 Adrenal Cortex Hormones

Mineralocorticoids regulate mineral homeostasis by signaling the kidneys to secrete certain electrolytes into the urine. The major mineralocorticoid is aldosterone. **Aldosterone** regulates the blood level of sodium ions (Na^+) and potassium ions (K^+) as well as blood pressure. When blood pressure drops, aldosterone is secreted from the adrenal cortex. Aldosterone acts on kidneys and

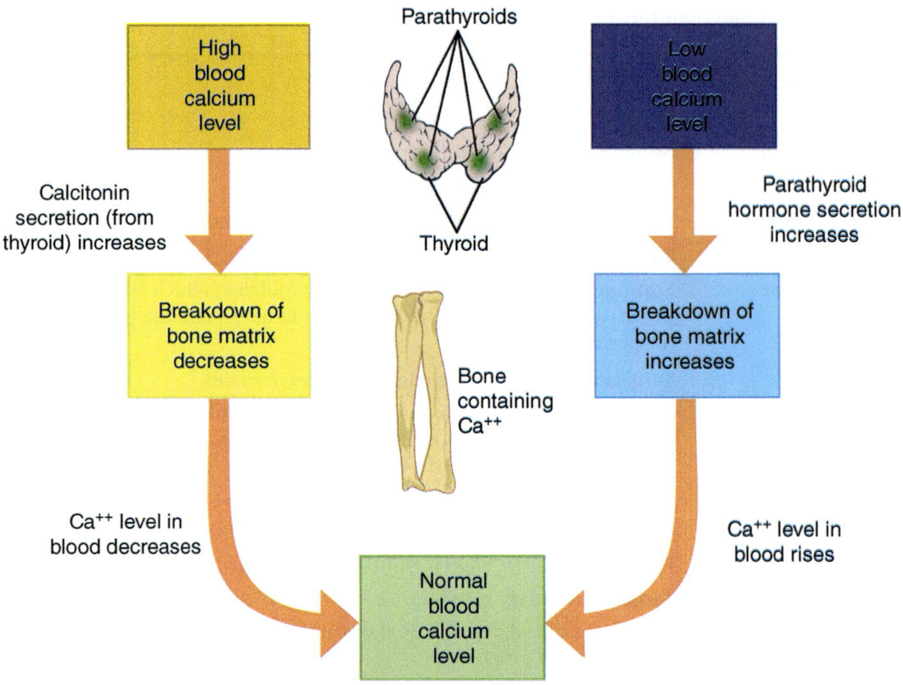

Figure 3.31 Blood calcium level regulation by thyroid and parathyroid activities.

increases the reabsorption of Na^+ into the blood. Due to the osmotic pressure, water follows Na^+ into the blood and the urea volume decreases. This means that less water is lost and, as a result, blood pressure increases.

Glucocorticoids regulate glucose homeostasis by stimulating gluconeogenesis and causing an increase in blood glucose concentration. Gluconeogenesis is the process of converting amino acids into glucose. These hormones also have anti-inflammatory, anti-immunity, and anti-allergy effects. One of the most important glucocorticoids is **cortisol** and it accounts for 95% of the glucocorticoid activity.

Androgens (a.k.a. **sex hormones)** stimulate sexual drive in females and get converted to estrogens, but they have negligible effects on males.

3.4.5.2 Adrenal Medulla Hormones

Epinephrine and **norepinephrine** together regulate fight-or-flight response of the body. These hormones are released under stressful situations and during exercise. They increase the blood pressure and cardiac output by increasing the heart rate and force of contraction. In addition, they increase blood flow to the heart and skeletal muscles. They also increase the blood glucose level.

3.4.6 Pancreatic Islets

The **pancreas** plays a major role in metabolism and contains both endocrine and exocrine cells. The pancreas contains two types of endocrine cells that secrete different hormones: **alpha cells** secrete glucagon and **beta cells** secrete insulin (Figure 3.33).

Glucagon increases blood glucose levels by accelerating liver glycogenolysis. Glycogenolysis is the conversion of glycogen (a stored form of carbohydrate) to glucose (simple sugar). **Insulin** decreases blood glucose levels by accelerating the movement of glucose out of the blood and into

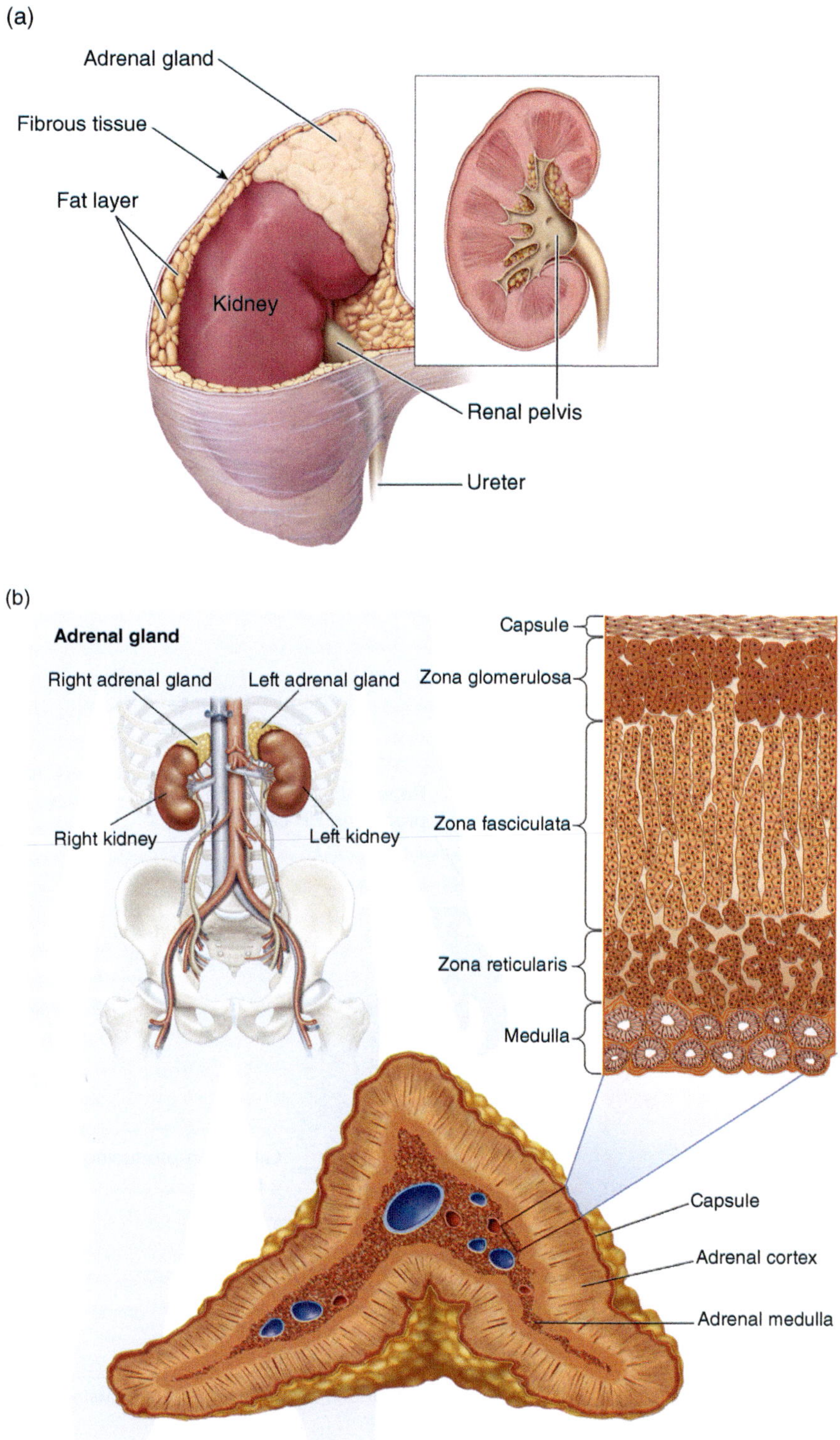

Figure 3.32 (a) Structure of the kidney. *Source:* Renal Cell Cancer Treatment (PDG®) was originally published by the National Cancer Institute. (b) Location and regions of the adrenal glands. *Source:* Reprinted with permission from Encyclopædia Britannica, © 2018 by Encyclopædia Britannica, Inc.

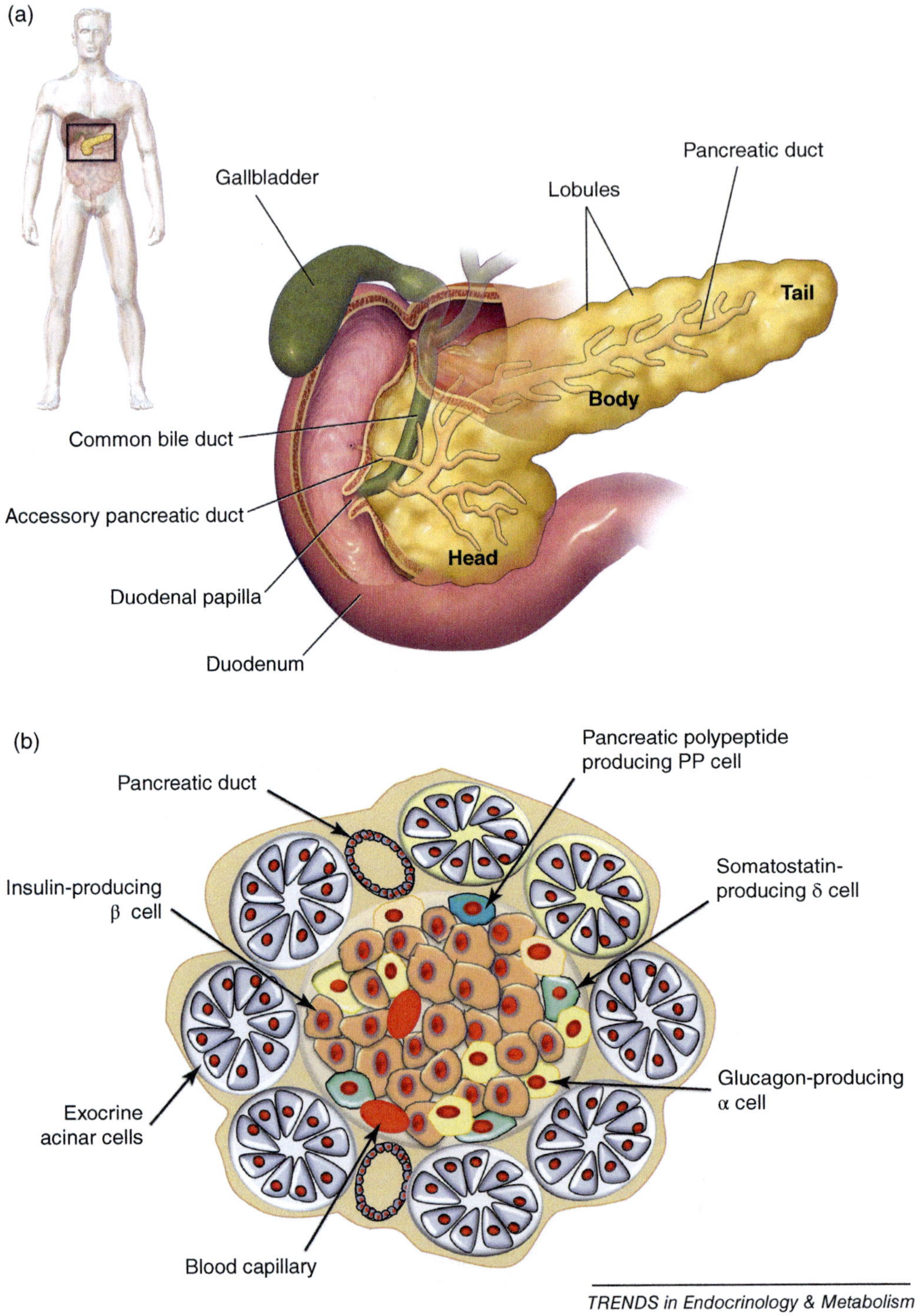

Figure 3.33 (a) Anatomy of the pancreas. *Source:* BruceBlaus [7], used under CC-BY 3.0 https://creativecommons.org/licenses/by/3.0/. (b) Pancreatic islet and endocrine cells. *Source:* Efrat and Russ [25]. Reprinted from Trends in Endocrinology & Metabolism, Copyright © 2012 Published by Elsevier, Inc., with permission from Elsevier.

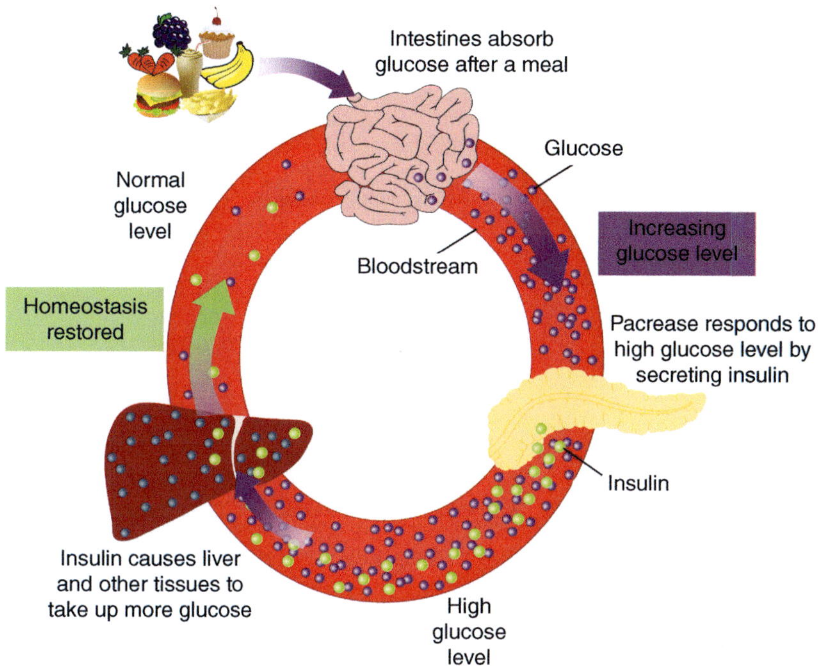

Figure 3.34 Negative feedback loop of insulin.

cells, particularly liver cells. Insulin is an important hormone since it is the only one that can reduce blood glucose levels.

The pancreas plays an important role in the negative feedback loop that reverses the direction of change in a physiological system (Figure 3.34). When the intestines absorb glucose after a meal, the blood glucose levels increase, causing the pancreas to respond by secreting insulin. The insulin signals the liver and other tissues to take up more glucose, which restores homeostatic levels of glucose.

3.5 Lymphatic System

The lymphatic system consists of a network of vessels and nodes (a.k.a. lymph vessels and lymph nodes) (Figure 3.35). The lymph vessels assist in transporting excess fluid away from interstitial spaces (i.e. spaces that surround tissue cells). One of the purposes of the lymphatic system is to monitor and regulate the flow of excess fluid in the body. However, the lymphatic system also plays a major role in defending the body against diseases and pathogens.

3.5.1 Lymph Vessels and Nodes

Lymph is a clear fluid similar to interstitial fluid. In fact, when interstitial fluid enters the lymphatic vessels, it is called lymph. **Lymph vessels** are separate from the circulatory system. Recall that blood pressure in the capillaries pushes water into the interstitial space at the arterial end of the capillary and pulls water back in at the venous end, but that a net amount of water goes into the interstitial space. Lymph capillaries have a special architecture that allows them to work like valves (Figure 3.36). Increased interstitial fluid pressure opens the lymph capillary and the capillary is filled with the fluid. Once inside the lymph capillary, this fluid cannot escape.

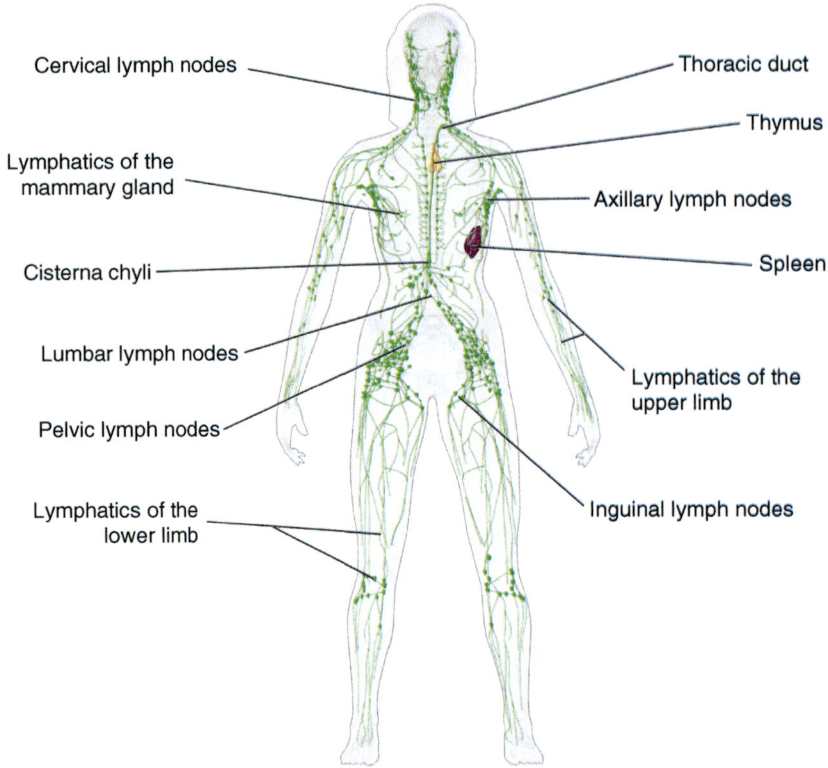

Figure 3.35 Lymphatic system organs and components. *Source:* BruceBlaus [7], used under CC-BY 3.0 https://creativecommones.org/licenses/by/3.0/.

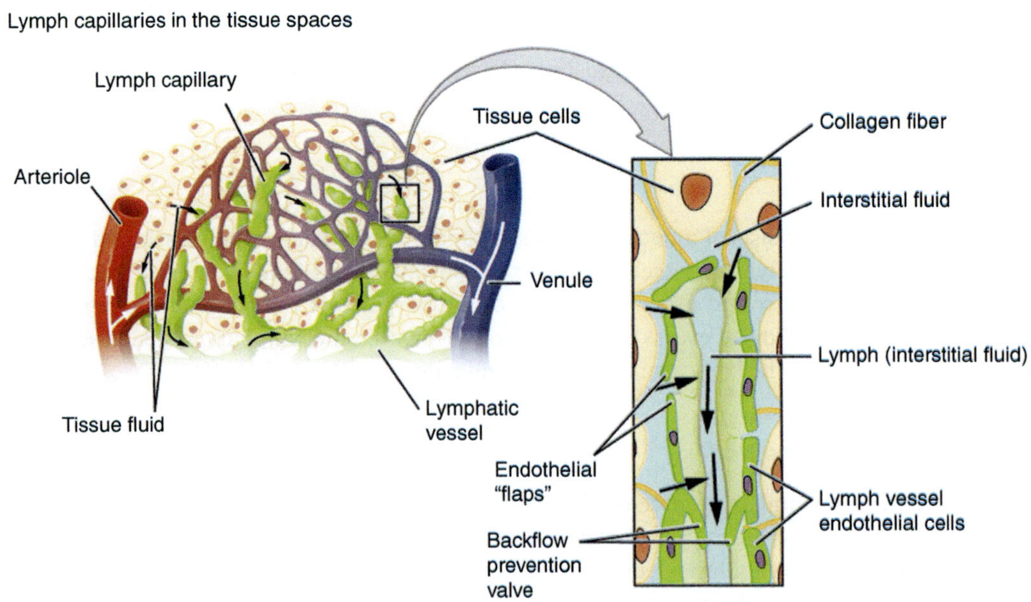

Figure 3.36 Lymphatic capillary network and lymphatic capillary structure. *Source:* OpenStaxCollege [26], used under CC-BY 3.0 https://creativecommones.org/licenses/by/3.0/.

Lymph vessels drain excess fluids from the tissue by carrying them back to the circulatory system through the subclavian vein (Figure 3.36). **Lymph nodes** are small oval-shaped organs located along lymphatic vessels (Figure 3.37). There are about 600 lymph nodes distributed throughout the human body (usually in groups) and these nodes are linked by lymphatic vessels (Figure 3.35). Lymph nodes can sample fluids and filter potentially harmful particles from the lymphatic system before returning them to the bloodstream. Lymph nodes are also sites of immune surveillance by macrophages and lymphocytes (B cells and T cells), which fight foreign invaders. The lymph nodes are also sites of lymphocyte production.

3.6 Immune System

The human body is protected by a number of forms of immunity, either nonspecific or specific (Figure 3.38). **Nonspecific immunity** (a.k.a. innate immunity) refers to the mechanisms by which the body defends itself against foreign pathogens in a manner that depends only on very general properties of those pathogens. Examples of nonspecific immunity include mechanical barriers (e.g. skin, mucous membranes that prevent toxins from entering through the respiratory tract, and tears that wash out toxins from the eye surface), chemical immunity (e.g. extreme acidic pH in the stomach and enzymes in various body fluids), phagocytosis, inflammatory response, and natural killer cells. **Specific immunity** (a.k.a. adaptive immunity) refers to mechanisms that the body

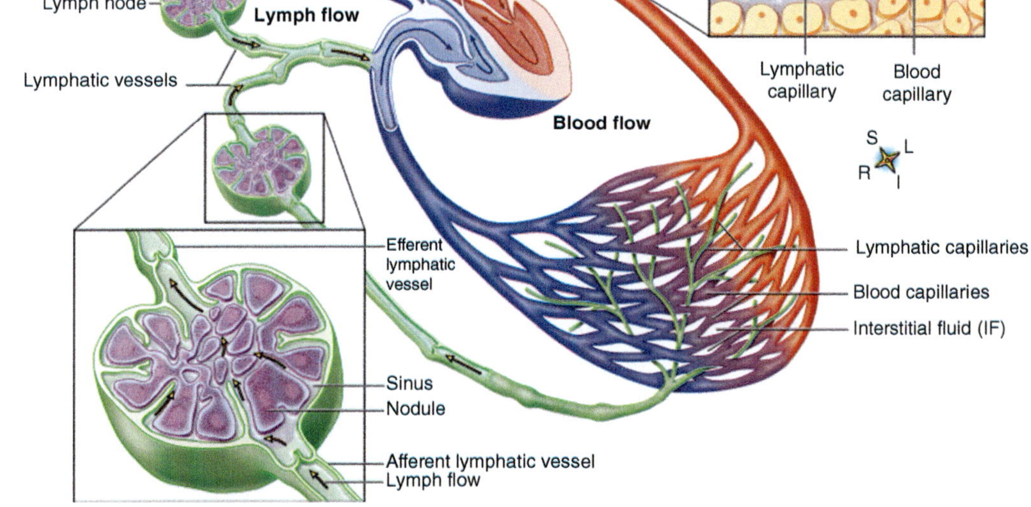

Figure 3.37 Lymph network connects to circulatory system at subclavian veins (inset shows a lymph node). *Source:* Thibodeau and Patton [27]. This article was published in Anatomy and Physiology Lymphatic System, Copyright © 2007 Published by Elsevier.

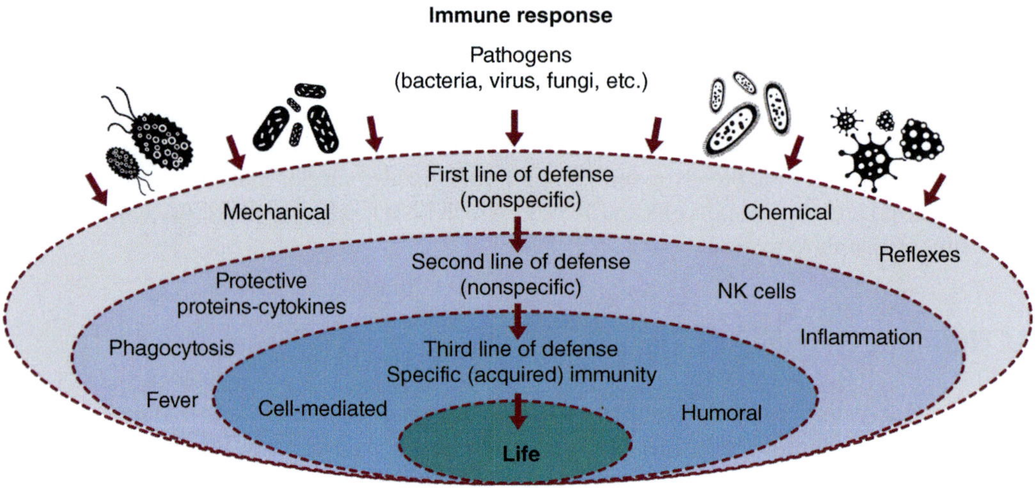

Figure 3.38 Nonspecific and specific immunity elements.

can use to recognize and protect itself with a prepared response against unique features of pathogens that were previously encountered.

3.6.1 Phagocytosis – Nonspecific Immunity

Phagocytosis protects the body from invading microorganisms such as bacteria. Phagocytic cells take invading pathogens into their own cell bodies and digest them (with acidic conditions and a variety of enzymes) by the process of phagocytosis (Figure 3.39). Examples of phagocytes include neutrophils (the most abundant white blood cell in the blood) and macrophages. The phagocytes recognize the entity as a "foreign body" and proceed to engulf and then digest them. In some cases, phagocytosis does not occur smoothly and certain bacteria or viruses (e.g. tuberculosis) can infect the phagocyte and use it as a host to reproduce.

3.6.2 Specific Immunity

Specific immunity describes a form of "tailored" protection against certain types of invading bacteria or other toxic materials. Using mechanisms of specific immunity, the body is capable of adapting to newly encountered "enemies." There is some sort of learning curve, as the target must be specific. Upon first exposure, the body fights to destroy the invading organism, which is often accompanied by symptoms such as high temperature (fever). Upon the second and subsequent exposures, no serious symptoms are exhibited because the body is "immune" (i.e. prepared to respond very rapidly to neutralize the invasion). However, specific immunity to one invader does not protect against another, or even another instance of the same type. This is why flu vaccines have to be given annually to protect against different strains of the flu virus. Exposure to a harmful agent can be categorized as either natural exposure or artificial exposure through immunization. The body does not differentiate between natural and artificial agents; it merely sees the foreign "body" and responds. However, unlike wild-type pathogens, immunization exposures do not usually cause the individual to get sick. This is because immunizations and vaccines are made from attenuated (e.g. noninfectious) forms of the given wild-type pathogen.

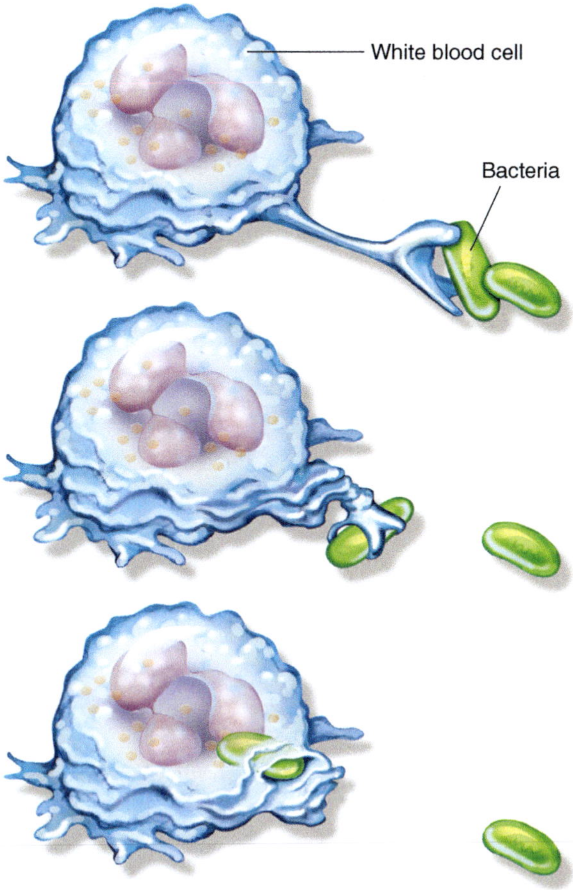

Figure 3.39 Phagocytosis by a neutrophil. *Source:* Thibodeau and Patton [28]. This article was published in Structure and Function of the Body, Copyright © 2008 Published by Elsevier.

3.6.2.1 Antibodies and Antigens

Antibodies are proteins that give the "specificity" to certain immunity functions. A single antibody is able to recognize and bind to a specific compound called its antigen. **Antigens** are individual molecules or small regions on the surfaces of pathogens like bacteria and viruses. Antigens are often protein molecules embedded on the surface membranes of invading or diseased cells such as microorganisms or cancer cells. Antibodies have a "Y" structure that includes two copies of the same variable region that has the ability to specifically bind to a unique antigen (Figure 3.40). All antibodies have the same constant region. Therefore, an antibody that binds to antigen A and an antibody that binds to antigen B will have the same constant region, but will have different variable regions that are specific to antigens A and B. Each antibody has two identical antigen-binding sites, meaning that each antibody can bind to two antigens of the same type (i.e. both arms can bind to antigen A).

3.6.2.2 Antibody Function

In the context of the immune system, antibodies aim to bind to an antigen and initiate a process that will prevent the antigen (or the invader that carries this antigen) from harming the body. This can be accomplished in a number of ways:

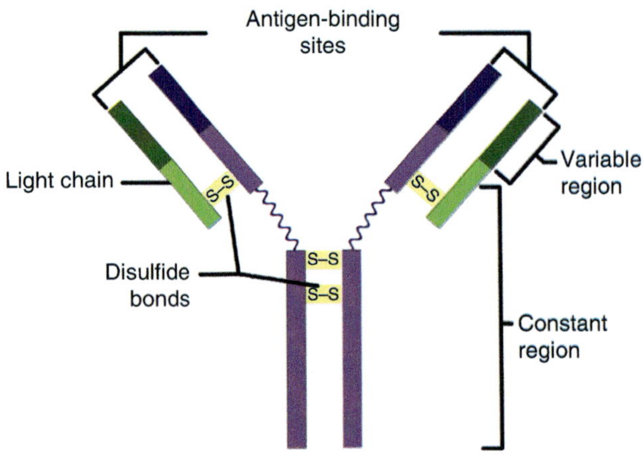

Figure 3.40 Structure of an antibody.

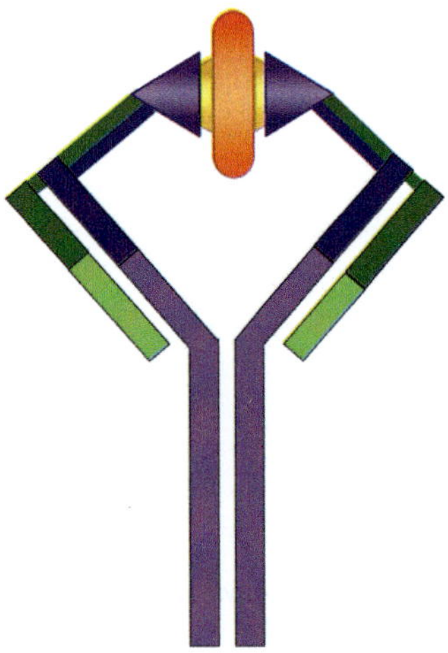

Figure 3.41 Antibody inactivates antigen.

Inactivating antigens: If the antigen is a small molecule toxin, the antibody can neutralize, or make the toxin nonpoisonous, by capping it (Figure 3.41). Capping the toxin makes it incapable of interacting with its target(s), which inhibits the toxin from producing its poisonous effect. This neutralization is accomplished in multiple ways including preventing the toxin from entering the cell, preventing the toxin from reaching its target due to size constraints, or blocking the active area of the toxin (i.e. the part of the toxin that makes it dangerous).

Clumping antigens together: If the antigens are molecules on the surface membranes of invading cells, the antigen-antibody complex may make the invading cells stick together in clumps (Figure 3.42). Macrophages or other phagocytes can rapidly destroy these clumps by ingesting and digesting large numbers of them at one time. One bacterium often has hundreds or even thousands of antigens on its surface, so many antibodies can attach to the same bacteria in order to deactivate it.

Facilitating phagocytosis: Certain antibodies help promote immunity through the attachment to phagocyte cells, promoting them to engulf the antibody-bacterium complex (Figure 3.43). This approach enhances the interaction between the phagocyte cell and its victim, and the object is

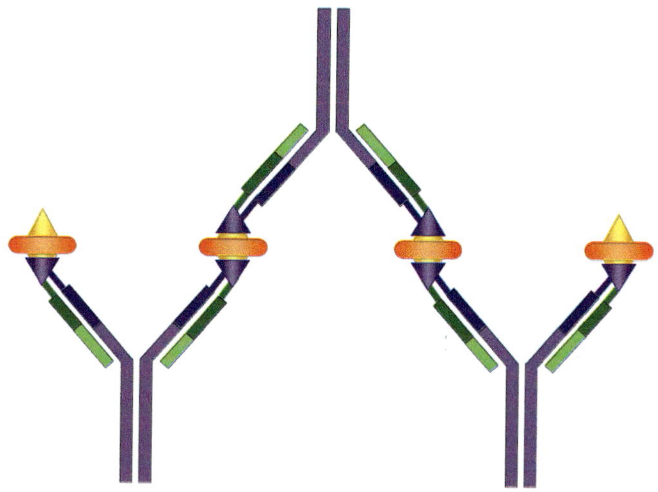

Figure 3.42 Antibodies clumping antigens together.

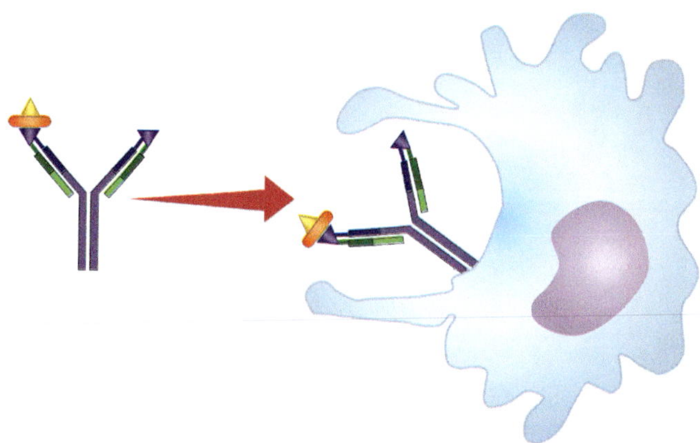

Figure 3.43 Antibodies can facilitate phagocytosis.

more easily ingested. Thus, the phagocyte may not recognize the target on its own, and the antibodies are a method of tagging the target and informing the phagocytes to destroy the target.

Complementing proteins: Sometimes as an antibody attaches to an antigen on an invading cell, the interaction will change the shape of the antibody molecule, slightly exposing two previously hidden regions called complement-binding sites. Complement proteins in the blood are naturally inactive, but interaction with the complement-binding sites on the antibodies activates them. The complement proteins arrange on the invading cell's membrane in doughnut-shaped rings, opening up a hole, and allowing Na^+ ions to enter the cell. This increases the salt concentration, causing water to rush into the cell (due to osmotic pressure) until the cell bursts (i.e. cell lysis) (Figure 3.44).

A rotavirus (the virus responsible for diarrhea) is shown in Figure 3.45. In this figure, the image on the left shows many antigens sticking out of the rotavirus, all of which antibodies can attach to. The image on the right shows the same rotavirus after exposure to antibodies. Notice that the shape of antibodies resembles the letter "Y" as illustrated in Figure 3.40. It is relatively easy for the immune system to detect viruses that have been coated in antibodies like this. In other cases, virus

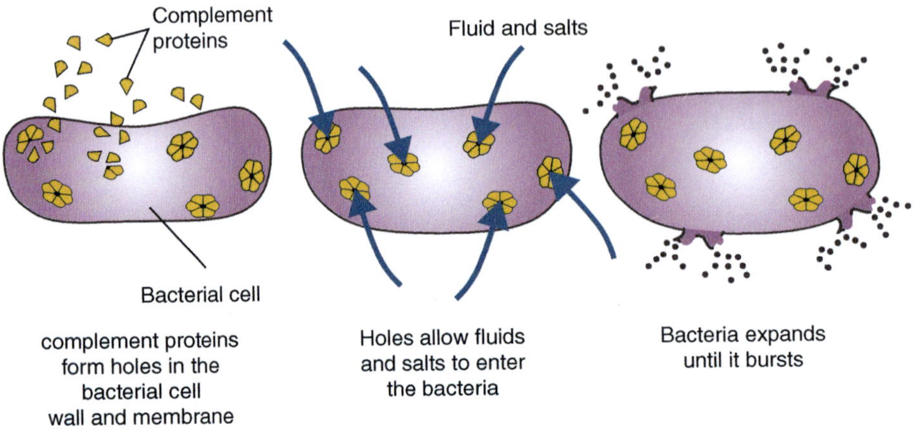

Figure 3.44 Antibodies creating holes with complement proteins to cause the cell to burst.

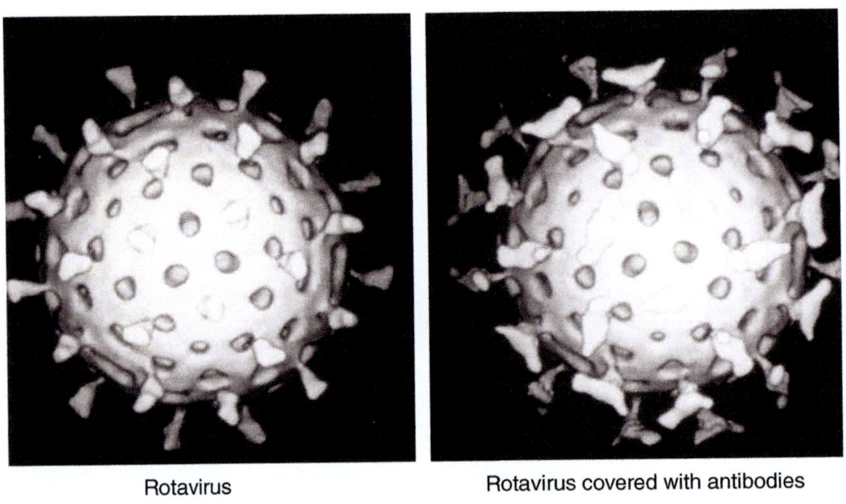

Figure 3.45 Antibodies binding to rotavirus antigens. *Source:* GrahamColm [29], used under CC-BY-SA 3.0 https://creativecommons.org/licenses/by-sa/3.0/.

recognition is not so simple. For example, HIV has a very thick coating of sugars that look like normal body cells. HIV also has a mechanism which continually changes its surface after replication so that immune system keeps seeing different surfaces and cannot mount the proper virus-specific response. A lot of current HIV research is aimed at determining the sites that remain constant on HIV so that drugs can target a part of the virus that does not change.

3.6.2.3 Lymphocytes

Lymphocytes are the most numerous cells of the immune system. Certain lymphocytes called B cells are responsible for antibody production. There are several million lymphocytes continuously circulating in body fluids and searching for any enemy cells that may have entered. Lymphocytes reside primarily in the lymph nodes and other lymphatic tissues (the thymus gland in the chest, and the spleen and liver in the abdomen). There are two major types of lymphocytes: B- and T-lymphocytes (a.k.a. B cells and T cells). Like phagocytes, lymphocytes help protect against

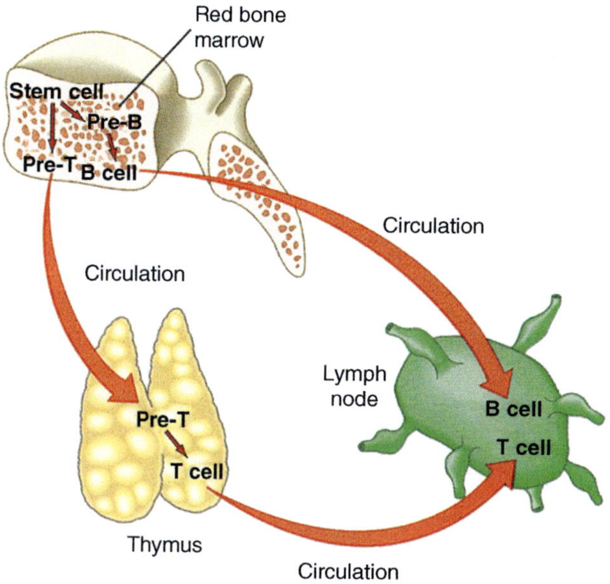

Figure 3.46 Origin of lymphocytes. *Source:* Thibodeau and Patton [30]. This article was published in Anatomy and Physiology, Copyright © 2007 Published by Elsevier.

infections. **B cells** secrete antibodies that destroy particular bacteria, viruses, or chemical toxins; **T cells** directly face and attack bacteria or cancerous cells.

All lymphocytes arise from stem cells in the bone marrow (Figure 3.46). The undifferentiated lymphocytes created in bone marrow go through a series of changes that differentiate them into either B cells or T cells. The location of differentiation depends on the cell type. Immature B-cells are differentiated in the bone marrow and transported into lymph nodes through the circulatory system. On the other hand, T-cells are differentiated in the thymus gland and then transported to the lymph nodes through the circulatory system.

3.6.2.4 B Cell Development

Stem cells in the bone marrow differentiate (i.e. turn into) **immature B cells** which are small lymphocytes that have synthesized and inserted into their membranes numerous copies of one specific kind of antibody. The immature B cells eventually leave the bone marrow and travel through the blood to lymph nodes. They undergo repeated mitosis (cell division) to form a family of many identical immature B cells (a.k.a. clones), all of which bear the same type of surface antibody molecules as their single ancestor cell. If, and only if, an immature B cell meets an antigen complementary to its antibody, then it turns into an **activated B cell** (not all immature B cells will undergo this change during their lifetime). An activated B cell then divides rapidly to form two clones of activated B cells: plasma cells and memory cells. **Plasma cells** secrete large amounts of the antibodies into the blood (up to 2000 antibodies per second per plasma cell), and they have a lifetime of a few days. **Memory cells** remain in "reserve" in the lymph nodes. If and when the same antigen is encountered again, memory cells very quickly develop into plasma cells, which then secrete large amounts of antibodies into the blood. You can see this development process in Figure 3.47. B cell production and maturation continue throughout a person's life.

As previously mentioned, specific immune responses differ from the first and second exposures to a pathogen. The **primary immune response** occurs the first time the body (and immature B

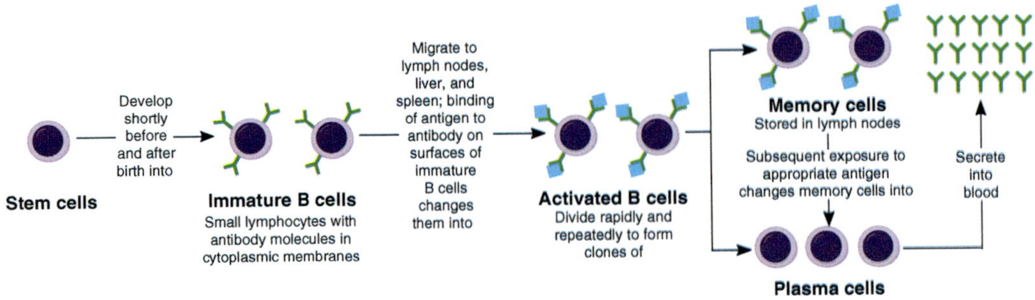

Figure 3.47 B-cell development stages.

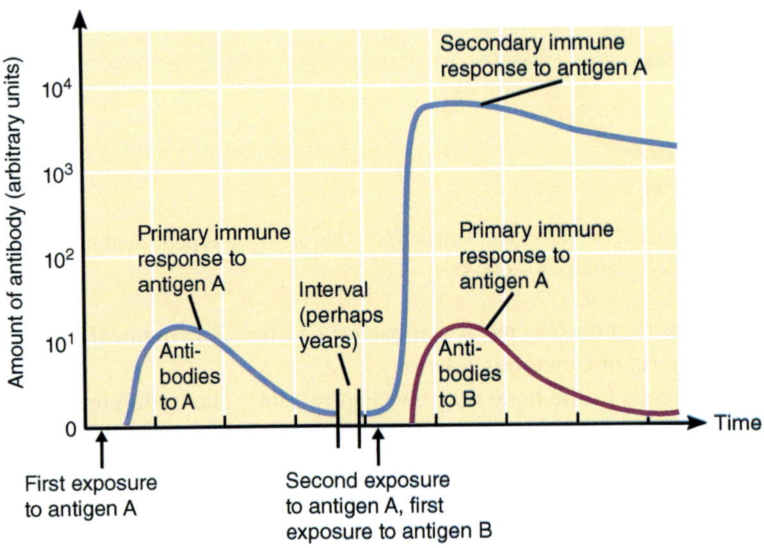

Figure 3.48 Primary vs. secondary immune response.

cells) is exposed to the antigen. After 3–6 days, plasma cells are created, and after 10 days, peak levels of plasma antibody are achieved, after which antibody levels decline. The **secondary immune response** occurs after re-exposure to the same antigen, which causes a much faster immune response. Memory B cells respond within hours by producing antibodies. Antibody levels peak in two to three days at much higher levels than in the primary response. Antibodies bind with greater affinity and their levels in the blood can remain high for weeks to months. A comparison between primary and secondary immune response is shown in Figure 3.48.

3.6.2.5 T Cell Development

T cells are developed when undifferentiated lymphocytes from the bone marrow travel to the thymus gland where they differentiate into T cells (this process occurs shortly before and after birth). The newly formed T cells then migrate to the lymph nodes, liver, and spleen. Most of an individual's T-cells are created before puberty, but T cells keep maturing and leaving the thymus throughout the life of the person. Each T cell membrane has many copies of one type of antibody. If a T cell comes into contact with its antigen, the T cell turns into a sensitized T cell (Figure 3.49).

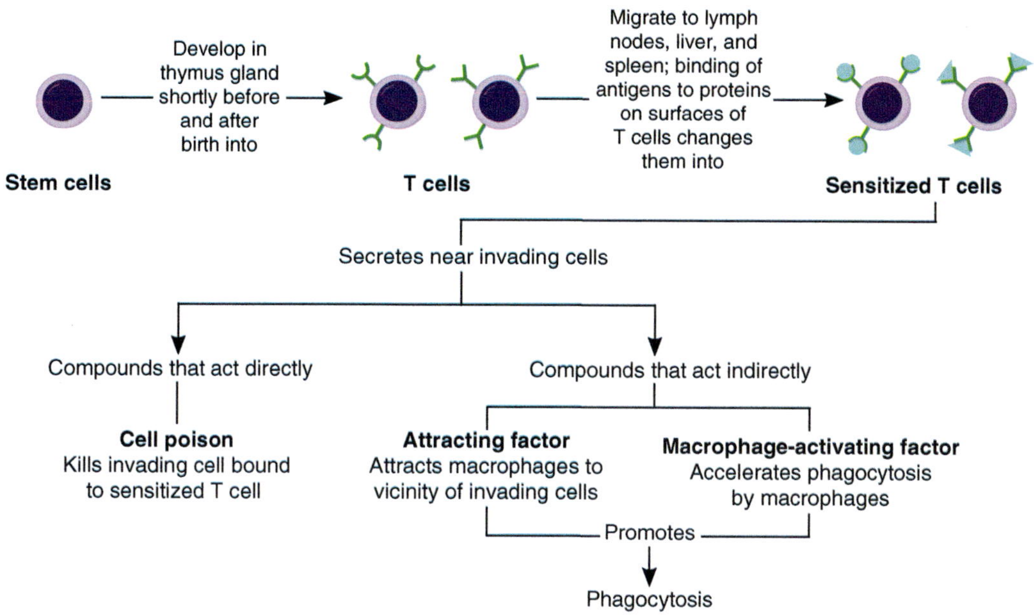

Figure 3.49 T cell development and sensitization. Sensitized T cell types.

Sensitized T cells produce cell-mediated immunity. There are three types of sensitized T cells: cytotoxic T cell, helper T cell, and memory T cell.

Cytotoxic T cells kill invading cells directly by releasing a lethal poison against the bound cell. **Helper T cells** indirectly fight the invader by releasing compounds that recruit macrophages, which then destroy the cells by phagocytosis. Attracting factors attract macrophages to the vicinity of invading cells, while macrophage-activating factors accelerate phagocytosis by macrophages. **Memory T cells** are T cells that remain after the first exposure and are ready for a fast secondary response.

3.6.2.6 Blood Types (Antibody–Antigen Interaction)

We can look at different blood types as an example of interactions between antibodies and antigens. Every person's blood can be one of four types: A, B, AB, or O. Type A blood contains A antigens on the red blood cells' surface, Type B blood contains B antigens, type AB blood contains both A and B antigens, and type O blood contains neither type of antigen (Figure 3.50). In addition, type A blood contains anti-B antibodies in the plasma, type B blood contains anti-A antibodies, type O contains both types of antibodies, and type AB blood contains neither type of antibodies. Thus, a person with type A blood cannot receive a blood donation of type B or AB blood, since the person's anti-B antibodies will bind to the type B antigens in the donor blood's red blood cells and cause agglutination (i.e. clumping) of the blood, which can have fatal results. Similarly, a person with type B blood cannot receive type A or AB blood, while a person with type O blood can only receive type O blood.

An example of blood agglutination is shown in Figure 3.51. Part (a) shows that no agglutination happens when both donor and receiver have type A blood. The reason is that a type A receiver would only have anti-B antibodies in the blood. Since anti-B does not attach to type A antigen, no clumping would occur. On the other hand, in part (b), donor blood is type A and the receiver is type B. The receiver in this case has anti-A antibodies and they stick to type A antigens on the surface of transfused

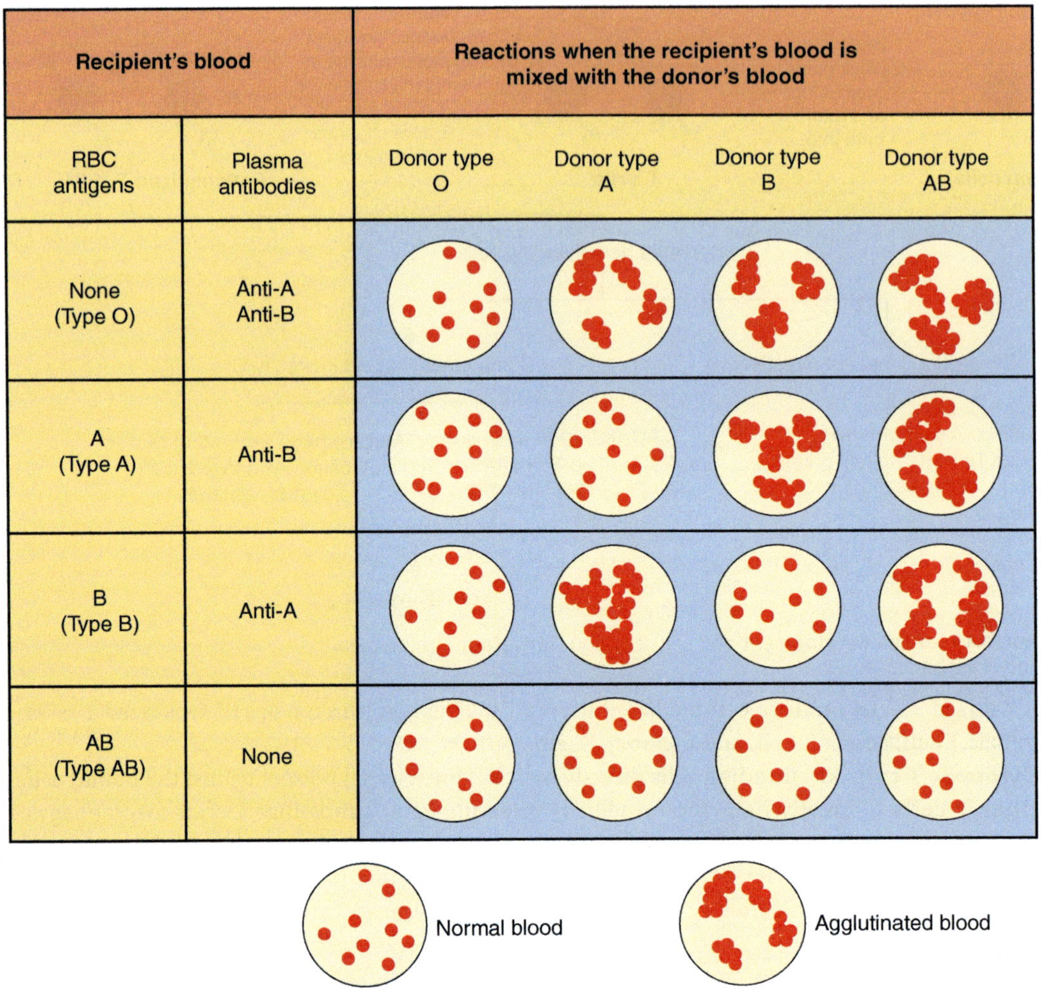

Figure 3.50 Blood type response to antigens.

RBCs. Following agglutination, the antibody–antigen complex activates complementing proteins to poke holes on the RBC surface. The end result is hemolysis (rupturing of RBCs). This may lead to serious complications because hemolysis causes release of hemoglobin into the bloodstream. Free hemoglobin can damage the kidneys by blocking the filtration process.

Did You Know?

Did you know that you can determine your blood type? All you need are anti-A and anti-B antibodies (commonly sold kits). Take two drops of blood from a person and spot them on a surface. Then, test one of the spots with anti-A antibodies and the other one with anti-B antibodies. Depending on the observed agglutination, the blood type can be determined as shown in Figure 3.52. If you have type A antigens on your RBCs, the blood will agglutinate with anti-A. If you have type B antigens on your RBCs, the blood will agglutinate with anti-B. If the blood only reacts with anti-A, then you are blood type A. If the blood only reacts with anti-B, then you are blood type B. If it reacts with both, you are AB, and if does not react at all, you are type O.

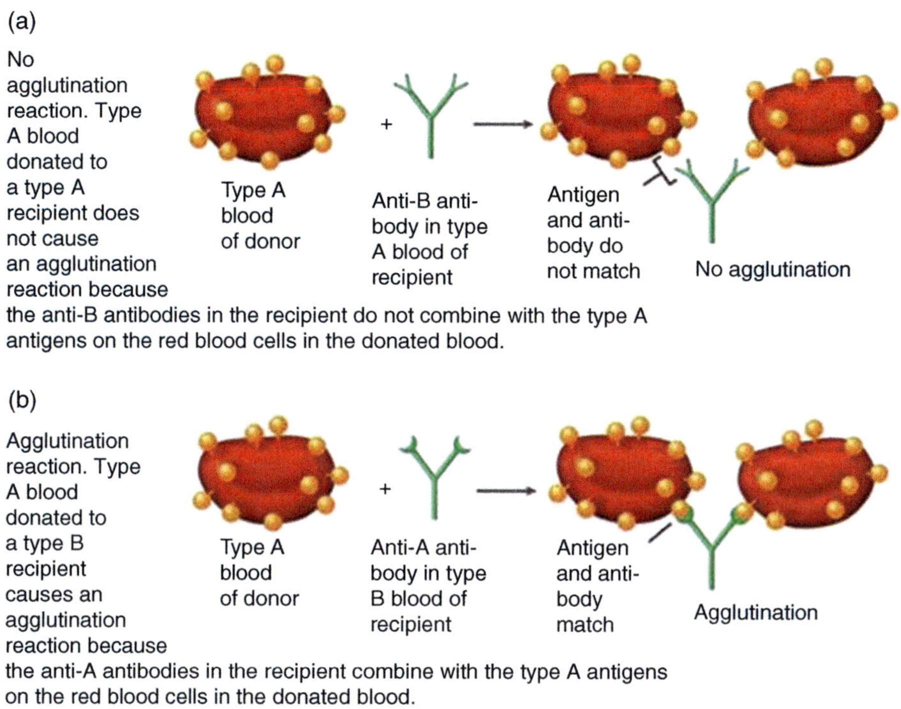

Figure 3.51 Illustration of blood agglutination. *Source:* Mader and Windelspecht [22].

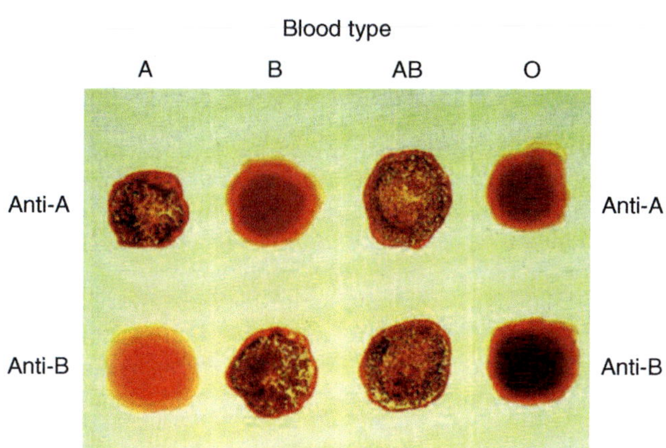

Figure 3.52 ABO blood reactions [31].

Problems

3.1 Explain how a signal propagates within a neuron and how it is delivered to adjacent neurons.

3.2 Match each component of the central nervous system in Column A with its main activity or function in Column B.

Column A	Column B
1) _____ Medulla oblongata	A. Crying while watching a very sad movie.
2) _____ Pons	B. After workout, your heartbeats increase.
3) _____ Midbrain	C. Someone kicks your knee by accident, and you feel your leg moves unconsciously.
4) _____ Hypothalamus	D. Alerting or arousal mechanisms.
5) _____ Thalamus	E. Performing on a balance beam.
6) _____ Cerebellum	F. Breathing.
7) _____ Cerebrum	G. Becoming hungry.
8) _____ Spinal cord	H. Relay for visual and auditory impulses

3.3 Explain what cerebrospinal fluid (CSF) is and list at least three functions of it.

3.4 Order the following structures based on their blood pressures (during diastole) from high pressure to low pressure:
A capillaries
B right atrium
C veins
D aorta
E arterioles
F venules

3.5 Place the following structures in their proper order in blood flow through the heart by putting a 1 in front of the first structure the blood would pass through and ending with a 11 in front of the last structure the blood would pass through. The starting point (1) was arbitrarily decided to be the right atrium.
A _____ left atrium
B _____ tricuspid valve (right atrioventricular valve)
C _____ right ventricle
D _____ pulmonary vein
E _____ aorta (and the aortic semilunar valve)
F _____ mitral valve (left atrioventricular valve)
G _____ left ventricle
H _____ pulmonary artery (and the pulmonary semilunar valve)
I _____ right atrium
J _____ circulatory arteries → circulatory capillaries → circulatory veins
K _____ lungs (pulmonary arteries → pulmonary capillaries → pulmonary veins)

3.6 Explain why a pressure difference must exist between the aorta and the right atrium.

3.7 Explain why a second messenger system is necessary for nonsteroid hormones but not for steroid hormones.

3.8 This hormone is released by the anterior pituitary and stimulates breast development during pregnancy necessary for eventual milk production:

A estrogen
B oxytocin
C prolactin
D progesterone

3.9 This hormone is released by the anterior pituitary and stimulates the secretion of mineralocorticoids for regulating electrolyte homeostasis

A Prolactin
B Cortisol
C TSH
D ACTH
E Aldosterone

3.10 What would be the effect on the body if the thyroid gland were removed?

3.11 The prefix "hypo" indicates underproduction of a hormone while the prefix "hyper" indicates overproduction. What are the definitions of the following terms and their effects on the body?

A Hyperthyroidism
B Hypothyroidism
C Hyperparathyroidism
D Hypoparathyroidism

3.12 If a doctor discovered a patient had very low levels of thyroxine (T4) but high levels of TSH, would the patient's problem be in the thyroid gland or the pituitary gland? Explain your answer.

3.13 The pancreas of a patient is not working properly. What would be the effect on this patient's blood glucose level in the following scenarios? Explain.

A The pancreas produces too little insulin.
B The pancreas produces too much insulin.
C The pancreas produces the right level of insulin, but the insulin contains a mutation that makes it ineffective.

3.14 Match each statement in Column B with the proper hormone in Column A.

Column A	Column B
1) _____ Parathyroid hormone (PTH)	A. Made by alpha cells in the pancreatic islets
2) _____ Mineralocorticoids	B. Made by the adrenal cortex, stimulates gluconeogenesis, thereby increasing glucose blood level
3) _____ Glucocorticoids	C. The hormone made by the placenta and detected by home pregnancy tests

Column A	Column B
4) _____ Human chorionic gonadotropins	D. Made in the anterior pituitary, stimulates secretion of mineralocorticoids for regulating electrolyte homeostasis
5) _____ Glucagon	E. Made in the adrenal cortex, regulates electrolyte concentrations in the blood
6) _____ Insulin	F. Made in the anterior pituitary, stimulates breast development during pregnancy necessary for eventual milk production
7) _____ Prolactin	G. Has the opposite effect of calcitonin
8) _____ ACTH	H. Made in the pancreas islets; decreases blood glucose levels

3.15 Name at least three hormones that affect the blood glucose concentration. Where are they produced in the body and what is their effect (increase or decrease) on the blood glucose level?

3.16 For each hormone listed below, name the location where it is produced in the body and its effect (increase or decrease) on blood glucose level?

A Insulin
B Glucagon
C Cortisol
D Epinephrine
E ACTH
F Growth hormone
G Thyroxine

3.17 Group the following immunity elements into two categories:

Specific immunity or Nonspecific immunity

A Skin
B Flu vaccine
C Extreme acidic pH in the stomach
D Tears
E B cells
F Antibodies
G Fever
H T cells
I Mucous membranes

3.18 Describe five ways that antibodies are used by the immune system to fight infection.

3.19 Describe the role of each of the following cell types in primary and secondary immune responses. How does vaccination play a role in primary and secondary immune responses?

A Immature B cell
B Memory cell
C Plasma cell

3.20 Sofia, a graduate student at Stanford University, heard that her friend, David, returned from a foreign country a few days ago, and she really wanted to see his pictures. She visited him immediately and heard about his experiences. A couple of days later, he told her that he was diagnosed with a local contagious disease by his doctor, and that she should self-quarantine for about 10 days to prevent further infection and ensure complete recovery. She was so disappointed because she planned to go and watch the Big Game 10 days later with her friends. A week later, she suddenly recalled what she learned in her Biochips and Medical Imaging course and decided to measure the concentration of her serum antibody against this infectious pathogen to figure out whether she had been infected. The measurement results showed that she had a high level of antibodies, thus she decided to stay home to avoid infecting other people, while blaming David for her first infection with this disease. However, after three weeks, she still felt tired. So, she measured the concentration of the antibodies again and found that the level was almost similar to what she measured three weeks ago. Do you think this is her first infection with this disease? Explain your reason.

3.21 Which of the following cell types are typically found in the bloodstream of a healthy individual (select all that apply)?

A Immature B cells
B T cells
C Neutrophils
D Red blood cell

3.22 Describe two ways in which T-cells are used by the immune system to fight invading cells.

3.23 If the following statement describes the development or functioning of a B cell, write a B in front of it. If it describes the development or functioning of a T cell, write a T in front of it.

____ produces antibodies

____ some develop into plasma cells

____ the main cell involved in cell-mediated immunity

____ the main cell involved in humoral immunity (i.e. secretion of antibodies to the blood)

____ develops in the thymus gland

____ moves to the site of the antigen and releases cell poison

____ once this cell is activated, it divides rapidly into clones of itself

____ releases a substance that attracts macrophages

____ some of these cells develop into memory cells

3.24 Explain the difference between blood clot formation and the process of blood agglutination (e.g. what happens when a blood type B is donated to a patient with blood type A).

3.25 (a) Explain the difference between blood clot formation and the process of blood agglutination (e.g. what happens when blood of type B is donated to a blood type A patient).

(b) E.T. came back to visit his friend, Elliott, but while coming to earth, his vehicle was broken and crushed in the backyard of your house. He was severely injured and needed some blood donation. You learned that E.T. has an ACO blood type system on his alien planet instead of ABO. Since this was a very urgent situation, you decided to transfuse your blood to him and finally he survived. What could be your blood type (list all possible types)?

References

1 Jmarchn, https://commons.wikimedia.org/wiki/File:Nervous_system_diagram-en.svg
2 BruceBlaus, https://commons.wikimedia.org/wiki/File:Glia.png and blausen.com
3 Thibodeau, G.A. and Patton, K.T. (2008). The Nervous System. In: *Structure and Function of the Body*, 13e, 188–212. Mosby.
4 Юкатан, https://commons.wikimedia.org/wiki/File:Patellar_reflex-ru.svg
5 Thibodeau, G.A. and Patton, K.T. The Senses. In: *Structure and Function of the Body*, 13e, 228–229. *Mosby*.
6 BruceBlaus (2016). https://sw.wikipedia.org/wiki/Picha:Brain_Anatomy.png and blausen.com
7 Blausen.com staff (2014). Medical gallery of Blausen Medical 2014. *WikiJournal of Medicine* 1 (2): https://doi.org/10.15347/wjm/2014.010.
8 Polarlys and Mikael Häggström, https://commons.wikimedia.org/wiki/File:Spinal_cord_tracts_-_English.svg
9 OpenStax College (2013). Anatomy & Physiology, Connexions. http://cnx.org/content/col11496/1.6/
10 Thibodeau, G.A. and Patton, K.T. The Nervous System. In: *Structure and Function of the Body*, 13e, 204. *Mosby*.
11 Thibodeau, G.A. and Patton, K.T. The Nervous System. In: *Structure and Function of the Body*, 13e, 205. *Mosby*.
12 Alan Hoofring (2001). National Cancer Institute, https://visualsonline.cancer.gov/details.cfm?imageid=4279
13 Doc James, http://en.wikipedia.org/wiki/File:4_vials_of_human_cerebrospinal_fluid.jpg
14 Madhero88, https://commons.wikimedia.org/wiki/File:SVG_Human_With_All_Organs.svg
15 OpenStax College, https://commons.wikimedia.org/wiki/File:1413_Structure_of_the_Eye.jpg
16 Thibodeau, G.A. and Patton, K.T. The Senses. In: *Structure and Function of the Body*, 13e, 238. *Mosby*.
17 Jacopo Werther, https://commons.wikimedia.org/wiki/File:Mantis_shrimp_(Odontodactylus_scyllarus).jpg
18 OpenStax (2016). Versioin 8.25 from the Textbook OpenStax Anatomny and Physiology. https://openstax.org/books/anatomy-and-physiology/pages/preface.
19 Mader, S. and Windelspecht, M. (2014). *Human Biology*, 13e. McGraw Hill Publishing.
20 Dcoetzee, https://commons.wikimedia.org/wiki/File:Blausen_0457_Heart_SectionalAnatomy.png
21 Blausen Medical Communications, Inc., https://commons.wikimedia.org/wiki/File:2101_Blood_Flow_Through_the_Heart.jpg
22 Mader, S. and Windelspecht, M. (2014). *Inquiry into Life*, 14e. McGraw Hill Publishing.

23 Thibodeau, G.A. and Patton, K.T. The Endocrine System. In: *Structure and Function of the Body*, 13e, 255–260.

24 This article was published in Structure and Function of the Body, 13th Edition, Gary A. Thibodeau and Kevin T. Patton, The Endocrine System, pp. 255–260, Copyright © 2008 Published by Elsevier

25 Efrat, S. and Russ, H.A. Making β cells from adult tissues. *Trends in Endocrinology & Metabolism* 23 (6): 278–285.

26 OpenStaxCollege (2013). Anatomy & Physiology, Connexions, http://cnx.org/content/col11496/1.6/

27 Thibodeau, G.A. and Patton, K.T. Lymphatic System. In: *Anatomy and Physiology*, 6e, 783. Elsevier.

28 Thibodeau, G.A. and Patton, K.T. Blood. In: *Structure and Function of the Body*, 13e, 288. *Mosby.*

29 GrahamColm, https://commons.wikimedia.org/wiki/File:Rotavirus_with_antibody.jpg

30 Thibodeau, G.A. and Patton, K.T. Immune System. In: *Anatomy and Physiology*, 6e, 811. Elsevier.

31 *Life: The Science of Biology* by Sadava et al. (2013) Figs.10-12, 16-6 pp. 225, 359. By permission of Oxford University Press, USA

Further Reading

Tortora, G.J. (2006). *Principles of Anatomy and Physiology, 11e. Wiley.*
http://bio1152.nicerweb.com/Locked/media/ch43/phagocytosis.html

4

Cancer

4.1 Epidemiology (Statistics)

Cancer is a type of disease in which a group of abnormal cells undergoes uncontrolled growth through cell division. Cancer can occur in many different areas in the body. As cancerous cells divide, they interact with their surroundings and their genome can work in various ways to allow them to grow more and more in an uncontrolled manner, ultimately forming a tumor. Cancer also has the ability to form new blood vessels to provide the tumor with nutrients and oxygen to support its rapid growth. Another characteristic of cancer, which is what differentiates cancerous tumors from benign tumors, is the ability to metastasize – sending cancer cells throughout the body that will spread to other organs and form new colonies there. In fact, about 90% of cancer deaths are due to metastasis.

Cancer is the second leading cause of death in modern countries, after cardiovascular diseases. About one in four Americans will die of cancer. There are more than 100 different types of cancer, which can affect nearly any organ in the body, with different subtypes for each affected organ. Figure 4.1 illustrates the number of new cases and deaths from the 12 leading types of cancer in 2017.

Certain cancers are more aggressive than others. For example, lung cancer has a 30% survival rate, while only 15% of prostate cancer patients will die from the disease. Some cancers are generally found either in men or in women, e.g. breast and ovarian cancers in women and prostate cancer in men. It should be noted that the diagram in Figure 4.1 shows the number of diagnosed cancer cases, but does not include people with cancer who were not diagnosed.

As different cancers evolve, it becomes essential for the research community to focus on specialized treatments and diagnostics specific to a particular type of cancer. For example, an early detection method for ovarian cancer is a major need, since it is a very deadly disease but highly curable if detected at the early stages. This is not true for some other types of cancer, which have limited treatment options even at the early stages, and thus may not benefit from early detection and intervention. Researchers must consider and understand cancers affecting each organ to determine if research in early diagnosis techniques is likely to be worth the effort. Cancer treatments or "cures" can occur at multiple levels. For example, early diagnosis of a certain cancer may result in a cure by surgical removal, while later stages could cause metastasis, necessitating a different approach for treatment or a "cure."

In the past few decades, multiple new treatments have been developed for certain types of cancer, such as stomach and uterine cancer. Lifestyle choices, such as careful dietary planning and exercise, can also help prevent cancer. These factors have reduced the death rate of cancer.

Biochips and Medical Imaging, First Edition. Adam de la Zerda and Shan Xiang Wang.

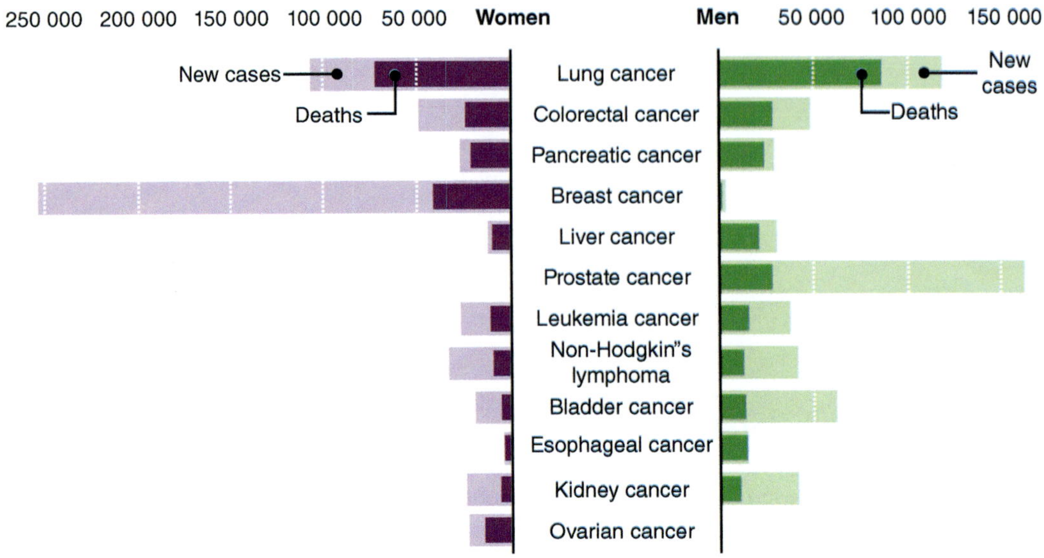

Figure 4.1 The 12 cancers that claimed the greatest number of lives in 2017. There were 1.69 million new cases and 600 920 deaths from cancer in the United States in 2017.

Figure 4.2 clearly shows that the death rate of stomach cancer has dropped significantly since the 1930s. This drop is largely attributed to the use of refrigerators and consumption of fresh fruits and vegetables; some bacteria on spoiled food (e.g. *Helicobacter pylori*) may cause the development of stomach cancer. However, lung cancer incidence has dramatically increased over the past few decades (Figure 4.2), while other cancers have decreased. The rise in lung cancer is primarily attributed to chemicals found in cigarettes such as tobacco, carbon monoxide, and ammonia.

Cancer imposed a huge cost to the US healthcare system (about $228 billion) in 2009. This includes $93 billion in direct medical costs (the total of all health expenditures) and $19 billion in indirect morbidity costs (the cost of lost productivity due to illness, etc.). Medical costs related to cancer are increasing rapidly, partly due to the availability of new treatments and diagnostics. Research into new treatments and diagnostics must consider cost as well – it must be cost-effective to diagnose and treat a large number of people.

4.2 What Causes Cancer

Cancer is caused by a combination of genetic mutations that can accumulate over time in certain cells within the human body. There are multiple mechanisms by which these mutations are accumulated. Some of these mutations are hereditary – an individual may be more prone to specific cancers because of the genes they inherit from their parents. Examples of hereditary susceptibility to cancer include Familial Adenomatous Polyposis to colon and rectum cancer and retinoblastoma, as well as BRCA1 mutations to breast and ovarian cancer. There are also certain chemicals that an individual may be exposed to through smoking, air/food/water pollution, drugs, pesticides, and hormones (e.g. estrogen) that can cause certain cancers. Chemicals (especially nonbiological chemicals) that can induce cancer are often called **carcinogens**. High-energy radiation from UV and X-rays (both environmental and cancer therapy) are also factors. Infectious agents can also increase an individual's genetic mutations. Certain infectious agents can insert genes into human

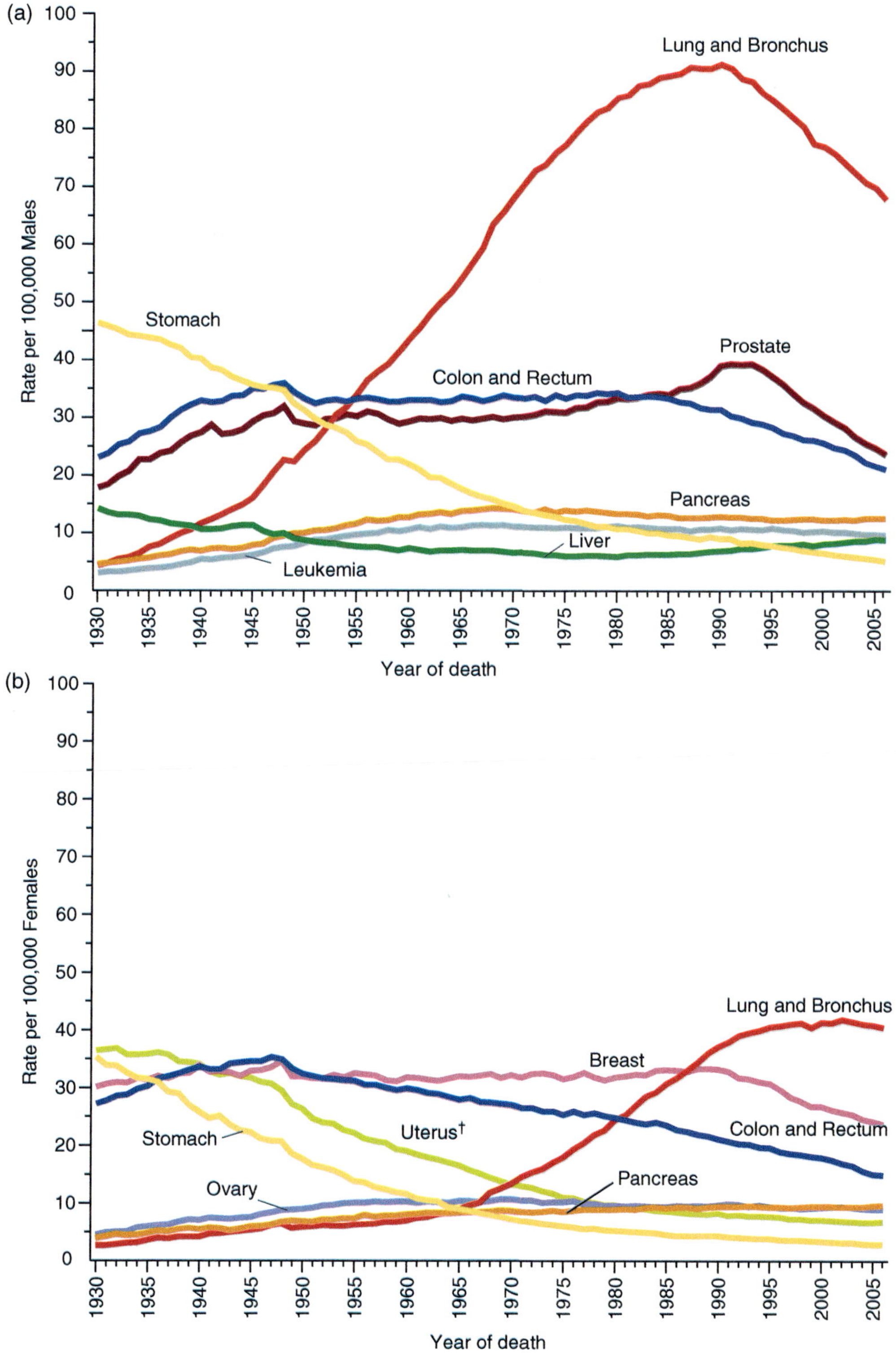

Figure 4.2 Cancer deaths over the years for (a) men and (b) women. *Source:* Jemal et al. [1].

cells, such as the Human Papilloma Virus (implicated in cervical and ovarian cancer), the Herpes Virus (implicated in Kaposi Sarcoma), and *H. pylori* (implicated in gastric cancer). These viruses and bacteria can provide researchers with the exact sequence of a gene that causes cancer. Moreover, smoking, dietary factors (excessive red meat, alcohol use, food colorings/additives, and frying), and obesity can increase the risk of cancer.

4.2.1 Bacteria and Stomach Cancer

The bacterium *H. pylori*, which can cause stomach ulcers, has been associated with the development of cancer. Thus, people infected with *H. pylori* are at increased risk for stomach cancer. Research is under way to define the genetic interactions between this infectious agent and its host tissues that lead to cancer development (Figure 4.3). First, *H. pylori* can penetrate the mucus layer of the host's stomach and adhere to the surface of gastric mucosal epithelial cells. Then *H. pylori* produces ammonia from urea using an enzyme called urease. This ammonia (which is basic) can neutralize gastric acid in the stomach and help *H. pylori* survive in the otherwise extreme pH of the stomach. *H. pylori* can then proliferate, migrate, and, finally, form an infectious focus that can cause the host to develop stomach ulcers. Gastric ulcerization is developed by destruction of mucosa, inflammation, and mucosal cell death. This physical damage to the tissues of the stomach can make the organ more susceptible to the development of cancer.

4.3 Oncogenesis (Cancer Development)

Oncogenesis (Figure 4.4) is the process during which normal cells develop into invasive cancer cells. Typically, in oncogenesis, normal cells undergo a mutation that inactivates the suppressor gene, followed by cell proliferation, then mutations inactivating DNA repair genes, then proto-oncogenes mutating to oncogenes, and, finally, more mutations, more genetic instability, and metastatic disease. A well-differentiated tumor resembles mature cells of the tissue of origin, while a poorly differentiated tumor is composed of primitive cells with little differentiation.

Benign tumors are well-differentiated while malignant tumors are poorly differentiated or undifferentiated ("anaplastic"). Note that a tumor is composed of multiple cell types, each of which may have different numbers and types of mutations!

4.3.1 Microscopic Appearance of Cancer Cells

A cancer tissue has several properties that help distinguish it from a healthy tissue when viewed under the microscope. For example, a doctor can look for a large number of irregularly shaped dividing cells, variation in nuclear size and shape, variation in cell size and shape, loss of specialized cell features, loss of normal tissue organization, and a poorly defined tumor boundary. These distinctions are depicted in Figure 4.5.

4.3.2 Biopsy Gives Tumor Grading

Microscopic examination can also provide information regarding the likely behavior of a tumor and its responsiveness to treatment. Cancers with highly abnormal cell appearance and large numbers of dividing cells tend to grow more quickly, spread to other organs more frequently, and be less responsive to therapy than cancers that are composed of cells with a more normal appearance.

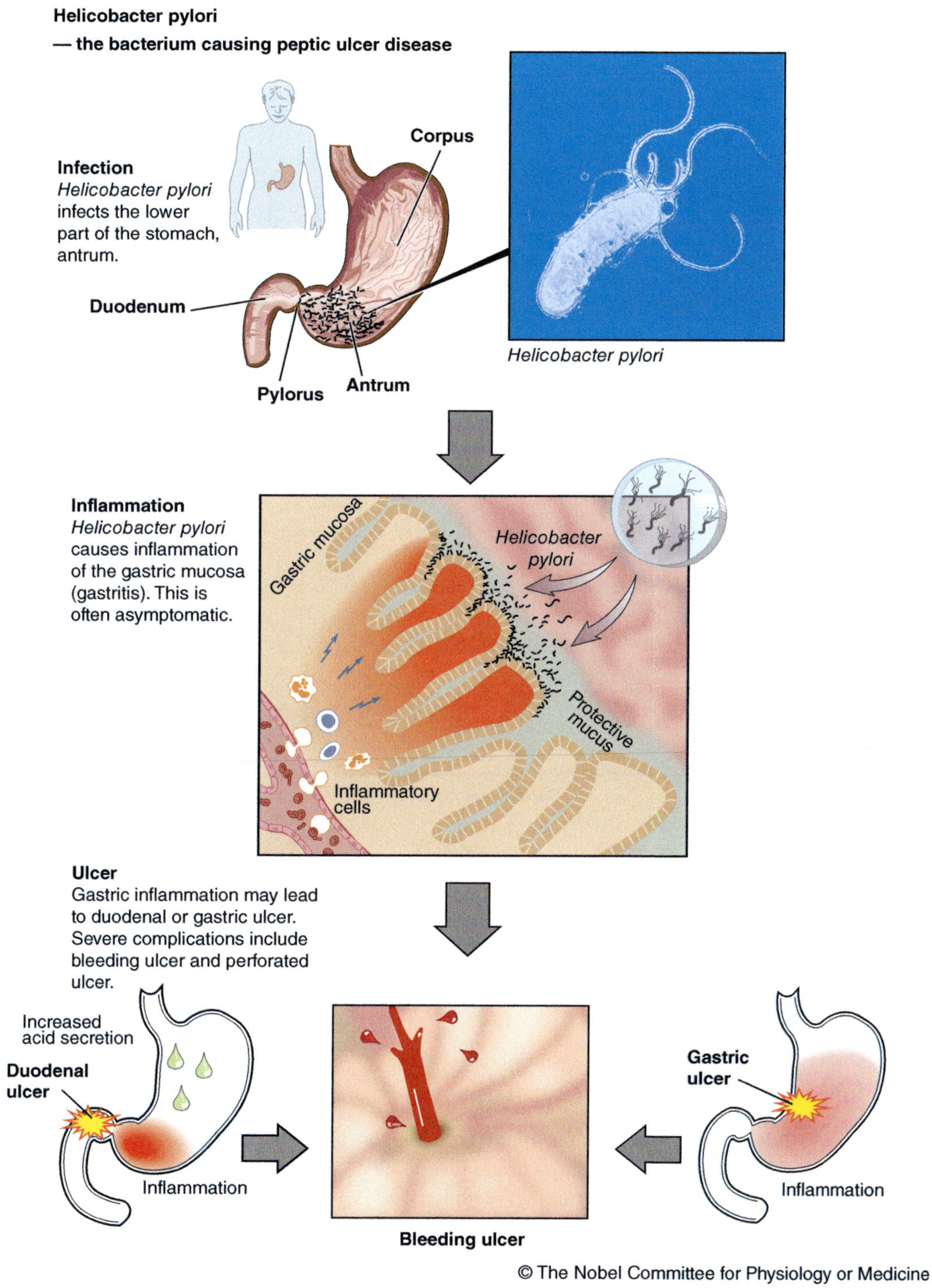

Figure 4.3 Diagram of gastric ulceration by *H. pylori*. *Source:* NobelPrize.org [2].

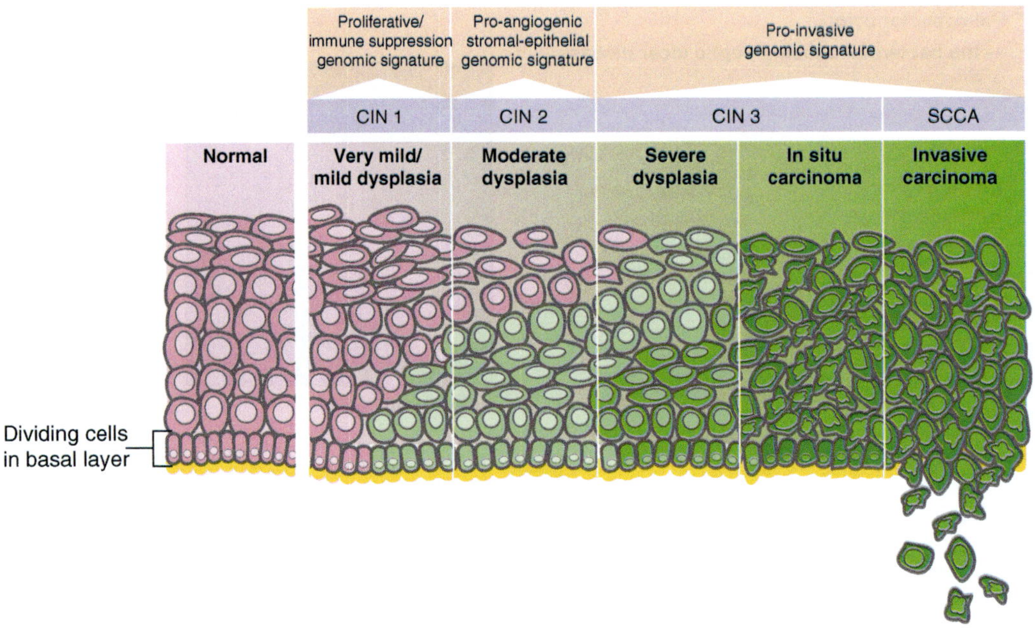

Figure 4.4 Oncogenesis. *Source:* National Cancer Institute.

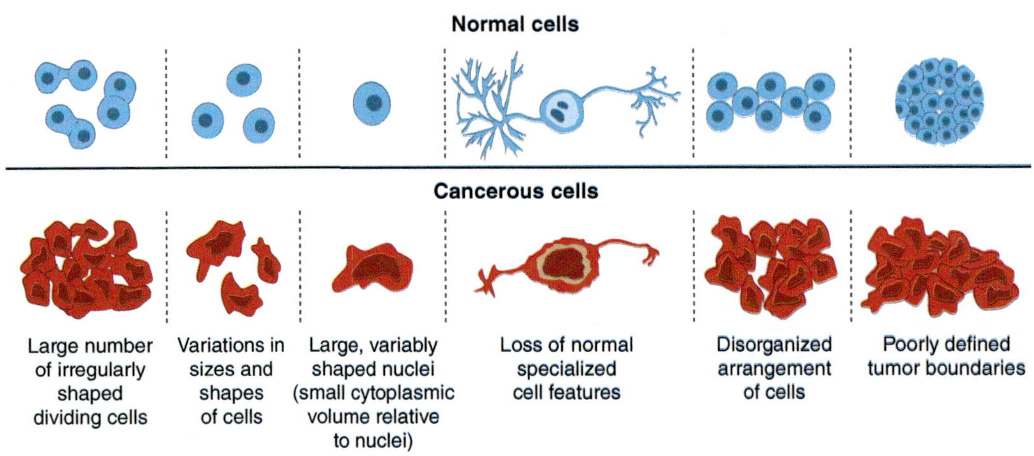

Figure 4.5 Microscopic appearance of normal and cancer cells.

Based on these differences in microscopic appearance, doctors assign a numerical "grade" to most cancers. In this grading system, a low number grade (grade I or II) refers to cancers with fewer cell abnormalities than those with higher numbers (grade III or IV). Patients with lower grade tumors typically have more favorable prognoses and survival rates (Figure 4.6).

4.3.3 Cancer Staging (TNM System)

After cancer has been diagnosed, doctors ask the following three questions to determine how far the disease has progressed: (i) How large is the tumor and how deeply has it invaded into surrounding tissues? (ii) Have cancer cells spread to regional lymph nodes? (iii) Has the cancer spread (metastasized) to other regions of the body?

Based on the answers to these questions, the cancer is assigned a "stage." Staging helps the doctor plan the appropriate treatment, estimate the patient's prognosis, and identify clinical trials that may be suitable for the patient. Staging also provides a common terminology that (i) allows health care providers and researchers to readily exchange information about patients, and (ii) provides a standard metric for evaluation and comparison of clinical trial results. Each stage is characterized by the distinct morphology of the tumor. A patient's chances for survival are better when cancer is detected at a lower stage (Figure 4.7).

4.3.4 Benign Versus Malignant Tumors

Tumors are classified as either benign or malignant depending on whether or not they can spread to other parts of the body by invasion and metastasis. Benign tumors cannot spread by invasion or metastasis; hence, they only grow locally. They are slow-growing, well-differentiated, noninvasive, and isolated. On the other hand, malignant tumors are capable of spreading by invasion and metastasis. By definition, the term "cancer" applies only to malignant tumors. Malignant tumors have variable, frequent, and abnormal mitosis, are undifferentiated or mixed differentiated, invasive, and infiltrative. As shown in Figure 4.8, benign tumors can develop into malignant tumors over time. This is often the result of additional genetic mutations within the tumor cells and the continued loss of structural cell organization.

4.4 The Six Hallmarks of Cancer

Our body cells have been programmed over the years to resist cancer; one example is the development of multiple regulatory systems

Tumor grades

G_X: Grade cannot be assessed
G_1: Well-differentiated
G_2: Moderately differentiated
G_3: Poorly differentiated
G_4: Undifferentiated

*Well-differentiated cells are good!

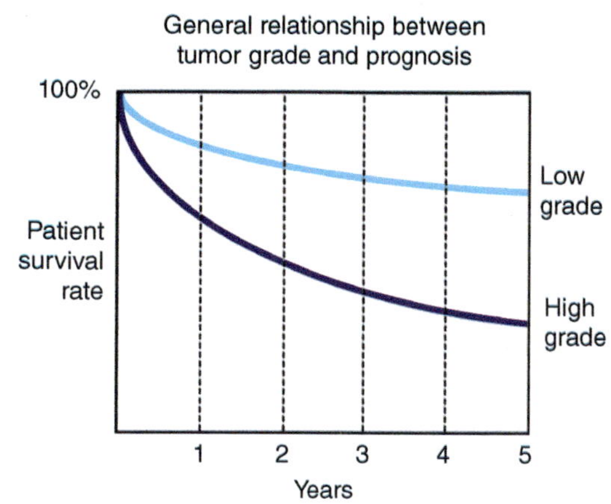

Figure 4.6 Tumor grade vs. prognosis.

Tumor stages*

0: Precancerous
1: Small localized cancer
2: Larger cancer and probable lymph nodes' involvement
3: Larger cancer and evident lymph nodes' involvement
4: Metastisis
TNM: Tumor? Node? Metastasis?

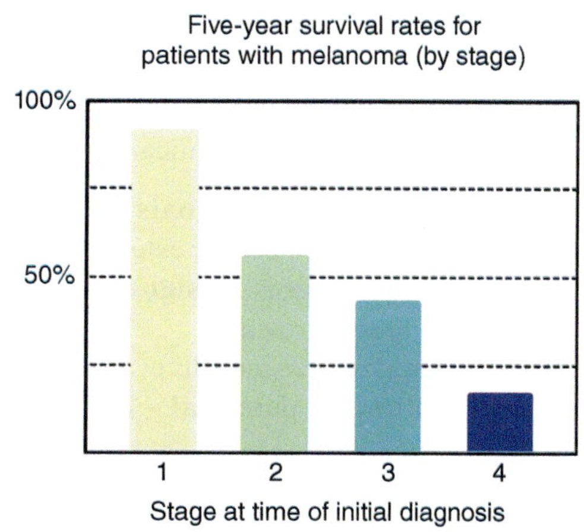

Figure 4.7 Five-year survival rates for patients with melanoma.

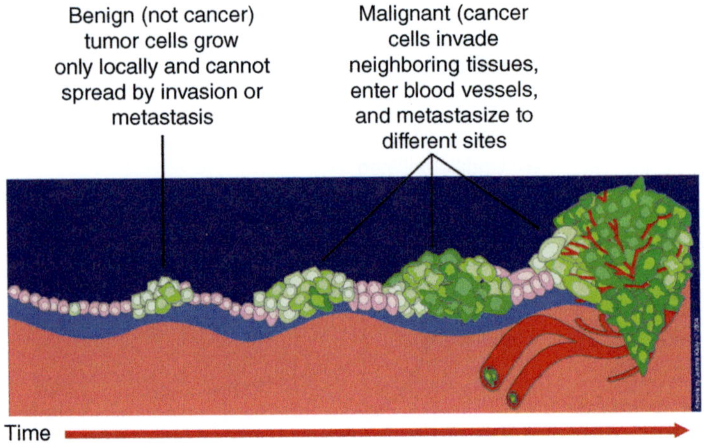

Figure 4.8 Benign versus malignant tumors. *Source:* Mader and Windelspecht [3].

within the cell. Such regulatory systems are present in processes like DNA replication and transcription, which involve proofreading mechanisms to ensure that no mistakes were made (i.e. no mutations were introduced).

For a cell to become cancerous, it must experience some changes in its genomic content that disable certain regulatory mechanisms and enable others. Changes to these mechanisms can produce defects in the regulatory circuits (pathways) that govern normal cell proliferation and homeostasis. These changes in the genomic contents are called mutations, and they can be caused by a number of factors. These factors can be intrinsic to cells (e.g. errors when replicating DNA during mitosis) or extrinsic to cells (e.g. carcinogenic materials or X-ray beams that cause mutations to DNA). Because there are many different mutations that alter these regulatory pathways and because we have hundreds of pathways, it may not be surprising that there are more than 100 distinct types of cancer. Since cancers of various types can be drastically different from one another in terms of genomic mutations, altered mechanisms, progression, and invasiveness to the host body, finding a generic treatment to cancer is difficult, if not impossible.

The mechanisms and proteins involved in cancer development are very complex and multiple pathways must be disrupted for a cell to become cancerous. Despite the enormous number of pathways involved in cancer development, it is believed that these altered pathways can be categorized by the presence of six essential characteristics. For a cell to be considered a cancerous cell, it must adapt all these **six hallmarks of cancer** (Figure 4.9). Each of these six hallmarks represents a different type of breach in our cell's anticancer mechanisms. The six hallmarks of cancer are:

1) **Self-sufficiency in growth signals** – cancer cells generate their own growth signals to stimulate mitosis without the need for external signals.
2) **Insensitivity to anti-growth signals** – cancer cells become insensitive to the environment that tells them to stop growing.
3) **Evading apoptosis** – cancer cells evade apoptosis.
4) **Limitless replication potential – long DNA ends** – cancer cells have limitless replication potential.
5) **Sustained angiogenesis** – cancer cells turn on different molecular switches that allow surrounding blood vessels to feed them with more oxygen and nutrients, allowing growth.
6) **Tissue invasion and metastasis** – cancer cells invade neighboring cells and spread throughout the body to new sites.

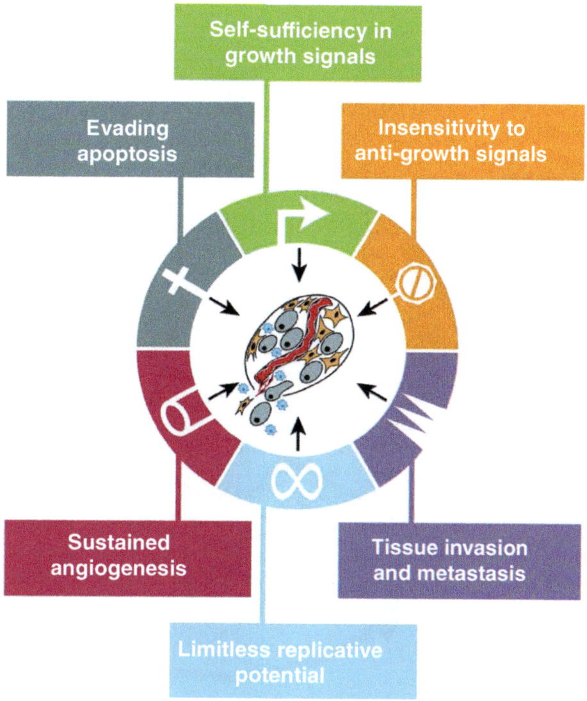

Figure 4.9 Six hallmarks of cancer. *Source:* Reprinted from Hanahan and Weinberg [4]. Copyright © 2000 Published by Elsevier Inc., with permission from Elsevier.

4.4.1 Self-Sufficiency in Growth Signals

Mitosis constitutes one portion of an entire cycle that is heavily regulated (Figure 4.10). Typically cells reside in a dormant stage called G_0 (a.k.a. resting state). Cells cannot decide to leave G_0 and start the cell division cycle on their own. **Growth signals** from other cells must first interact with receptors on the cell membrane, signaling the cell to start the division cycle. These growth factors are typically either released by other cells or are anchored to other cells' membranes. Growth factors released by other cells can diffuse in the interstitial space and find their target cells to signal growth processes. Growth factors that are anchored to other cells' membranes can activate such processes directly through cell-to-cell interactions. The growth signals instruct the cell to replicate, and the cell responds by transitioning into the cycle of active cell division. This cycle consists of the G_1 (growth) stage when the cellular content, excluding the chromosomes, is duplicated, followed by the S stage (synthesis), where each of the 46 chromosomes is duplicated by the cell. Finally, in the G_2 stage, the cell performs error checks on the duplicated chromosomes and makes any necessary repairs before mitosis starts (for a review of the cell cycle, refer to Chapter 1).

In contrast to normal cells, cancer cells can generate their own growth signals (Figure 4.11), which then affect themselves, in a process called **autocrine growth stimulation**. The term "**autocrine**" describes the cell's ability to affect itself by producing its own signals. Healthy cells typically develop mechanisms that prevent growth signals that they secrete from affecting themselves. They achieve this by either producing growth signals that do not interact with their own receptors (i.e. growth factors cannot bind to the receptors on the cell that produced them) or by shutting down the receptors (i.e. telling them not to listen to the growth signals). In cancer cells, these protection mechanisms are shut down. Therefore, cancer cells have self-sufficiency in growth signals regardless of their surrounding environment. Moreover, cancer cells' growth signals can also signal surrounding cells to start growing.

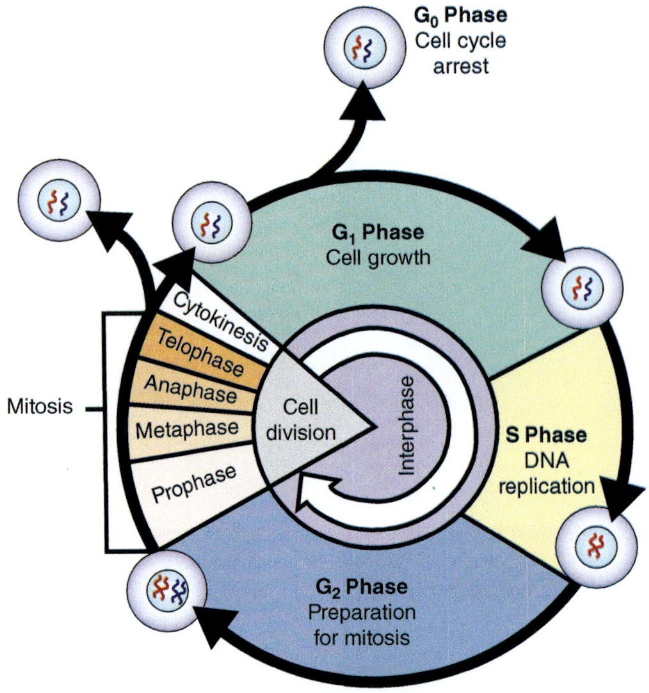

Figure 4.10 Cell cycle.

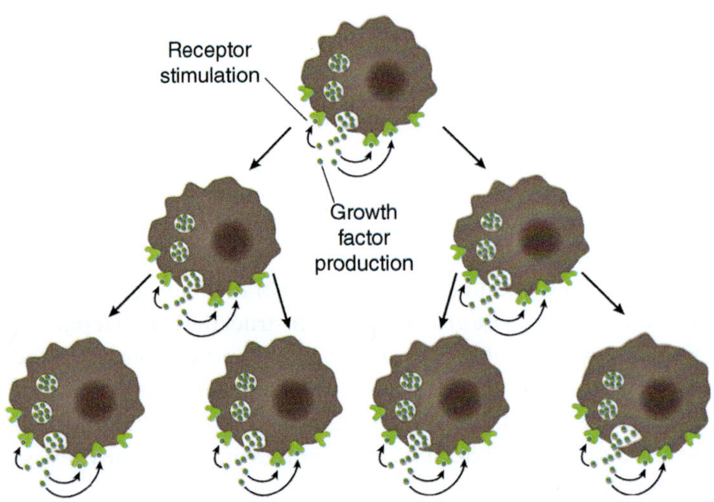

Figure 4.11 Autocrine growth stimulation of cancer cells. *Source:* Image courtesy of Jim Strommer.

4.4.2 Insensitivity to Anti-Growth Signals

Normal cells respond to anti-growth signals. **Anti-growth signals** interfere with the cell division cycle by forcing a cell out of the cell cycle into the G_0 state or by inducing a cell to enter a post-mitotic state where it can no longer proliferate. Cancer cells have developed multiple ways to interfere with anti-growth signals. For example, E2F is a transcription factor – a protein that controls the expression of many genes by binding to one or more promoters at the beginning of genes and encouraging those genes to be transcribed. The genes whose transcription is controlled by E2F are genes that encode proteins essential for progression from the G_1 to the S phase in the cell division cycle. Therefore, E2F is a critical factor that allows the cell to complete the cell division cycle. Rb is an anti-growth agent that works by blocking E2F; thus, Rb prevents the completion of the cell cycle. However, some cancer cells produce E7 – an oncogene product that inactivates Rb. Because E7 inactivates Rb, the E2F promoter becomes active and allows the cell to transition from G_1 to S phase. For example, one of the Human Papilloma Viruses (HPVs) infects the host cell with this E7 oncogene (Figure 4.12). Note that oncogene products like E7 can be derived from either viral infection or random mutations within the cell.

4.4.3 Evading Apoptosis

Apoptosis, the programmed cell death process that occurs in all healthy cells, is triggered either by sensors that monitor the intracellular environment (e.g. the p53 protein that monitors DNA damage) or by sensors that monitor the extracellular environment (e.g. to monitor external signals that indicate the cell needs to undergo apoptosis). For example, if external radiation caused DNA damage in a cell, the p53 protein would induce apoptosis in this cell since DNA damage could lead to cell damage or even cancer. The machinery for apoptosis is encoded in the DNA of all cells in the body. Once apoptosis is triggered, the cell follows a precise series of steps: cellular membranes are disrupted, the nuclear skeleton is broken, chromosomes are degraded, and the nucleus is fragmented. The entire process takes 30–120 minutes to complete. In the end, the remaining cell fragments are engulfed by nearby cells (Figure 4.13) and degraded, typically within 24 hours. The p53 protein is sometimes called the anticancer protein because it randomly samples DNA at all times and can detect certain types of damage (e.g. simple mutations such as nucleotide-pair mismatches). The protein p53 is not the only protein that can look for errors in DNA. There are more complex proteins that are capable of scanning for multiple types of DNA errors.

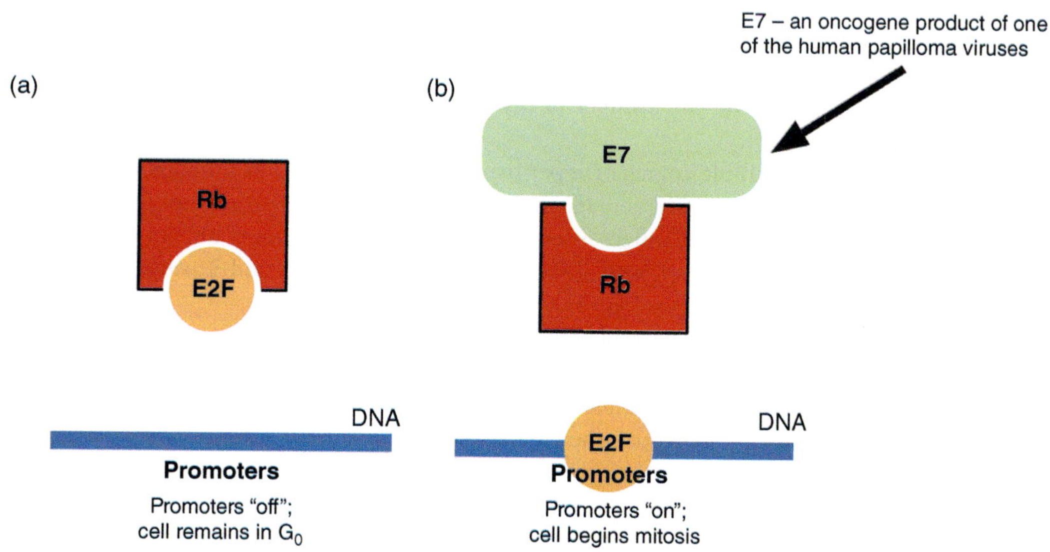

Figure 4.12 An example of anti-growth signal insensitivity. (a) Rb (anti-growth signal) inactivates E2F (transcription factor) by binding to it and, as a result, a cell cannot produce proteins required for mitosis. (b) E7 (oncogene product) inactivates Rb. Inactivated Rb cannot bind to E2F and, as a result, E2F promotes production of proteins required for mitosis.

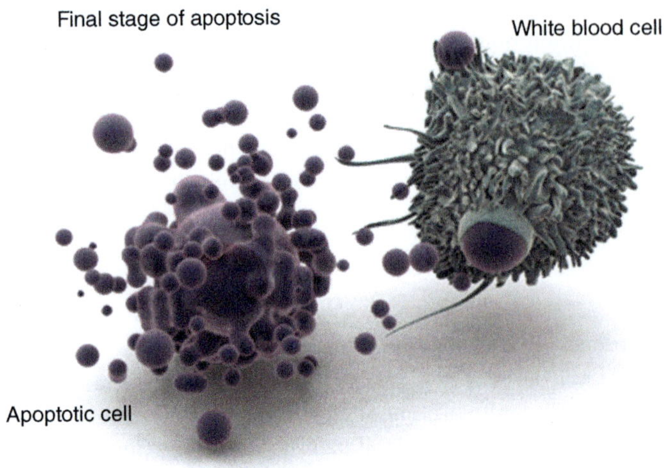

Figure 4.13 After the death of a cell, the remains are engulfed by other cells. *Source:* National Library of Medicine [5].

In general, the growth of a group of cells depends on two factors: the cell proliferation rate and the cell attrition (death) rate. Cancer cells have acquired mechanisms of resistance to apoptosis that allow them to avoid the death process. This ability is likely present in all types of cancers.

4.4.4 Limitless Replication Potential

Every cell division cycle causes the DNA of the cell to shorten by 50–100 base pairs at the end of each chromosome. These sequences at the ends of the DNA are called **telomeres**. To protect the genome, an enzyme called **telomerase** can add "extra" base pairs at the ends of the chromosomes and lengthen the telomeres. Telomerase is active during embryogenesis as well as in cells that need to undergo many cell division cycles, such as stem cells in the bone marrow, but is otherwise inactive in adult cells. Therefore, chromosomal DNA becomes shorter with each successive cell division cycle, which sets a limit on the number of cell divisions a cell can undergo before critical genes are damaged.

A telomere consists of multiple copies of repetitive DNA: $(TTAGGG)_n$ in humans, where n is 1500–2000, resulting in an average telomere length of about 10 kb in newborns. Once the telomere is too short (around 2–3 kb), the cell enters a senescent state and is no longer able to divide. The discovery of the telomere mechanism was made by Blackburn, Greider, and Szostak, who were awarded the 2009 Nobel Prize in Physiology or Medicine for this discovery.

Cancer cells bypass the normal cell's replication limit in one of the two ways: either by upregulating telomerase (i.e. increasing expression levels of telomerase in the cell), which is done by 90% of cancers or by inventing a new mechanism that maintains long telomeres. Therefore, when a cancer cell's telomeres become too short, the cancer cell can artificially add more base pairs to elongate the telomeres.

An illustration of the limitless replication potential of cancer cells is shown in Figure 4.14. In Figure 4.14a, normal cells are shown during different cycles of replication. Initially, their chromosomes have long telomeres (represented with green flag). After one mitotic cycle, the telomeres get shorter (represented by yellow flag). After the third cycle, the telomere length is too short for further replication (represented by red flag). Once this stage is reached, cells stop replicating. In cancer cells (Figure 4.14b), when the telomere length reaches a certain level (represented by yellow flag), the

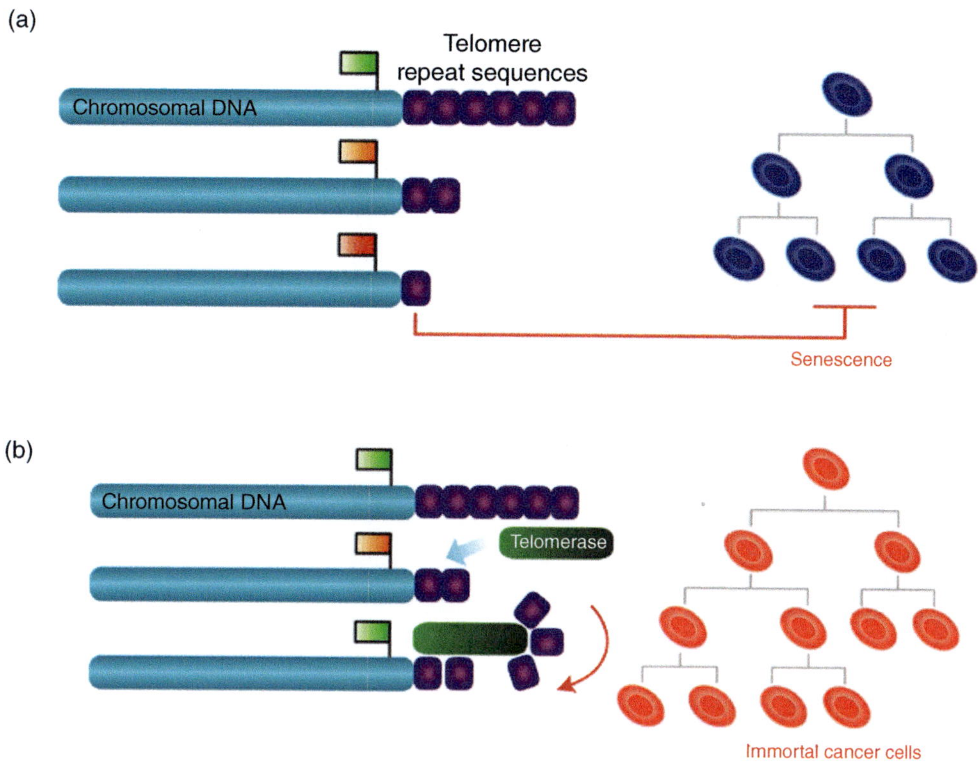

Figure 4.14 (a) Replication in healthy cells. (b) Limitless replication potential of cancer cells. *Source:* Figure 1 from Keith et al. [6]. © Cambridge University Press.

cancer cell activates telomerase, which extends the telomere regions of the chromosomes. This allows the cancer cell to replicate infinitely because it is able to avoid telomere length limitations.

4.4.5 Sustained Angiogenesis

Cancer cells can initiate **angiogenesis**, the growth of new blood vessels. During the normal growth of tissues, angiogenesis is transitory and carefully regulated, and during other times, the angiogenic switch is turned off. However, in order to receive oxygen and nutrients from the vasculature, any body cell must reside within 100 μm of a capillary blood vessel. When a tumor reaches a size of about 1 mm^3, it acquires the ability to induce angiogenesis (i.e. turn "on" the angiogenic switch), and cells within the tumor will start to secrete over 20 possible angiogenesis-inducing factors into the extracellular matrix (i.e. the area between cells in a tissue). These factors then instruct nearby blood vessels (typically capillaries) to expand and develop new vasculature that grows toward the tumor. One such important factor is **Vascular Endothelial Growth Factor (VEGF)**, shown in Figure 4.15.

These newly developed blood vessels are different in many ways from healthy blood vessels. On a molecular level, they overexpress receptors on their internal and external surfaces such as **Vascular Endothelial Growth Factor Receptors** (**VEGFR**, not to be confused with VEGF) and the integrin family of receptors. It is possible to molecularly target these receptors using antibodies and small protein fragments called peptides (more information on molecular targeting will be provided in the chapters on *in vivo* imaging).

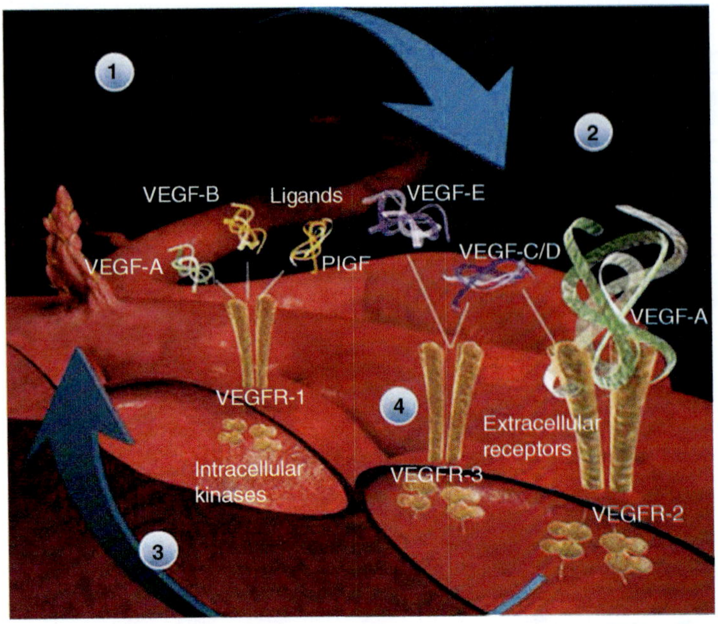

Figure 4.15 Sustained Angiogenesis. *Source:* Genentech, Inc. Reprinted with permission.

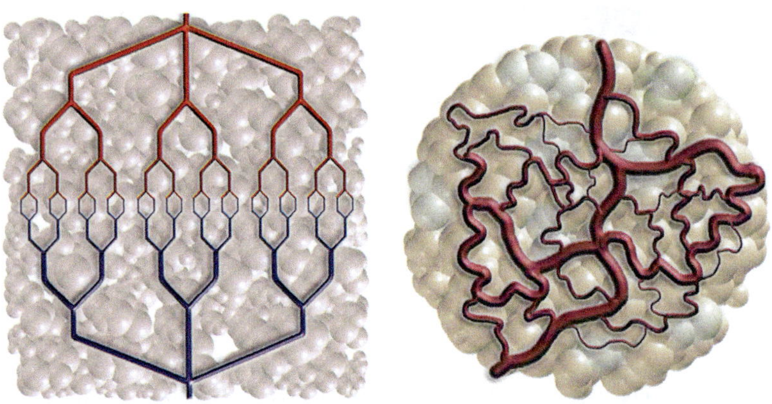

Figure 4.16 Angiogenesis by cancer leads to abnormal vasculature. *Source:* Jain [7]. Reprinted by permission from Springer Nature. Copyright © 2001 by Springer Nature.

On a more mechanical level, an important characteristic of the new tumor blood vessels is that they are made of disrupted cell layers (because tumor-induced angiogenesis is poorly regulated compared to healthy angiogenesis). This disrupted structure renders tumor blood vessels leaky, allowing small particles in the bloodstream to leak into the tumor bed. This effect is known as the **Enhanced Permeability and Retention effect (EPR effect)**. The new tumor blood vessels have a characteristic irregular shape, are typically tortuous, and may even contain internal loops (Figure 4.16).

Understanding the process of angiogenesis led to the development of an important class of cancer drugs that work by inhibiting angiogenesis (a.k.a. antiangiogenic therapy). The concept behind this approach is as follows: by cutting off the tumor's blood supply, the tumor's ability to grow will be severely limited. For example, antibodies against VEGF have proven effective in treating several cancer types by preventing VEGF from reacting with its receptor partner – VEGFR. If VEGF receptors on the newly formed blood vessels are not interacting with their counterpart, VEGF, then the blood vessels regress and the tumor shrinks to about 1 mm^3 in size and becomes dormant.

4.4.6 Tissue Invasion and Metastasis

Cancer cells can invade adjacent or distant tissues, where they start new colonies in a process called invasion and metastasis (Figure 4.17). The cancer cells release extracellular protease enzymes which operate outside the cell and allow them to disassociate from neighboring cells by cleaving proteins that form cell-junctions (cell–cell bonds that help keep the tissue together as one piece). This makes the tumor cells more fluid and independent of their environment. The tumor cells are then free to travel throughout the extracellular space, reach the vasculature, and enter the circulatory system. Through the circulatory system, the cancer cells reach distant tissues in the body, where they reside and form new colonies of cells with similar characteristics as the original tumor.

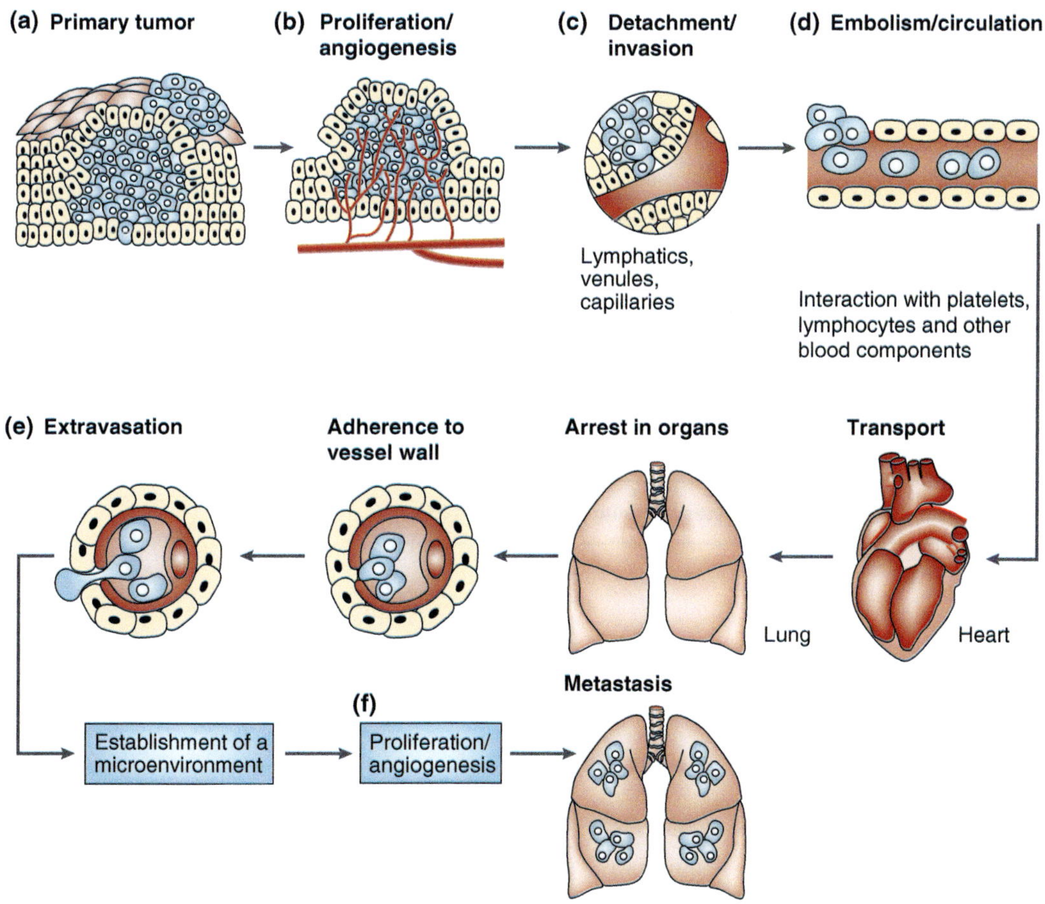

Figure 4.17 Illustration of the process of metastasis. *Source:* Fidler [8]. Reprinted/adapted/translated by permission from Springer Nature: on behalf of Cancer Research UK. Copyright © 2003 by Springer Nature.

The difference between benign tumors and malignant (cancerous) tumors is their ability to invade and metastasize. In fact, 90% of cancer deaths are caused by metastasis. However, treating a cancer at the metastatic stage is very difficult and is often unsuccessful. In the clinic, it is not uncommon to find cancer patients with over 50 metastasis sites spread throughout their bodies.

4.5 Conclusion

For cells to acquire all six hallmarks of cancer through random genomic mutations is highly unlikely as the process of mutations is highly inefficient. The primary reason for its inefficiency is the random nature of the mutations, which can occur at any location along the genome. Moreover, multiple DNA monitoring and repairing enzymes (e.g. p53 protein), and multiple checkpoints during the cell division cycle, detect such genomic mutations and act accordingly (either by correcting the mutation or by initiating programmed cell death). Still, cancer is more frequent than one would expect based on the incident rate of random mutations. The reason is that mutations to a mechanism responsible for capturing mutations (such as the protein p53) inhibit their function, thereby rendering the cell more vulnerable to future mutations, which can inhibit other anticancer mechanisms and so forth. Table 4.1 shows the percentage of p53 mutations associated with different types of cancer.

Problems

4.1 **A** Prostate cancer is a very slowly progressing cancer. Based on Table 4.2, explain why five-year survival rates may not be a good measure for estimating the efficacy of early detection of prostate cancer.

Table 4.1 Distribution of cancers and p53 mutations.

Type of cancer	Percentage of cases involving p53 mutations (%)
Lung	70
Stomach	45
Breast	20
Colon	60
Liver	20
Prostate	10–30
Cervix/Uteri	Special
Head/Neck	60
Esophagus	40
Leukemia	10
Lymphoma	30
Ovary	60
Bladder	60

Table 4.2 Five-year survival rates (%) for various types of cancer based on stage at diagnosis.

	All stages	Local	Regional	Distant		All stages	Local	Regional	Distant
Breast (female)	90	99	85	27	Oral cavity and pharynx	65	84	64	39
Colon and rectum	65	90	71	14	Ovary	47	93	73	29
Colon	64	91	72	14	Pancreas	8	32	12	3
Rectum	67	88	70	15	Prostate	99	>99	>99	30
Esophagus	19	43	23	5	Stomach	31	67	31	5
Kidney[a]	74	93	67	12	Testis	95	99	96	73
Larynx	61	77	45	34	Thyroid	98	>99	98	56
Liver[b]	18	31	11	3	Urinary bladder[c]	77	70	35	5
Lung and bronchus	18	56	29	5	Uterine cervix	67	92	57	17
Melanoma of the skin	92	99	63	20	Uterine corpus	81	95	69	16

Rates are adjusted for normal life expectancy and are based on cases diagnosed in the SEER 18 areas from 2007 to 2013, all followed through 2014.
[a] Includes renal pelvis.
[b] Includes intrahepatic bile duct.
[c] Rate for in situ cases is 96%.
Local: an invasive malignant cancer confined entirely to the organ of origin. **Regional:** a malignant cancer that (i) has extended beyond the limits of the organ of origin directly into surrounding organs or tissues; (ii) involves regional lymph nodes; or (iii) has both regional extension and involvement of regional lymph nodes. **Distant:** a malignant cancer that has spread to parts of the body remote from the primary tumor either by direct extension or by discontinuous metastasis to distant organs, tissues, or via the lymphatic system to distant lymph nodes.
Source: American Cancer Society [9].

B If you could design a diagnostic tool to detect any one type of cancer, regardless of its stage, which type of cancer would it be? Use Table 4.2 and Figure 4.1 ("Cancer statistics") to support your answer. You may assume that the five-year survival rates listed in Table 4.2 represent true overall survival rates (not just over five years). You may also assume in your answer that 100% of the patients are diagnosed with cancer at the late "Distant" stage.

Hint: The objective of your diagnostic device is to reduce the mortality from cancer as much as possible.

4.2 Match each function in Column B with the proper item in Column A.

Column A	Column B
1) ____Telomerase	A Added DNA strands at the end of each chromosome.
2) ____G_0	B Programmed cell death.
3) ____Telomeres	C Mechanism where a cell produces growth signals that, upon release, stimulate the cell to undergo cell division.
4) ____Apoptosis	D Receptors that are upregulated on the surface of new blood vessels (neovascularization).
5) ____Integrins	E Enzyme that acts on DNA to add the sequence TTAGGG at its end.
6) ____Autocrine growth stimulation	F A resting state in the cell division cycle.

4.3 Telomeres shorten upon cell division. If we assume that cells never die in a perfect environment, what is the minimum number of cycles of cell division that can happen until a cell reaches the senescent state (using numbers given in the chapter)? If you start with a single cell, how many cells can you obtain after this number of cycles? Do you think this is reasonable given that there are about 30 trillion cells in the human body?

4.4 A cell is highly unlikely to acquire all six hallmarks of cancer through the random process of genomic mutations since these mutations occur with low probability at random locations along the genome. Explain why cancer is more prevalent than one would expect, given this inefficient mutation process.

4.5 The p53 protein is sometimes called the "anticancer" protein. Explain its role in preventing cancer and which hallmark(s) of cancer are affected by it (you only need to give examples that are mentioned in the chapter).

4.6 Explain the rationale for the following new cancer treatments and which hallmark(s) they are affecting:

A an inhibitor of matrix metalloproteinases (a protease that cleaves surface receptors or other extracellular matrix proteins)

B antibodies that block the function of VEGF

C antibodies that block the function of growth signals

4.7 **A** Sofia wants to develop a new therapy for killing cancer cells. Recalling what she learned in class, she decided to treat some cancer cells with a drug, doxorubicin, which is known to damage DNA. She was fascinated by the result because she found that apoptosis occurred in almost all the cells. What is the main protein or pathway involved with this? Explain its role.

B David visited Sofia's lab and said that a small subset of the cells probably survived due to depletion of the drug. To test this, Sofia collected and cultured the survived cells, and treated them again with the same drug. However, this time very few cells died. Explain the reason for this and which hallmarks are primarily involved.

References

1 Jemal, A., Siegel, R., Xu, J., and Ward, E. (2010). Cancer statistics. CA: A Cancer Journal for Clinicians 60: 277–300.

2 NobelPrize.org. (2018). Press release. *Nobel Media AB* 2018. https://www.nobelprize.org/prizes/medicine/2005/press-release/.

3 Mader, S. and Windelspecht, M. (2014). *Human Biology*, 14e. New York: McGraw Hill Publishing.

4 Hanahan, D. and Weinberg, R.A. (2000). The hallmarks of cancer. *Cell* 100 (1): 57–70.

5 National Library of Medicine (US) (2018). How do genes control the growth and division of cells?. Help Me Understand Genetics page. Genetics Home Reference [Internet]. Bethesda (MD): The Library. https://ghr.nlm.nih.gov/primer/howgeneswork/genesanddivision.

6 Keith, W., Bilsland, A., Evans, T., and Glasspool, R. (2002). Telomerase-directed molecular therapeutics. *Expert Reviews in Molecular Medicine* 4 (10): 1–25.

7 Jain, R.K. (2001). Normalizing tumor vasculature with anti-angiogenic therapy: a new paradigm for combination therapy. *Nature Medicine* 7 (9): 987–989.

8 Fidler, I.J. (2003). The pathogenesis of cancer metastasis: the 'seed and soil' hypothesis revisited. *Nature Reviews Cancer* 3 (6): 453–458.

9 American Cancer Society (2018). *Cancer Facts and Figures 2018*. Atlanta: American Cancer Society, Inc.

Further Reading

http://www.biology-pages.info/T/TumorSuppressorGenes.html.

5

Cardiovascular Diseases (CVDs)

5.1 Epidemiology and Introduction

Cardiovascular disease (CVD) refers to the class of diseases that involve the heart and/or the blood vessels, especially the veins and arteries leading to and from the heart. While the term CVD technically applies to any disease affecting the cardiovascular system, it is usually used to refer to conditions related to atherosclerosis (hardening of artery), like arterial disease.

CVD is the leading cause of death in the US, surpassing even cancer (Figure 5.1). Examples of CVD include heart attack, stroke, and heart failure. In recent news (2010), two high-profile American figures have been afflicted with CVD: US diplomat Richard Holbrooke passed away from a torn aorta, despite 20 hours of surgery, and former President Bill Clinton was hospitalized due to blockage in one of his quadruple bypass channels, and had two stents installed. CVD imposes a significant burden on the US: for example, in 2006, CVD caused 831 thousand deaths compared to 560 thousand deaths from cancer. Fortunately, the survival rate of CVD patients in the US has improved significantly in recent decades, largely due to improvements in diagnostic, treatment, and prevention techniques (Figure 5.2). However, CVD is an emerging problem in developing countries including China and India.

There are several important concepts that are commonly used in CVD, cancer, and other disease statistics. Mortality is the total number of deaths from a given disease in a population during a specific interval of time (usually a year). If normalized by the population, it is called the mortality rate or death rate. Prevalence is the total number of cases of a given disease existing in a population at a specific point in time. It is also given as a percentage of the population. The prevalence of CVD in the US from 2007 to 2010 is depicted in Figure 5.3. Incidence is the total number of new cases of a given disease that develop in a population at a specific time period, usually a year. It is also given as a percentage of the population during the period. The incidence of CVD in the US is depicted in Figure 5.4. The survival rate is defined as the portion of the population remaining alive at a specified time after a life-threatening event or diagnosis of a disease. A survival plot, a.k.a. Kaplan–Meier plot, shows the portion of diagnosed patients who are still alive over a certain time period.

Biochips and Medical Imaging, First Edition. Adam de la Zerda and Shan Xiang Wang.

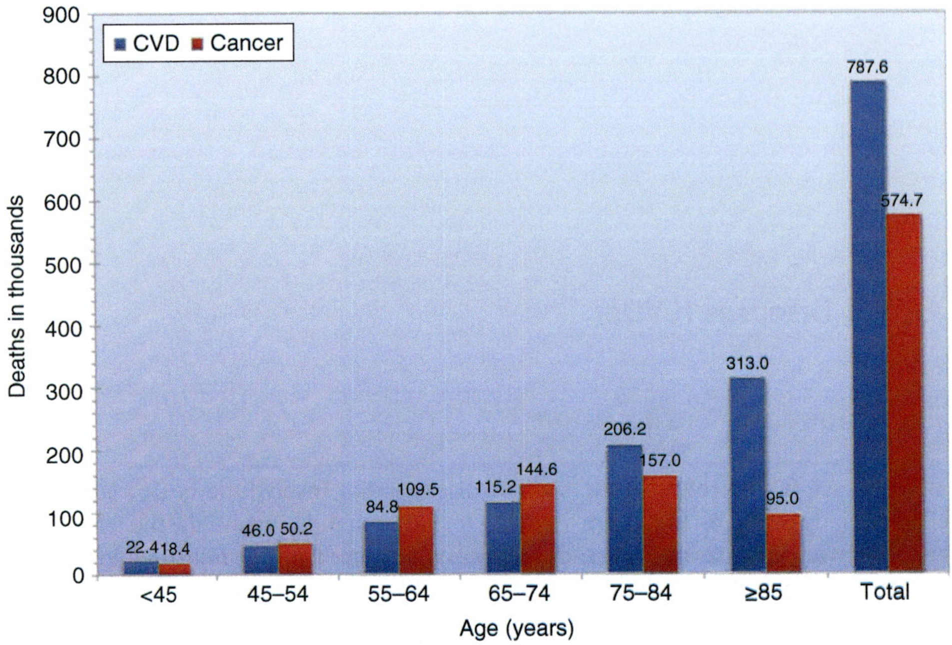

Figure 5.1 Deaths from CVD versus deaths from cancer in the US in 2010 (by age group). *Source:* Go et al. [1]. Republished with permission of Wolters Kluwer Health, Inc. from "Heart Disease and Stroke Statistics—2014 Update." Copyright © 2013 American Heart Association, Inc.

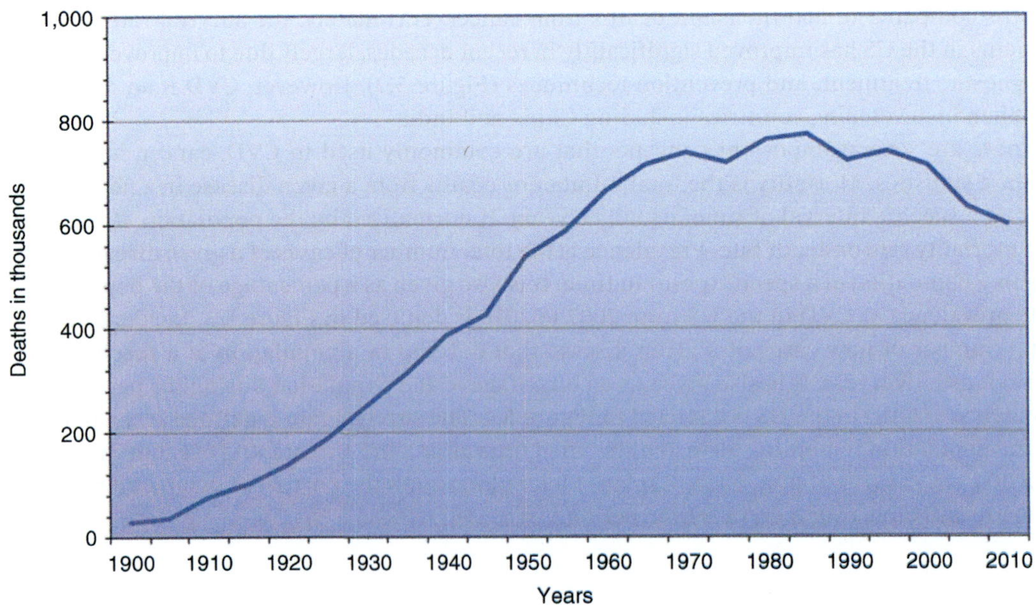

Figure 5.2 Annual deaths due to CVD since 1900. *Source:* Go et al. [1]. Republished with permission of Wolters Kluwer Health, Inc. from "Heart Disease and Stroke Statistics—2014 Update." Copyright © 2013 American Heart Association, Inc.

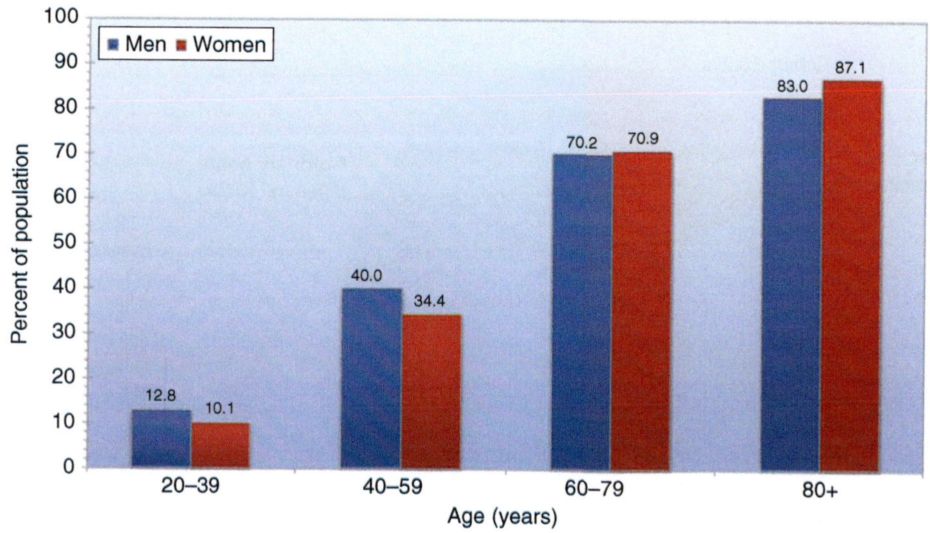

Figure 5.3 Prevalence of CVD in men and women from 2007 to 2010. *Source:* Go et al. [1]. Republished with permission of Wolters Kluwer Health, Inc. from "Heart Disease and Stroke Statistics—2014 Update." Copyright © 2013 American Heart Association, Inc.

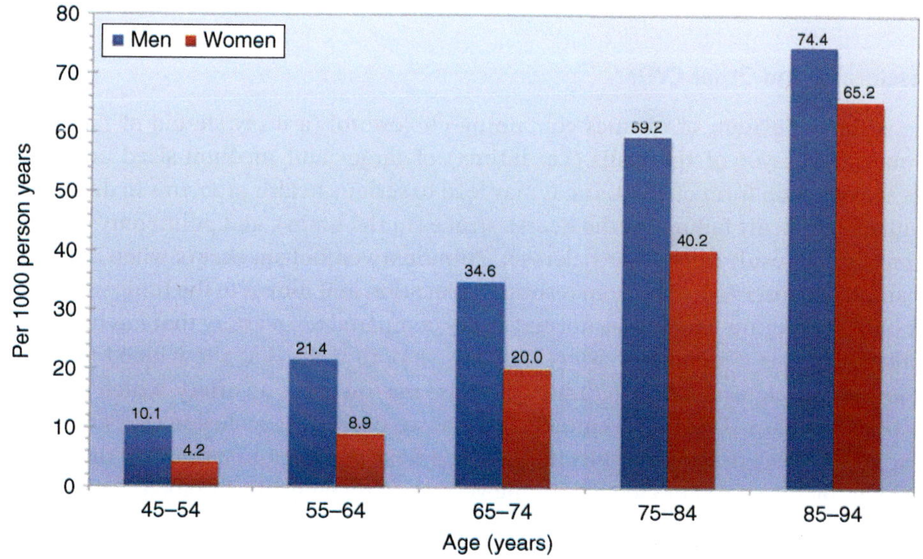

Figure 5.4 Incidence of CVD in men and women from 1980 to 2003. *Source:* Go et al. [1]. Republished with permission of Wolters Kluwer Health, Inc. from "Heart Disease and Stroke Statistics—2014 Update." Copyright © 2013 American Heart Association, Inc.

5.2 Types of CVD

There are several conditions that are collectively referred to as CVDs. The relative contributions of each of these conditions to the total CVD deaths in the US in 2010 are shown in Figure 5.5. The causes, diagnoses, and treatment of several of the major types of CVD are discussed in detail below.

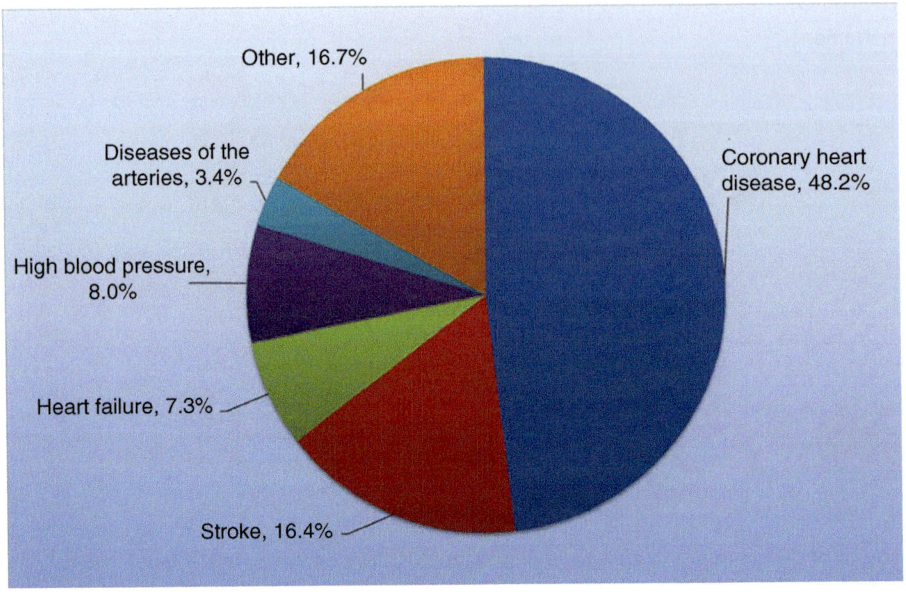

Figure 5.5 Deaths due to different types of CVD in the US (2010). *Source:* Go et al. [1]. Republished with permission of Wolters Kluwer Health, Inc. from "Heart Disease and Stroke Statistics—2014 Update." Copyright © 2013 American Heart Association, Inc.

5.2.1 Atherosclerosis and Other CVDs

Atherosclerosis is the deposition of plaques containing cholesterol (a waxy steroid of fat) and lipids on the innermost layer of the walls (i.e. intima) of large- and medium-sized arteries. Atherosclerosis is a common form of CVD, and it may lead to serious health problems in different organs. Heart attack and heart failure (in the heart), stroke (in the brain), and pulmonary embolism (in the lung) can all result from atherosclerosis. Pulmonary embolism occurs when a blood clot formed by atherosclerosis dislodges from its original location and moves to the lung, where it blocks the flow of blood. Figure 5.6 shows a normal artery compared to an artery that has become narrowed by atherosclerosis. The normal artery has very smooth walls that allow blood to flow easily. In contrast, atherosclerotic plaque buildup can cause narrowing of an artery, which results in abnormally low blood flow. This can eventually lead to two problems: occlusion (i.e. stenosis) in which the narrowed artery diameter results in less blood flow, or the more serious condition of thrombus, in which the formation of clots inside the vessels completely blocks blood flow, causing a heart attack or stroke.

5.2.2 Coronary Artery Disease

Coronary artery disease (CAD), also called coronary heart disease (CHD), is a condition in which plaque builds up inside the coronary arteries, which supply the heart muscle with oxygen-rich blood. While atherosclerosis refers to the buildup of plaque throughout the vessel system, which can have effects at distant sites, CAD is a subtype of atherosclerosis that refers to plaque that forms in the coronary arteries, which specifically affects the heart muscle.

Many CAD patients have no symptoms, which makes estimation of incidence very difficult. One early warning sign of CAD is angina (i.e. chest pain), which had a prevalence of about 15.8 million

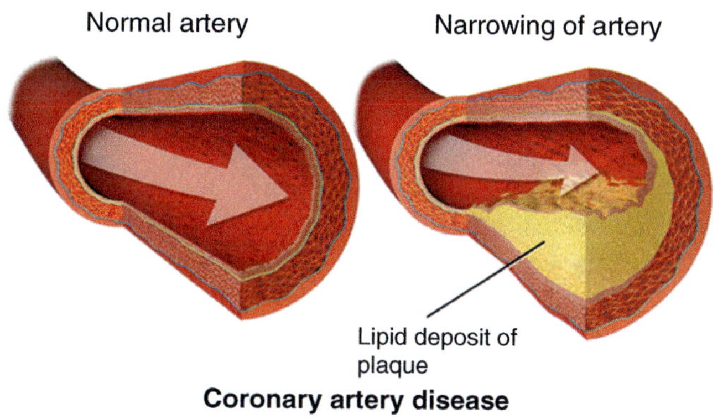

Figure 5.6 Schematic of a normal artery versus an artery narrowed by atherosclerosis. *Source:* Blausen.com staff [2]. Used under CC-BY 3.0 http://creativecommons.org/licenses/by/3.0/.

in 2006. Angina can occur in either stable or unstable forms. Stable angina is typically brought on by stress or exercise, while unstable angina may be sudden or more variable. Angina is typically the result of ischemia since the heart lacks oxygen supply due to decreased blood flow. The overall progression of heart disease can be summarized as follows: high blood pressure (a macroscopic symptom) and/or high cholesterol or other factors, which can lead to atherosclerosis, then ischemia, and, finally, heart attack (death of heart muscle) and heart failure. In some cases, ischemia can even lead directly to heart failure. Both heart attack and heart failure can result in death.

CAD can lead to a myocardial infarction (abbreviated as MI or AMI, where A stands for acute), a.k.a. heart attack, where tissue necrosis (death) occurs in the heart muscle due to lack of blood. An example of MI is the blockage of the left coronary artery (LCA) or right coronary artery (RCA) (Figure 5.7). Heart attacks have an incidence of about 1.2 million per year, of which 40% are fatal. Half of all heart attack deaths occur within one hour of symptom onset (e.g. intense chest pain), before the patient can receive hospital treatment. This high mortality rate highlights the importance of heart disease prevention and early diagnosis of angina and other symptoms of CAD.

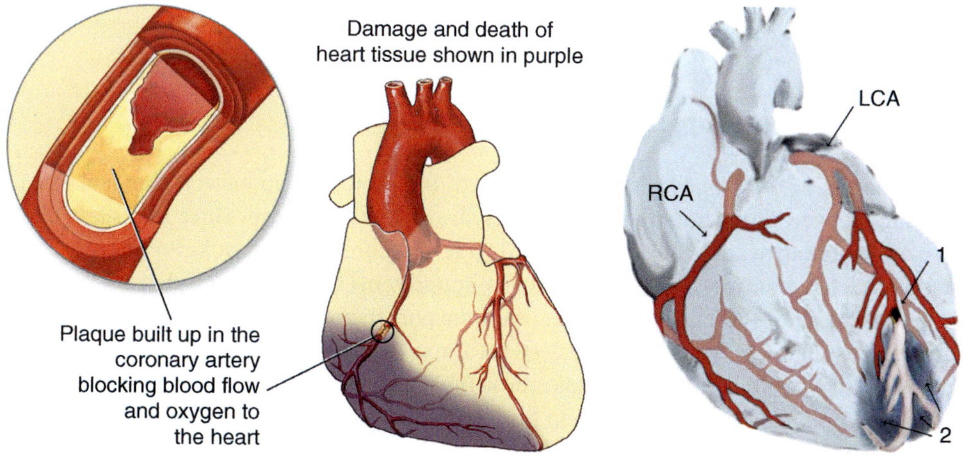

Figure 5.7 Blockage of right coronary artery (RCA) and left coronary artery (LCA). *Sources:* Republished with permission of ADAM Images and Heuser [3]. Used under CC BY-SA 3.0 http://creativecommons.org/licenses/by-sa/3.0/.

5.2.3 Arrhythmia

Arrhythmia (dysrhythmia) refers to any change from the normal sequence of electrical impulses that cause the heart to beat. The electrical impulses may happen too quickly, too slowly, or erratically, causing the heart to beat too quickly, too slowly, or erratically. When the heart does not beat properly, it cannot pump blood effectively, and, in turn, the lungs, brain, and all other organs cannot work properly and may be damaged or shut down. The prevalence of arrhythmia is 14.4 million, or 5.3% of the US population. There are four types of arrhythmia: bradycardia (too slow), tachycardia (too fast), fibrillation (quivering), and premature contraction (early beat).

5.2.4 Cardiac Arrest

Cardiac arrest is the sudden, abrupt loss of heart function. The victim may or may not have been diagnosed with heart disease, but cardiac arrest most commonly arises from coronary heart disease. Most cardiac arrests that lead to sudden death occur when the electrical impulses in the diseased heart become rapid (ventricular tachycardia), chaotic (ventricular fibrillation), or both. This irregular heart rhythm (arrhythmia) causes the heart to suddenly stop beating. Some cardiac arrests are due to extreme slowing of the heart (bradycardia).

5.2.5 Heart Failure

Heart failure is a common condition that usually develops slowly as the heart muscle weakens and must work harder to keep blood flowing through the body. It refers to a condition where the heart is unable to pump enough blood to the body's tissues rather than where the heart suddenly stops. People with heart failure often complain of feeling tired. Heart failure, characterized by myocardial thickening (also known as hypertrophic cardiomyopathy, illustrated in Figure 5.8), develops following an injury to the heart, such as the damage caused by a heart attack, long-term high blood pressure, or an abnormality of one of the heart valves. Heart failure is often not recognized until its more advanced stages, commonly referred to as congestive heart failure (CHF). In CHF, fluid may leak into the lungs, feet, legs, and, in some cases, the liver or abdominal cavity. The incidence of CHF is 550 thousand per year in the US.

5.2.6 Atherosclerotic Plaque Formation

Lipids are transported in the bloodstream in the form of lipoproteins. Lipoproteins are spherical particles that have a hydrophilic outer surface and a hydrophobic inner core. Since lipids and cholesterol are not soluble in water, they get carried inside the core of water-soluble lipoproteins. There are two major types of lipoproteins: low-density lipoprotein (LDL) and high-density lipoprotein (HDL). LDLs take cholesterol from the liver and transport them to the body cells. As you may recall from previous chapters, cells need cholesterol for various functions (e.g. cell membrane repair and steroid hormone synthesis). Cholesterol in LDLs is often called "bad cholesterol" because it may build up and cause narrowing in the arteries. HDLs work in the opposite direction; they transport cholesterol from the cells to the liver. The liver excretes this cholesterol as bile into the intestines. Cholesterol carried by HDLs is often called "good cholesterol" because it helps remove excess cholesterol from the bloodstream.

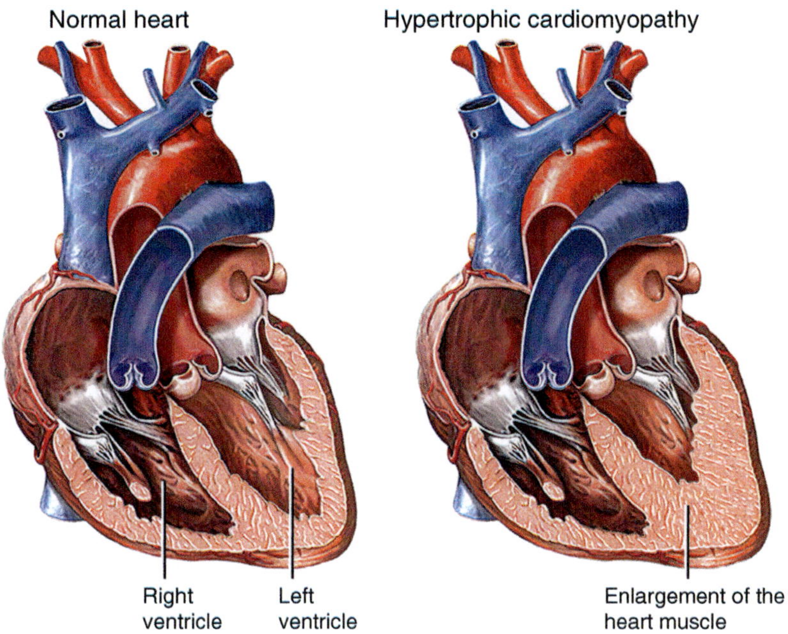

Figure 5.8 Schematic of healthy heart (left) and a heart with myocardial thickening (right), which is characteristic of early heart failure. *Source:* Republished with permission of A.D.A.M. Images.

The causes of plaque formation are still not fully understood. Generally, a plaque begins to form as LDLs start to build up in the innermost layer of arteries (Figure 5.9a, b). The lipids and proteins in this buildup get oxidized and become toxic to the surrounding blood vessel cells. As a response to this, blood vessels dilate and become more permeable so that macrophages can access these oxidized LDLs. Macrophages ingest LDLs through phagocytosis. Unfortunately, macrophages cannot degrade oxidized LDLs, which therefore simply accumulate within the macrophages. Macrophages that become filled with oxidized LDL particles are called foam cells (because of their foamy appearance under a microscope). Eventually, foam cells burst and deposit more oxidized cholesterol in the artery wall, exacerbating the original problem. This further deposition attracts more macrophages in the region and the plaque gets thicker and thicker over time due to this positive feedback loop.

The macrophages trapped in the plaque secrete chemicals that migrate from the smooth muscle cells of the middle layer of the artery to the inner layer. These chemicals induce the formation of a fibrous cap over the plaque and push plaque away from the lumen (the central space in an artery through which blood flows) of the vessel (see Figure 5.9d–e).

Very few heart attacks are caused by stenosis (occlusion) because usually the plaques expand away from the bloodstream. In many cases, the main reason for heart attack is the rupture of fibrous cap due to inflammation (Figure 5.9f). Stable plaques are abundant in smooth muscle cells and have strong caps. Vulnerable plaques, on the other hand, have more foam cells and often have weaker caps that rupture more easily. Rupture of the thin fibrous cap causes the occlusion to become a thrombus.

5.2.7 Thrombus

Thrombus formation can be an eventual consequence of long-term plaque buildup in a blood vessel to which the body responds by covering the plaque with a thin layer or fibrous "cap." When this

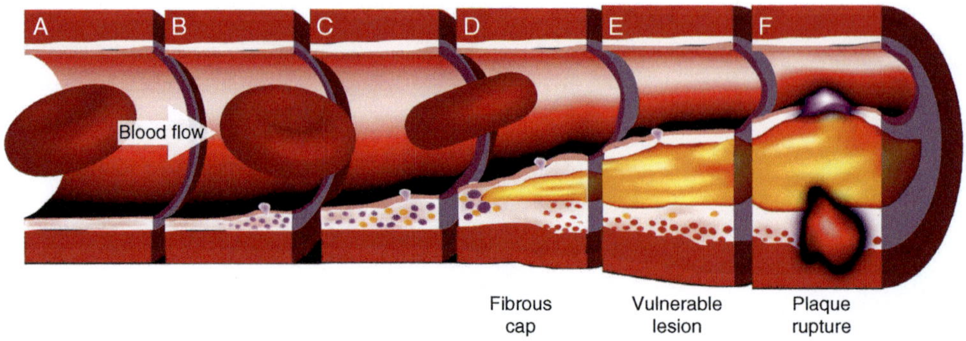

Figure 5.9 Schematic of plaque formation. *Source:* Wu [4]. Republished with permission of Future Medicine Ltd., from "Early Detection of Acute Coronary Syndrome and Risk Stratification by Multi-marker Analysis." Copyright © 2007 by Future Medicine Ltd.; permission conveyed through Copyright Clearance Center, Inc.

fibrous cap ruptures (described above), the inside of the plaque is exposed to the blood and this exposure sends chemical signals to nearby blood cells. These signals can induce platelets to come to the rupture site and form a blood clot. This blood clot can cause ischemia (i.e. the lack of blood supply downstream of the blood clot that results in tissue damage), and, if severe clotting occurs, infarction (i.e. tissue death) can occur at any site downstream of the blood clot, such as the brain, heart, or lung. Interstitial collagen fibrils, derived from smooth muscle cells, crucially determine the integrity of the plaque's fibrous cap. Ultimately, inflammation in the intima produces molecular signals that inhibit new collagen production in smooth muscle cells and render them unable to repair and maintain the collagen that runs straight to the plaque's fibrous cap.

In addition to ischemia and infarction, an embolus can also occur. An embolus is a blood clot that detaches from the vessel wall and travels in the circulatory system. An embolus can cause blockage in another artery (e.g. pulmonary arteries in lungs) away from the origin. If vessels in the neck or head are affected, ischemia or infarction of the brain tissue can follow, resulting in a stroke.

5.2.8 Stroke

Stroke is a cerebrovascular disease (i.e. disease related to the blood vessels supplying the brain) that is caused by thrombus or an embolus in blood vessels supplying the brain. Stroke is a leading cause of death in older Americans, with 600 thousand patients in 2006, of which 15% died shortly after the stroke occurred. Stroke is also the leading cause of adult disability. Infarction due to stroke results in brain damage and can have varying effects and long-term damage depending on the area of infarction. About two-thirds of stroke survivors develop a permanent disability, such as limb weakness, speech impediment, or partial or total paralysis due to nervous system damage.

5.3 Diagnosis of CVDs

There are many methods to diagnose CVD, including the three examples to be discussed in this chapter: coronary angiography (an imaging technique), blood tests, and electrocardiogram (ECG or EKG – German spelling). Heart attack symptoms such as chest pain are responsible for

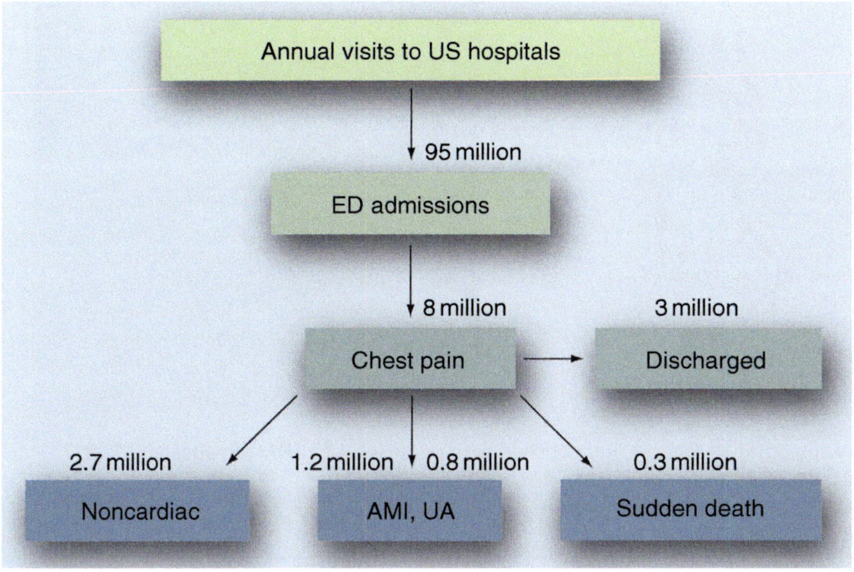

Figure 5.10 Annual visits to emergency departments in the US due to cardiac symptoms. *Source:* Wu [4]. Republished with permission of Future Medicine Ltd., from "Early Detection of Acute Coronary Syndrome and Risk Stratification by Multi-marker Analysis." Copyright © 2007 by Future Medicine Ltd.; permission conveyed through Copyright Clearance Center, Inc.

a significant portion of the 95 million annual admissions to hospital emergency departments (ED). Of the 8 million patients presented with chest pain, about 5 million will be admitted. Of these 5 million, 2.7 million are admitted for noncardiac reasons, 1.2 million for acute MI (AMI), 0.8 million with unstable angina (UA), and 0.3 million with sudden death (Figure 5.10). Therefore, hospitals require accurate diagnostic tests for CVD that can be done quickly and with reasonable cost so that noncardiac patients can be ruled out.

5.3.1 Coronary Angiography

In coronary angiography, a catheter is inserted through a blood vessel up to the heart and a contrast agent is injected near the problem area (Figure 5.11). Since blood looks the same as tissue in an X-ray image, the contrast agent enables standard X-ray or CT (computer tomography) imaging to take pictures and image any occlusions (indicated by the arrow on the radiograph in Figure 5.11) that are present in the blood vessels.

5.3.2 Important Concepts in AMI Diagnosis

There are two key concepts needed to understand the following sections on AMI diagnosis. First, a host of cardiac disorders result in left ventricle dysfunction (LVD) followed by CHF. Second, biomarkers are anything that can be used as an indicator of a particular disease state or some other physiological state of an organism. For example, the concentration measurements of certain proteins in the blood reflect the severity or presence of MI. Some of the more commonly used cardiac protein biomarkers in the blood are shown in Figure 5.12.

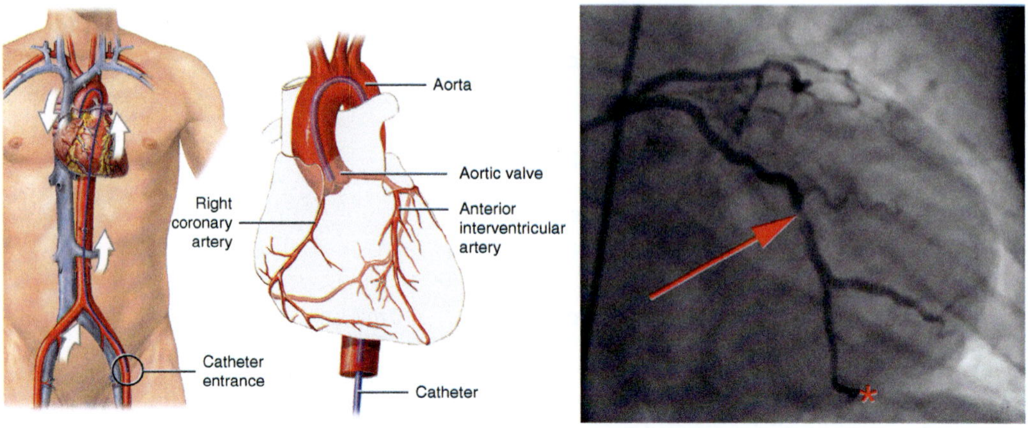

Figure 5.11 Coronary angiography. *Sources:* Republished with permission of ADAM Images and Todt et al. [5]. Used under CC-BY 2.0 http://creativecommons.org/licenses/by/2.0/.

PAPP: Pregnancy-Associated Plasma Protein	cTn: Cardiac Ttroponin (released following MI)	Mb: Myoglobin (released after muscle injury)	CK: Creatine Kinase
CK-MB: Isoform of Creatine Kinase	IMA: Ischemia-Modified Albumin	BNP: B-type Natriuretic Protein	LDH: Lactate Dehydrogenase

Figure 5.12 Cardiac protein biomarkers.

5.3.3 Blood Tests

Blood tests measure the concentrations of cardiac protein biomarkers, which are then used to determine MI presence and progression. In the initial plaque vulnerability stage, a protein called PAPP is present in blood, which is later followed by the presence of IMA protein during ischemia, then cTn protein during necrosis (heart muscle death), and, finally, BNP protein during muscle overload. Thus, different biomarkers can indicate the stage of heart disease, as shown in Figure 5.13. However, these biomarkers are not always specific and can result in false positives (healthy person tested sick) and false negatives (diseased person tested healthy). For example, a heart attack causes an increase in both cTn and Mb concentrations, but Mb increase occurs after any muscle injury. Thus, cTn is a more specific biomarker than Mb since it occurs only with heart muscle death.

Diagnosis of MI through blood tests is based on protein concentrations. In single-plex diagnostics, a biomarker concentration in blood is measured and compared to an established cutoff value. For example, cTn concentrations above $30\,\text{pg}\,\text{ml}^{-1}$ are often considered to indicate MI. The biomarker concentration distribution of non-diseased and diseased populations usually overlaps, making a perfect cutoff impossible. To avoid both missing cases and misdiagnosing cases of MI, physicians also look at time-ordered sets of protein concentrations in the blood (i.e. protein concentrations taken at multiple time points). They then use both the cutoff value and temporal pattern to diagnose MI (they also look at EKG patterns discussed later in the chapter). Examples of time-ordered set patterns in a cTn assay are shown in Figure 5.14. MI is ruled out if the patient's cTn concentration stays constant, even if the concentration is above the 99th percentile upper reference limit (URL) (i.e. cutoff value). MI is ruled in if the patient's cTn concentration either rises or falls over a nine-hour period and if at least one of the values is above the cutoff value.

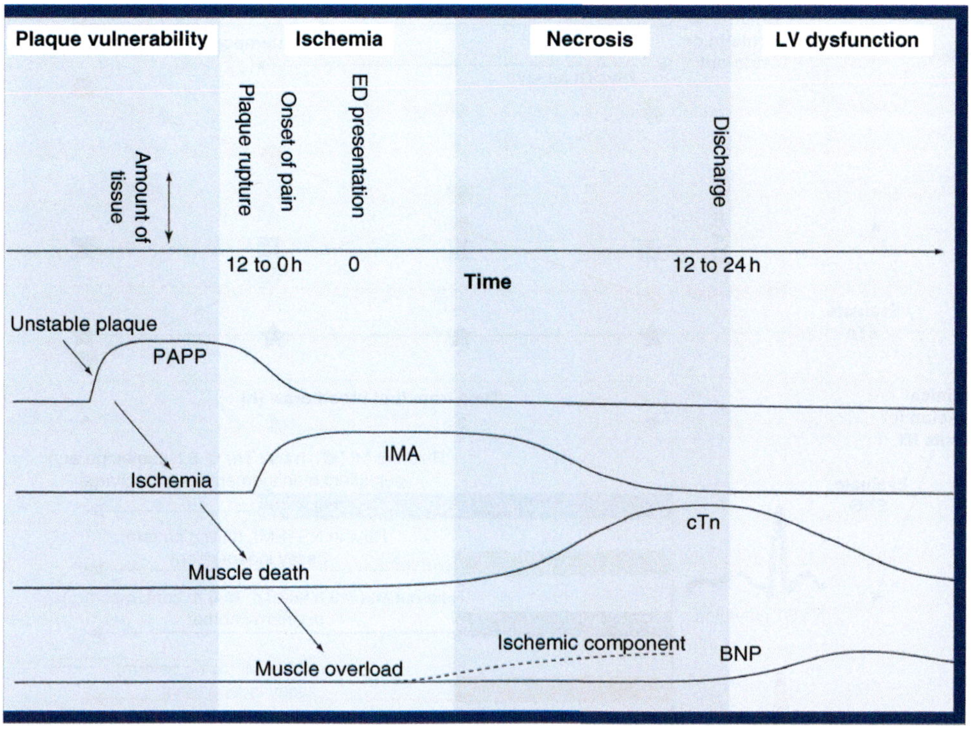

Figure 5.13 Biomarkers present in different stages of myocardial infarction. PAPP is a metalloproteinase which is released into blood during plaque vulnerability. Plaque rupture leads to myocardial ischemia and a modified albumin (IMA). Prolonged ischemia leads to myocardial necrosis and release of cTn. After 12–24 hours, there can be left ventricular dysfunction and myocardial muscle overloading, causing the release of BNP. *Source:* Wu [4]. Republished with permission of Future Medicine Ltd., from "Early Detection of Acute Coronary Syndrome and Risk Stratification by Multi-marker Analysis." Copyright © 2007 by Future Medicine Ltd.; permission conveyed through Copyright Clearance Center, Inc.

In a multivariate index assay (MIA), an algorithm based on multiple protein concentrations is used to establish an indicator (index). The indicator function (as seen in Figure 5.15) is at a minimum before the overlapping region, is linear during the overlapping region, and is at a maximum after the overlapping region. A linear function is created between these two limits, and a cutoff level of detection for the disease is determined. These indicator functions for multiple protein concentrations are then combined into an "index":

$$\text{MMX} = \sum_{a} \left[w_a \times I_a \left(C_a \right) \right],$$

where C_a is the concentration of analyte a, I_a is the indicator function of a, and w_a is the weighting factor of a.

Did You Know?

Blood tests are not just used for cardiac diseases. Prostate cancer screening is based on a blood test of prostate-specific antigen (PSA) concentrations. Biopsy is recommended if PSA $\geq 4\ \text{ng ml}^{-1}$, and biopsy is considered if PSA $> 2.5\ \text{ng ml}^{-1}$ or PSA velocity (increase in concentration per unit time) $\geq 0.35\ \text{ng ml}^{-1}\text{year}^{-1}$ when PSA $\leq 2.5\ \text{ng ml}^{-1}$. The cTn test (described above) is more specific (i.e. has less false positives) for heart attack than the PSA test for prostate cancer. A more in-depth treatment of molecular diagnosis will be given in Chapter 12.

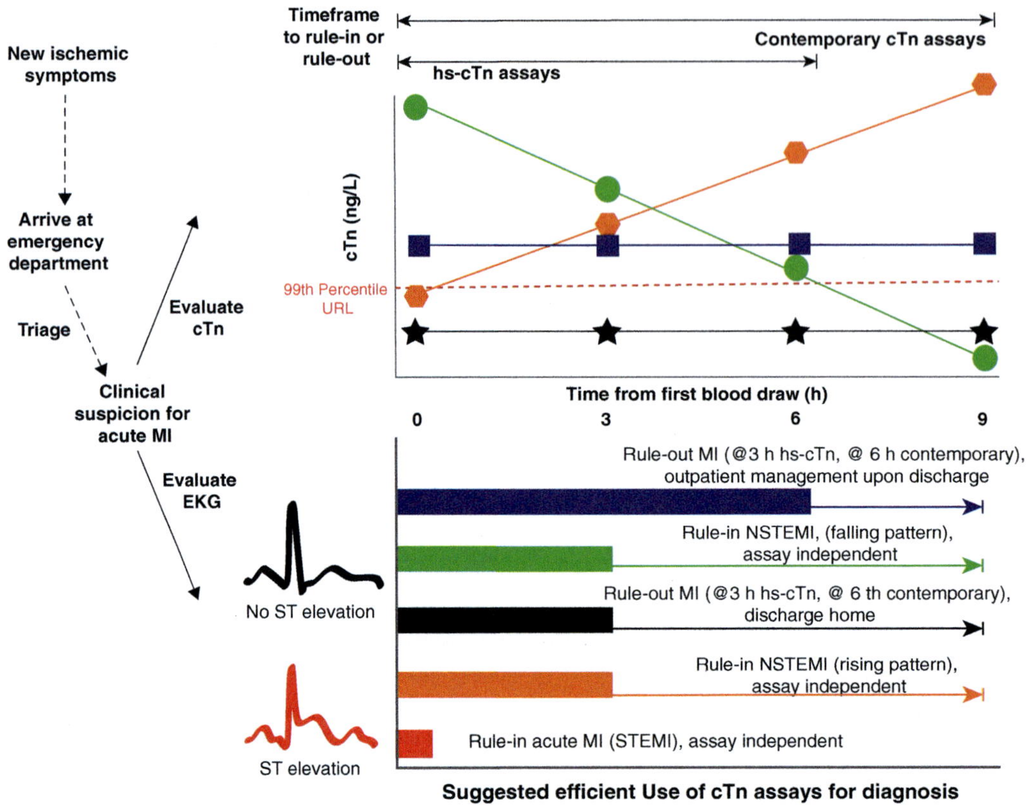

Figure 5.14 Time-ordered sets of cTn assay and corresponding diagnosis. *Source:* Love and Apple [6]. Republished with permission of American Association for Clinical Chemistry. Copyright © 2014 American Association for Clinical Chemistry.

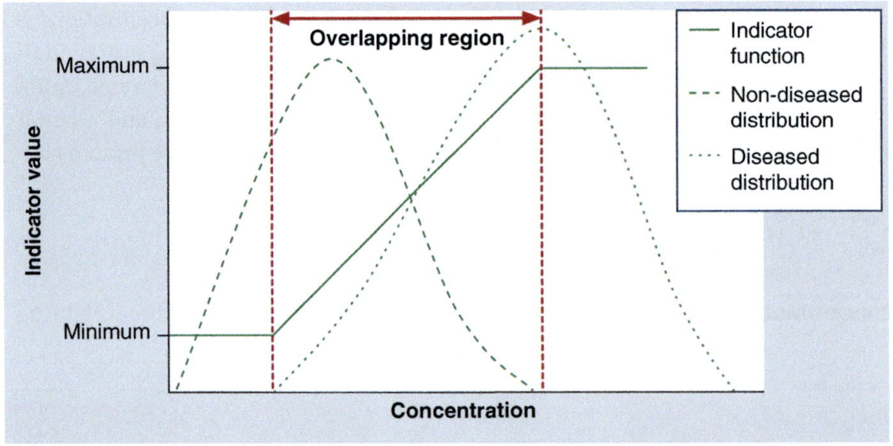

Figure 5.15 Defining indicator function. Notice that indicator function is at a minimum until the diseased distribution starts. The indicator reaches a maximum when non-diseased distribution ends. *Source:* Wu [4]. Republished with permission of Future Medicine Ltd., from "Early Detection of Acute Coronary Syndrome and Risk Stratification by Multi-marker Analysis." Copyright © 2007 by Future Medicine Ltd.; permission conveyed through Copyright Clearance Center, Inc.

5.3.4 Electrocardiogram (ECG/EKG)

The electrocardiogram (ECG or EKG) is not only the oldest but also the most commonly used cardiovascular lab procedure. Willem Einthoven, who received the Nobel Prize in Physiology or Medicine in 1924, invented ECG. It is performed by placing electrodes on the patient's chest (Figure 5.16) and measuring the current flow in the chest caused when the heart muscle depolarizes during each heartbeat. Every heart muscle cell at rest contains a charge across its cell membrane, which reduces to zero during depolarization, which then activates the cell's contraction mechanisms. A normal ECG period is about 1 second, which corresponds to 60 heartbeats per minute (bpm). A normal adult resting heart rate is 60–100 bpm. This rate depends on the level of fitness. Athletes usually have lower resting heart rate due to stronger heart muscles. For example, cyclist Lance Armstrong is known to have a resting heart rate of 32 bpm.

Figure 5.17 shows a typical ECG of a healthy heart. The heart wall is completely relaxed (polarized) at the base line. Then the P wave occurs when the AV node (atrioventricular node) and atrial walls depolarize. The QRS complex occurs as the atria repolarize (Q and S) and the ventricular walls depolarize (R). The T wave appears when the ventricular walls repolarize. After the ventricles are completely repolarized, we are back at the baseline of the ECG.

In people with CVDs, the ECG pattern is altered in some distinct ways. Examples of ECG patterns for various conditions are shown in Figure 5.18.

5.4 Treatment of CVDs

There are a number of different treatments for heart attacks, including drugs, balloon angioplasty, stents, and bypass. Atorvastin (Lipitor®) is a drug that targets plaque. It consists of a calcium salt from the statins drug class and is used to lower blood cholesterol and to stabilize plaque through

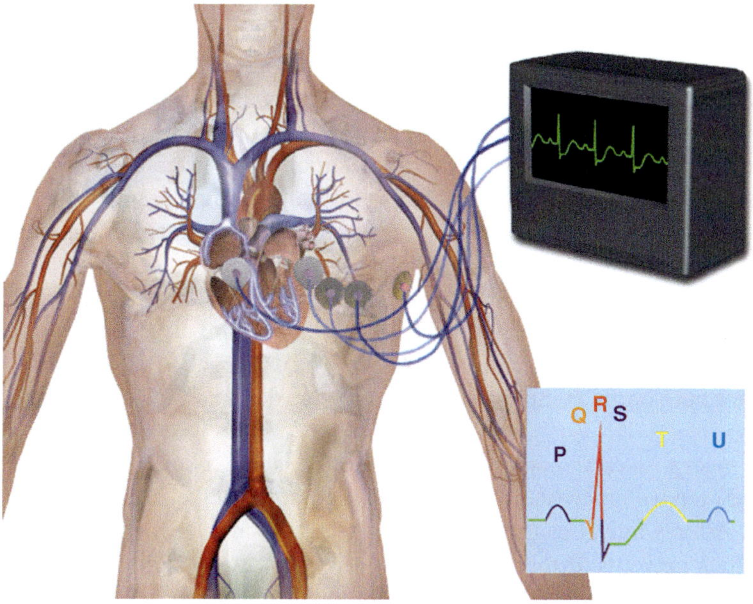

Figure 5.16 ECG placement. *Source:* Blausen.com staff [7]. Used under CC-BY 3.0 http://creativecommons.org/licenses/by/3.0/.

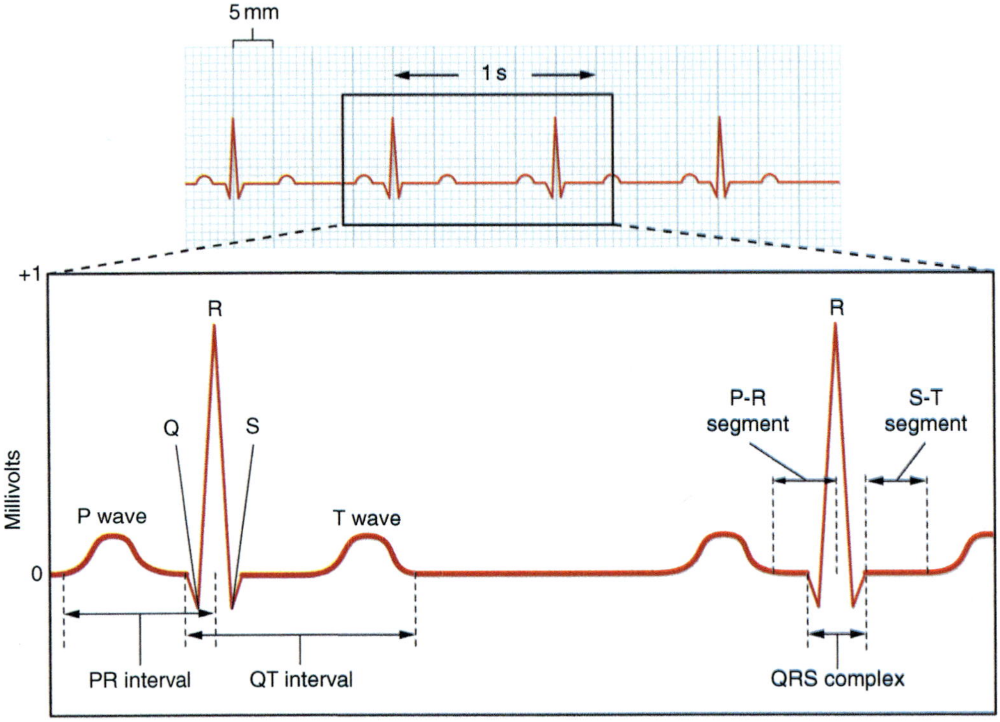

Figure 5.17 Typical ECG of a healthy person. *Source:* OpenStax College [8]. Used under CC-BY 3.0 http://creativecommons.org/licenses/by/3.0/.

anti-inflammatory and other mechanisms. Warfarin (Coumadin) is an anti-coagulation drug, which inhibits clot formation by antagonizing vitamin K cycling. These are prescribed prior to the onset of MI. Tissue plasminogen activator (tPA) is a thrombolytic drug that uses a protease to dissolve blood clots and has been approved for use in certain heart attack or stroke patients. Clot-dissolving agents such as tPA have been shown to potentially reduce the amount of damage to the heart muscle and save lives. However, they must be given within a few hours after MI symptoms begin to be effective, therefore few MI patients qualify for this treatment. Moreover, tPA must be administered through an intravenous (IV) line in the arm by hospital personnel, and patients treated within 90 minutes after the onset of chest pain is 1/7 as likely to die, compared to patients who receive therapy later.

Balloon angioplasty is a surgical procedure in which a balloon is inserted near the obstructed artery with a catheter and then inflated to break up atherosclerotic plaque and clear the arterial blockage (Figure 5.19). The balloon is then deflated and withdrawn. The drawback to balloon angioplasty is that the plaque is not necessarily completely removed at the site, and plaque can later regrow at the same site.

Another similar technique incorporates angioplasty with a coronary stent, a device consisting of a wire cage that is mounted on a balloon catheter, then implanted in the vessel and expanded when the balloon is inflated. After removal of the balloon, the stent remains in the vessel and keeps the vessel expanded, which prevents further narrowing of the artery wall (Figure 5.20). An advanced version of stents (drug-eluting stents) can also continuously deliver drugs to prevent the regrowth of plaque.

Superventricular tachycardia (SVT): Heart rate may reach up to 280 bpm. In this case, the P wave is greater than 100 bpm.	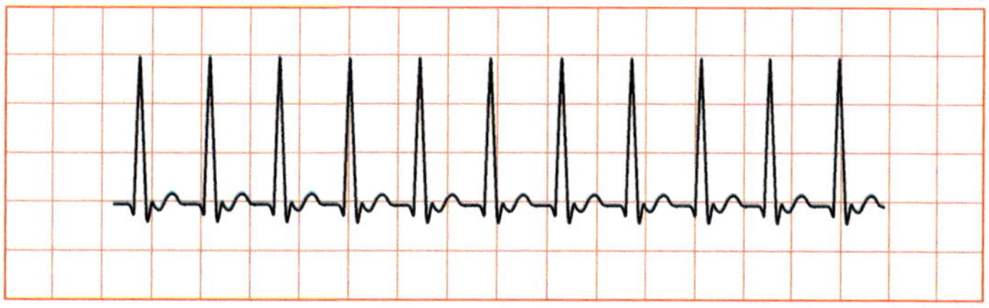
Sinus bradycardia: The P wave rate is less than 60 bpm. This means that waves appear farther apart from each other.	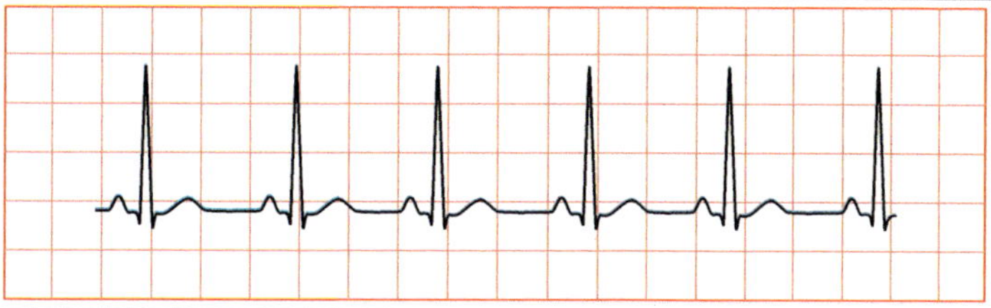
Premature atrial contraction: A premature P wave followed by a longer P-P interval on ECG.	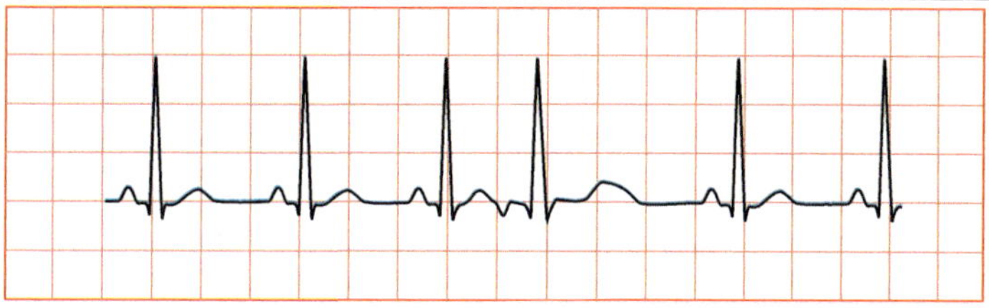
Premature ventricular contraction: Contraction of the ventricles before the atria. It causes wide QRS complex on ECG.	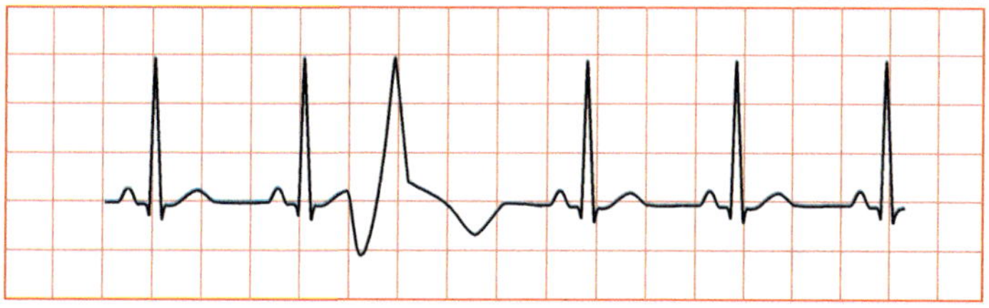
Atrial fibrillation: The rapid and irregular contraction of atria. It causes a lack of P waves and irregular spacing of R peaks in ECG	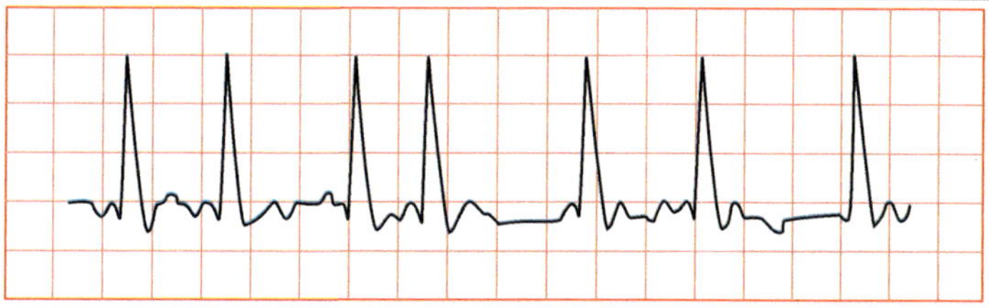
Myocardial infarction: Shows as an ST elevation in ECG (measurement of ST elevation not covered in this course)	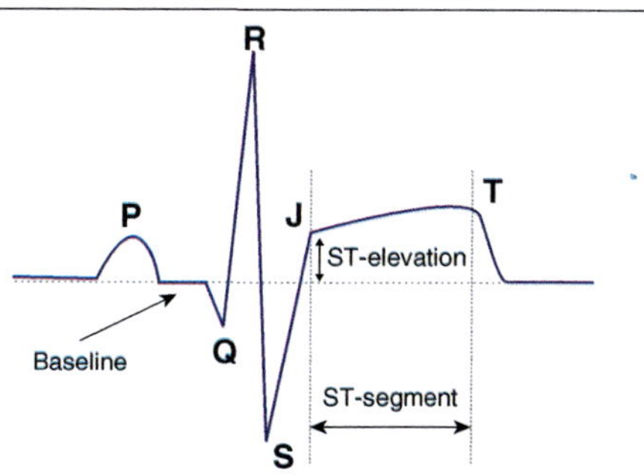

Figure 5.18 An example of ECG patterns.

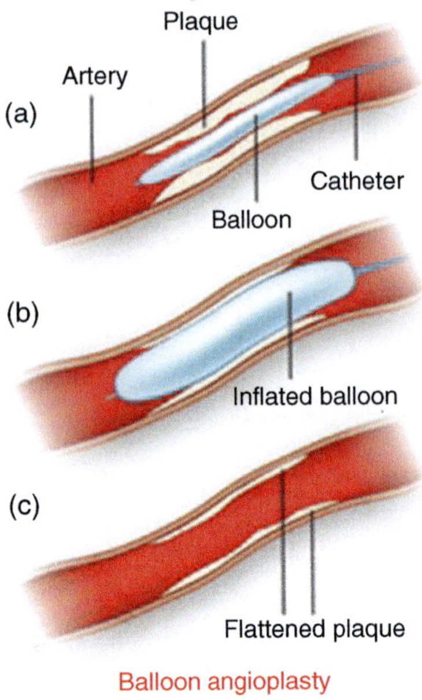

Figure 5.19 Balloon angioplasty. *Source:* Courtesy of Texas Heart Institute.

Another treatment option is a coronary artery bypass graft (CABG), which is a more complicated surgical procedure than angioplasty. A graft blood vessel is removed from elsewhere in the body (usually the leg) and used to bypass the occlusion and restore normal blood flow around the blockage site (Figure 5.21). During this procedure, the heart is temporarily stopped to allow the surgery to proceed. CABG can involve a single bypass or up to quadruple bypass.

5.5 Conclusion

CVDs impose a huge burden as the single leading cause of death in the modern world. Promising advances have been made in the form of new treatments and diagnostics in the past few decades. Coupled with increased prevention awareness, the death rate due to CVD has decreased in recent decades. The overall progression of heart disease can be summarized as follows: high blood pressure and/or high cholesterol levels, which can lead to atherosclerosis, then ischemia, and, finally, heart attack (death of heart muscle) and heart failure. In some cases, ischemia can even lead directly to heart failure. Both heart attack and heart failure can result in death. Researchers continue to develop low-cost, rapid blood tests that can diagnose heart attacks, so that treatment can be targeted and improved for MI patients.

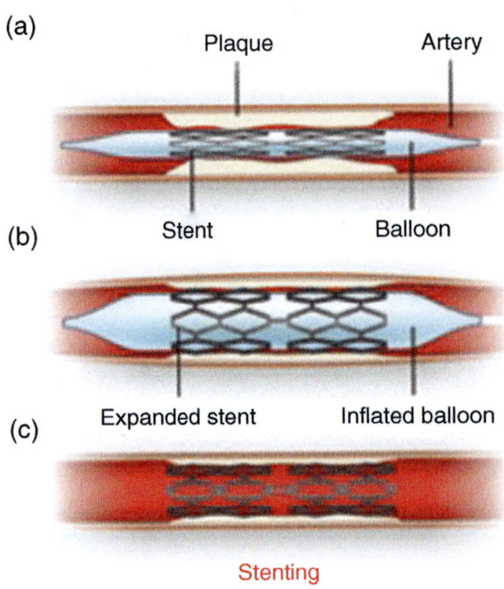

Figure 5.20 Coronary stent angioplasty procedure. *Source:* Courtesy of Texas Heart Institute.

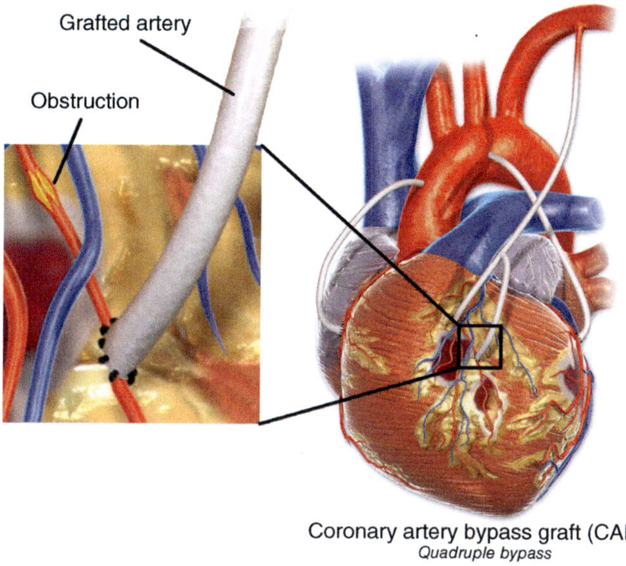

Figure 5.21 Coronary artery bypass graft. *Source:* Adapted from Blausen.com staff [9]. Used under CC-BY 3.0 http://creativecommons.org/licenses/by/3.0/.

Problems

5.1 What are the various stages in the progression of heart disease? Explain the significant characteristics of each stage.

5.2 Match each term in Column A with its appropriate meaning in Column B:

Column A	Column B
7) ___Occlusion	A. Clot in blood vessels supplying the brain
8) ___Thrombus	B. Tissue damage due to lack of blood supply
9) ___Embolus	C. Narrowed artery; leads to less blood flow
10) ___Stroke	D. Tissue death due to lack of blood supply
11) ___Ischemia	E. Blood clot that travels and causes blocks in other blood vessels
12) ___Infarction	F. Clots that completely block blood flow

5.3 Inflammation in the intima is believed to weaken the integrity of the fibrous cap in a vulnerable plaque because inflammatory signals from the intima inhibit new collagen production in smooth muscle cells, making them unable to repair and maintain the collagen in the fibrous cap.
A True
B False

5.4 Which of the features below is NOT associated with vulnerable plaques?
A Large lipid core
B Large number of inflammatory cells

C Abundance of smooth muscle cells
D Thin fibrous cap

5.5 Which of the following biomarkers is not related to heart attack? Explain your choice.
A High cholesterol level
B High androgen level
C High myoglobin level
D High troponin level

5.6 Which of the enzymes below is most likely to be associated with ischemia prior to the onset of myocardial infarction (MI)?
A PAPP
B IMA
C cTn
D BNP
E Myoglobin

5.7 Briefly explain the following diagnosis techniques and their use:
A Coronary angiography
B ECG

5.8 Compare the following treatment options for myocardial infarction (MI) patients by describing their advantages and disadvantages:
A Balloon angioplasty with coronary stent
B Coronary artery bypass graft

References

1 Go, A.S., Mozaffarian, D., Roger, V.L. et al. (2014). Heart disease and stroke statistics – 2014 update: a report from the American Heart Association. *Circulation* 129 (3): e28–e292. https://doi.org/10.1161/01.cir.0000441139.02102.80.
2 Blausen.com staff (2014). Medical gallery of Blausen Medical 2014: coronary artery disease. *WikiJournal of Medicine* 1 (2) https://doi.org/10.15347/WJM/2014.010. https://commons.wikimedia.org/wiki/File:Blausen_0259_CoronaryArteryDiseas e_02.png and blausen.com.
3 Heuser, J. (2006). AMI scheme.png. https://commons.wikimedia.org/wiki/File:AMI_scheme.png.
4 Wu, A.H.B. (2007). Early detection of acute coronary syndromes and risk stratification by multimarker analysis. *Biomarkers in Medicine* 1 (1): 45–57.
5 Todt, T., Maret, E., Alfredsson, J. et al. (2012). Relationship between treatment delay and final infarct size in STEMI patients treated with abciximab and primary PCI. *BMC Cardiovascular Disorder* 12 (9). https://doi.org/10.1186/1471-2261-12-9 http://en.wikipedia.org/wiki/File:NERC-map-en.svg.
6 Love, S. and Apple. F. (2014) "Cardiac troponin – serial ordering recommendations: for today and tomorrow." *Clinical Laboratory News*. https://www.aacc.org/publications/cln/articles/2014/may/cardiac-troponin.

7 Blausen.com staff (2014). Medical gallery of Blausen Medical 2014: electrocardiography. *WikiJournal of Medicine* 1 (2) https://doi.org/10.15347/WJM/2014.010. https://commons.wikimedia.org/wiki/File:Blausen_0339_Electrocardiogram.png and blausen.com.
8 OpenStax College (2013). Electrocardiogram Illustration from Anatomy & Physiology, Connexions Web site. http://cnx.org/content/col11496/1.6/ https://commons.wikimedia.org/wiki/File%3A2022_Electrocardiogram.jpg (accessed 19June 2013).
9 Blausen.com staff (2014). Medical gallery of Blausen Medical 2014: quadruple coronary artery bypass. *WikiJournal of Medicine* 1 (2) https://doi.org/10.15347/WJM/2014.010. https://commons.wikimedia.org/wiki/File:Blausen_0154_CABG_Quadruple.png.

Further Reading

Nabel, E.G. (2003). Cardiovascular diseases. *The New England Journal of Medicine* 349: 60–72.
Zhang, X.H., Lu, Z.L., and Liu, L. (2008). Coronary heart disease in China. *Heart* 94: 1126–1131.
Tortora, G.J. (2006). *Principles of Anatomy and Physiology*, 11e. Hoboken, NJ: Wiley.

6

DNA Chips and Sequencing

6.1 Introduction to DNA Chips and PCR

A DNA chip, a.k.a. DNA microarray, is a technology used to detect the presence of a particular DNA sequence in a sample. A microarray is a high-density array of molecules attached to a solid support, usually numbering thousands or tens of thousands of molecules per array. "Chip" is a more loosely used term equivalent to microarray, but chips may have any density of molecules, perhaps as few as 10.

6.2 Polymerase Chain Reaction (PCR)

Prior to performing biochip experiments, it is often necessary to perform polymerase chain reaction (PCR) to produce a large number of copies of a specific DNA region of interest. By creating many copies of the same DNA fragment, PCR amplifies the sample signal so that it can be sensed by a DNA microarray. The target region for PCR is typically a small segment of a very long DNA molecule, chosen by specific primers. The PCR process involves a number of thermal cycles, typically around 30, each consisting of three steps: a denaturing step (where the DNA template strand is separated into single-stranded DNA molecules), an annealing step (where the primers are attached to the single-stranded DNA template), and the extending step (where DNA polymerase synthesizes a new DNA strand complementary to the DNA template strand). In subsequent thermal cycles, the template strand and the newly formed strand are both used as templates, and thus DNA strands can be amplified exponentially with the number of thermal cycles. This amplification typically has an efficiency (E) of less than 100%. For 30 cycles at 100% efficiency, one expects 1.07 billion copies of the target DNA to be created. However, if 30 cycles produce only one million copies, then the efficiency is given by:

$$(1+E)^{30} = 10^{6} \rightarrow E = 58.5\%$$

The basic principles of PCR were covered in Chapter 2.

6.2.1 Fluorescence and Fluorophores

Fluorescence is the emission of light from an atom or a molecule in response to absorption of an energetic photon. This process occurs in three steps: excitation, relaxation, and emission

Biochips and Medical Imaging, First Edition. Adam de la Zerda and Shan Xiang Wang.

(Figure 6.1a). Excitation is the absorption of photons by the electrons in the fluorescent molecule (fluorophore, see Figure 6.1b for examples). When electrons absorb photons, they move into a higher energy state (a.k.a. excited state). The excited state exists for a finite time (typically 1–10 ns). During this time, the fluorophore undergoes conformational changes and is also subject to a multitude of possible interactions with its molecular environment. These processes have two important

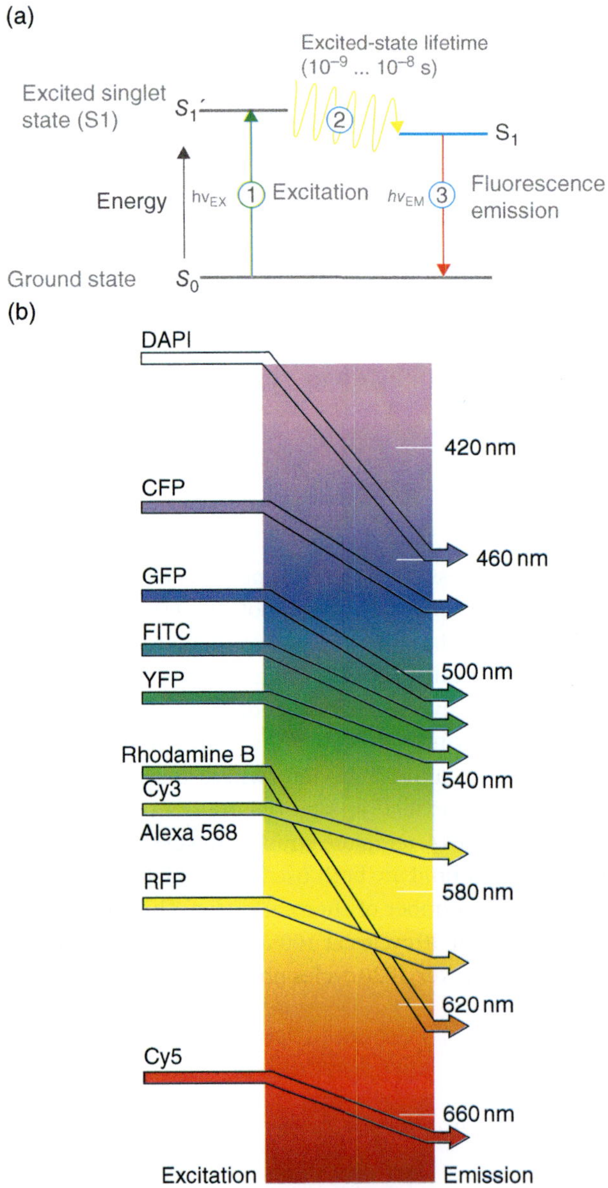

Figure 6.1 (a) Energy state of a fluorophore. Steps 1, 2, and 3 refer to excitation, relaxation, and emission, respectively. *Source:* Geb [1]. Republished with permission of Dr. Christop Geb from Leica Science Lab. Copyright © 2018 by Leica Microsystems. (b) Excitation and emission spectrum of some popular fluorophore dyes. *Source:* Alberts [2]. Republished with permission of Garland Science – Books. Copyright © 2007 by Garland Science; permission conveyed through Copyright Clearance Center, Inc.

consequences. First, the energy of S_1' is partially dissipated, yielding a relaxed singlet excited state (S_1) from which fluorescence emission originates. This is called relaxation. Second, not all the molecules initially excited by absorption (Stage 1) return to the ground state (S_0) by fluorescence emission. Other processes such as collisional quenching, fluorescence resonance energy transfer (FRET), and intersystem crossing may also depopulate S_1. Electrons in the relaxed S_1 state return to the ground state S_0 and lose energy in the form of an emitted photon. This step is called emission. The fluorescence quantum yield, which is the ratio of the number of fluorescence photons emitted (in emission) to the number of photons absorbed (in excitation), is a measure of the relative extent (and efficiency) to which these processes occur.

Fluorescent probes like TaqMan and Molecular Beacon are widely used in real-time PCR processes. Both of these probes have a reporter fluorophore and a quencher. The fluorophore and quencher interact via FRET. FRET is a mechanism describing energy transfer between two chromophores (coloring molecules) (Figure 6.2). A donor chromophore, initially in its electronic excited state, may transfer energy to an acceptor chromophore (in close proximity, typically less than 10 nm) through nonradiative dipole–dipole coupling. This mechanism is termed "Förster resonance energy transfer" and is named after the German scientist Theodor Förster. When both chromophores are fluorescent, the term "fluorescence resonance energy transfer" is often used instead, although the energy is not actually transferred by fluorescence. In order to avoid an erroneous interpretation of the phenomenon that is always a non-radiative transfer of energy (even when occurring between two fluorescent chromophores), the name "Förster resonance energy transfer" is preferred to "fluorescence resonance energy transfer." However, the latter enjoys common usage in scientific literature. FRET is analogous to near field communication in that the radius of interaction is much smaller than the wavelength of light emitted. In the near field region,

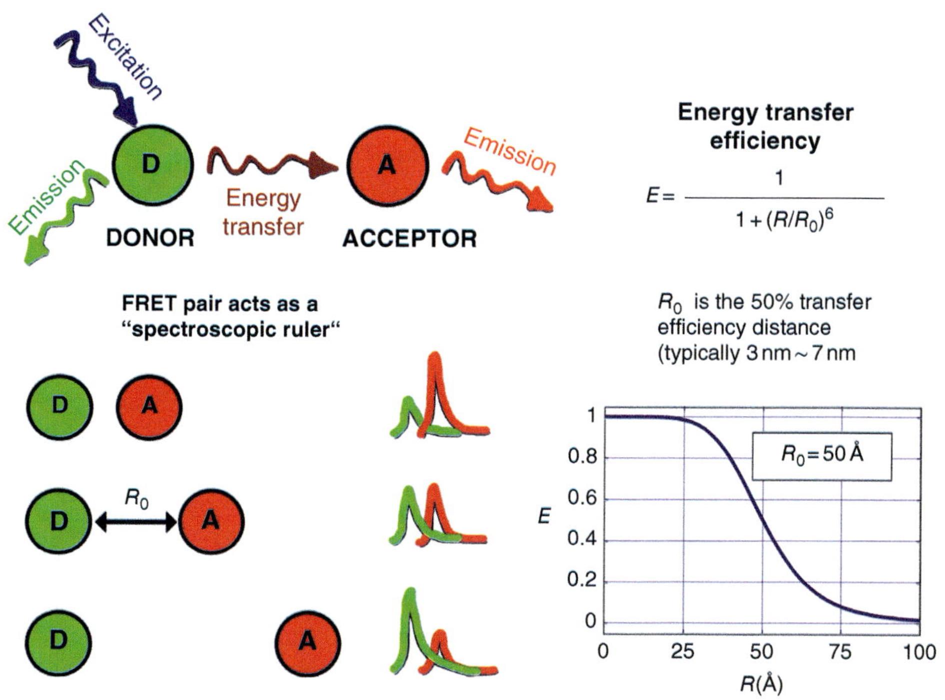

Figure 6.2 FRET mechanism.

the excited chromophore emits a virtual photon that is instantly absorbed by a receiving chromophore. These virtual photons are undetectable since their existence violates the conservation of energy and momentum, and hence FRET is known as a radiationless mechanism.

6.2.2 Reverse Transcription PCR (RT-PCR)

Reverse transcription PCR (RT-PCR) is a technique used in genetic studies that enables the detection and quantification of mRNA. It is a very sensitive method that demonstrates whether or not a specific gene is being expressed in a given sample. If the mRNA is present, then the addition of reverse transcriptase, deoxynucleoside triphosphates (dNTPs), and primers will allow the mRNA sequence to be reverse transcribed into a complementary strand of DNA (cDNA). This cDNA strand can then be replicated with primers, dNTPs, and Taq Polymerase by using the standard PCR process, which produces millions of copies of the single-stranded DNA in a short time. Finally, the PCR products (i.e. the cDNA strands) are separated based on size by agarose gel electrophoresis and the molecular weight band corresponding to the target mRNA is scanned for the expression of the associated gene. Alternatively, the PCR products can be quantified optically by fluorescence labeling either at the end of the PCR process or in real time.

Reverse transcription allows us to use PCR (DNA amplification) to indirectly detect a given RNA sequence. For example, some viruses such as influenza, hepatitis C, and polio have only RNA as their genetic material. In order to detect the small amounts of RNA in a viral sample, we need to amplify it. Since we can amplify DNA using PCR, we first create a complementary DNA and then amplify this cDNA to detect the existence of RNA in original sample.

The ability to detect RNA is also important for understanding which genes are being expressed in the cell. All the cells in our body have the same DNA and the same genes. When a gene is expressed, mRNAs are transcribed from those genes. Because diseased cells often experience altered gene expression relative to healthy cells, we can differentiate healthy and diseased cells using RT-PCR.

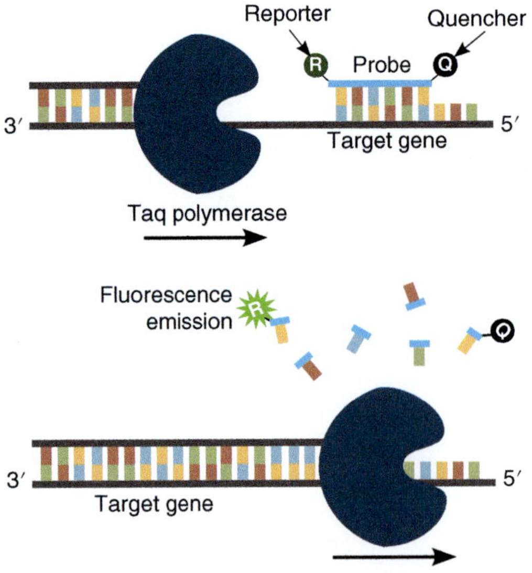

Figure 6.3 Real-time PCR schematic.

6.2.3 Real-Time PCR

In real-time PCR, a.k.a. quantitative PCR (qPCR), the accumulation of PCR product can be detected in "real time" (i.e. as it happens) as opposed to regular PCR in which an assay is performed after the sample amplification is completed. PCR product is detected in real time due to copies that have fluorescently labeled probes (Figure 6.3). Standard curves of the amount of amplification product versus the number of amplification cycles can be plotted. Since the number of amplification cycles needed to reach a certain threshold level of signal depends on the number of starting molecules, standard curves can be obtained from known samples, which allow unknown DNA samples to be quantified by comparing the sample's qPCR plot to the standard curves. The threshold level must be set to achieve a balance between reliability and sensitivity. A low threshold results in low reliability and reproducibility due to background noise, while a high threshold results in low sensitivity.

Figure 6.4 shows an example of a real-time PCR run along with a standard curve (top left). The horizontal axis (x-axis) is the number of PCR cycles performed and the vertical axis (y-axis) is the signal level in relative fluorescence units (RFU). The threshold level is selected where the amplification curve is still exponential. For example, in this case, we can choose our threshold as 0.2 RFU. If we follow the red sample, we can see that it crosses the threshold around 27 cycles. On the other hand, the blue sample crosses the same threshold around 31 cycles. We can use these values to estimate the amount of DNA in the original sample. We use the standard curve for this estimation. The horizontal axis (x-axis) of the standard curve is the concentration (in log scale) and the vertical axis (y-axis) is the number of cycles required to reach the defined threshold value. It is thus easy to find the concentration in the original sample if the number of cycles is known. If the original sample is dilute (few DNAs to begin with), it takes more cycles to reach the threshold value and indeed the standard curve tells us that a higher number of cycles corresponds to a lower concentration.

Did You Know?

There are multiple methods of quantitative PCR. A widely used version of qPCR, sometimes called TaqMan PCR, relies on the 5′-3′ exonuclease activity of Taq polymerase, a type of DNA polymerase harvested from Taq bacteria that is thermally stable at the high temperatures required for PCR. During the PCR process, Taq polymerase extends a DNA segment corresponding to a target gene (Figure 6.3). Then, the polymerase will digest a probe with reporter fluorophore and quenching labels that was bound to the target gene. After the breakdown of the probe, the reporter fluorophore is separated from the quencher and thus the reporter will emit light that can be optically detected. Hence, as PCR proceeds further, more light output will be detected from the probes. The name TaqMan comes from the Taq polymerase and the computer game Pac-Man. It was named after Pac Man because the digestion of the probe by the polymerase resembles the actions of the main character of the game.

Real-time PCR probes are sequence-specific probes that come in different arrangements: e.g. TaqMan has a straight probe that connects a reporter fluorophore and a quencher. It is an irreversible reaction as the straight probe is digested by the polymerase in each cycle if it is annealed to the target gene. In contrast, Molecular Beacons use probes with a hairpin structure. The hairpin extends and closes reversibly in each cycle of PCR and it is not digested by polymerase (Figure 6.5).

6.3 DNA and RNA Chip Technology

6.3.1 Advantages of DNA Chip Technology

A DNA chip can monitor up to tens of thousands of nucleic acids in parallel so that many target genes can be detected simultaneously. This is done with an assay that can read out the relative abundance of nucleic acid sequences, most commonly for mRNA expression profiling. Typically, a fluorescent microarray is used to determine relative abundance of DNA sequences. Fluorescent microarrays are measured with a confocal laser scanner that detects the fluorescent intensity, or ratio of intensities, at a particular location on the array.

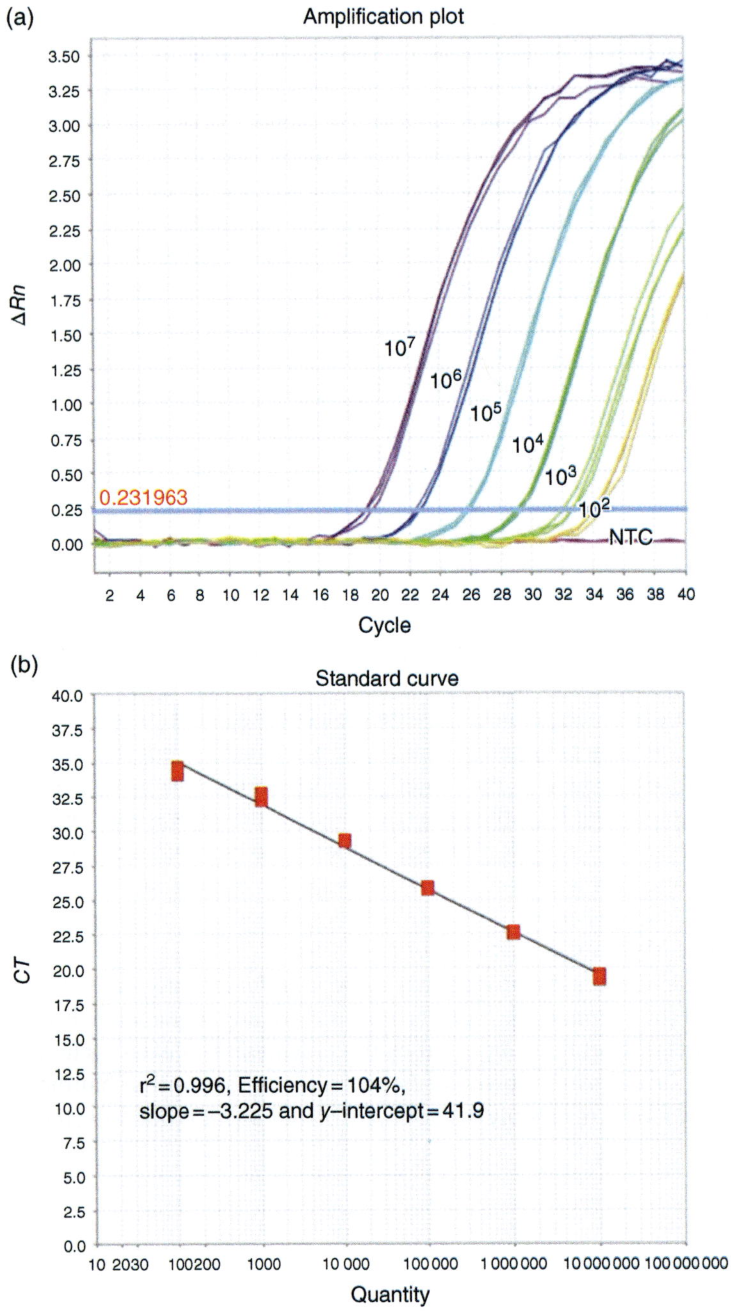

Figure 6.4 Quantitative PCR plot. *Source:* Hajano et al. [3]. Reprinted with permission of the publisher, John Wiley and Sons, Inc. Copyright © 2016 by British Society for Plant Pathology.

6.3.2 Single Color DNA Microarray

The Affymetrix GeneChip is a single-color DNA microarray that uses fluorescent tags to detect the presence of a DNA sample. First, the microarray is prepared by synthesizing probes onto a solid support in situ. Second, the DNA sample is amplified by a PCR process, which creates sufficient

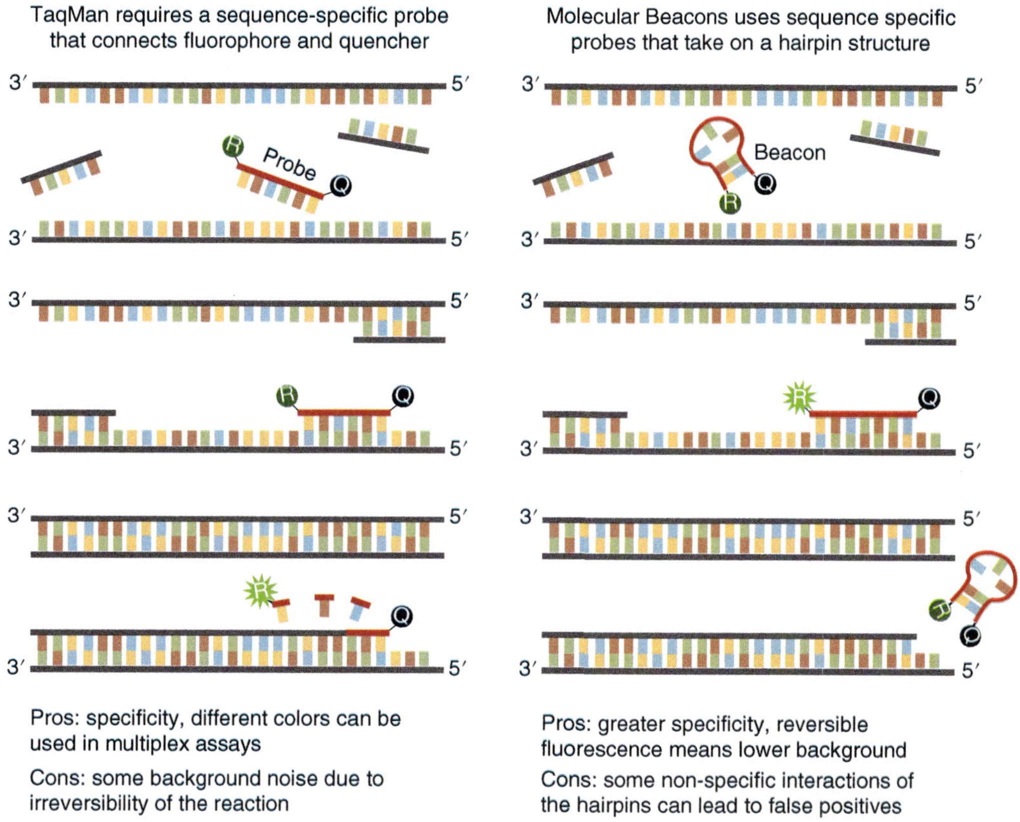

Figure 6.5 Comparison of qPCR probe.

sample for detection. Third, a labeling reaction attaches fluorescent tags onto the test samples. (Note that steps 2 and 3 could be done in a single PCR process.) Finally, when the test samples are added to the microarray, the samples will hybridize with the complementary probes and cause fluorescent light at specific sites that can be detected and quantified (Figure 6.6). The GeneChip is a single-color microarray, so it can only handle one sample at a time.

6.3.3 DNA Chip Fabrication and Technologies

Microarrays can be constructed in a variety of ways (Figure 6.7), but most fall into one of two categories. Using printing pins or inkjets, droplets containing many copies of a sequence of DNA can be directly spotted on a solid substrate. Contact printing involves wetting a printing pin with the DNA solution and tapping it to the microarray surface. Inkjetting ejects uniform droplets of solution onto the substrate. An alternative, known as in situ fabrication, builds the DNA sequence at each site one nucleotide at a time. This is done using either inkjets or photolithography. In inkjetting, solutions of nucleotides are ejected from the nozzle onto the substrate and then chemically fixed to the surface. The next set of nucleotides are jetted onto the first and chemically fixed to those. The process is repeated until the desired set of DNA strands is complete. In photolithography, light at 365 nm is shined through a mask to illuminate a subset of regions on a substrate, which is coated with a photosensitive capping chemical. The light releases the capping chemical, exposing parts of the substrate and rending them capable of coupling to nucleotides. A solution

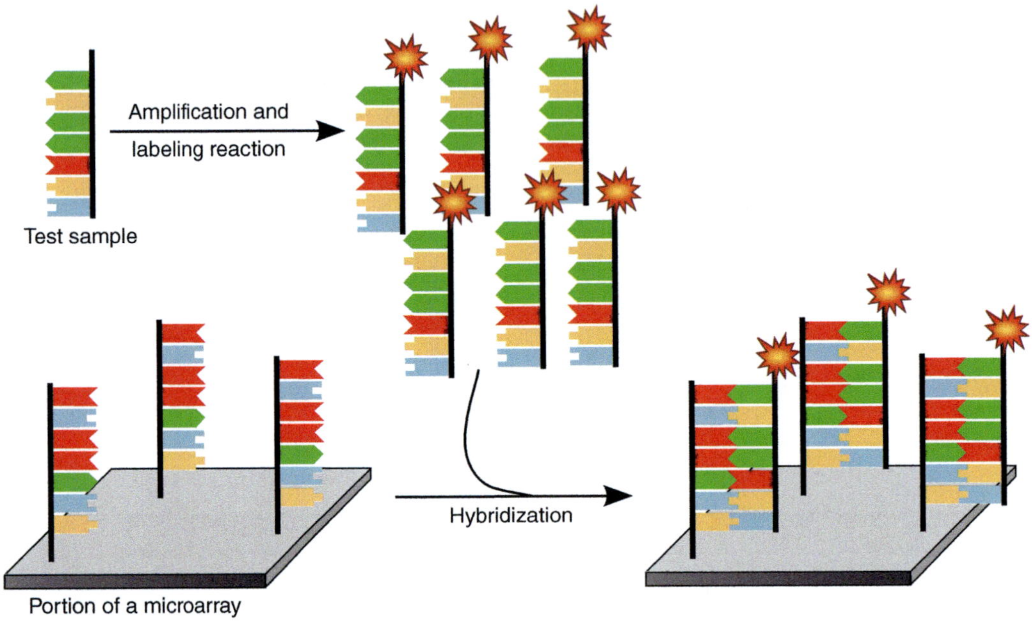

Figure 6.6 GeneChip microarray. *Source:* Courtesy of Chris Webb.

containing a single type of nucleotide attached to a photosensitive chemical is then washed over the substrate. The nucleotides attach to the unprotected sites, adding their own capping layer. The process is repeated, building up sequences of DNA.

Microarray fabrication requires a very clean substrate, which is most commonly glass, silicon coated with SiO_2, or gold. The SiO_2 surface is often functionalized by an alkylsilanization process (Figure 6.8, left half), so that various terminal functional groups can be introduced to the surface for DNA or protein immobilization. Microarrays with gold substrates typically use gold-thiol coupling to form a self-assembled monolayer (SAM) with a functional group at the end (Figure 6.8, right half).

6.3.4 Target Sequence and Tiling Probes

Affymetrix utilizes its DNA chips for single nucleotide polymorphism (SNP) detection. When samples of a single DNA strand are compared across different people, there will be some nucleotide variation from person to person at the same locus (a location on the DNA strand). A PCR primer is designed to target the same location of DNA strands from many people. For example, if a target sequence is . . .tttcca<u>gacagactcctatggtgacttctct</u>ggaaaa. . ., the perfect match (PM) probe (25 bases long, called 25-mer) and the underlined target region (Allele 1) are completely complementary, while the mismatch (MM) probe differs from PM probe just by one base (A changed to T in the middle base position of the 25-mer probe), as shown in Figure 6.9. Each assay column corresponds to different alleles, and the PM probes for different alleles are arranged in the same row. The measurements are interpreted by first throwing out the high and low probes (outliers), and excluding any PM-MM values that are more than three standard deviations from the mean. The remaining PM-MM values and their corresponding targets are counted as detected alleles.

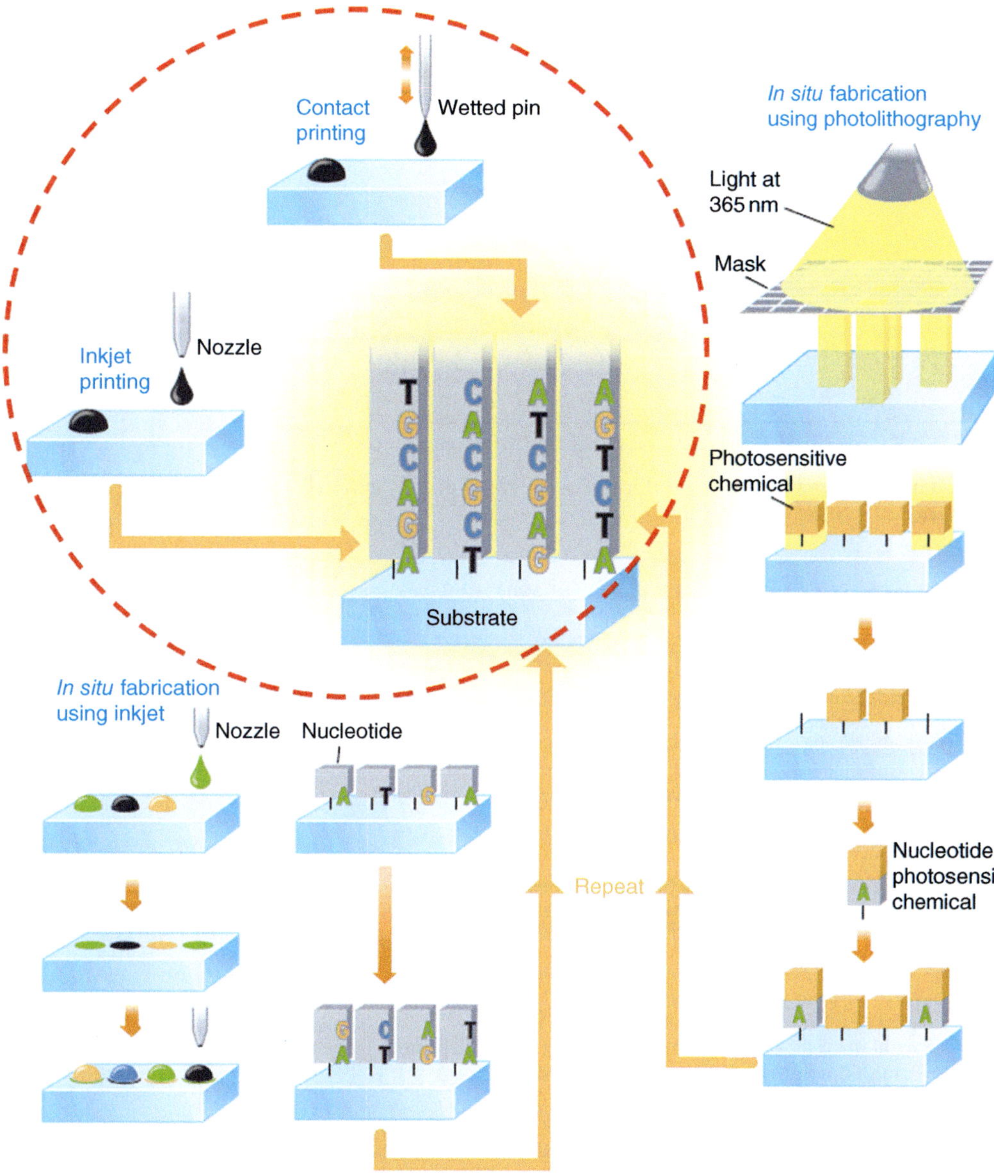

Figure 6.7 DNA chip fabrication techniques. *Source:* Moore [4]. Reprinted, with permission of IEEE. Copyright © 2001 IEEE.

6.3.5 DNA and RNA Mass Detection

Looking at a target gene can aid in subtyping cancer. However, diseases due to infectious agents can be identified as foreign genetic material (DNA or RNA) within a patient sample. One method to identify the host organism of the foreign genetic material (i.e. the organism that is causing the disease) is to count the number of each type of nucleotide base (A, C, G, and T or U) in a specific region of the foreign genetic material. Counting the number of bases provides a "fingerprint" for several different microorganisms. That is, by determining the number of each type of nucleotide

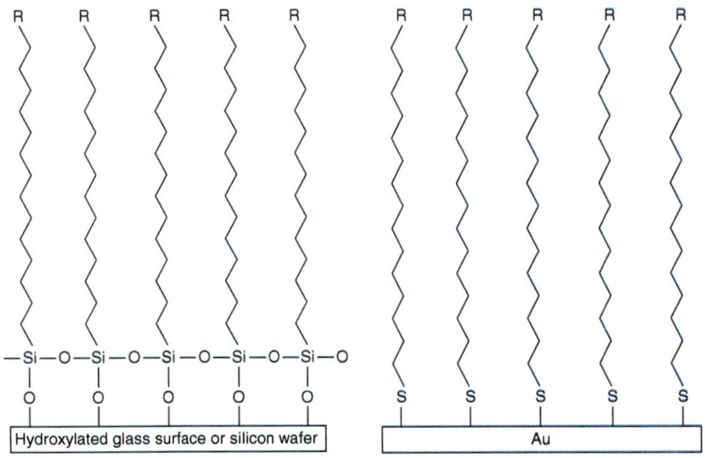

Figure 6.8 Functionalized microarray surfaces. *Source:* Wu et al. [5]. Reprinted by permission of the publisher, Taylor & Francis.

Target sequence (129 bases, >37 bases shown)

...tttccagacagactcctatggtgacttctctggaaaa...

Probe pair for one allele

ctgtctgaggataccactgaagaga **Perfect match (PM)**

ctgtctgaggattccactgaagaga **Mismatch (MM)**

Microarray Image (partial)

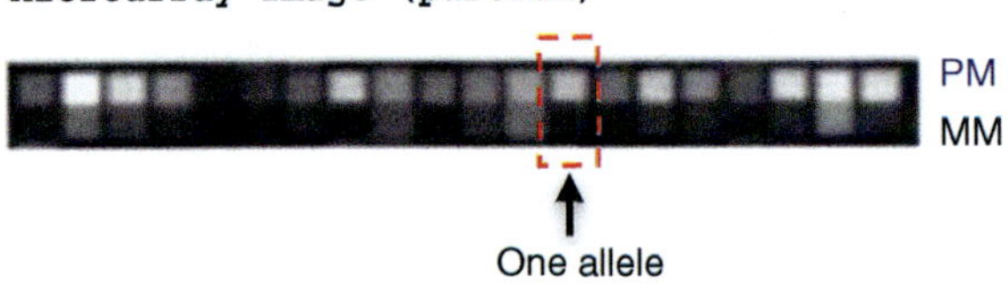

Figure 6.9 Partial microarray image. *Source:* Kunz et al. [6]. Reprinted by permission of the publisher, John Wiley and Sons, Inc. Copyright © 2004 by Blackwell Munksgaard.

base in a specific region, one can identify the host microorganism. To count the number of bases, the foreign genetic material is first amplified via PCR. Special primers called broad-range primers are used. Broad range primers are designed to target very select sequences of DNA or RNA that provide a "fingerprint" of the organism. These sequences contain two regions, a conserved region and a variable region (Figure 6.10). The conserved region is a sequence of DNA that is present in a broad range of organisms (e.g. bacteria that can be tinted with a Gram stain, which gives information about the structural makeup of the cell wall). The conserved region narrows down the potential microorganism to a general category (e.g. gram-positive or gram-negative). The variable region then identifies a specific species within a category. For example, the variable region can identify *Staphylococcus aureus* from gram-positive bacteria; Methicillin-resistant *S. aureus* (a.k.a. MRSA) has been the culprit of many hospital outbreaks. After amplification by PCR with broad-range primers, the DNA samples are run through a mass spectrometer. In a mass spectrometer, the samples are ionized and then passed through a magnetic field. The now-charged samples are deflected in the magnetic field based on their mass. Therefore, the mass spectrometer measures the weight of each sequence of DNA. Based on this weight, one can deduce the number of each type of base present in the sample as each base has a different molecular weight.

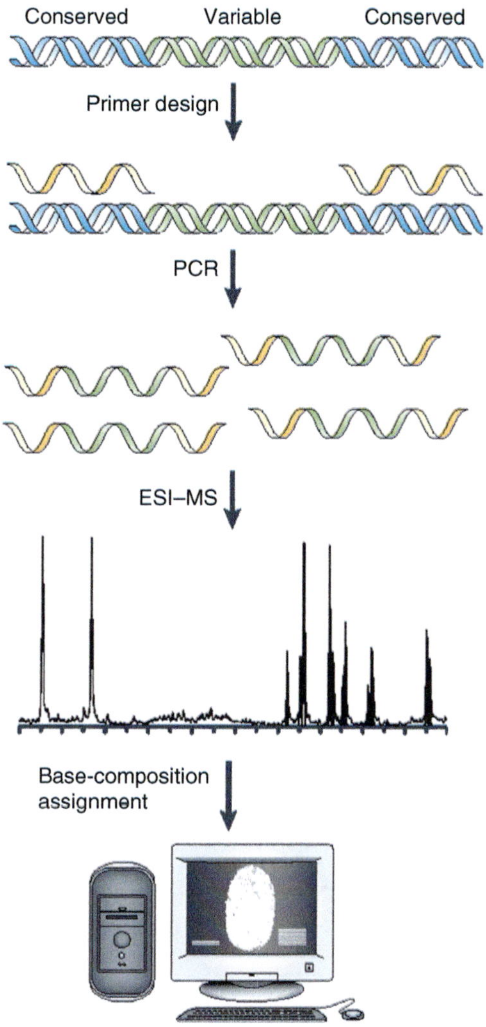

Figure 6.10 Steps for identifying infectious agents based on molecular weight of DNA. *Source:* Ecker et al. [7]. Reprinted by permission from the publisher, Springer Nature. Copyright © 2008 by Nature Publishing Group.

6.3.6 Spotted cDNA Chips (Microarrays)

Spotted cDNA chips are used to detect the relative gene expression of different samples, e.g. those of tumor cells versus normal cells (Figure 6.11). First, probes are spotted on the chips. Second, samples of mRNA strands are extracted from a pool of cell lines and tumor cells. Third, reverse transcription PCR is performed on the mRNA samples to produce many copies of cDNA strands. Fourth, these cDNA strands are labeled with green and red dyes, respectively, and then incubated in a DNA microarray. A red spot on the chip indicates the presence of mRNA in the tumor cell, while a green spot indicates the presence of mRNA in the pool of cell lines. In other words, red color indicates that the tumor cells expressed the corresponding mRNA strand. The specific mRNA is identified by the location on the microarray since a unique probe set was placed at every spot. Occasionally, a yellow spot is produced, which indicates that both the cell lines and tumor cells expressed the same gene and produced a mixture of green and red colors. Analysis of the exact color can determine the relative expression of each type of mRNA. Spotted cDNA chips often use two colors so that two samples can be processed simultaneously.

6.3.7 Gene Expression Profiling with RNA Samples

A microarray can also be used for gene expression profiling with RNA samples, without the need for reverse transcription PCR to amplify the signals (Figure 6.12). One option uses two mRNA samples from two different people on a single chip, as in the spotted cDNA chip. Another option is to use two single-color chips, one for each person's RNA sample. Then data processing can be used to read and quantify the measurements, which results in reliable and reproducible results.

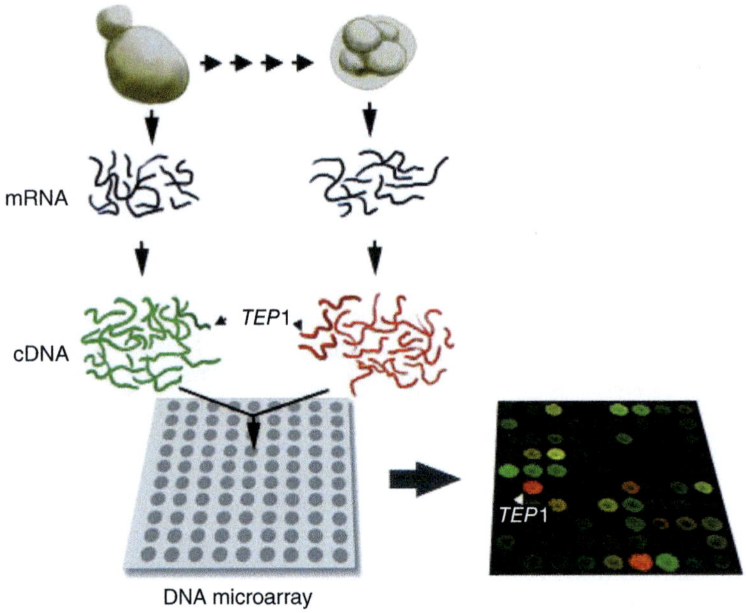

Figure 6.11 Spotted DNA microarray process. *Source:* Brown and Botstein [8]. Reprinted by permission from the publisher, Springer Nature. Copyright © 1999 by Nature America Inc.

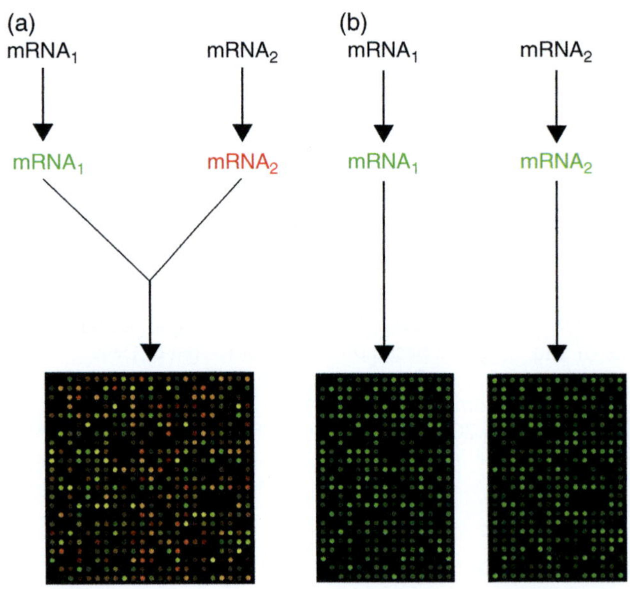

Figure 6.12 Gene expression profiling with RNA. (a) Two-channel microarray. (b) Single-channel microarrays.

Two-color microarrays or two-channel microarrays are typically hybridized with cDNA prepared from two samples to be compared (e.g. diseased tissue vs. healthy tissue) and are labeled with two different fluorophores. Fluorescent dyes commonly used for cDNA labeling include Cy3, which has a fluorescence emission wavelength of 570 nm (corresponding to the green part of the light spectrum), and Cy5 with a fluorescence emission wavelength of 670 nm (corresponding to the red part of the light spectrum). The two Cy-labeled cDNA samples are mixed and hybridized to a single microarray that is then scanned in a microarray scanner to visualize fluorescence of the two fluorophores after excitation with a laser beam of a defined wavelength. Relative intensities of each fluorophore may then be used in ratio-based analysis to identify upregulated and downregulated genes.

Several popular single-channel systems are the Affymetrix "Gene Chip", Illumina "Bead Chip", Agilent single-channel arrays, the Applied Microarrays "CodeLink" arrays, and the Eppendorf "DualChip" and "Silverquant." One strength of the single-dye system lies in the fact that an aberrant sample cannot affect the raw data derived from other samples because each array chip is exposed to only one sample (as opposed to a two-color system in which a single low-quality sample may drastically impinge on overall data precision even if the other sample was of high quality). Another benefit is that data are more easily compared to arrays from different experiments so long as batch effects have been accounted for. A drawback to the one-color system is that when compared to the two-color system, twice as many microarrays are needed to compare samples within an experiment.

6.3.8 Nanostring Multiplex RNA Assay

An RNA assay is a technology used to detect and quantify the presence of a particular mRNA segment in a sample. An RNA assay can provide useful information about the gene expression of a particular sample of cells. The Nanostring multiplex RNA assay is capable of detecting many different types of mRNA strands simultaneously. This nCounter system is capable of sensitive, precise, and quantitative measurements with no amplification required. First, the mRNA sample is incubated with multiple types of reporter and capture probes, which correspond to different mRNA segments. During the incubation process, the mRNA segments of interest undergo hybridization. After excess reporter and capture probes are removed, the remaining reporter and capture probe complexes are bound to a surface and oriented. Finally, the surface is imaged and reporter probes are decoded. The measurement output indicates both the gene that was expressed as well as the number of copies of each mRNA segment that was detected. The Nanostring multiplex RNA assay has been perfected to multiplex up to 400 mRNA strands simultaneously.

6.3.9 Important Concepts

Sensitivity or limit of detection is the smallest signal that can be reliably detected and is affected by the signal-to-noise ratio and whether the signal is biological or electrical. Specificity is determined by how well the system can discriminate between similar biomolecules and between the analyte and impurities. Dynamic range is the linear range of detection. In order for detection to occur, the signal must be above the background. For a signal to be above the background, the signal minus the local background must be positive and must be above some threshold. This threshold, the limit of detection, is often defined as two or three standard deviations of the local background.

6.4 DNA Sequencing

6.4.1 Sanger Method of DNA Sequencing

The Sanger method is the traditional process for DNA sequencing in which the nucleotide sequence that makes up a strand of DNA is identified. First, the DNA molecule to be sequenced is digested into many smaller segments of different length. Second, deoxynucleotides and dideoxynucleotides are added to the solution, which will be incorporated into the DNA strands during chain elongation in a PCR-like process. Because all four normal nucleotides are present, chain elongation proceeds normally until, by chance, DNA polymerase inserts a dideoxynucleotide instead of the normal deoxynucleotide. If the ratio of normal nucleotide to the dideoxy versions is high enough, some DNA strands will succeed in adding several hundred nucleotides before insertion of the dideoxy version halts the process. The result is DNA strands with random length, which can be separated by electrophoresis. The dideoxynucleotides of successively longer fragments are then identified; a laser is used to activate the fluorescent dideoxynucleotides and a detector distinguishes the colors. Thus, the original sequence of the template strand is obtained (Figure 6.13).

6.4.1.1 Sanger Sequencing by Capillary Electrophoresis

The ABI Prism 310 genetic analyzer is a machine that performs a modified version of the Sanger DNA sequencing. It performs a non-gel form of electrophoresis by applying a large electric field on the capillary causing the DNA segments to migrate through the capillary, segments of different lengths will reach the end at different times. The DNA segments can then be ordered by length based on the timing of their arrival at the outlet of the capillary. Finally, a fluorescence detector can identify the DNA sequences using the Sanger Sequencing method (Figure 6.14).

6.4.2 Shotgun Sequencing

The chain termination method of DNA sequencing can only be used for fairly short strands (100–1000 base pairs), longer sequences must be subdivided into smaller fragments, and subsequently reassembled to give the overall sequence. In shotgun sequencing, multiple overlapping "reads" for the target DNA are obtained by performing several rounds of random fragmentation and sequencing (Table 6.1). Computer programs then use the overlapping ends of different reads to assemble them into a continuous sequence. Multiple rounds are needed to overcome sequencing errors and ambiguity of repetitive sequences from different loci. In the Human Genome Project (1990–2003), most of the genome was sequenced at 12× or greater coverage, meaning that each base in the final sequence is present in 12 reads on average.

6.5 Conclusion

DNA microarrays are widely used to detect the presence of a DNA or RNA segments in a sample. Using a high-density array of probes attached to a solid support, a DNA chip can monitor up to tens of thousands of nucleic acids in parallel so that many target genes can be detected simultaneously. PCR or RT-PCR can be used for signal amplification of DNA and mRNA samples, respectively, and quantitative PCR is widely used to quantitate a few unknown DNA sequences in a sample. DNA sequencing of an entire genome can be performed either by the traditional Sanger method or several different types of next-generation sequencing techniques.

6.6 Additional Information

6.6.1 Southern, Northern, Western, and Eastern Blotting

Northern blotting of mRNA is used to identify a target mRNA of interest (Figure 6.15). First, the RNA is separated by agarose gel electrophoresis in which an electric field will separate an unknown

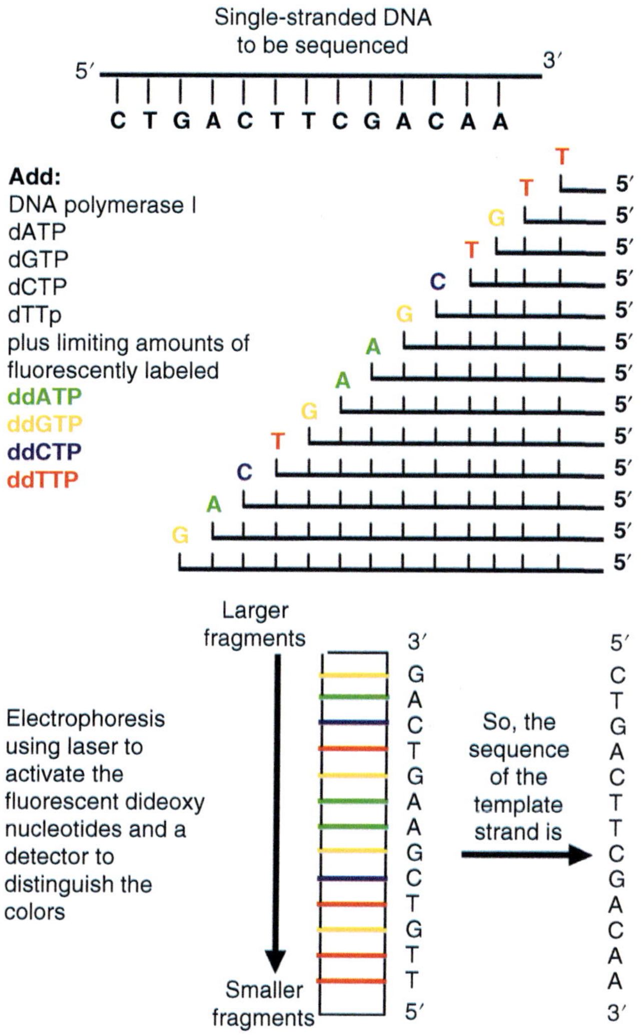

Figure 6.13 DNA sequencing by Sanger method. *Source:* Kimball [9]. Used under CC-BY 3.0 http://creativecommons.org/licenses/by/3.0.

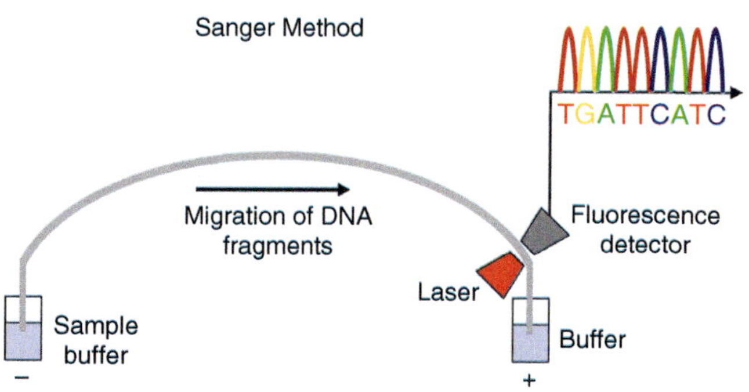

Figure 6.14 Capillary electrophoresis. *Source:* Lakdawalla [10]. CC0-1.0 public domain https://creativecommons.org/publicdomain/zero/1.0.

Table 6.1 Shotgun method.

Strand	Sequence
Original	A G C A T G C T G C A G T C A T G C T T A G G C T A
First shotgun sequence	A G C A T G C T G C A G T C A T G C T - - - - - - -
	- - - - - - - - - - - - - - - - - - - T A G G C T A
Second shotgun sequence	A G C A T G -
	- - - - - - C T G C A G T C A T G C T T A G G C T A
Reconstruction	A G C A T G C T G C A G T C A T G C T T A G G C T A

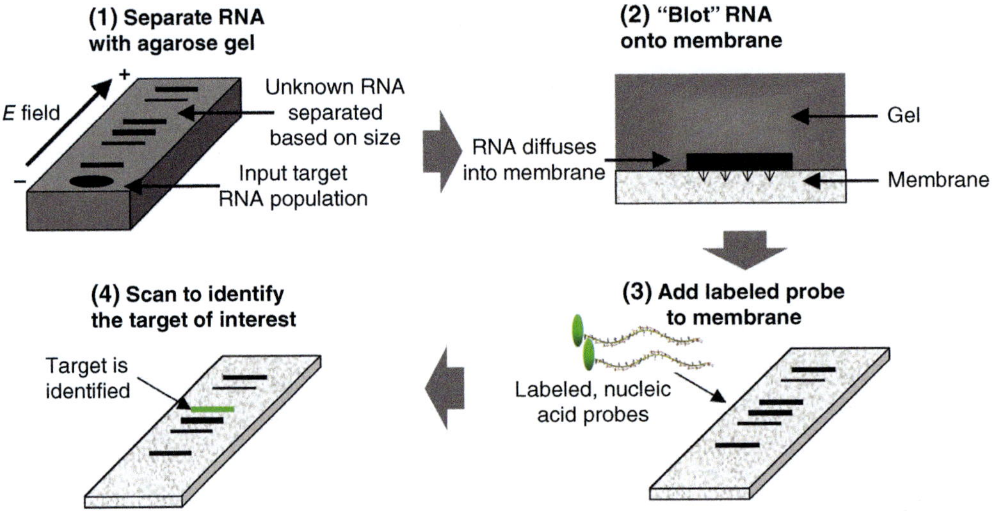

Figure 6.15 Northern blotting technique. *Source:* Conzone and Pantano [11]. Reprinted with permission from Elsevier. Copyright © 2004.

RNA sample into separate bands based on molecular weight. Second, the RNA is blotted (transferred) onto a membrane, which causes the RNA to diffuse into the membrane. Third, labeled nucleic acid probes are added to the membrane. Finally, the membrane is scanned to identify the band corresponding to the target RNA of interest. Similar blotting procedures can be done to detect DNA (Southern blotting) or protein (Western blotting). For Southern blotting, an additional denaturation step (to yield single-stranded DNA) is added before the blotting step. In Western blotting, the proteins can be separated based on isoelectric point, molecular weight, electric charge, or a combination of these factors based on the sample preparation method and the nature of the gel. Since Western blotting is identifying proteins, it utilizes labeled antibodies as opposed to labeled nucleic acid probes. Finally, there are several detection mechanisms for Western blots including colorimetric, chemiluminescent, radioactive, and fluorescent. A drawback to Northern blotting is its low sensitivity, thus a large number of RNA molecules are needed. Likewise, Southern blotting or Western blotting is not very sensitive either. An interesting fact about the naming is that Southern blotting was first developed by Edwin Southern for DNA detection. Northern blotting (for RNA), Western blotting (for proteins), and Eastern blotting (for protein modifications) were named after Southern blotting based on the similarity of the technique.

Problems

6.1 In practice, during each thermal cycle of PCR, the number of DNA strands multiplies by a factor of $1+E$, where E is the PCR efficiency ($0 \leq E \leq 100\%$). If E is a constant throughout the entire PCR process and we know that the number of DNA strands has increased by a factor of one million, find the value of E.

6.2 In real-time PCR, the efficiency in a thermal cycle is $E = 75\%$ and it is constant throughout all PCR cycles. We also know that each fluorophore produces signal S. Assuming that we start with a single piece of double-stranded DNA, find the signal amplitude after 15 thermal cycles when the probe is a molecular beacon versus Taqman.
Note: You can further assume that the fluorescent intensities do not reach saturation amplitude in 15 cycles.

6.3 **A** In a real-time PCR, all the reactions reach some saturated fluorescent intensity after a certain number of cycles. Using Google or any appropriate reference tool, find at least two reasons for this saturation phenomenon.
B Explain how the fluorescence in real-time PCR based on molecular beacon is indeed "reversible."

6.4 You are trying to design a probe for your own qPCR (quantitative PCR). Which of the probes in Table 6.2 do you think is the best (in terms of signal-to-noise ratio)? Hint: The size of a nucleobase is 3.3 Å.

Table 6.2 Parameters for three different qPCR probes.

	Minimum number of nucleobases to anneal	R_0 (Förster distance) (nm)
SuperProbe	18	6.0
Probe Leland	20	6.7
ThermoProbe	24	7.2

6.5 Jane tried to measure the number of copies of p53 mutated genes in her cancer cells by using qPCR. To do that, she obtained known p53 mutated DNA at a concentration of one million copies per milliliter. Three more samples were prepared by diluting this sample 10-fold serially (10×, 100×, and 1000×). She transferred 10 μl of each sample to individual reaction wells and DNA isolated from the cancer cells to another well. To evaluate the background signal level of the system, she measured some buffer solutions that contain DNA and probes without any polymerase. The fluorescent intensities of the five background signal measurements were 1.1, 0.9, 1.0, 1.1, and 1.0. According to the manufacturer of the qPCR kit, the efficiency is 0.5 and each reporter generates a fluorescent intensity of 10^{-6} upon separation from the quencher. After 30 cycles, she found that the pH of the reagents was accidentally changed and the efficiency dropped to 0.1, but the brightness of the reporter remained the same. The experiment was terminated after 40 cycles.
A What signals will she obtain from the four standard samples? Please sketch a graph (fluorescent intensity vs. amplification cycle) and clearly indicate your threshold,

which can be defined as the mean background level plus two standard deviations. You may want to use a log scale for fluorescent intensity, which ranges from 10^{-1} to 10^4.

B If the signal from the cancer cell DNA becomes higher than your threshold after 20 cycles, how many copies of p53 mutated DNA are in the cancer cell sample?

6.6 Your advisor asked you to design a DNA microarray to detect one segment of the sequence of human immunodeficiency virus (HIV). The target sequence is 5′ ACT GGC GAA AGG GAT TGG CAC 3′.

A You plan to have a 21-mer prefer match (PM) probe as well as its mismatch (MM) probe as a control for cross-hybridization. What is the probe pair for this virus sequence? Please indicate the 5′ and 3′ ends clearly.

B With the DNA microarray, you realized that you can also detect corresponding mRNA by using reverse transcription polymerase chain reaction (RT-PCR). Now, you plan to test the central dogma by developing an immunoassay for the peptide translated from this mRNA. What is the target peptide you need to detect? You may assume a start codon and end codon are located at the 5′ end and 3′ end of this sequence, respectively. Would a sandwich assay or direct assay be better for detecting this peptide? Explain your rationale.

6.7 What is the advantage of gene expression profiling with cDNA chips where RNA is reverse transcribed compared to microarray where RNA samples are used directly?

References

1 Geb, C. *Basic Principles of Luminescence*. Leica Science Lab.

2 Alberts, B. *Molecular Biology of the Cell*, 5e. Garland Science.

3 Hajano, J., Zhang, H.B., Ren, Y.D. et al. (2016). Screening of rice (Oryza sativa) cultivars for resistance to rice black streaked dwarf virus using quantitative PCR and visual disease assessment. *Plant Pathol* 65: 1509–1517. https://doi.org/10.1111/ppa.12534.

4 Moore, S.K. (1 Mar 2001). Making Chips to Probe Genes. IEEE Spectrum: Technology, Engineering, and Science News, IEEE Spectrum. http://spectrum.ieee.org/biomedical/diagnostics/making-chips-to-probe-genes.

5 Wu, P., Castner, D.G., and Grainger, D.W. (2008). Diagnostic devices as biomaterials: a review of nucleic acid and protein microarray surface performance issues. *J Biomater Sci Polym Ed.* 19 (6): 725–753.

6 Kunz, M., Ibrahim, S.M., Koczan, D. et al. (2004). DNA microarray technology and its applications in dermatology. *Experimental Dermatology* 13: 593–606. https://doi.org/10.1111/j.0906-6705.2004.00243.x.

7 Ecker, D.J., Sampath, R., Massire, C. et al. (2008). Ibis T5000: a universal biosensor approach for microbiology. *Nature Reviews Microbiology* 6 (7): 553–558. https://doi.org/10.1038/nrmicro1918. http://www.nature.com/nrmicro/journal/v6/n7/abs/nrmicro1918.html.

8 Brown, P.O. and Botstein, D. (1999 Jan). Exploring the new world of the genome with DNA microarrays. *Nat Genet.* 21 (1 Suppl): 33–37.

9 Kimball, J.W. Online biology textbook. Kimball's Biology Pages © John W. Kimball. http://www.biology-pages.info/D/DNAsequencing.html

10 Abizar Lakdawalla, https://commons.wikimedia.org/wiki/ File:CE_Basic.jpg. CC0-1.0 public domain https://creativecommons.org/publicdomain/zero/1.0/.

11 Conzone, S.D. and Pantano, C.G. Glass slides to DNA microarrays. *Materials Today* 7 (3): 20–26.

7

Next-Generation Sequencing and FET-Based Biochips

7.1 Introduction to Next-Generation Sequencing

Previously, we have seen that Sanger sequencing can be used to determine and quantify DNA sequences. However, this conventional sequencing method has limitations in throughput, scalability, and speed. To overcome these, next-generation sequencing (NGS) can enable high-throughput decoding of DNA molecules up to the scale of the entire human genome.

7.1.1 Conventional Versus Next-Generation Sequencing

The workflows of conventional and next-generation (or second-generation) sequencing are shown in Figure 7.1. With high-throughput shotgun Sanger sequencing (Figure 7.1a), genomic DNA is fragmented and cloned to a plasmid vector, which is then used to transform E. coli. For each sequencing reaction, a single bacterial colony is picked and its plasmid DNA is isolated. During each cycle of a single sequencing run, a sequencing reaction takes place within a microliter-scale volume, generating a ladder of ddNTP-terminated, dye-labeled products, which are subjected to high-resolution electrophoretic separation within one of 96 or 384 capillaries. As fluorescently labeled fragments of discrete sizes pass a detector, the four-channel emission spectrum is used to generate a sequencing trace. Sanger sequencing can be applied to read DNA sequences with lengths up to about 1000 bp and costs about $0.50 per kilobase.

The concept of cyclic-array sequencing (Figure 7.1b) can be summarized as the sequencing of a dense array of DNA features by iterative cycles of enzymatic manipulation and imaging-based data collection. First, common adaptors are ligated to fragmented genomic DNA, which is then subjected to one of several protocols that results in an array of millions of spatially immobilized PCR colonies or "polonies." Each polony consists of many copies of a single shotgun library fragment. As all polonies are tethered to a planar array, a single microliter-scale reagent volume (e.g. for primer hybridization and then for enzymatic extension reactions) can be applied to manipulate all array features in parallel. Similarly, imaging-based detection of fluorescent labels incorporated with each extension can be used to acquire sequencing data on all features in parallel. Successive iterations of enzymatic interrogation and imaging are used to build up a contiguous sequencing read for each array feature. Note that not all next-generation methods rely on optical-based data; rather, some detect electrical signal associated with nucleotide addition. Methods based on both types will be discussed in this chapter.

Biochips and Medical Imaging, First Edition. Adam de la Zerda and Shan Xiang Wang.

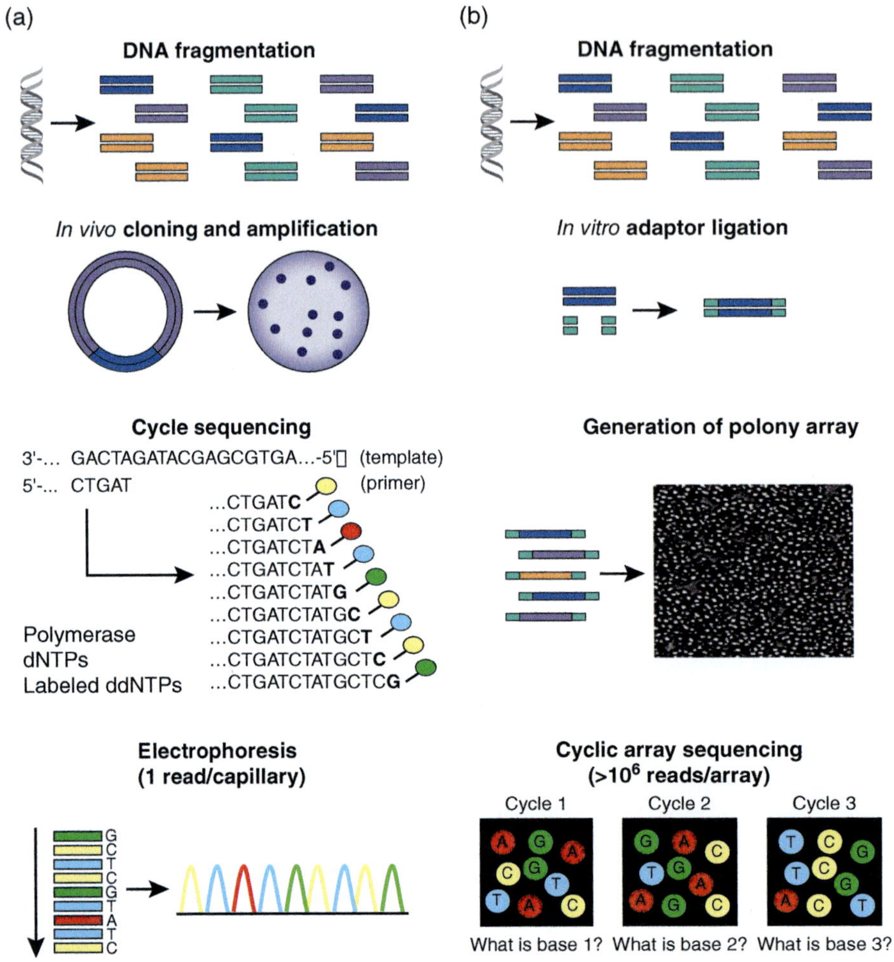

Figure 7.1 (a) Conventional and (b) second-generation DNA sequencing schemes. *Source:* Shendure and Ji [1]. Reprinted by permission from Springer Nature. Copyright 2008 by Springer Nature.

7.2 Optical-Based Methods

7.2.1 Illumina/Solexa Genome Analyzer

The Illumina/Solexa Genome Analyzer platform is an example of NGS technology, which can sequence in parallel many adaptor-flanked fragments up to several hundred base-pairs (bp) in length. Amplified sequencing features are generated by bridge PCR (Figure 7.2). In this approach, both forward and reverse PCR primers are tethered to a solid substrate by a flexible linker (i.e. "bridged"), such that all amplicons arising from any single template molecule during the amplification remain immobilized and clustered to a single physical location on an array. The resulting "clusters" each consist of ~1000 clonal amplicons. Several million clusters can be amplified to distinguishable locations within each of the eight independent "lanes" that are on a single flow-cell (such that eight independent libraries can be sequenced in parallel during the same instrument run). After cluster generation, the amplicons are single-stranded (linearized) and a sequencing primer is hybridized to a universal sequence flanking the region of

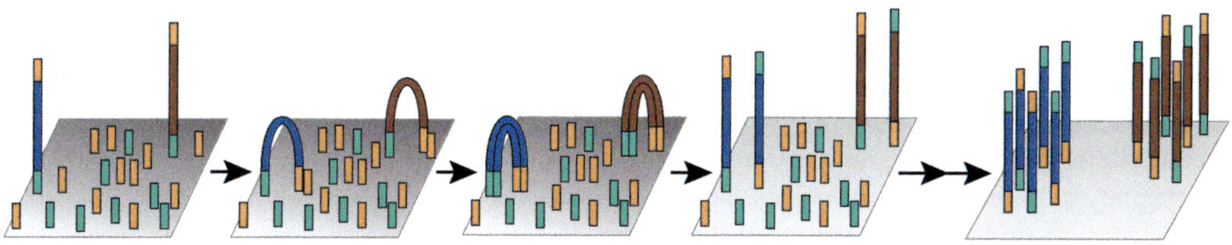

Figure 7.2 Illumina/Solexa – bridge PCR. *Source:* Shendure and Ji [1]. Reprinted by permission from Springer Nature. Copyright 2008 by Springer Nature.

interest. Each cycle of sequence interrogation consists of a single-base extension with a modified DNA polymerase and a mixture of four nucleotides. These nucleotides are modified in two ways. They are "reversible terminators" in that a chemically cleavable moiety at the 3′ hydroxyl position allows only a single-base incorporation to occur in each cycle; and one of four fluorescent labels, also chemically cleavable, corresponds to the identity of each nucleotide. After single-base extension and acquisition of images in four channels, chemical cleavage of both groups sets up for the next cycle. Read lengths up to 36 bp are currently routine; longer reads are possible but may incur a higher error rate.

The Illumina/Solexa platform is an example of sequencing by synthesis, where a complementary strand is built based on the sequence of a template strand, which is extended in cycles (Figure 7.3). During each cycle, sequencing reagents are added one at a time and the first base that is incorporated will generate a corresponding signal that will give the next nucleobase in the sequence. In general, the enzyme driving the sequencing by synthesis can be either a polymerase or a ligase and data are acquired by imaging the full array of fluorescently labeled nucleotides at each cycle.

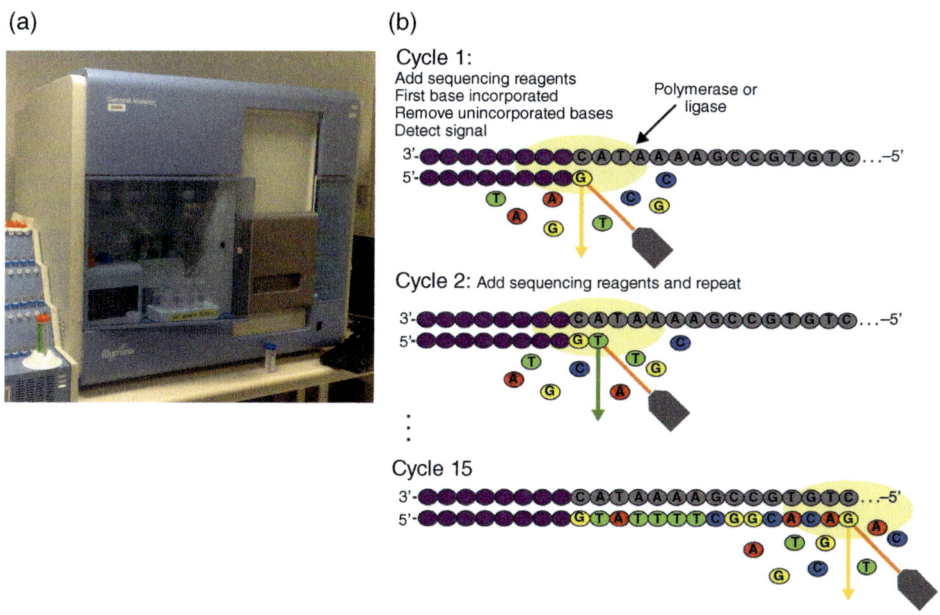

Figure 7.3 (a) Illumina/Solexa machine. *Source:* Jon Callas [2]. Used under CC-BY-2.0 http://creativecommons.org/licenses/by/2.0/. (b) Schematic of detection by synthesis.

7.2.2 454 Pyrosequencing

454 Life Sciences (acquired by Roche) was the first to implement an NGS method – 454 pyrosequencing (Figure 7.4). While the system is no longer in circulation, it is nonetheless informative to understand the methodology. Rather than tagging individual nucleotides, the 454 system detects a single signal common to all nucleotides. The nucleotides are added iteratively to ensure that only one type of nucleotide is responsible for the detected signal. The 454 system relies on template-bound beads, which are placed into a PicoTiterPlate along with an enzyme cocktail. The incorporation of a nucleotide triggers an enzyme cascade that ends with the conversion of luciferin into oxyluciferin, for which the by-product is light. Iterating through the nucleotides and measuring the light signal allows for the sequence to be tracked. As shown in the right side of Figure 7.4, when multiple of the same bases are incorporated in a row (i.e. homopolymer regions), the signal is proportional to the length of the region.

7.2.3 SOLiD

Similar to the Illumina and 454 systems, the SOLiD system by Thermo Fisher relies on optical detection for sequencing. However, sequencing is done by ligation rather than by synthesis (Figure 7.5). Ligation is initiated with the binding of an anchor sequence (purple) to a known adapter sequence (red). The SOLiD platform then utilizes fluorophore-labeled two-base-encoded probes, which are composed of known nucleotides in the first two positions (blue) followed by degenerate or universal bases (pink). After a probe has been added, the terminal degenerate bases and fluorophore are cleaved leaving five bound nucleotides. The process is repeated ten times until two out of every five bases are identified. The strand is then reset by removing all of the ligated bases. This entire process is then repeated four times each with an anchor sequence that has been

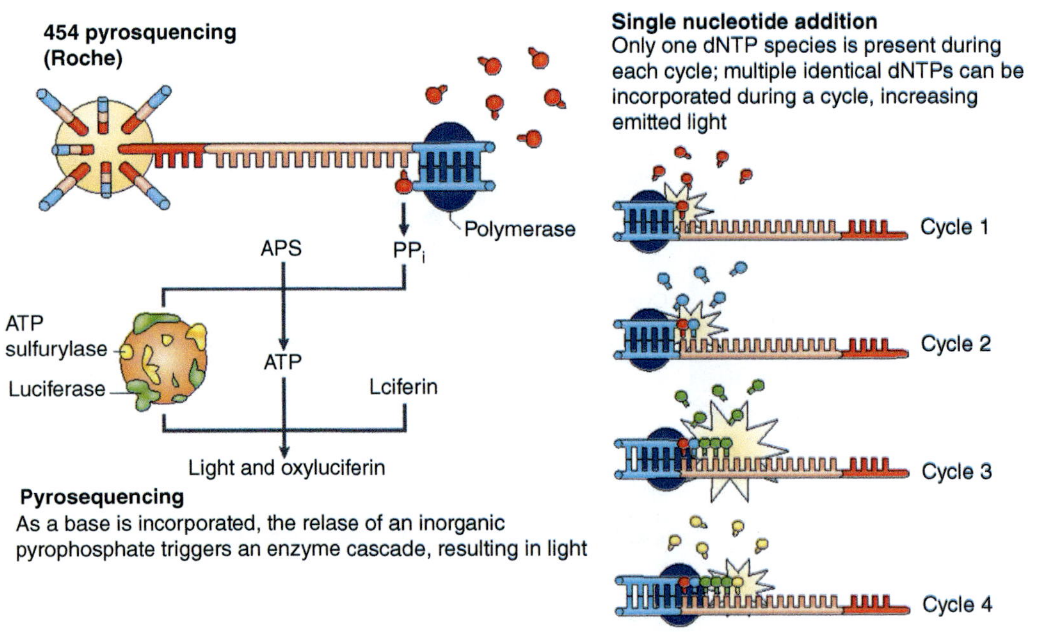

Figure 7.4 Schematic of 454 pyrosequencing technique. *Source:* Goodwin [3]. Reprinted by permission from Springer Nature. Copyright 2016 by Springer Nature.

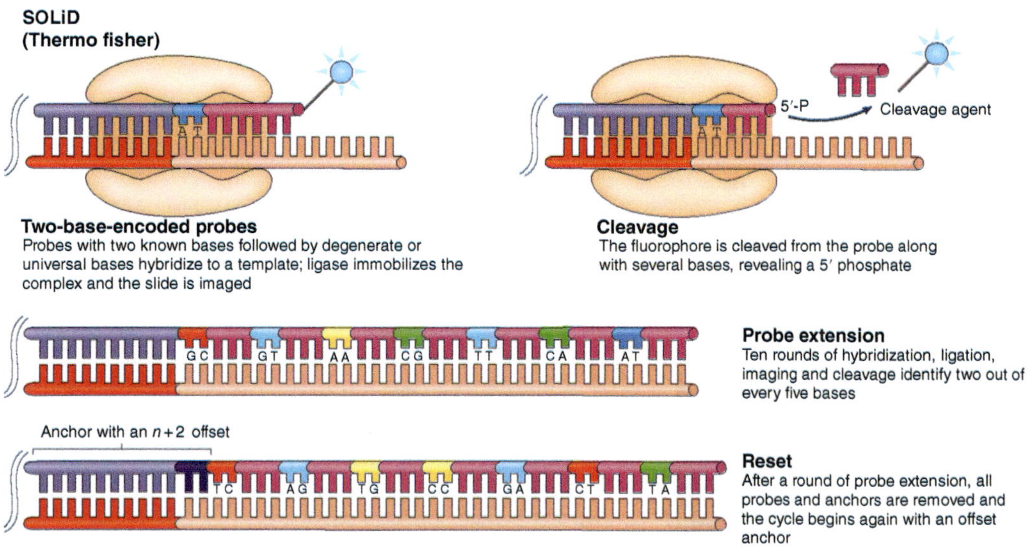

Figure 7.5 Method utilized by SOLiD, which is based on fluorophore-labeled two-base-encoded probes. *Source:* Goodwin [3]. Reprinted by permission from Springer Nature. Copyright 2016 by Springer Nature.

extended by a single base (i.e. with anchor offsets of $n+1$, $n+2$, $n+3$, and $n+4$). Since the SOLiD system works with pairs of bases, there are 16 possible signals (i.e. 16 possible dinucleotide combinations); these 16 signals cannot be individually associated with spectrally resolvable fluorophores. Therefore, only four fluorescent signals are used, each of which represents four possible dinucleotide combinations. To determine the sequence of individual bases, the signals must be deconvoluted during data analysis (the overlap of the several runs allows for this deconvolution).

7.2.4 HeliScope

The Helicos Genetic Analysis System is similar to Illumina in that it performs sequencing based on single nucleotide addition. However, the system is unique because it does not require any clonal amplification making the system capable of single molecule sequencing. To achieve a resolution down to single molecule, the system utilizes a proprietary substrate to capture single DNA molecules on the surface (no amplification required) and then uses an extremely sensitive fluorescence detection system (based on evanescent wave microscopy and single-pair FRET) to interrogate the molecules (Figure 7.6). The use of "virtual" terminators prevents the addition of more than one base at a time. Single molecule sequencers are attractive because of their promise to deliver low error rates by avoiding amplification bias, intensity averaging, and phasing or synchronization problems.

7.3 Electronic-Based Methods

7.3.1 Charge Perturbation Detection in DNA Synthesis

Another next-generation sequencing by synthesis (SBS) method is based on charge perturbation detection, shown in Figure 7.7. First, a surface is coated with gold and isolated from the chip by an insulation layer below the self-assembled monolayer (SAM). Given an input template strand, a

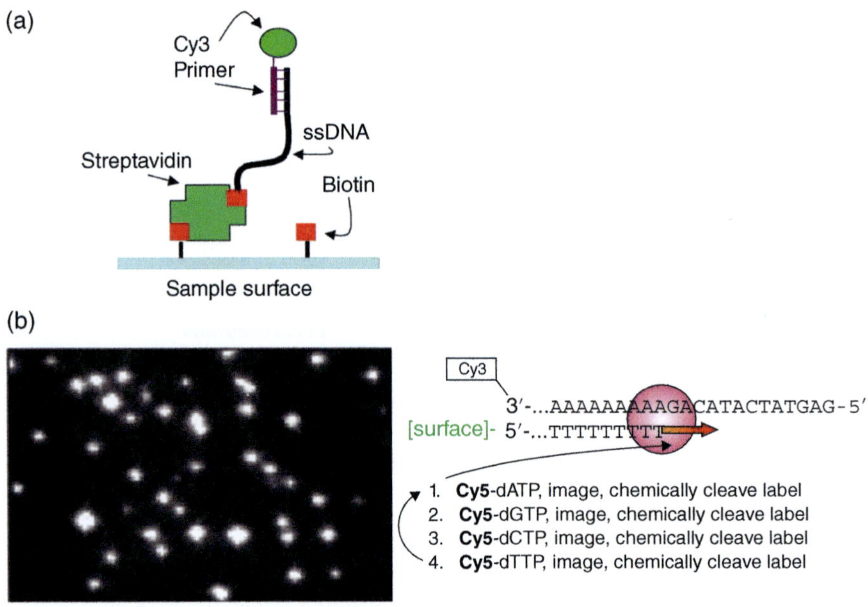

Figure 7.6 (a) Schematic of single molecule conjugation to a proprietary surface. *Source:* Braslavsky et al. [4]. Reprinted by permission from National Academy of Sciences. Copyright (2003) by National Academy of Sciences, USA. (b) Example data from the HeliScope system and illustration of the sequencing by synthesis process. *Source:* Shendure and Ji [1]. Reprinted by permission from Springer Nature. Copyright 2008 by Springer Nature.

complementary DNA strand can be synthesized one base at a time. First, precursors (dNTP·Mg complexes) are added. Second, the DNA strand is extended by reacting with the dNTP; during this process, the hydrogen atom at the 3′ end of the DNA strand being extended will be dissolved into solution as an H^+ ion, leaving behind a net negative charge contributed from the phosphate. Third, the negative charge will induce a compensating positive charge in the gold by charge neutrality. Finally, the positive charge results in a negative current pulse in the underlying circuit, which can be detected and measured.

These steps are repeated for each of the four different nucleotide bases which are added one at a time in order to identify the bases in the template DNA sequence. One of the dNTPs will match the template base and thus generate a current pulse, the other three will not. Then, the whole process is repeated at the next template base, until the entire template sequence is complete with the double helix.

7.3.2 Ion-Sensitive FET (ISFET)

The ion-sensitive FET (ISFET), whose structure is based on a field-effect transistor (FET), can be used to measure ion concentrations in solution. Figure 7.8 shows the schematics of two FET devices: the metal-oxide semiconductor FET (MOSFET) and the ISFET.

In a MOSFET with a p-type bulk and n-type source and drain regions, when a positive voltage is applied to the gate electrode, electrons (minority carriers) are attracted to the surface of the semiconductor. This thin layer of electrons will form a conducting channel between the source and the drain near the silicon dioxide interface. The conductivity of the channel can then be modulated by adjusting the strength of the electrical field between the gate electrode and the silicon, perpendicular to the substrate surface.

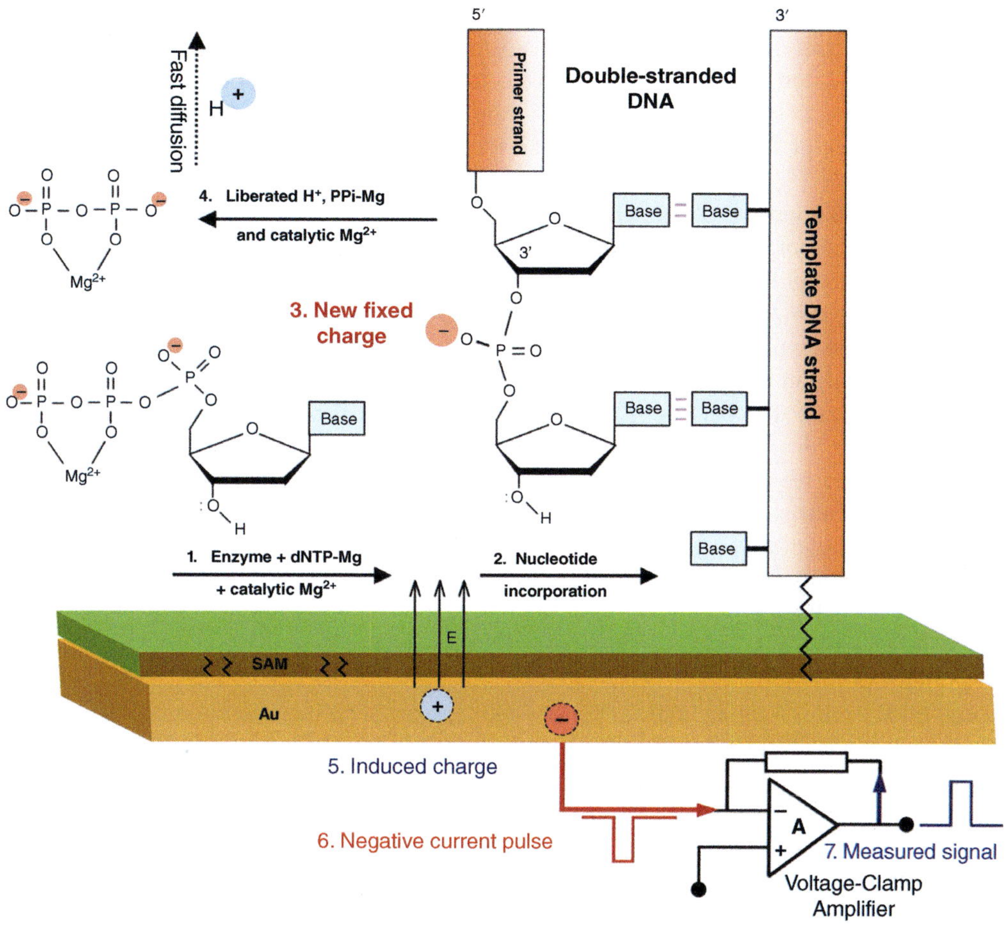

Figure 7.7 CMOS-integrated DNA sequencing based on charge perturbation detection. *Source:* Pourmand et al. [5]. Reprinted by permission from National Academy of Sciences. Copyright (2006) by National Academy of Sciences, USA.

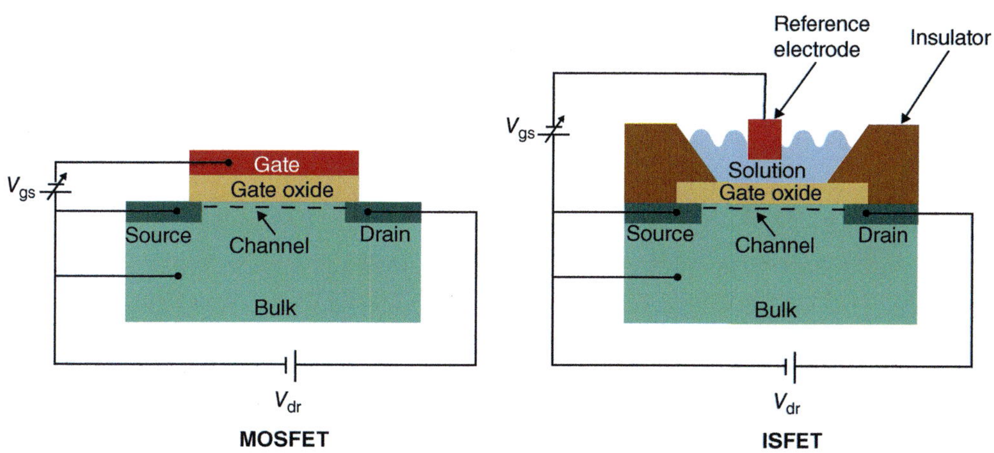

Figure 7.8 MOSFET and ISFET sensor designs.

The ISFET's structure is very similar to that of the MOSFET, except that the gate metal electrode is replaced by an electrolyte solution which is contacted by a reference electrode, and the silicon dioxide gate oxide is placed directly in an aqueous electrolyte solution. When the ion concentration (such as H^+ ion) changes, the current through the transistor will change accordingly, and thus the pH change (in the case of H^+ ion) can be measured accurately.

7.3.2.1 ISFET-qPCR Biochip

The ISFET can be incorporated into the ISFET-qPCR biochip device (Figure 7.9), which is capable of quantifying DNA amplification via the local change in pH generated by the H^+ release during DNA elongation. The device has potential for deep multiplexing. As the DNA polymerase (brown spheres) elongates the template DNA (red), protons are released. The presence of protons changes the local pH, triggering an increase in output voltage in the integrated circuit (IC) proportional to the amount of synthesized DNA. The IC contains heaters, temperature sensors, control circuits, and sensing ISFETs.

The ISFET-qPCR device is an integrated circuit with on-chip ISFETs, heaters, temperature sensors, and control circuitry (Figure 7.10). The cross-section of the biochip shows the ISFETs (floating gate, source [S] and drain [D]), temperature sensors (yellow squares), and digitally controlled resistive heater elements (blue squares) all embedded under the silicon nitride (Si_3N_4) sensing surface of the chip. All components are fabricated as part of the CMOS-manufacturing process flow. The chip is beneath a flow cell which creates separate reaction chambers, each of which may contain a unique primer set.

As exemplified in the chamber containing the wild-type primers, incorporation of nucleotides into the nascent nucleic acid strand results in proton production and a decrease in the pH. The protons accumulate at the Si_3N_4-sensing surface, which results in an increase in the charge distribution in the channel of the ISFET. This increase in charge distribution increases the integrated circuit (IC) output signal voltage when the ISFET is biased at a fixed current. The on-chip heaters and temperature sensors allow fine and fast temperature control of the wells for PCR thermal cycling.

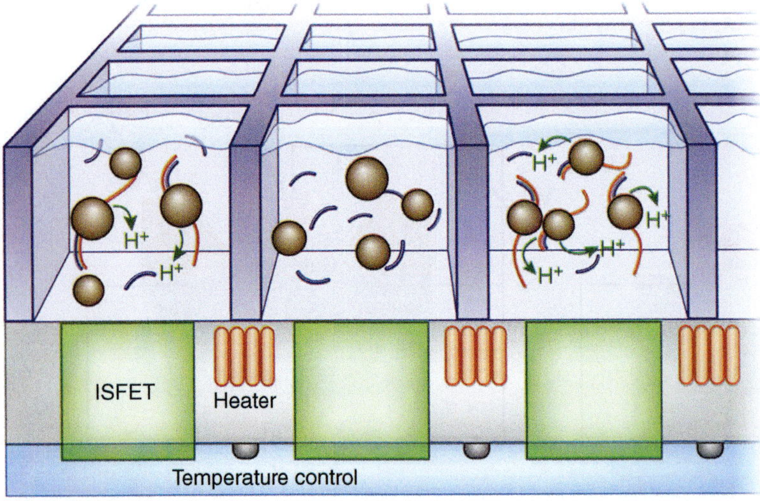

Figure 7.9 ISFET-qPCR biochip for pH-based detection of DNA amplification. *Source:* Guiducci and Spiga [6]. Reprinted by permission from Springer Nature. Copyright 2013 by Springer Nature.

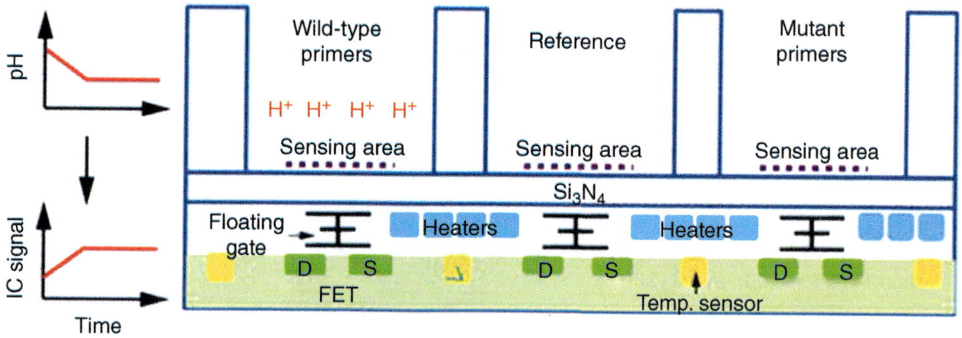

Figure 7.10 Schematic of ISFET-qPCR biochip. *Source:* Toumazou et al. [7]. Reprinted by permission from Springer Nature. Copyright 2013 by Springer Nature.

The strength of semiconductor-based parallel analytical devices derives from two main features: the fully electrical nature of the sensing principle and the possibility to scale up the number of sensors per chip by orders of magnitude with almost no technological effort.

7.3.2.2 SNP Typing

The ISFET can be incorporated into an integrated chip for detection of single nucleotide polymorphisms or SNP typing. This is a label-free, nonoptical, real-time method for detecting and quantifying target sequences by monitoring pH signatures of native amplification chemistries. The chip has ISFET sensors, temperature sensors, resistive heating, signal processing, and control circuitry all integrated to create a full system-on-chip platform. Using this platform and PCR with allele-specific primers, unique single-nucleotide polymorphism (SNP) variants, such as those found in homozygous wild-type, heterozygous, and homozygous mutant samples of human saliva, can be genotyped and discriminated between (Figure 7.11). This semiconductor technology may soon enable the creation of devices for cost-effective, portable, and scalable real-time nucleic acid analysis. In reaching this goal, there are still a few hurdles to overcome. In particular, the results thus far have been qualitative genotyping. To enable quantitative results, it needs to be shown that the technique is specific even in complex matrices. Interestingly, the main inventor of the device became interested in SNP typing after learning that his then 12-year-old son's kidneys were failing and the family learned that he is genetically predisposed to renal failure.

7.3.3 Ion Torrent Chip

The Ion Torrent chip technology is also based on the sequencing by synthesis method, during which a complementary strand is built based on the sequence of a template strand. The operating principle of the Ion Torrent chip is as follows. Single-strands of unknown DNA sample are attached to beads. The beads are then loaded into the microwells of an Ion Torrent chip along with the primers and enzymes that are required for DNA synthesis (see Figure 7.12a and b). Next, different types of dNTPs are added (dATP, dCTP, dGTP, and dTTP). These dNTPs are added to the wells one type at a time and if they are complementary to the current location of the unknown DNA, they get captured. Adding dNTPs to the sequence gives off a proton (H^+) and decreases the pH of the well. We detect this pH change using a metal-oxide-sensing layer at the bottom of the well. A pH change induces a change in surface potential of the metal-oxide-sensing layer and a change in potential of the source terminal of the underlying FET. If repeats are present in the

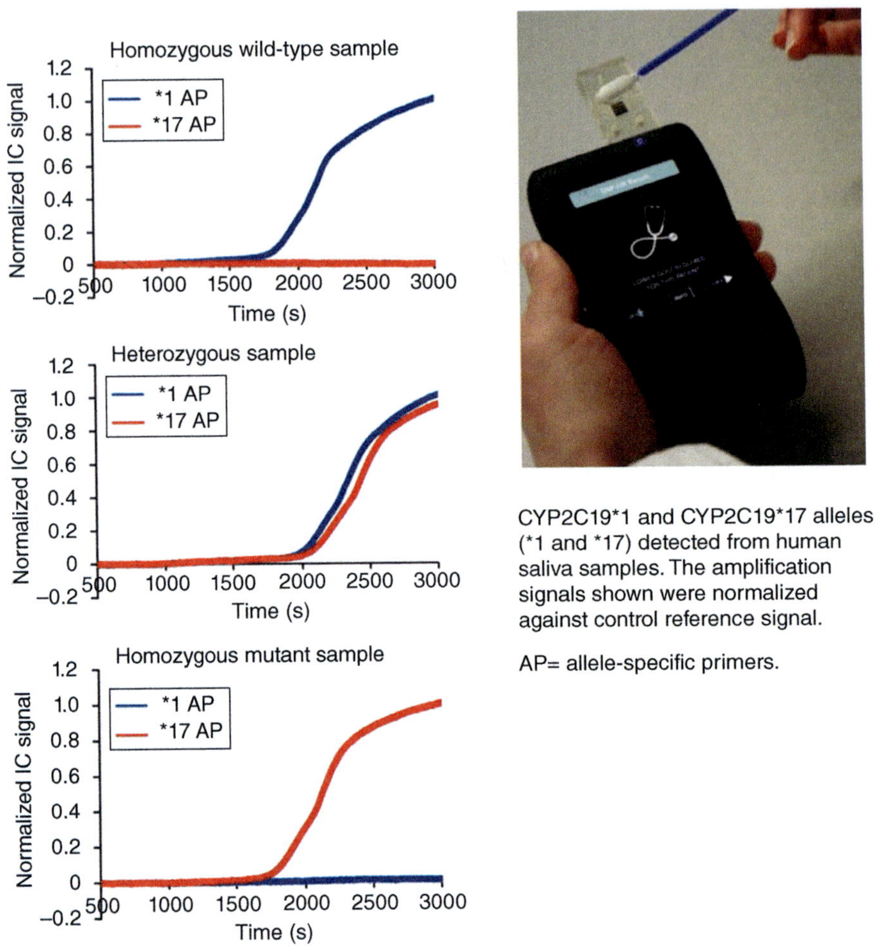

Figure 7.11 SNP typing using an ISFET sensor. *Source:* Toumazou et al. [7]. Reprinted by permission from Springer Nature. Copyright 2013 by Springer Nature and Courtesy of DNA Electronics. Copyright 2018 by DNA Electronics.

template sequence, multiple dNTP molecules will be incorporated in a single cycle, producing a corresponding number of released H^+ ions and a proportionally higher signal. We repeat the process with different types of dNTPs over and over again until the complementary strand for each unknown DNA is synthesized.

The Ion Torrent chip is built using semiconductor CMOS technology, which integrates the sensor array, sensor interface, and sensor readout all into one compact die in a ceramic package (Figure 7.13). As of 2011, it took 1000 such Ion Torrent chips to sequence one entire human genome. Figure 7.14 shows a scanning electron micrograph of a large array of 1.3 μm wells on a 1.68 μm pitch fabricated in the 110 nm CMOS technology node. This geometry allows for a two-transistor ion chip of 165 M sensors and supporting electronics to fit on a 23.7 mm × 20.0 mm die. According to Jonathan Rothberg, the inventor of the Ion Torrent, the “Ion Torrent marries simple chemistry to incredibly powerful, proprietary semiconductor technology – it's Watson meets Moore.”

Figure 7.15a depicts the workflow and detection method of the Ion Torrent chip, and Figure 7.12b illustrates the data collection and base calling method of the chip. Considering

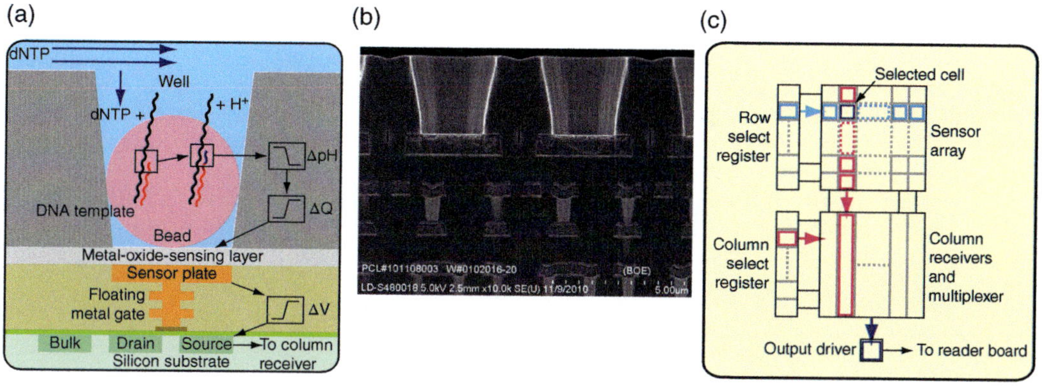

Figure 7.12 (a) Schematic of an Ion Torrent well. (b) Electron micrograph showing the arrangement of wells and underlying circuitry. (c) Sensors are arranged in a two-dimensional array and read sequentially by row/column select registers. *Source:* Rothberg et al. [8]. Reprinted by permission from Springer Nature. Copyright 2011 by Springer Nature.

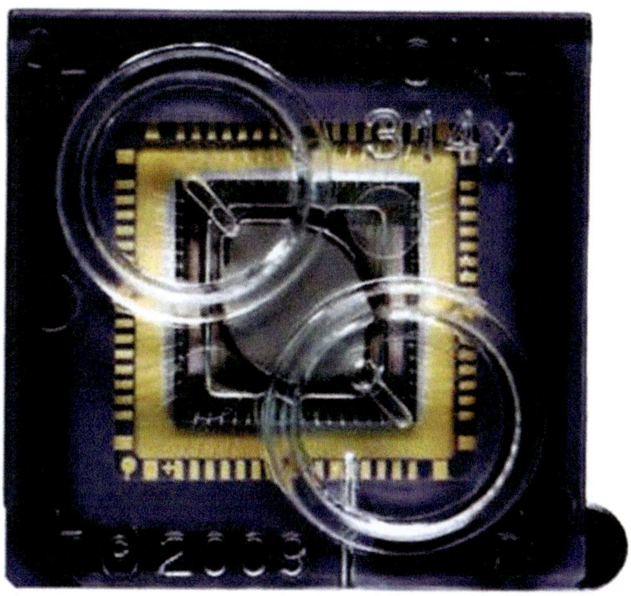

Figure 7.13 Ion Torrent chip. *Source:* Rothberg et al. [8]. Reprinted by permission from Springer Nature. Copyright 2011 by Springer Nature.

the 50 × 50 microwell portion of the chip, a grid of boxes with varying intensities can be seen. These intensities represent the strength of the incorporation reaction in individual sensor wells in one flow. To perform the base calling procedure, these intensity values can be expressed in a bar chart where each colored bar indicates the corresponding number of bases incorporated during that nucleotide flow cycle. The Ion Torrent's millions of microwells and hundreds of flow cycles combine to give the massively parallel sequencing capability typical of NGS technologies, which have driven down the cost of sequencing very long genomes to as low as $1000 in 2014.

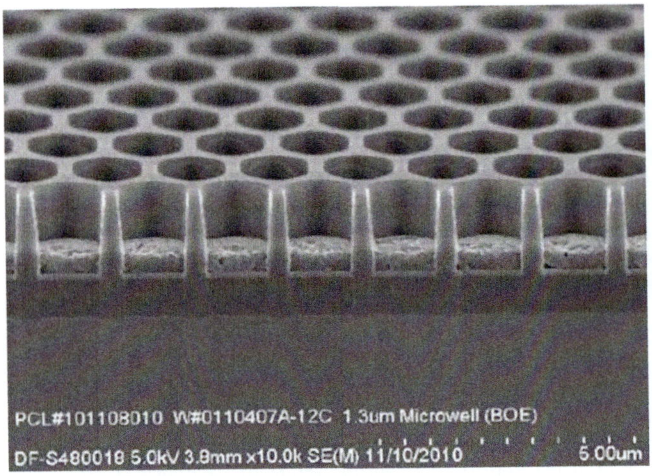

Figure 7.14 SEM image of Ion Torrent microwells. *Source:* Rothberg et al. [8]. Reprinted by permission from Springer Nature. Copyright 2011 by Springer Nature.

Did You Know?

Research indicates that the current achievable read lengths are insufficient for analyzing many complex elements within our genome. These elements often contain long repetitive elements, copy number alterations and structural variations that are relevant to evolution, adaptation, and disease. To overcome this challenge, long-read technologies are being explored. These technologies have read lengths that exceed several kilobases. The MinION from Oxford Nanopore Technologies (Figure 7.16) is one example of a long-read technology. A leader and a hairpin are ligated to the two ends of DNA that has been fragmented to 8–10 kb. The leader directs the DNA into a pore, which has current being passed through it. As the DNA is passed through the pore, the current is modulated according to the sequence of the bases. This temporal tracing is called the squiggle space. Unlike other sequencing technologies, the signal does not change for each individual base read. Rather the signal is a function of substring within a base sequence called a k-mer. For the nanopore, the length of the k-mer ranges from 5 to 6 bases. Because the signal is based on k-mers and not individual bases, the nanopore system has more than 1000 possible signals as opposed to the typical 1–4 possible signals. With so many possible signals, the nanopore technology suffers from a large error rate – up to 30% for a single read. To overcome this, the system is capable of reading the same sequence many times over, which results in a consensus sequence with significantly reduced error.

7.4 Conclusion

NGS technologies enable high-throughput decoding of DNA molecules up to the entire human genome, and allow highly multiplexed and parallel sequencing, which overcomes conventional sequencing's limitations in throughput, scalability, and speed. In addition, FETs and CMOS fabrication technology can be combined in platforms such as the ISFET and the Ion Torrent chip to allow very high throughput at low manufacturing costs and sensitive detection of electronic signals. Some relevant parameters of various NGS technologies are summarized in Table 7.1.

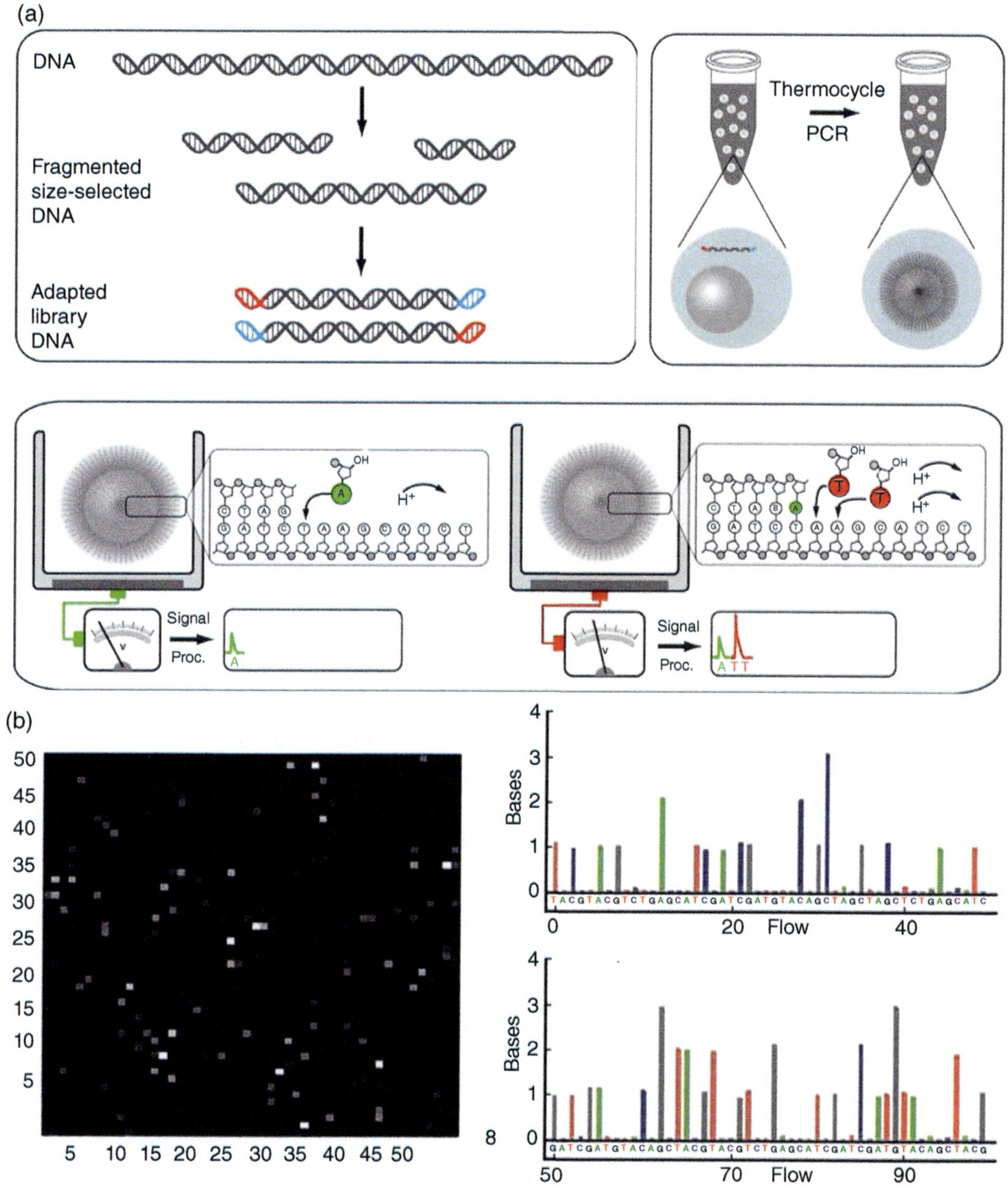

50 × 50 wells of the ion chip. The brightness represents the intensity of the incorporation reaction in individual sensor wells in one flow.

The first 100 flows from one well. Each colored bar indicates the corresponding number of bases incorporated during that nucleotide flow.

Figure 7.15 (a) Workflow and detection method and (b) data collection and base calling methods of Ion Torrent chip. *Source:* Rothberg et al. [8]. Reprinted by permission from Springer Nature. Copyright 2011 by Springer Nature.

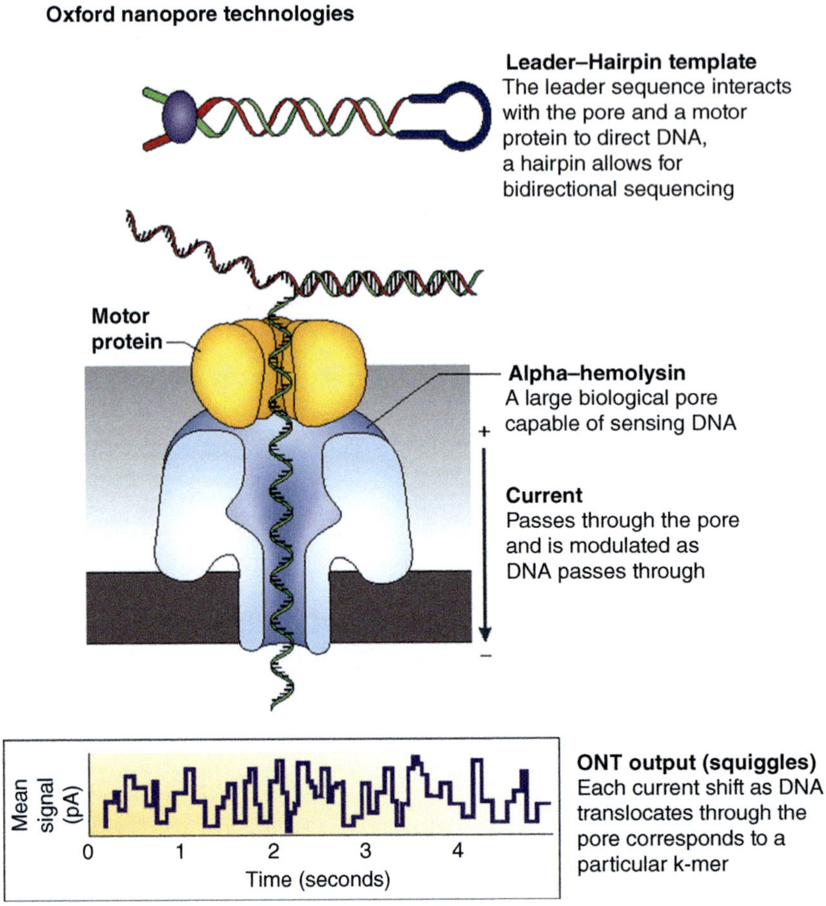

Figure 7.16 Illustration of Nanopore Technologies including the leader-hairpin structure, the pore structure, and an example temporal tracing of the current shifts. *Source:* Goodwin [3]. Reprinted by permission from Springer Nature. Copyright 2016 by Springer Nature.

Table 7.1 Several relevant parameters for various next-generation sequencing platforms:

Platform	Read length (bp)	Throughput	Runtime	Error	Cost per Gb (USD)
SOLiD 5500xl	75	240 Gb	10 days	≤ 0.1%	70
Illumina MiSeqv3	300	13.2–15 Gb	21–56 hours	0.1%	110
Illumina HiSeqX	150	800–900 Gb per flow cell	< 3 days	0.1%	7
454 GS FLX Titanium XL+	Up to 1000	700 Mb	23 hours	1%	9500
Ion S5 540	200	10–15 Gb	2.5 hours	1%	300
Pacific BioSciences RS II	~20 kbp	500 Mb – 1 Gb	4 hours	13% single pass, ≤ 1% circular consensus read	1000
Oxford Nanopore MK 1 MinION	Up to 200 kbp	Up to 1.5 Gb	Up to 48 hours	~12%	750

Source: Goodwin et al. [9]. Adapted from Springer Nature. Copyright 2016 by Springer Nature.

Problems

7.1 What is the main disadvantage of conventional Sanger sequencing? Name a next-generation sequencing technique that overcomes this disadvantage and briefly explain its operating process.

7.2 ISFET-based DNA sensors can be used for DNA detection or DNA sequencing based on charge perturbation. However, the charge perturbation in water solution can be shielded by opposing charge redistribution characterized by the so-called Debye length beyond which charge perturbation cannot be detected by an ISFET. It is known that the Debye length is inversely proportional to the square root of the ionic strength in the water solution.
If an ISFET sensor is immersed in 1X phosphate buffer solution (PBS) with an ionic strength of 162.7 mM and a pH of 7.4, the Debye length is 0.76 nm.

A What is the new Debye length if the 1X PBS is diluted to 0.01X (100-fold) with an ionic strength of 1.627 mM and a pH of 7.4?

B If the single-stranded DNA probe at the surface of ISFET must be located inside the Debye length to sense charge perturbation due to single base extension with the probe as the template, how many bases can the probe contain for it to be an effective probe?

C The Ion Torrent device utilizes ISFET for DNA sequencing in microwells with custom-made beads. Why the DNA fragments to be sequenced here can be much longer than the corresponding Debye length of the underlying ISFET?

7.3 In an Ion Torrent device, fragmented DNAs are conjugated with the beads and located in different wells. The graphs in Figure 7.17 are the first 40 flow signals obtained from two

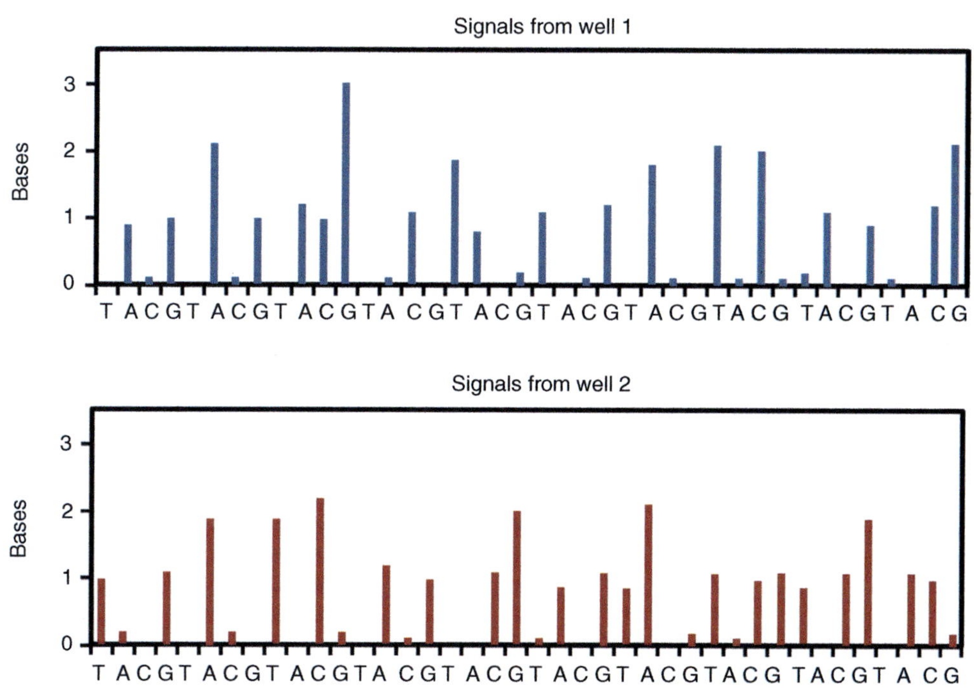

Figure 7.17 Flow signals from two different wells of an Ion Torrent device.

different wells. What are the sequences of the DNA fragments in the wells? If you can reconstruct a part of the original sequence based on them, what is that?

7.4 Epstein–Barr Virus (EBV), also known as human herpesvirus 4, is a member of the herpes virus family. It is one of the most common human viruses. EBV is found all over the world. Most people get infected with EBV at some point in their lives. EBV spreads most commonly through bodily fluids, primarily saliva. EBV can cause infectious mononucleosis, also called mono or the kissing disease. A portion of EBV genomic sequence is shown in Figure 7.18.
If the 38-base sequence above is analyzed in a reaction well by an Ion Torrent Sequencer, plot the readout voltage waveform (flow signals) as a function of flow input, i.e. the input nucleotides added to the reaction well in the order of T A C G T A C G T A C G. . . . . . To save time, you only need to show flow signals for the first 20 bases from the left.

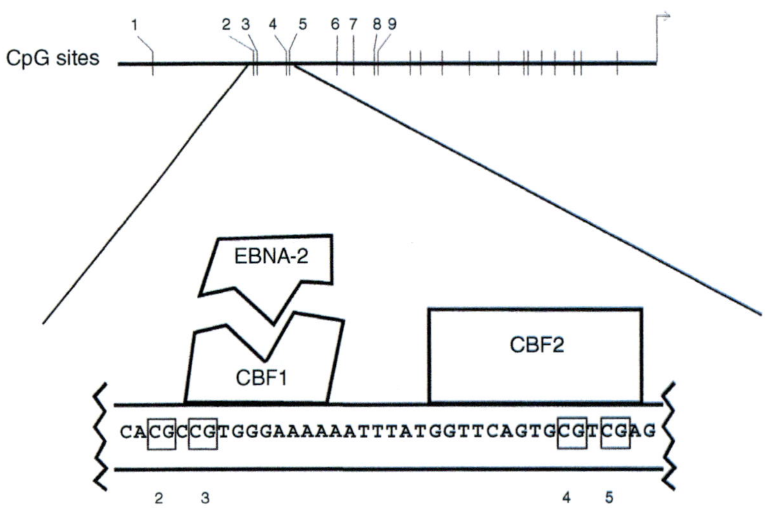

Figure 7.18 Portion of the genomic sequence of the Epstein–Barr virus. *Source:* Robertson and Ambinder [10]. Republished with permission of American Society of Hematology. Copyright 1997 by American Society of Hematology; permission conveyed through Copyright Clearance Center, Inc.

7.5 Huntington's disease is an awful genetic disease for which there is no cure. The disease-causing version of the gene has too much DNA, not too little, and the protein produced, known as huntingtin, is thus too big (huntingtin gene = Huntington disease gene). One part of every huntingtin gene contains a stretch in which the genetic letters C, A, and G are repeated several times in that order. This translates into a chain of identical amino acids within the huntingtin protein (the amino acid in question is glutamine). In most people, the number of repeats ranges from 9 to 35. These people are healthy. Those with 36 or more repeats are, however, at risk of developing Huntington's disease, and those with more than 40 will definitely develop it, unless they die beforehand of something else.

A You are tasked to design a DNA microarray to detect people who are at risk of developing Huntington's disease. Is it possible to use the Affymetrix platform for this task? If not, why? If yes, how? Each probe in Affymetrix must be a 25-mer, but a tiling probe design strategy has been developed to cover target sequences much longer than 25-mer.

B If you are free to use any DNA microarray technology, design the DNA probe you would use for the above task.

C Now you are given an Ion Torrent NGS machine for the same task. Plot the base readout waveform as a function of base-specific nucleotide (flown to the well in each cycle) from the ISFET sensor in one well, which contains the sequence from the huntingtin gene, for a person with risk of developing the disease. Note that the maximum number of bases that the Ion Torrent NGS machine can read out is 100.

D If a person is at the borderline of risk, how can the Ion Torrent NGS machine tell if the person is at risk or not?

References

1 Shendure, J. and Ji, H. (2008). Next-generation DNA sequencing. *Nature Biotechnology* 26: 1135–1145. http://www.nature.com/nbt/journal/v26/n10/pdf/nbt1486.pdf.

2 Jon Callas (2008).Illumina gene sequencing machine https://commons.wikimedia.org/wiki/File:Illumina_Genome_Analyzer_II_System.jpg (accessed 26 September 2008).

3 Goodwin, S., McPherson, J.D., and McCombie, W.R. (2016). Coming of age: ten years of next-generation sequencing technologies. *Nature Reviews Genetics* 17: 333–351.

4 Braslavsky, I., Hebert, B., Kartalov, E., and Quake, S.R. (2003 Apr 1). Sequence information can be obtained from single DNA molecules. *PNAS* 100 (7): 3960–3964.

5 Pourmand, N., Karhanek, M., Persson, H.H. et al. (2006 Apr 25). Direct electrical detection of DNA synthesis. *PNAS* 103 (17): 6466–6470.

6 Guiducci, C. and Spiga, F.M. (2013). Another transistor-based revolution: on-chip qPCR. *Nature Methods* 10: 617–618. http://www.nature.com/nmeth/journal/v10/n7/pdf/nmeth.2525.pdf.

7 Toumazou, C., Shepherd, L.M., Reed, S.C. et al. (2013). Simultaneous DNA amplification and detection using a pH-sensing semiconductor system. *Nature Methods* 10: 641–646.

8 Rothberg, J.M., Hinz, W., Rearick, T.M. et al. (2011). An integrated semiconductor device enabling non-optical genome sequencing. *Nature* 475: 348–352.

9 Goodwin, S., McPherson, J.D., and McCombie, W.R. (2016). Coming of age: ten years of next-generation sequencing technologies. *Nature Reviews Genetics* 17: 333–351.

10 Robertson, K.D. and Ambinder, R.F. Methylation of the Epstein-Barr virus genome in normal lymphocytes. *Blood: Journal of the American Society of Hematology, 9* 11: 4481.

Further Reading

MacLean, D., Jones, J.D.G., and Studholme, D.J. (2009). Application of'next-generation' sequencing technologies to microbial genetics. *Nature Reviews Microbiology* 7 (4): 287–296.

Vivien Marx (2013). The Author File: Chris Toumazou http://www.nature.com/nmeth/journal/v10/n7/pdf/nmeth.2550.pdf.

8

Protein Assays and Chips

8.1 Introduction

Immunoassay is a laboratory technique that makes use of binding between an antigen and its homologous antibody in order to identify and quantify the specific antigen or antibody in a sample. A protein assay is a technique to identify or quantify proteins. A protein assay is a broader term that refers to a technique to identify or quantify any proteins.

There are many different protein assay technologies that can identify and quantify multiple antibodies and other proteins simultaneously, which can be used to detect for a variety of biomarkers of interest. These include ELISA (enzyme-linked immunosorbent assay), protein array, bead array, and ECL (electrochemiluminescence) assay. All four technologies can be used in an immunoassay, which is a laboratory technique that makes use of the binding between an antigen and its homologous antibody in order to identify and quantify the specific antigen or antibody in a sample.

8.2 ELISA

ELISA, which stands for enzyme-linked immunosorbent assay, is a type of immunoassay with three components: antibody, solid phase (sorbent), and enzymatic amplification. The antibody allows for specific detection of an analyte of interest. The solid phase (sorbent) allows one to wash away all the material that is not specifically captured. Enzymatic amplification allows a small capture of analyte to be converted into a visible color change that can be quantified using an absorbance plate reader. ELISA has many different uses, including: measuring antibody or antigen levels (e.g. allergies and vaccines), detecting viruses (e.g. hepatitis, HIV, and venereal diseases), detecting hormonal changes (e.g. hCG for pregnancy tests), and detecting circulatory inflammatory markers (e.g. cytokines, which are related to many diseases such as cancer and heart attacks). ELISA is the most common method used for these purposes because it is sensitive, quantitative, and reproducible. The sensitivity of ELISA varies depending on the detected analyte. ELISA's predecessor is radioimmunoassay, a related technique developed in the 1950s, which uses radioactive labels for signal transduction. The main inventor of the radioimmunoassay, Rosalyn Yalow, won the Nobel Prize in Medicine in 1977. ELISA is often commercialized in kit form for common markers, e.g. cardiac troponin (cTn).

Biochips and Medical Imaging, First Edition. Adam de la Zerda and Shan Xiang Wang.

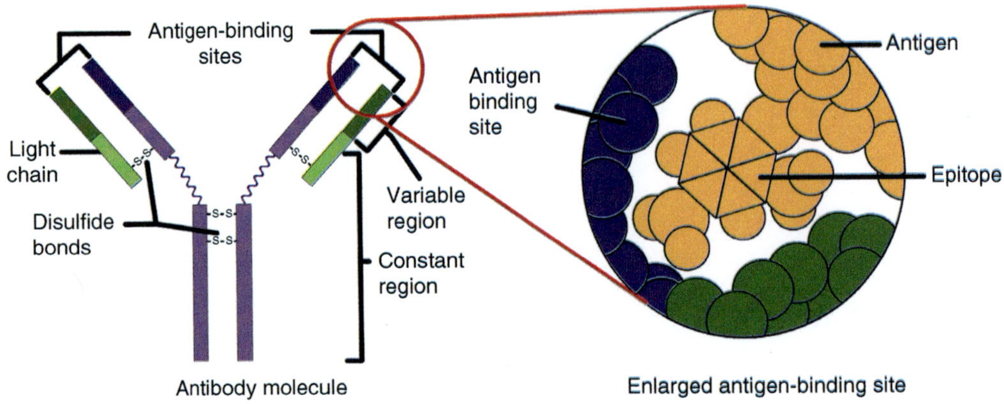

Figure 8.1 Antibody structure and antigen-binding specificity. An epitope is a surface region of an antigen that is capable of eliciting an immune response and of combining with a specific antibody.

8.2.1 Antibodies

Antibodies (or immunoglobulins) are large Y-shaped proteins that are typically used by the body's immune system to identify and fight foreign objects, such as viruses and bacteria. Antibodies contain a hypervariable region with high specificity, i.e. bonding only to specific antigens with a lock-key model (Figure 8.1), which can occur with many different bonding mechanisms (hydrogen bonding, ionic bonding, hydrophobic absorption, and van der Waals forces). An antibody and its antigen have an affinity, or association constant (K_a), which is the ratio of on rate, k_{on} (in $M^{-1}s^{-1}$), and off rate, k_{off} (in s^{-1}), in a reaction. A higher value of K_a indicates a higher affinity between antibody and antigen. The Langmuir isotherm formula gives an expression at equilibrium conditions for the fraction of antibodies reacted with matched antigens (which are provided in solution) at a concentration of [Ag] (i.e. the fraction of surface coverage):

$$\theta = \frac{[\mathrm{Ag}]}{[\mathrm{Ag}] + K_d},$$

where K_d is the dissociation constant defined as:

$$K_d \equiv \frac{1}{K_a} \equiv \frac{k_{off}}{k_{on}}.$$

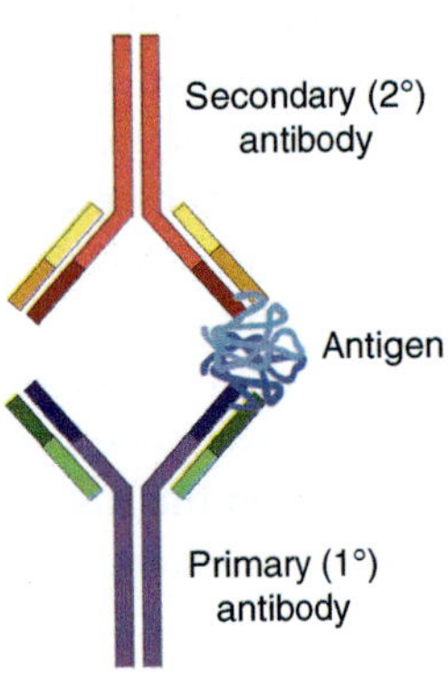

Figure 8.2 Sandwich complex formed in ELISA.

8.2.2 Sandwich ELISA

The sandwich complex (Figure 8.2) is the most commonly used and most sensitive form of ELISA. To form the sandwich complex, a primary antibody is first coated onto a microplate. Second, antigen is added to the plate, causing the antibody and antigen to bind together. Third, a secondary antibody is added, which binds to a different location (epitope) on the antigen to form a sandwich structure. The primary antibody is called the capture antibody because it captures antigen molecules and the secondary antibody is called the detection antibody because it is the source of the detected signal (via conjugated fluorescent dyes, etc.).

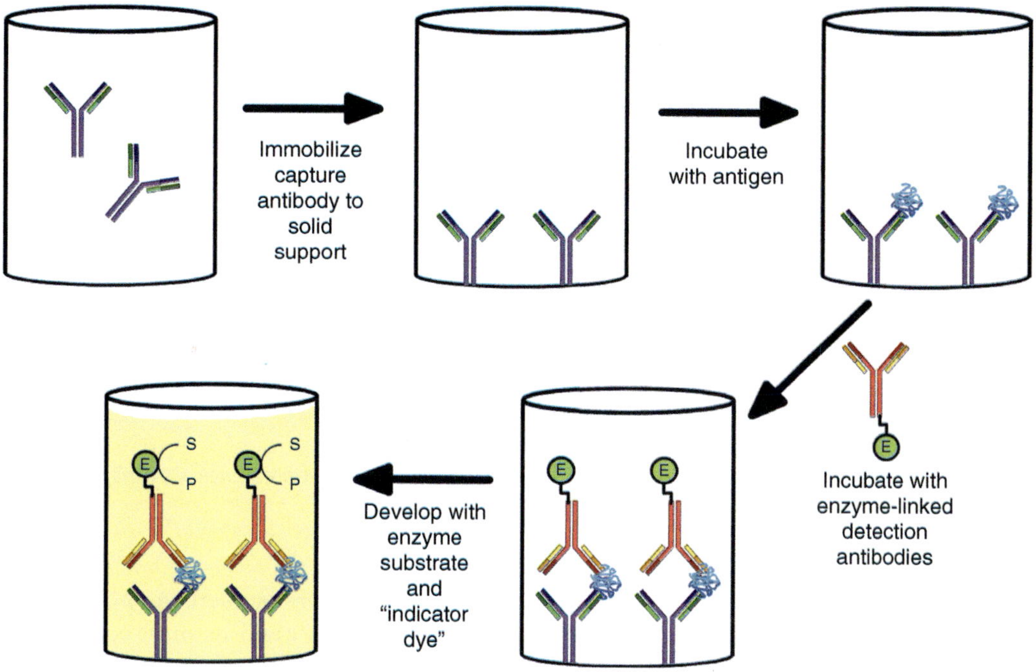

Figure 8.3 Steps in performing a sandwich ELISA.

A sandwich ELISA is performed as follows (Figure 8.3). First, a capture antibody is immobilized to a solid support. Second, an antigen is incubated to bind with the capture antibody. Third, an enzyme-linked secondary antibody is incubated to form a complete sandwich structure. Fourth, the assay is developed with enzyme substrate and "indicator dye," which causes the enzyme to catalyze a chemical reaction that produces a color change in that location. Finally, the color change is read out by optics, which can be very sensitive to one specific wavelength. Standard curves of an antigen, such as human CRP (a cardiac marker), can be generated by performing ELISA on a series of samples with known concentrations and plotting the optical density versus concentration. The standard curve can then be used to convert from measured optical density of an unknown sample to an antigen concentration (Figure 8.4).

8.2.3 Enzyme with Chromogenic Substrates

Enzymes are catalysts that speed up certain reactions. Molecules that they act on are called substrates and the resulting molecules of this reaction are called products. Enzymes convert substrates into products. If a product's color is different from its substrate's, that substrate is called a chromogenic substrate. An example of this is recombinant DNA validation discussed in Chapter 2. Remember that β-galactosidase breaks down a colorless X-gal sugar and the resulting products give blue color after being oxidized. In this example, β-galactosidase is the enzyme and X-gal is its chromogenic substrate. There are many enzymes with chromogenic substrates but when choosing one for ELISA, there are several important characteristics to consider. First of all, the colored products must have a high molar extinction coefficient so that a strong color change can be detected. Second, there must be a strong binding between the enzyme and substrate. Third, there should be (ideally) a linear relationship between the concentration of the

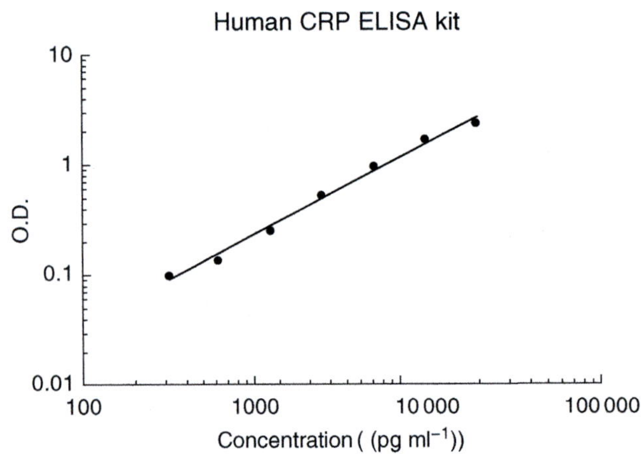

Figure 8.4 Standard curve of optical density versus target protein concentration. *Source:* Courtesy of Boster Bio, Copyright © 1993–2018 by Boster Biological Technology.

enzyme and the color intensity, in either linear or log–log scale (Beer–Lambert Law). The most commonly used enzyme in ELISA is horseradish peroxidase (HRP) and its most commonly used chromogenic substrates are TMB, 4-CN, and DAB. The number of enzyme molecules is proportional to the number of sandwich complexes. In the chromogenic reaction, enzymes are not consumed but substrates are.

8.2.4 Lateral Flow Pregnancy Test

One of the well-known applications of sandwich ELISA is the lateral flow pregnancy test. During pregnancy, a hormone called human chorionic gonadotropin (hCG or HCG) is secreted from the placenta. The hCG hormone is measured in milli-international units per milliliter (mIU ml^{-1}). An hCG level of less than 5 mIU ml^{-1} is considered negative for pregnancy and anything above 25 mIU ml^{-1} is considered positive for pregnancy. There are two common types of hCG tests. A qualitative hCG test detects if hCG is present in the blood. A quantitative hCG test (or beta hCG) measures the amount of hCG actually present in the blood.

Lateral flow tests are simple devices intended to detect the presence (or absence) of a target analyte in a sample. Most commonly, these tests are used for home testing, point-of-care testing, or laboratory testing because the results are acquired in a timely fashion and do not require quantitative analysis. The testing mechanism is illustrated in Figure 8.5. First, the sample with analytes is introduced to the sample pad. The sample starts moving toward the wicking pad due to capillary flow. On its way to the test line, the sample crosses the conjugate pad. The conjugate pad contains tags with antibodies. If the sample contains analytes, then these tagged antibodies capture them and continue moving along with the capillary flow. Once they reach the test line, analytes are captured and fixed on the test line antibodies. This creates the ELISA sandwich structure and accumulation of tags causes the test line to light up (meaning pregnant). As the capillary flow continues, control line antibodies capture the control tags causing the control line to light up. The control line indicates that the test was completed successfully. If there are no analytes in the original sample, there will not be any accumulation of tags on the test line and only the control line will light up (meaning not pregnant).

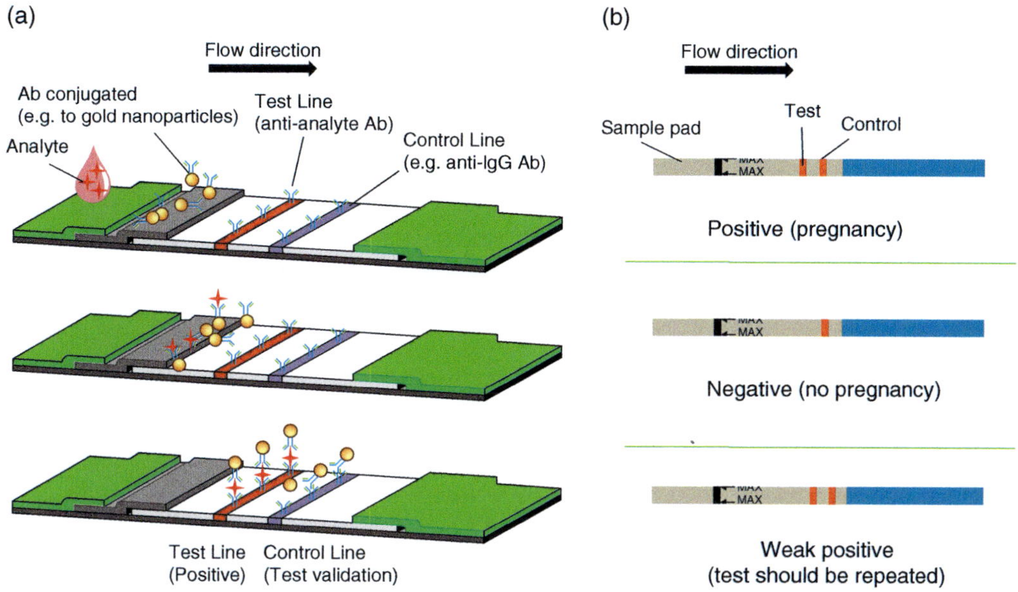

Figure 8.5 Lateral flow ELISA assay for pregnancy test: (a) 3-dimensional view of the assay process, (b) cross-sectional view of the assay process. *Source:* Koczula and Gallotta [1]. Republished with permission conveyed through Copyright Clearance Center, Inc.

8.3 Protein Arrays

8.3.1 History of Protein Assay Technology

Technology platforms have gradually advanced to enable higher multiplex capability and parallel analysis of different samples and analytes. Protein assay technology started with test tubes, then advanced to microwell plates with 96 or more microwells, then protein microarrays (protein chips or planar arrays), which are similar to DNA microarrays, and, finally, to xMAP technology which uses a microsphere-based liquid array to produce a multi-analyte profile (Figure 8.6).

Multiplex assays (shown in Figure 8.7) are useful because they have the ability to simultaneously detect multiple biomarkers or intracellular signaling modifications. Antibodies are often used in sandwich immunoassays and are either immobilized on chips as "planar arrays" or conjugated to microbeads as "suspension arrays." A planar array or chip can spot different antibodies in spatially distributed locations (spots), similar to spotting DNA strands on a chip. A bead array is based on microbeads or nanobeads, in which many kinds of beads are coated with different antibodies and mixed together. In either configuration, one reaction is sufficient to monitor all the different antibodies present in different spots or beads.

8.3.2 Spotted Antibody Microarray

Spotted antibody microarrays can be used to perform multiple sandwich ELISA on a chip. First, antibodies are spotted as an array on a solid support, with different antibodies located in different locations (often with replicates for quality control). Second, antigen samples are incubated on the chip, during which the antigen-bonding reactions occur on all matching spots simultaneously. Third, incubation with a biotinylated detection antibody and then labeled streptavidin are

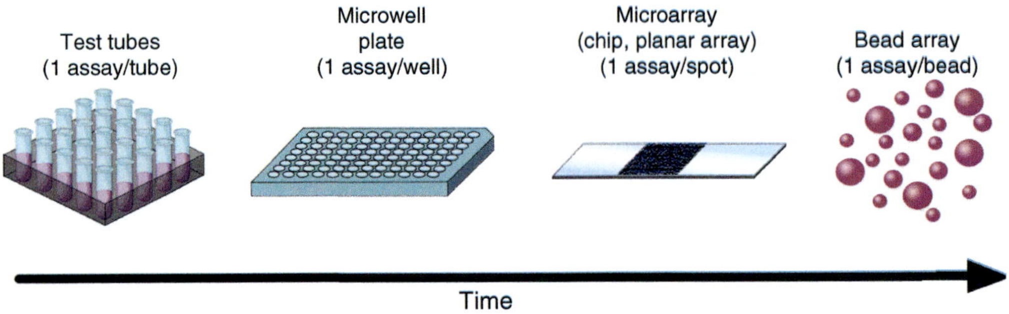

Figure 8.6 Evolution of protein assay technology.

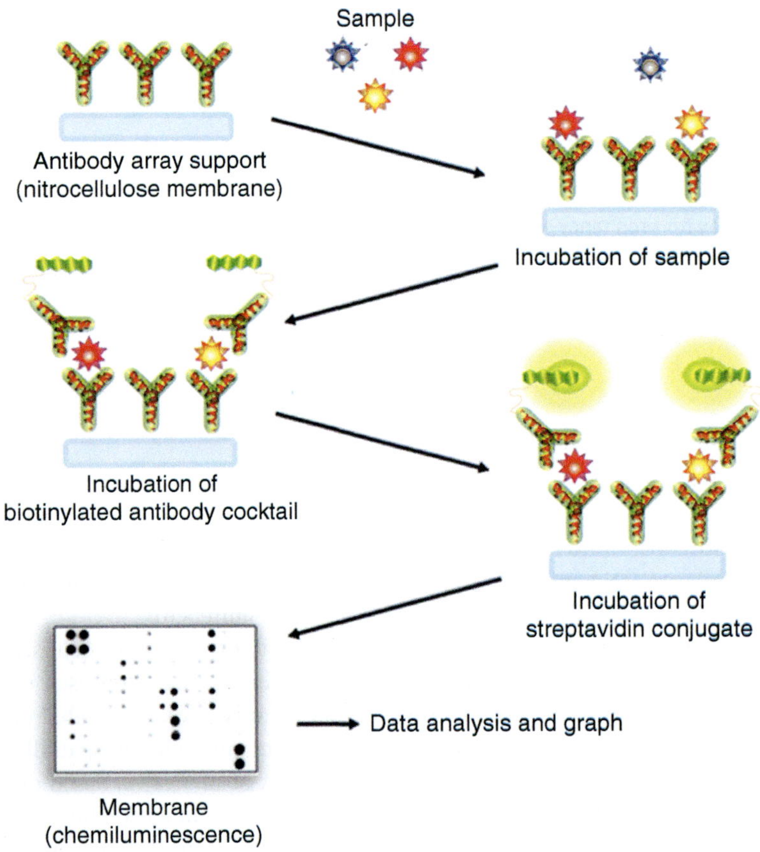

Figure 8.7 Multiple sandwich ELISA on a chip. *Source:* Courtesy of RayBiotech, Copyright © 2007–2018 by RayBiotech, Inc.

performed to complete the sandwich complex. Finally, substrate is added to bind with the enzyme and the resulting color change is read out with a CCD camera or optical scanner.

8.3.3 Streptavidin and Biotin

Leveraging the interaction between streptavidin and biotin is often used for labeling. The structures of streptavidin and biotin are shown in Figure 8.8. Streptavidin–biotin coupling is a strong

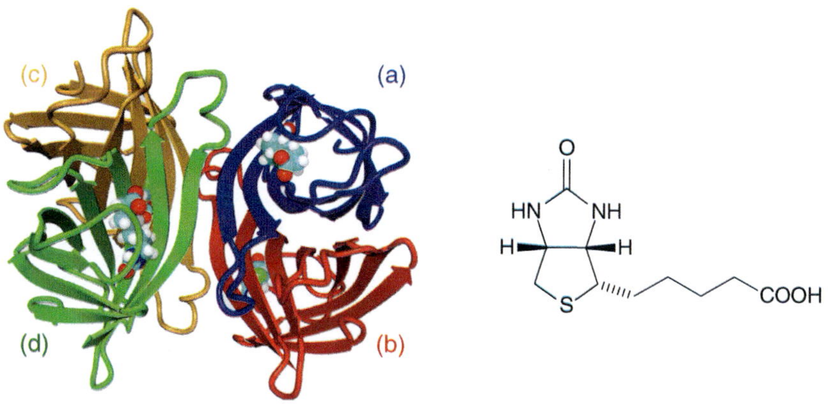

Figure 8.8 (Left) Streptavidin (tetramer) with two bound biotin molecules. *Source:* O'Sullivan [2]. Used under the Creative Commons Attribution License. (Right) Chemical structure of biotin. *Source:* https://http://commons.wikimedia.org/wiki/File:Biotin_structure.svg. By User: Mysid [Public domain], from Wikimedia Commons.

interaction that is slightly weaker than a covalent bond. Biotinylated detection antibodies readily couples with streptavidin-HRP conjugates. Another use is biotinylated DNA which readily couples with streptavidin-HRP conjugates.

Did You Know?

Researchers are planning to use immunoassay chips to test for life on Mars. The Viking Mission in 1976 consisted of the first and only search for life on Mars. While the tests appeared inconclusive, it was later determined that even if there were life on Mars, the tests would not have been able to find it. Since then, wide arrays of tests for biological materials have been developed; in particular, the immunoassay can detect for hundreds of types of proteins, DNA, and other biological materials. With such a wide variety of tests available, researchers are left with the question of what biomolecules should they be looking for on Mars. Potential ideas include proteins that would be useful for surviving on Mars (e.g. cold-adapted enzymes that would allow organisms to survive in Mars frigid temperatures or enzymes to repair DNA since Mars suffers from strong radiation effects) and pervasive biomolecules (e.g. ATP, which is used by all living organisms on Earth for metabolic activity). The strong ionizing radiation felt on Mars could potentially completely destroy biomolecules, so rovers (such as Curiosity pictured in Figure 8.9) must take samples from far below the surface when testing for life on Mars.

8.3.4 Important Concepts

Positive control is the probes (or sensors) that are supposed to give a large signal. For antibody microarrays, positive control is achieved by putting control probes on the chip and adding its antigen to the sample. Thus, for every test, the sample should have a positive control antigen which should give a strong signal. If the positive control does not give a signal, it is an indicator that something is wrong and the test is not valid. Negative control is the probes (or sensors) that are supposed to give no signal. The corresponding signal measured by negative control is often called background. A common negative control is bovine serum albumin (BSA). When the sensor is coated with BSA, the antigens in the sample cannot reach the sensor and, as a result, the sensor

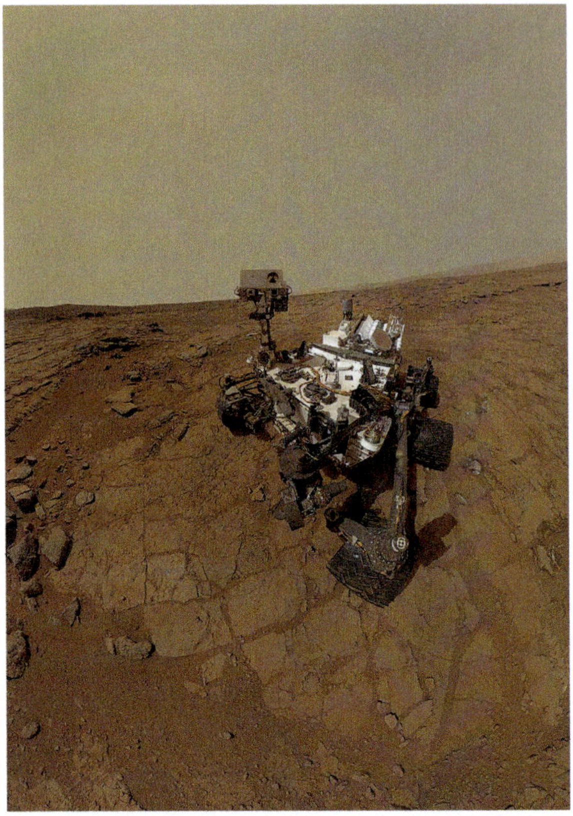

Figure 8.9 Curiosity self-portrait. *Source:* Image Credit: NASA/JPL-Caltech/MSSS. Curiosity Rover's Self Portrait at "John Klein" Drilling Site.

gives no signal. Again, similar to the positive control example, if the negative control gives a high signal, then the test is considered not valid. Zero analyte level refers to the mean signal of positive probes (or sensors) for a sample with zero analyte matching the positive probes. Zero analyte level usually constitutes a more stringent background signal than the negative control level mentioned previously and both levels should be fairly close to each other in a good protein assay. The intra-chip CV (coefficient of variation) is the standard deviation of signals from replicate probes normalized by the mean, which is used to measure variation across different probes within chip. The inter-chip CV is the standard deviation of mean signals of a given marker from replicate chips normalized by the average of mean signals, which is used to measure variation across different chips. Recall that the sample standard deviation is calculated with an $N-1$ value in the denominator instead of N, which gives a better representation for a small number of samples (replicate probes or chips). The CVs required for molecular diagnostics depend on the application and can vary widely. Generally speaking, a $CV < 20\%$ is considered good for research uses, while a $CV < 10\%$ is often required for FDA approval.

8.3.5 Forward and Reverse Phase Protein Arrays

Antibody microarrays are usually used in forward-phase format in which specific antibodies are immobilized on slides or beads, then incubated with a sample (serum, plasma, whole blood, cell culture media, etc.). This format is limited by antibodies which can function when immobilized, as well as the cross-reactivity of antibodies. Protein microarrays can be used in reverse-phase in which a large number of lysate or serum samples are immobilized on slides as microspots, then probed with specific antibodies. This method is limited by the number of analytes that can be analyzed on a single slide. The differences between forward and reverse phase assays are depicted in Figure 8.10.

8.3.6 Spotted Antigen Peptide Microarray

Spotted antigen/peptide microarrays, like the ones shown in Figure 8.11, are ideal for detection of autoimmune diseases. Autoimmunity is the immunity against the body's own cells or proteins. The healthy immune system protects the body from infection or disease by attacking the invader organisms or substances. In autoimmunity, white blood cells attack and destroy the body's healthy tissue by producing antibodies (autoantibodies) against the body's tissue. This leads to many types of autoimmune diseases such as rheumatoid arthritis (RA), type-I diabetes, Graves' disease, and multiple sclerosis. Spotted antigen/peptide microarrays can be used as follows. First, peptides or antigens are printed onto a slide. Second, the array is incubated with autoimmune serum from a patient with excessive antibodies. Third, the incubated protein array is labeled with fluorophore-labeled secondary antibodies. Finally, the output is read with an optical scanner or CCD camera. The data provided can determine if the antibodies corresponding to the spotted locations exist in the patient. For example, a spotted antigen microarray can detect the presence of rheumatoid arthritis in a patient by detecting upregulation of hnRNP-B1 antibody. Influenza A and Pneumovax antigens are used as positive controls to form green circles for most types of autoimmune serums. A spotted antigen microarray can be used to distinguish different autoimmune diseases.

8.3.7 Bead Array (Luminex)

A protein bead array uses a bead-based sandwich structure to perform an immunoassay. First, beads are coated with capture antibodies. Second, the beads are incubated with sample analytes,

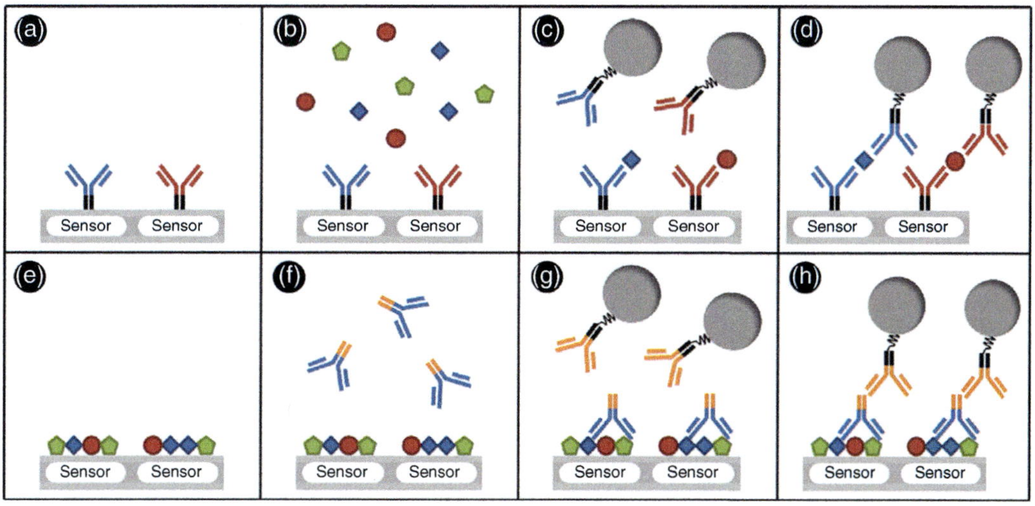

Figure 8.10 Forward phase protein array (panels (a)–(d)) versus reverse phase protein array (panels (e)–(h)). *Source:* Lee et al. [3]. Reprinted by permission of Taylor & Francis.

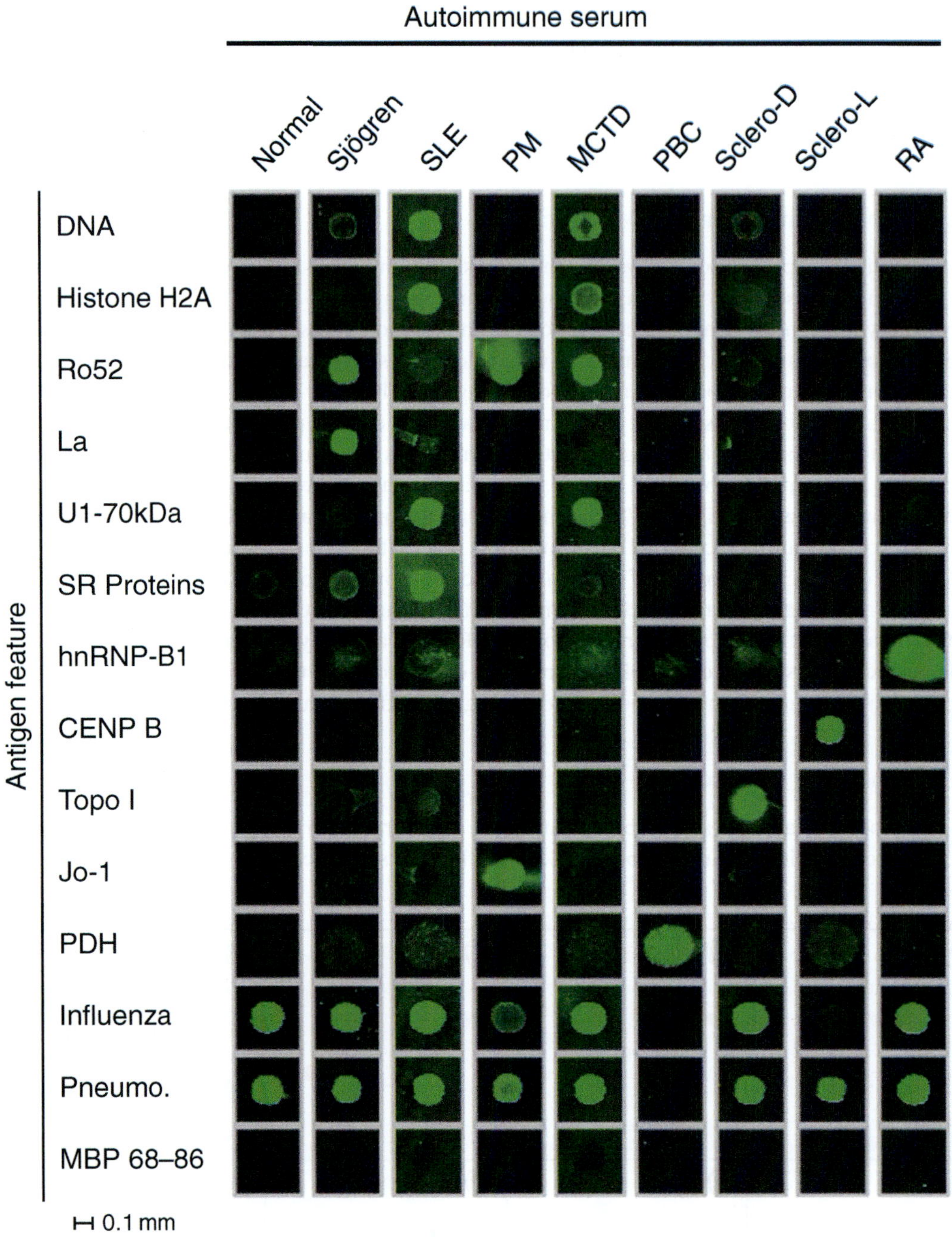

Figure 8.11 Example of an antigen array for autoimmune diseases. Source: Robinson et al. [4]. Reprinted by permission from Springer Nature: Nature Medicine. Copyright © 2002 by Springer Nature.

which will be captured if the analyte matches the capture antibody. Third, fluorescence-labeled detection antibodies are added to complete the sandwich structure. Finally, a two-step measurement is performed (Figure 8.12): the first laser stimulates fluorescence in the beads, which identifies which antibody is conjugated to that bead (e.g. red color), then a second laser quantifies the

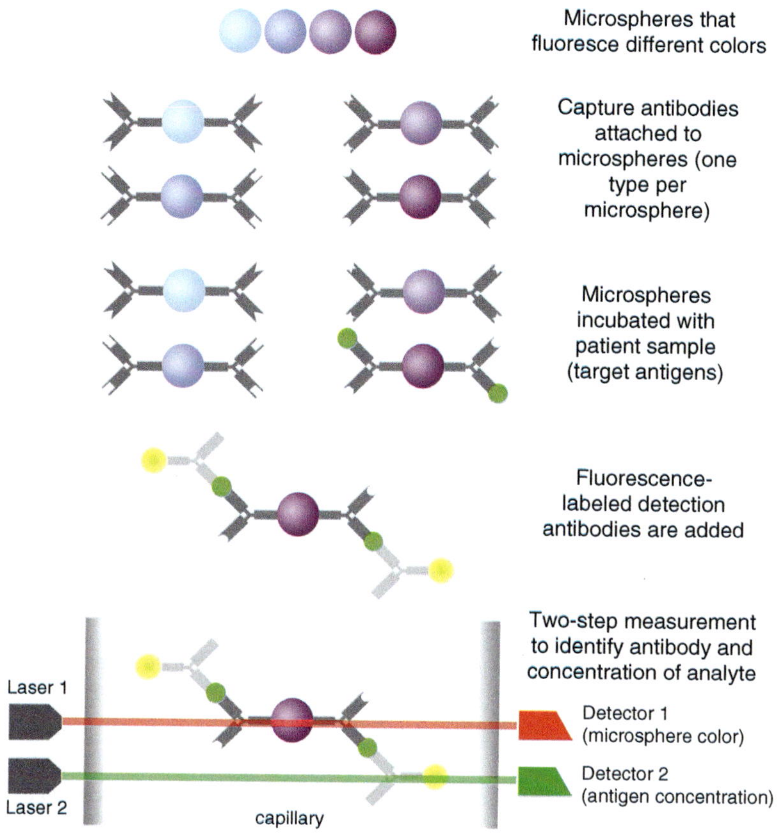

Figure 8.12 Dual laser readout used in bead array (Luminex) assay.

detection antibody (green color), which is related to the concentration of analyte by the corresponding standard curve (Figure 8.13).

The Luminex technology (xMAP) uses a protein bead array with microspheres, which are uniquely color-coded using blends of two dyes with different fluorescent intensities. Using this method, over 100 distinct microsphere sets can be created, allowing up to 100 simultaneous tests. Multiplex standard curves show a good dynamic range from less than 50 to more than 8000 MFI (median fluorescent intensities), and a limit of detection of about $4\,\mathrm{pg\,ml^{-1}}$ for certain cytokines.

8.3.8 Cytokines

Cytokines are secreted proteins which transduce messages in the immune system. One subcategory of cytokines is chemokines which transduce cell taxis information, such as mobilization, adherence, extravasation, infiltration, and egress. There are over 120 cytokines, of which more than 50 are chemokines. Cytokines and chemokines are present in a wide variety of body fluids such as plasma, cerebrospinal fluid, bronchoalveolar fluid, amniotic fluid, synovial fluid, middle ear effusion fluid, urine, and exhaled breath condensate. As an example, cytokine regulation of antibody isotype switching in B cells can be measured to monitor a patient's health. Some common isotypes of antibodies include IgM, IgG1, IgG2a, IgG3, IgA, and IgE. IL-4 is one of the most common cytokines, which inhibits production of IgM, IgG3, and IgG2a antibodies, and induces IgG1

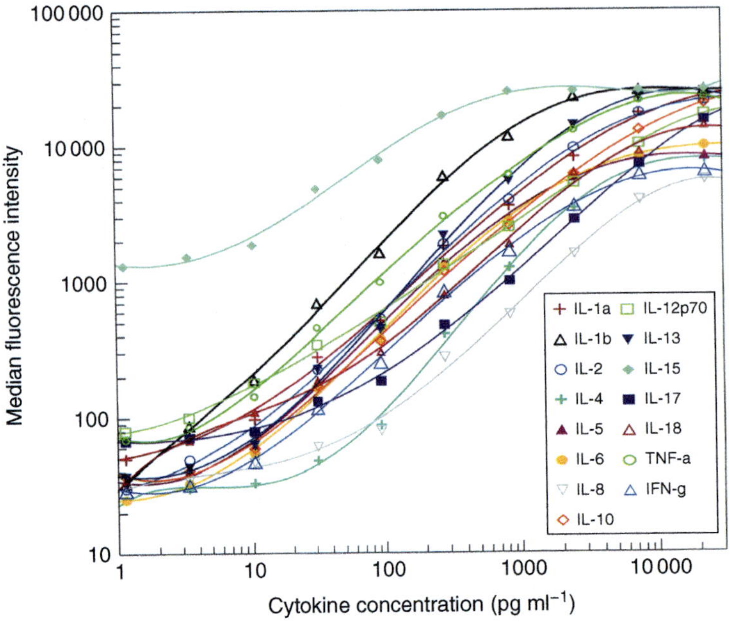

Figure 8.13 Multiplexed standard curves for various cytokines from Luminex assay. *Source:* de Jager et al. [5]. Republished with permission of American Society for Microbiology. Copyright © 1994; permission conveyed through Copyright Clearance Center, Inc.

and IgE antibodies. If we know IgG1 and IgE antibodies are being upregulated by the body (i.e. expressed more), then very likely IL-4 is also upregulated.

8.4 Conclusion

There are many different protein assay technologies that can identify and quantify multiple antibodies and other proteins simultaneously, which can be used to detect a variety of biomarkers of interest. The ELISA assay is the "gold standard" of protein assays, despite its single-plex capability and modest sensitivity because it is widely available in commercial kits for common analytes. Protein chips (based on fluorescence) have much higher multiplexing capability (up to 10 000s-plex) and are cross-reaction limited, and allow for the simultaneous assaying of thousands of samples and analytes; however, typically they are not as sensitive as ELISA and only provide semi-qualitative detection. The Luminex/Bead arrays provide up to 50-plex capability with sensitivity comparable to or less than ELISA.

8.5 Additional Information

8.5.1 Example of Chromogenic Assay

Chromogenic assays rely on the production of a colored reaction product to measure enzymatic activity. Figure 8.14 shows an example of a chromogenic assay for measuring the activity of the enzyme Factor Xa. In the body, Factor Xa acts on the protein prothrombin (coagulation factor II). Factor Xa makes cuts in the protein right after a specific amino acid sequence (Ile-Glu-Gly-Arg). There are two

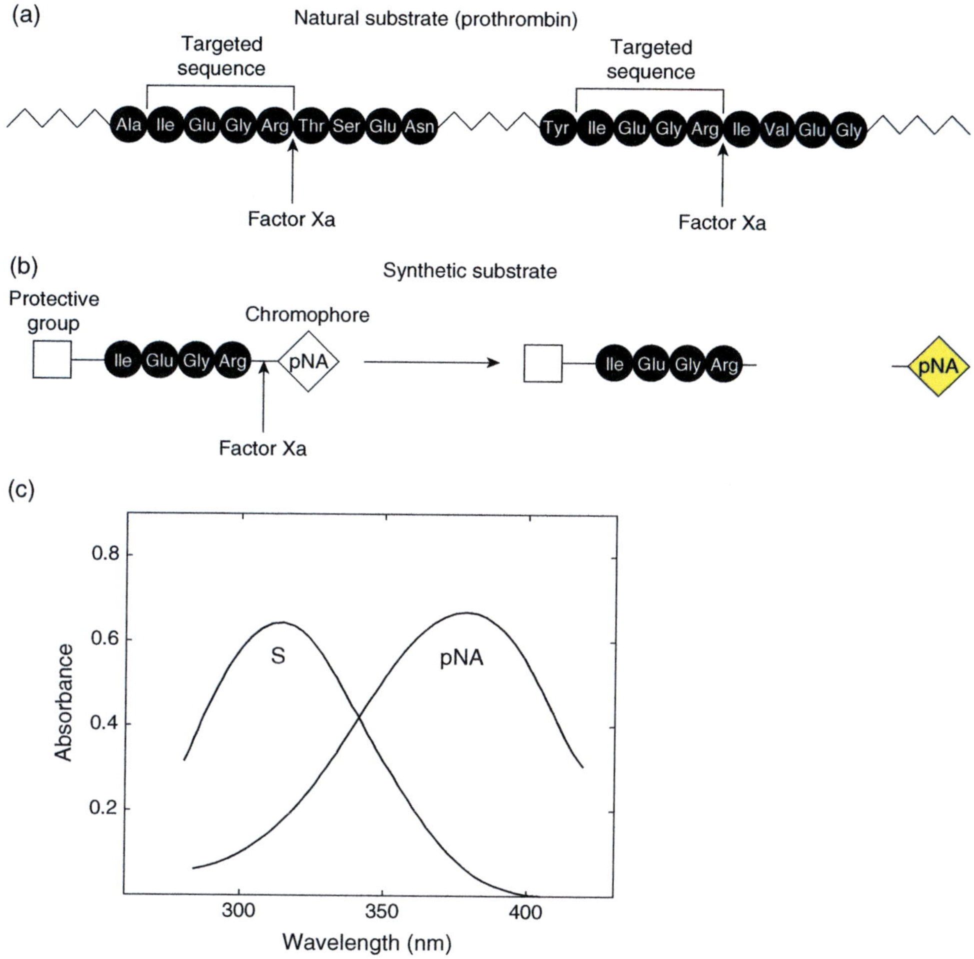

Figure 8.14 (a) In the body, Factor Xa cuts two specific locations in the protein prothrombin. (b) A synthetic substrate which is used to measure the enzymatic activity of Factor Xa through the production of a colored reaction product. (c) Absorption spectra of substrate prior to cleaving (S) and pNA.

such locations on prothrombin, as indicated in Figure 8.14a. Using this natural process, one can develop a synthetic substrate, which changes color upon reacting with Factor Xa. One such substrate is shown in Figure 8.14b. A protective group is attached to the beginning of the specific amino acid sequence, which is terminated with a chromophore (para-nitroaniline [pNA]). Enzymatic activity of Factor Xa cleaves the pNA, which causes a color change. The absorption spectrum of the substrate prior to cleaving and that of pNA are different, as shown in Figure 8.14c. Typically, the reaction is observed at 405 nm where the pNA is highly absorbing, but the substrate is not.

Problems

8.1 Human epididymal secretory protein E4 (HE4, also known as WAP four-disulphide core domain protein 2 or WFDC2) is a new promising biomarker for ovarian cancer. Its molecular weight is 25 kD (kiloDalton). Convert the HE4 molar concentration of 100 pM (mole/liter) to a concentration in another commonly used unit, ng ml^{-1} (nanogram per milliliter).

8.2 Vascular endothelial growth factor (VEGF) is a signal protein that stimulates vasculogenesis and angiogenesis. Its molecular weight is 20 kDa (kiloDalton). Convert the molar concentration of VEGF at 100 pM (picomole/liter) to a concentration in another commonly used unit, ng ml^{-1} (nanogram/milliliter).

8.3 The equilibrium condition for antigen (Ag) – antibody (Ab) reaction is as follows:

$$\text{Ag} + \text{Ab} \leftrightarrow \text{Ag} \cdot \text{Ab}$$

$$K_\text{d} \equiv \frac{[\text{Ag}]_\text{eq}[\text{Ab}]_\text{eq}}{[\text{Ag} \cdot \text{Ab}]_\text{eq}},$$

where $[\ldots]_\text{eq}$ is a concentration at equilibrium.

Derive the Langmuir isotherm formula of $\theta = \dfrac{[\text{Ag}]_\text{eq}}{[\text{Ag}]_\text{eq} + K_\text{d}}$ at equilibrium.

Hint: The summation of antigen-bound and unbound antibody concentrations is always constant.

8.4 We are designing a protein chip, which includes three capture antibodies for three analytes A, B, and C. The antibodies have dissociation constants of 1 μM, 1 nM, and 1 pM, respectively. At the detection limit, we have to capture at least 2000 molecules of each analyte to make a positive determination. Each capture antibody spot occupies an area of $10\,000\,\mu\text{m}^2$, and has an active antibody density of $10\,000$ antibodies μm^{-2}. All the antibodies on the spot are considered capable of reacting with the matched antigens.

A Based on the Langmuir isotherm formula, estimate the minimum concentrations: [A], and [C] that can be detected. The volume of the reaction well is 20 μL.

B What is the fraction of each analyte in the original sample which is actually (captured and) contributing to the signal?

8.5 We are designing a protein chip, which includes a capture antibody for analyte A. The antibody has a dissociation constant of 10 nM. At the detection limit, we must capture at least 200 000 molecules per antibody spot of this analyte to make a positive determination. Each capture antibody spot occupies an area of $100\,\mu\text{m}^2$, and has an active antibody density of $10\,000$ antibodies μm^{-2}. All the antibodies on the spot are considered capable of reacting with the matched antigens.

A Based on the Langmuir isotherm formula, estimate the minimum concentration $[A]$ that can be detected (assume the sensors are read after the association curve saturates).

B The time dependence of coverage θ is given by:

$$\theta = \frac{[A]}{[A] + K_\text{d}}\left(1 - \text{e}^{-(k_\text{on} \cdot [A] + k_\text{off})t}\right)$$

The on and off rates for biding between the antibody and analyte A are $k_\text{on} = 10^4\,\text{M}^{-1}\,\text{s}^{-1}$ and $k_\text{off} = 10^{-4}\,\text{s}^{-1}$. Assume initially all the ligands are unoccupied, and the analyte concentration is 100 nM (this is not the answer for (a)), calculate the incubation time needed such that the sensor can reach the detection limit for testing positive.

C If you were developing a portable sensor device for Point-of-Care applications and the device is designed to display results in five minutes after sample insertion, calculate the minimum and maximum sensor coverage if the analyte concentration ranges from 10 nM to 1 μM. For simplicity, assume the binding between the immobilized capture antibody and the target analyte is the only rate-limiting step (any other steps happen instantaneously).

D Based on what you know about binding kinetics, what can you do to increase the sensitivity of the portable device? Explain your answer.

8.6 You ordered a sandwich ELISA kit designed to detect antibodies against Virus X antigen in human serum to test whether an individual has been successfully vaccinated and has immune protection against Virus X infection.

A Which of the following would be included in the kit as reagents required to run this assay? The manufacturer only includes the least number of reagents you need to be able to run the assay. Assume the manufacturer provides the concentrations of all reagents in the kit.

1) Virus X antigen
2) Antibody against Virus X antigen
3) Substrate
4) HRP-labeled detection antibody against antibody to Virus X antigen
5) HRP-labeled detection antibody against Virus X antigen
6) Plates coated with Virus X antigen
7) Plates coated with antibody against Virus X antigen
8) Unconjugated HRP

B Using the kit, you obtain the standard curve of the ELISA kit and the assay results for three sera (sera = plural of serum, the signals in the plot and table are the optical densities given by the ELISA plate reader, and the standard curve is applicable to all dilution factors listed), as shown in Figure 8.15 and Table 8.1.

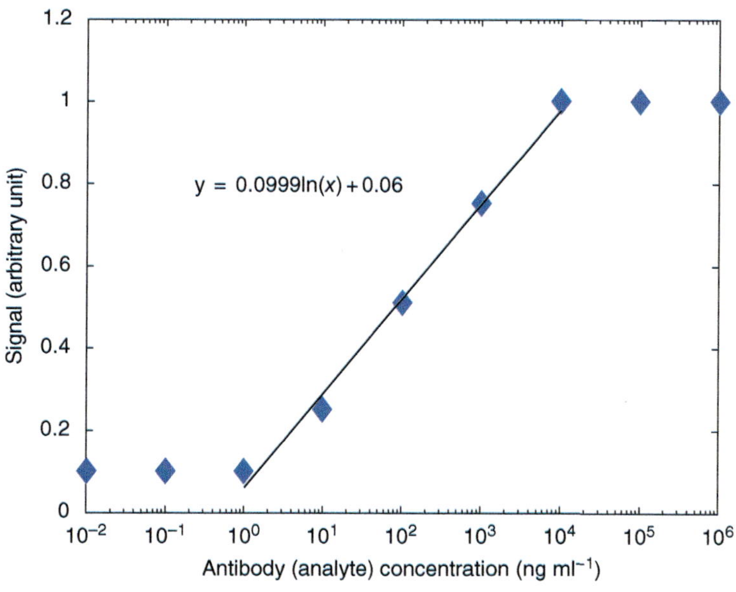

Figure 8.15 Standard curve of an ELISA kit.

Table 8.1 Results obtained with ELISA kit.

			Dilution factor				
Zero-analyte	**Negative control**	**Patient**	**1:1**	**1:10**	**1:100**	**1:1000**	**1:10000**
0.056	0.103	P1	1.02	1.001	0.88	0.65	0.42
0.068	0.096	P2	1.00	0.96	0.99	0.76	0.53
0.060	0.096	P3	0.104	0.102	0.093	0.093	0.091

What is the difference between the negative control and the zero analyte control?

C The assay is missing positive control. How would you do the positive control if you have access to additional materials?

D If you measure an undiluted sample and obtain a readout signal of 0.55, is the signal within the dynamic range of the assay? What is the concentration of the antibody in the sample? What is the antibody concentration if your readout signal is 1.01? Hint: You can utilize the fitting equation of the standard curve, which is valid only within the dynamic range of the assay.

E If the concentration of the antibody is above 3.3 mM ($MW_{\text{antibody}} = 150$ kDa), the patient is very likely protected against Virus X infection. Which (if any) of these patients are protected?
Explain your reasoning.

8.7 Both DNA microarrays and protein assays, especially enzyme-linked immunosorbent assay (ELISA), rely on the "amplification" scheme to detect a very low concentration of analyte of interest. Explain how this scheme is incorporated in DNA microarrays and ELISA.

8.8 We ran a triplicate of ELISA wells to quantify cTn concentrations in a patient with chest pain at Stanford's emergency department. The concentrations were 31.5, 37.0, and 33.5 pg ml^{-1}, respectively. The local cutoff for hospital admission is 30 pg ml^{-1}, i.e. patients with [cTn] ≥ 30 pg ml^{-1} are recommended for admission to the cardiac department.

A What are the mean and CV of the cTn levels measured? Please use "sample" standard deviation in calculating CV.

B What is the CV if you use conventional standard deviation?

C Would you recommend admitting or discharging this patient based on the cTn test alone?

Hint: The "sample" standard deviation of n samples $\{x_i, i = 1, \ldots, n\}$ is

$$\sqrt{\frac{\sum_{i=1}^{n}\left(x_i - x\right)^2}{n-1}},$$

where x is the mean. The conventional standard deviation has the same expression above except that $n-1$ is replaced by n.

8.9 What is the difference between forward and reverse phase protein arrays?

8.10 The autoimmunity protein array discussed in the chapter can be implemented in either forward phase or reverse phase format. If we want to detect possible RA and SLE in five human samples, propose your experiments in both formats. You only need to describe the essential steps.

8.11 Match each DNA or protein assay technology in Column A with an appropriate measurement task in Column B.

Column A	Column B
13) ___Real-time PCR with reverse transcription	**A** The genetic signature of a new pandemic virus.
14) ___DNA microarray	**B** A microRNA (miRNA), which is a short ribonucleic acid (RNA) molecule with only 22 nucleotides long, circulating in blood with very low concentrations (<1 fM).
15) ___DNA sequencing	**C** The prevalence of different strains (with distinct genetic signatures) of HIV, HCV, HPV, influenza, avian influenza, SARS, and human herpes virus, in 10 000 people randomly selected from a large population.
16) ___Sandwich ELISA	**D** Expression level of 20 different autoantibodies in an autoimmune patient.
17) ___Planar antibody array	**E** Expression level of 40 different antigens in five Alzheimer disease patients. Most of the protein concentration levels are known to be above 4 $pg\,ml^{-1}$.
18) ___Luminex/xMAP (sandwich assay)	**F** Expression level of 100 different antigens in 100 cancer patients to validate if some of these antigens are good cancer biomarkers.
19) ___Planar antigen array	**G** HE4 protein level (40–2000 pM) in blood to diagnose ovarian cancer.

References

1 Koczuła, K. and Gallotta, A. Lateral flow assays. *Essays in Biochemistry* 60: 111–120.

2 O'Sullivan, V.J., Barrette-Ng, I., Hommema, E. et al. (2012). Development of a tetrameric streptavidin mutein with reversible biotin binding capability: engineering a mobile loop as an exit door for biotin. *PLoS ONE* 7 (4): e35203.

3 Lee, J.R., Magee, D.M., Gaster, R.S. et al. (2013). Emerging protein array technologies for proteomics. *Expert Review of Proteomics* 10 (1): 65–75.

4 Robinson, W.H., DiGennaro, C., Hueber, W. et al. (2002). Autoantigen microarrays for multiplex characterization of autoantibody responses. *Nature Medicine* 8: 295–301.

5 de Jager, W., te Velthuis, H., Prakken, B.J. et al. (1994). Simultaneous detection of 15 human cytokines in a single sample of stimulated peripheral blood mononuclear cells. *Clinical and Vaccine Immunology Journal* 10 (1): 133–139.

Further Reading

Dill, L. and Grodzinski (2009). *Microarrays: Preparation, Microfluidics, Detection Methods, and Biological Applications*. Springer.

Robinson, B., Goldberger, O., and Maecker, H., Stanford University.

Roth, C., Rutgers University.

Sewter, C., Serologicals/Luminex.

Shena, M. (ed.) (2005). *Protein Microarrays*. Jones and Bartlett Publishers.

Forster, R.J., Bertoncello, P., and Keyes, T.E. (2009). Electrogenerated chemiluminescence. *Annual Review of Analytical Chemistry* 2: 359–385.

Diapharma 5.25.21. http://chromogenicsubstrates.com/tech/chromogenic_substrates_university.htm

NASA Content Administrator, Curiosity Rover's Self Portrait at 'John Klein' Drilling Site, Cropped, 12 February 2013. http://www.nasa.gov/mission_pages/msl/multimedia/pia16764.html

McKay, C.P. and García, V.P. (2014). How to search for life on Mars. *Scientific American*, June 1. http://www.scientificamerican.com/article/how-to-search-for-life-on-mars/?print=true.

9

Label-Free Affinity-Based Biosensors

9.1 Introduction

In general, affinity-based biosensors (Figure 9.1) all center on similar operating principles of binding kinetics. However, they differ in terms of how they transduce ligand-binding events into detectable signals. Generally, a recognition element or recognition elements containing antibodies or other ligands are incubated with a sample containing the target analytes and sometimes a matrix (any media such as blood with analyte embedded in it, which contains many other proteins that are not target analytes). To achieve good specificity, the recognition element is required to possess a high affinity to the target analyte and low affinity to nontargeted analytes and other molecules in the matrix. To achieve good sensitivity, the biosensor should be able to detect very low concentrations of target analyte. Once the target analyte is captured, different transduction mechanisms can be used (e.g. optical, electrical, mechanical, or magnetic detection) to measure various properties of the analyte.

9.1.1 Label-Free Biosensors

As the name implies, "label-free" biosensors are based on inherent signals associated with biomolecules, a binding process, or a biochemical reaction. Thus, no labeling for detection purpose is employed. For example, hemoglobin is an iron-containing oxygen-transport protein in red blood cells and it can be detected with a magnetometer without labeling. Most biosensors in use are "labeled" biosensors that rely on conjugating analyte complexes with signal-generating labels such as fluorescent, colorimetric, or magnetic molecules or particles.

9.2 Surface Plasmon Resonance (SPR) Sensor

Surface plasmon resonance (SPR) biosensors use the phenomenon of resonance due to surface plasmons (collectively oscillating free electrons) to detect target analytes. The cross section of an SPR biosensor is shown in Figure 9.2. An SPR biosensor is constructed from a transparent material such as glass that is coated by a gold film, which is the reflection layer that also provides surface plasmons (the quantized energy of the collective wave motion of surface electrons). Next, a linker layer is placed on top of the gold film, followed by a dextran layer, and finally capture probes

Biochips and Medical Imaging, First Edition. Adam de la Zerda and Shan Xiang Wang.

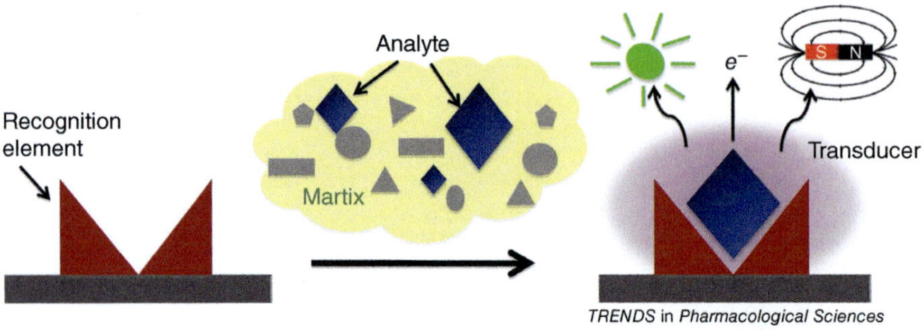

Figure 9.1 Affinity-based biosensors are all based on the affinity between a recognition element and analyte. *Source:* Mach et al. [1]. Reprinted from Trends in Pharmacological Sciences. Copyright © 2011, with permission from Elsevier.

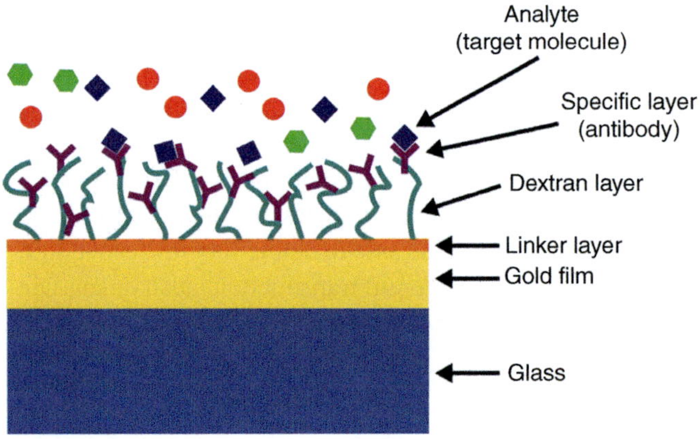

Figure 9.2 Cross section of an SPR biosensor. Immobilized capture antibodies couple to analytes in solution.

(e.g. antibodies as shown) are immobilized on top, which can couple with the target analyte molecules as shown. The coupling of the target analyte with an immobilized capture molecule causes a change in resonance that can be detected by a sensor. There are three ways for the ligand to couple with the analyte: direct coupling of ligand to surface, indirect coupling in which the ligand captures another molecule (e.g. a specific IgG) that then captures the analyte, or membrane anchoring where the interacting ligand is on the surface of a capture liposome (which can amplify the signal by capturing many analytes at one location).

9.2.1 Surface Functionalization

SPR biosensors have at least two common methods of surface functionalization: CM-5 (as shown in Figure 9.2) and SA (Figure 9.3). The CM-5 sensor chip features a carboxymethylated (CM) dextran-coated surface, which allows covalent coupling to a specific ligand (e.g. DNA or antibody) via a variety of functional groups, such as NH_2, SH, CHO, and COOH. The SA sensor chip uses a streptavidin (SA)-coated dextran surface, which can bind to a biotinylated ligand that then captures analyte in solution.

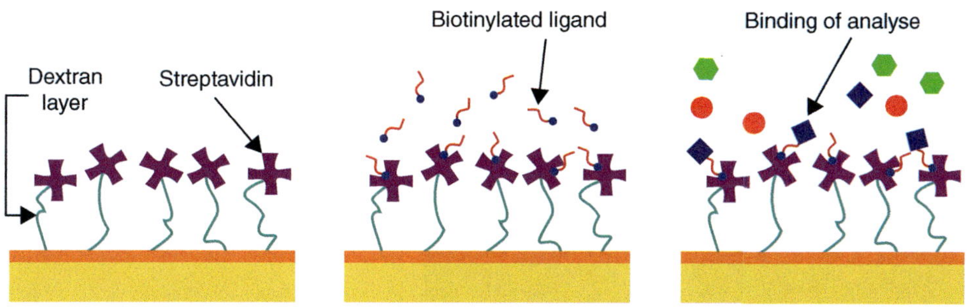

Figure 9.3 Streptavidin sensor chip.

9.2.2 Total Internal Reflection

Total internal reflection (TIR) of the light entering a prism occurs at angles of incidence that are greater than a certain critical angle (Figure 9.4). Although no photons exit the reflecting surface in TIR, their electric field extends about a quarter wavelength beyond the surface, in the form of evanescent waves decaying exponentially from the surface. If a thin gold film is placed on the reflecting surface, then the photons can interact with free electrons in the gold surface, possibly exciting SPR (Figure 9.5). When the SPR condition is satisfied, photons can be converted into plasmons, and the reflected light is greatly reduced. The SPR condition specifies that the horizontal components of the incident light wave vector and the surface plasmon wave vector are equal. This allows energy of incident light to be converted to plasmons by momentum conservation in the horizontal direction and is observed by a minimum reflection. This occurs when the incident light wave vector k_{i} is equal to the surface plasmon wave vector k_{p}:

$$k_{\mathrm{i}} = \frac{2\pi n}{\lambda} \sin\theta = k_{\mathrm{p}}.$$

9.2.3 Effect of Binding on SPR

Plasmons create an evanescent electric field extending into the medium surrounding the film. This electric field is affected by changes in the medium from binding of an analyte, due to a change in plasmon velocity. This velocity change, in turn, alters the incident light wave vector required for SPR and minimum reflection. It is this change that is measured by the SPR biosensors.

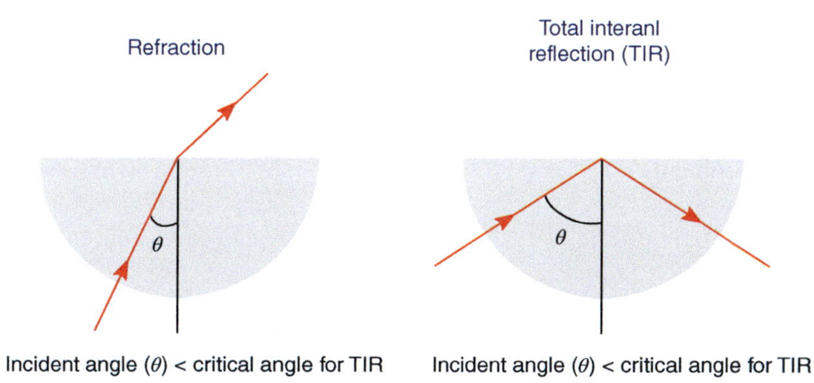

Figure 9.4 Refraction versus total internal reflection.

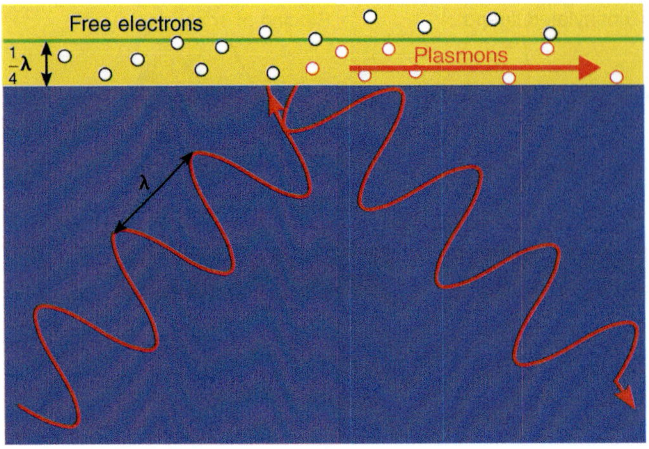

Figure 9.5 Incident light to plasmons.

9.2.4 Measurement of Binding

Light is shined from the back of the sensor and binding is measured as a change in the refractive index at the surface of the sensor due to SPR. The change in refractive index is essentially the same for a given mass concentration change which allows mass/concentration deductions to be made. Binding events are measured in real time, allowing separate on and off rates to be deduced.

9.2.5 How Does BIACore Measure This?

The BIACore SPR sensor uses angular scanning in which the sensor is oriented upside down and fixed wavelength light is directed at the sensor surface with a variable incidence angle (Figure 9.6a). Antigen-binding events are detected as changes in the particular angle where SPR creates extinction of light (i.e. the angle corresponding to minimum light intensity in the graph shown below) as shown in Figure 9.6b. This difference in minimum reflection angle serves as the resonance signal, which increases over time as more analyte molecules are bound.

The progress of an interaction is monitored as a sensorgram. Analyte binds to the surface-attached ligand during sample injection, resulting in an increase in signal during association. At the end of the injection, the sample is replaced by a continuous flow of buffer and the decrease in signal now reflects dissociation of interactant from the surface-bound complex. A response of 1000 RU (kRU or Kilo Resonance Unit, an arbitrary normalized unit of resonance signal) corresponds to a change in surface concentration of ~1 ng mm^{-2}. Finally, regeneration occurs when all analytes are detached by applied heat or oxygen plasma, and the sensor is regenerated by refunctionalizing for subsequent experiments.

9.2.6 SPR Measurements

As shown in Figure 9.7, the SPR sensor signal is linear with the concentration of analyte in solution measured in gram per liter. The same response is obtained for different proteins. Each shape corresponds to a different type of protein. Note that the concentration in solution is proportional to the surface concentration of analyte (often measured in nanograms per mm^2).

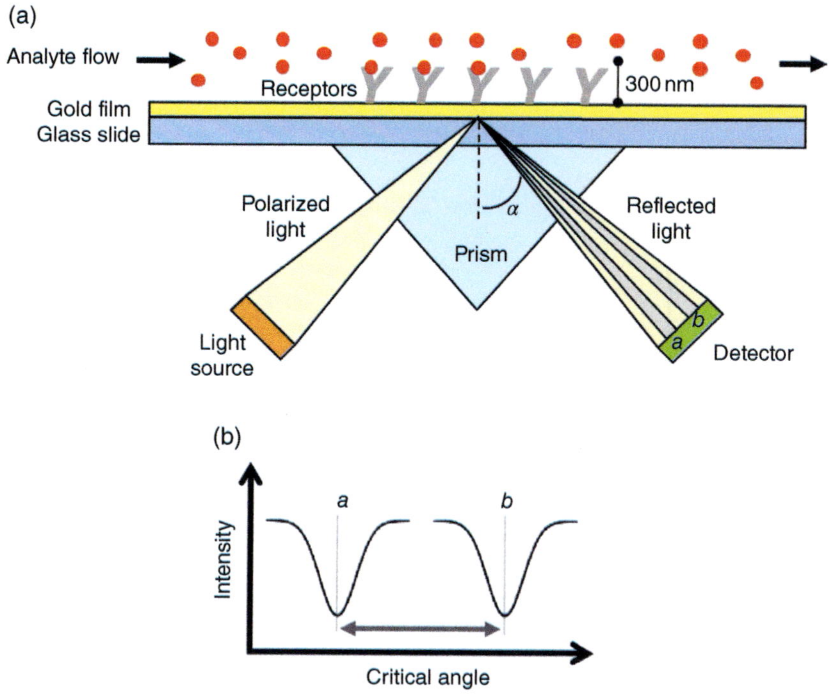

Figure 9.6 (a) BIACore SPR sensor configuration. (b) Change in critical angle of incident light upon binding of analyte to receptor molecule. *Source:* Patching [2]. Reprinted from Biochimica et Biophysica Acta (BBA) – Biomembranes. Copyright © 2014, with permission from Elsevier.

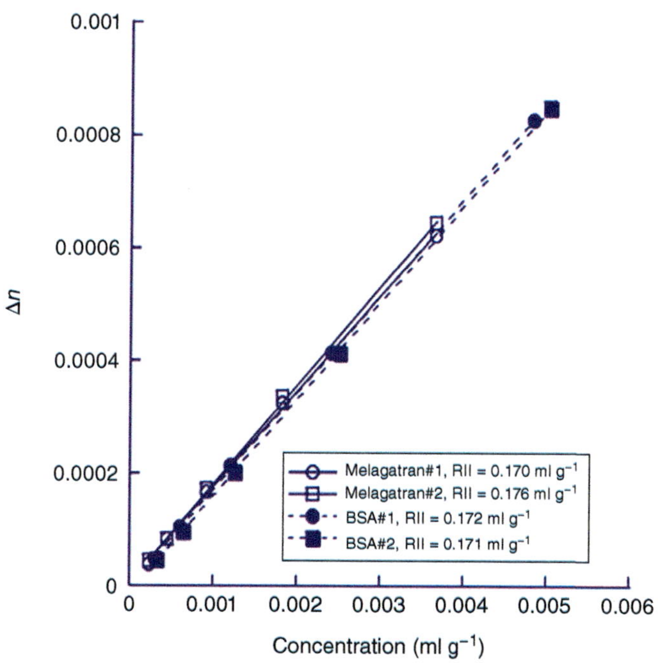

Figure 9.7 SPR sensor signal versus concentration of analyte in solution for various proteins. *Source:* Pol et al. [3]. Reprinted from Analytical Biochemistry. Copyright © 2016, with permission from Elsevier.

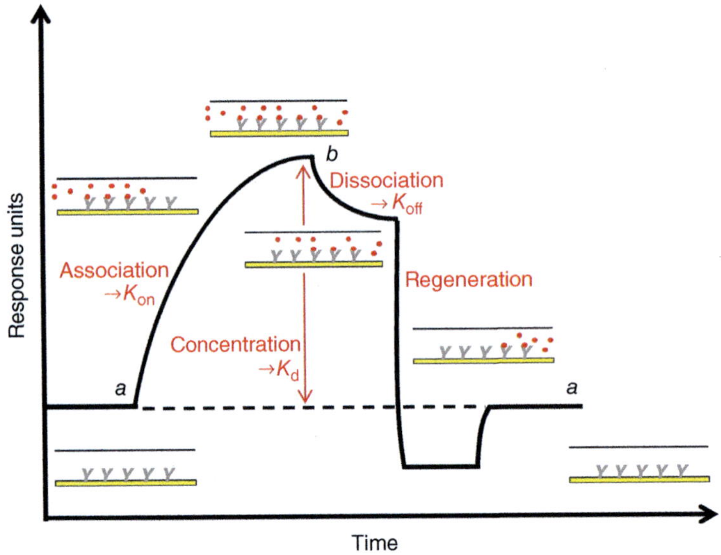

Figure 9.8 Kinetic interpretation of a SPR sensorgram (a and b on the graph correspond to changes in critical angle shown in Figure 9.6b). *Source:* Patching [2]. Reprinted from Biochimica et Biophysica Acta (BBA) – Biomembranes. Copyright © 2014, with permission from Elsevier.

SPR sensor measurements with different analyte concentrations can be used to generate binding kinetics curves (Figure 9.8), which can be used to measure the on rate (k_{on}), off rate (k_{off}), association constant (K_a), and disassociation constant (K_d). The kinetics equations are summarized below:

$$L + A \leftrightarrow LA,$$

where L = ligand, A = analyte.

$$\frac{\mathrm{d}[LA]}{\mathrm{d}t} = k_{on}[L][A] - k_{off}[LA].$$

At equilibrium,

$$k_{on}[L][A] = k_{off}[LA],$$

$$K_d = \frac{[L][A]}{[LA]} = \frac{k_{off}}{k_{on}} = \frac{1}{K_a}.$$

9.2.7 Flow Cell Design

SPR sensors can be incorporated into a flow cell design where the surface is divided into four channels (Figure 9.9), which can be used individually (F1 to F4) or in a number of combinations (e.g. in series with added signals). If the four chambers are functionalized with different recognition molecules, a 4-plex experiment can be performed. Alternatively, the four chambers can be functionalized with the same recognition molecules to measure the average signal across the four chambers.

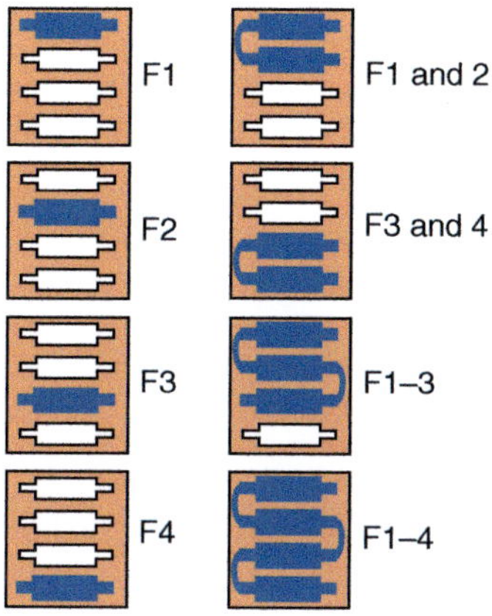

Figure 9.9 Flow cell designs.

The microfluidic channel design features laminar flow, which results in low reagents consumption, efficient mass transport, and low sample dispersion (i.e. moving at differing velocities). This gives highly reproducible injections, with CV values typically less than 1%. Also, the sample can be recovered from the microfluidic chip if needed.

9.3 Nanowire Field-Effect (FET) Sensors

Field-effect sensors rely on a FET structure to measure a change in conductance in response to analyte detection. Given a p-type Si channel, a positive applied voltage would result in hole depletion, which can be observed as a decrease in conductance. Similarly, a silicon nanowire-based FET sensor (Figure 9.10) is configured with antibody receptors that can capture target analyte molecules. When the sensor is exposed to a solution containing a macromolecule (e.g. protein) with a net positive charge in aqueous solution, specific binding will lead to an increase in the surface positive charge and a decrease in conductance for a p-type nanowire device. Nanowire FET sensors are among the most sensitive biosensors available, with a sensitivity of fM level for protein and DNA detection. Nanowire sensors can also be arranged in arrays for multiplexing capability.

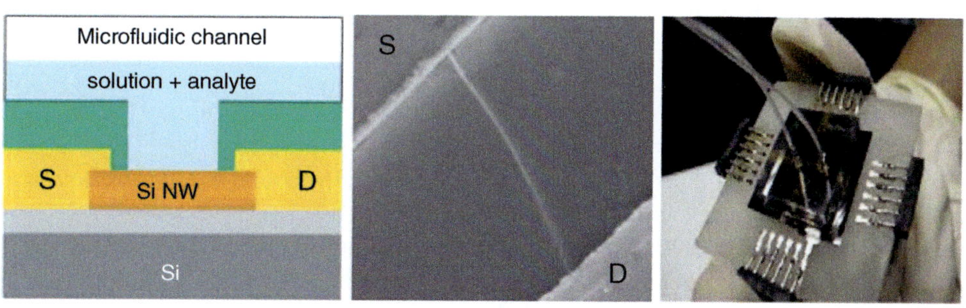

Figure 9.10 Cross sectional diagram and scanning electron microscopy image of a single Si nanowire sensor device, and a prototype nanowire sensor biochip with integrated microfluidic sample delivery. *Source:* Patolsky and Lieber [4]. Reprinted from Materials Today. Copyright © 2005, with permission from Elsevier.

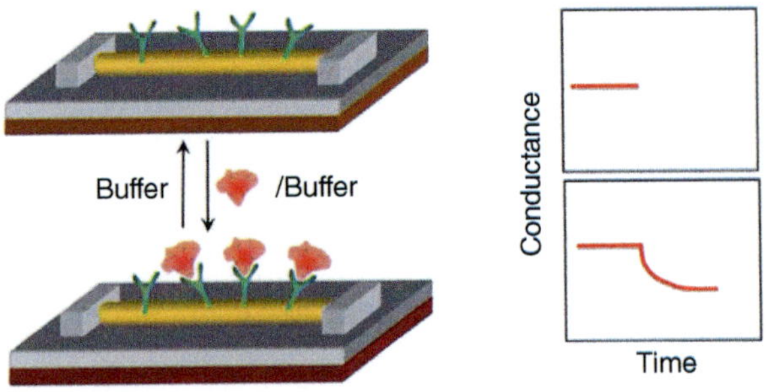

Figure 9.11 P-type Si nanowire-based FET. *Source:* Patolsky and Lieber [4]. Reprinted from Materials Today. Copyright © 2005, with permission from Elsevier.

Nanowire sensors can detect proteins and nucleic acids in solutions. If proteins are positively charged (when the pH value they are in is lower than their isoelectric point, pI), attachment of proteins near a p-type gate can turn the FET off by pushing away the holes from the channel region. This causes a decrease in the conductance.

A p-type Si nanowire-based FET is shown in Figure 9.11. The green moieties are antibodies fixed on the nanowire and the red substances are positively charged proteins. When the nanowire captures positively charged proteins, the positive charge pushes the holes from the channel and reduces the conductance between drain and source.

Similarly, nanowire sensors can detect negatively charged nucleic acids (e.g. DNA and RNA). DNA and RNA carry a net negative charge due to their phosphate backbone. When they get captured by a p-type Si nanowire-based FET, they pull holes to the channel region and increase the conductance between source and drain. This is similar to applying negative voltage to the gate of a pMOS and turning it on.

9.4 Cantilever Sensors

Cantilever sensors can detect chemical vapors or solution-phase analytes at very low concentrations based on the surface stress changes generated by the interactions between probe and target molecules on cantilever surfaces. The magnitude of the surface stress change depends on the type of interaction taking place, which includes hydrogen bonding, electrostatic forces, van der Waals forces, etc. Stoney's formula gives the deflection at the end of a cantilever, Δh, as a function of the surface stress change, $\Delta\sigma$:

$$\Delta h = \frac{3(1-v)L^2}{Et^2} \cdot \Delta\sigma,$$

where L and t are the length and thickness of the cantilever, respectively, and E and v are Young's modulus and Poisson's ratio of the cantilever material.

By measuring the cantilever deflection caused by the binding of target analyte molecules (Figure 9.12), the surface stress change can be found by using Stoney's formula, giving the target vapor (or analyte) concentration. The cantilever deflection can be detected optically by shining a beam of collimated light onto the cantilever, which produces a reflected light spot on a CCD image plane that moves up and down with cantilever deflection (Figure 9.13). Cantilever sensors can also be arranged in an array for multiplexing capability.

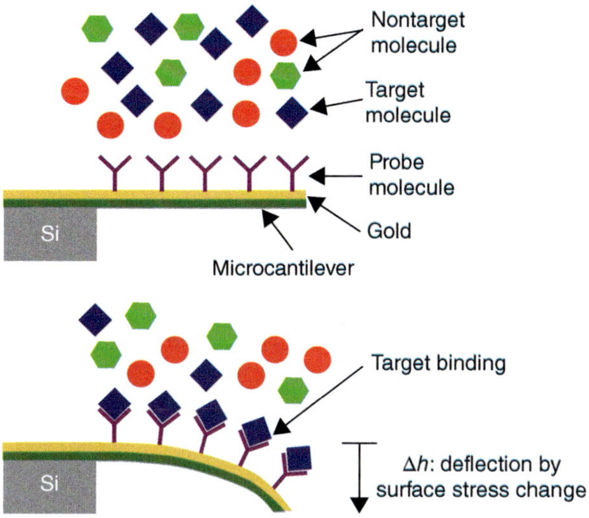

Figure 9.12 Cantilever sensor.

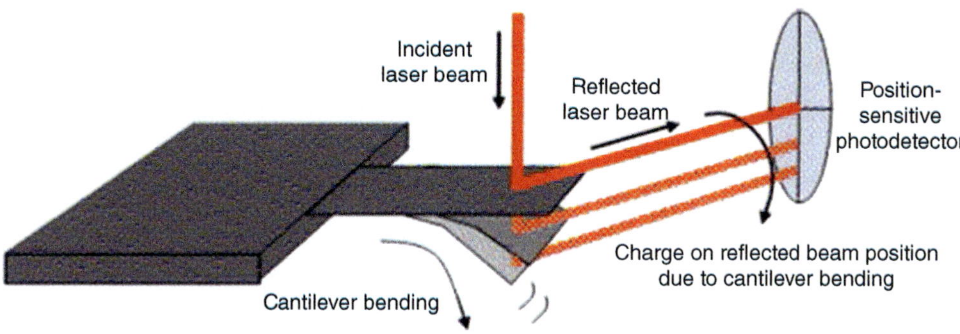

Figure 9.13 Measurement of cantilever sensor deflection by CCD. *Source:* Carrascosa et al. [5]. Reprinted from TrAC Trends in Analytical Chemistry. Copyright © 2006, with permission from Elsevier.

9.5 Electrochemical Sensors

Electrochemical biosensors are sensors that use electronics to detect a chemical reaction in response to the presence of a target analyte. Similar to ELISA, electrochemical biosensors typically feature a sandwich structure with a capture antibody, target analyte, and detection antibody. After the sandwich structure is formed, an enzyme such as horseradish peroxidase (HRP) induces added tetramethylbenzidine (TMB) substrate to undergo an oxidation reaction, which expels an electron. These electrons are then translated into an electrical signal that can be measured and quantified.

9.5.1 Electrochemical Biosensors for DNA/Protein

Figure 9.14a shows an array of 16 electrochemical biosensors, each made up of a gold film with a working electrode in the middle, surrounded by a reference gold electrode (circular electrode). A voltage is applied between the two electrodes of each sensor and the resulting current is measured in the presence of target analyte. Since each sensor is independent, up to 16 analytes can be

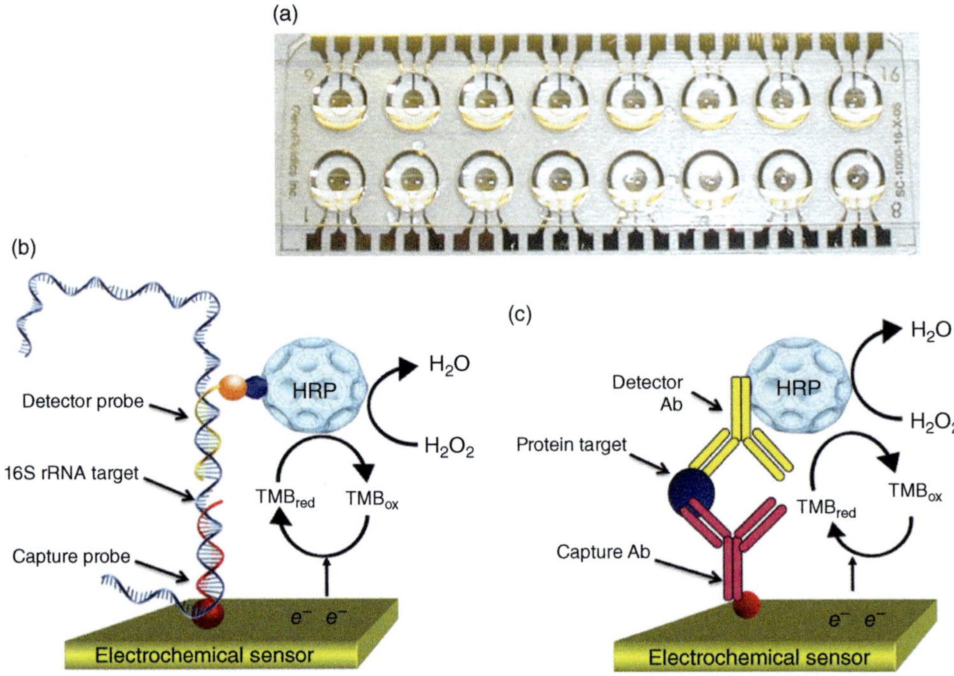

Figure 9.14 (a) Array of electrochemical sensors. *Source:* Gau et al. [6]. Reprinted from Methods. Copyright © 2005, with permission from Elsevier. (b) Nucleic acid detection. (c) Protein detection. *Source:* Mohan et al. [7]. CC0 1.0 public domain.

detected with one recognition molecule for each working electrode. Electrochemical biosensors can be used for detection of either nucleic acids (Figure 9.14b) or proteins (Figure 9.14c). For nucleic acid detection, a target strand is first captured with the capture probe, which then attracts a detector probe labeled with HRP enzyme. The enzyme will then catalyze an oxidation–reduction reaction, where TMB substrate is oxidized by peroxide and loses electrons in the process. This reaction is circular so that the signal will be amplified many times for one target (note the difference between signal amplification by HRP and sample amplification by PCR).

9.5.1.1 What Is 16S rRNA?

Ribosomes, which are organelles (~25 nm in size) and act like enzymes, move along the messenger RNA (mRNA) strand, reading the code contained in its sequence of nucleotide bases and stringing the right amino acids together based on the code to build protein chains, i.e. translating mRNA into proteins. Ribosomes are composed of two subunits (small subunit and large subunit) that come together to read the mRNA and create the peptide chain (Figure 9.15). Each of these subunits is made of ribosomal RNA and protein. Ribosomal ribonucleic acid (rRNA) is the RNA component of the ribosome. The orange-colored part is one single RNA molecule called 16S rRNA. The blue part is a collection of 21 proteins that are bound to the RNA.

16S rRNA is a type of rRNA that does not vary much from one organism to another. What variations there are occur in predictable locations. So, 16S rRNA is like a fingerprint: comparing certain locations on a 16S rRNA molecule with a database of known organisms allows the identification of organisms whose 16S rRNA signature is known. This is somewhat similar to single nucleotide polymorphism (SNP), which is used like a fingerprint for individuals, but on an interspecies scale (i.e. same within species but slightly different between different species).

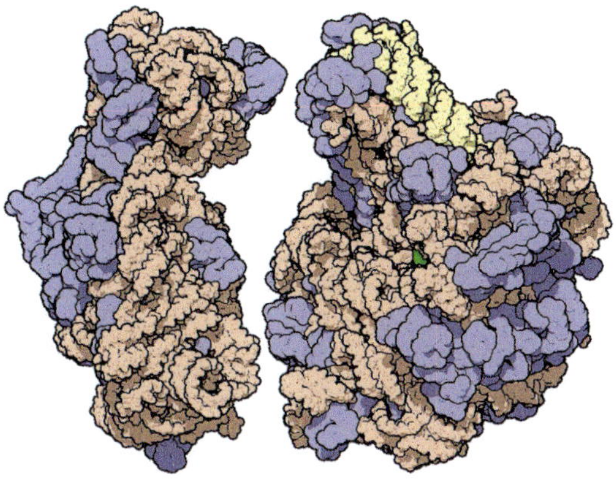

Figure 9.15 Subunits of ribosome. *Source:* Berman et al. [8]. Courtesy of PDB-101, rcsb.org. CC0 1.0 public domain.

9.5.2 Cyclic Voltammetry

The readout of the electrochemical sensor can be done by cyclic voltammetry, which uses alternate forward and reverse voltage scans applied to the working electrode with respect to the reference electrode to produce a hysteresis curve (Figure 9.16). The forward scan (with the working electrode increasingly negative) produces a negative current peak for any analytes that can be reduced through the range of the potential scanned. The current will increase as the potential reaches the reduction potential of the analyte, but then falls off as the concentration of the analyte is depleted close to the electrode surface. When the applied potential is reversed (with the working electrode increasingly positive) during the reverse scan, it will reach the potential that will reoxidize the product formed in the first reduction reaction, and produce a current of reverse polarity from the forward scan. As a result, information about the electrochemical reaction rates of the compounds is obtained.

9.6 Multiplex Detection of Polymicrobial UTI (Urinary Tract Infection)

Multiplex analyte detection is often useful, such as for detection of polymicrobial urinary tract infection (UTI). In order to detect commonly observed bacteria in UTI patients, first a sample is obtained from the patient and cultured, after a few days, the bacteria will grow into colonies

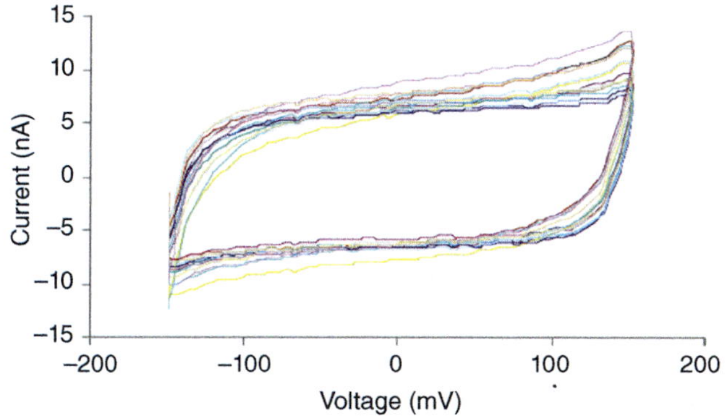

Figure 9.16 Cyclic voltammetry. *Source:* Reprinted with permission from Liao et al. [9]. Copyright © 2006 IEEE.

(a)

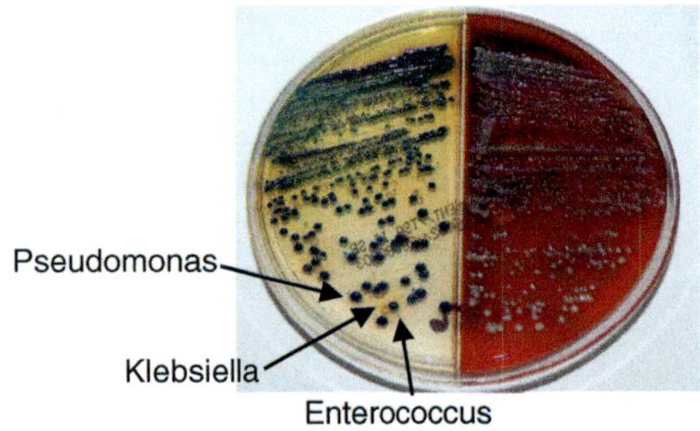

(b)

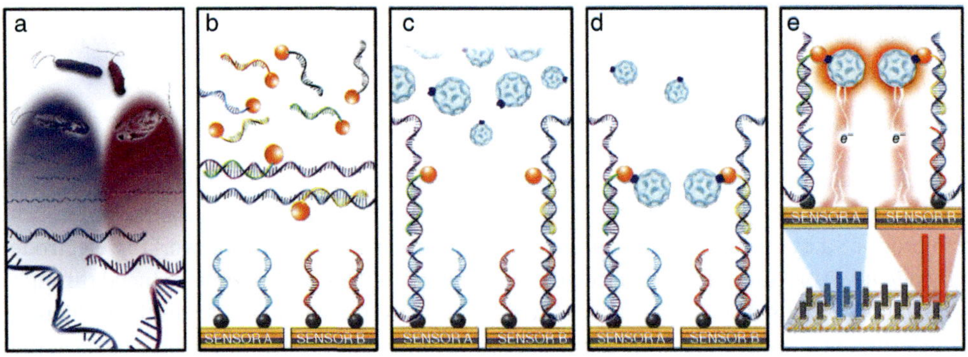

Figure 9.17 (a) Colonies on a petri dish. *Source:* Courtesy of Dr. Joseph Liao. (b) Multiple analyte detection. *Source:* Mach et al. [1]. Reprinted from Trends in Pharmacological Sciences. Copyright © 2011, with permission from Elsevier.

(Figure 9.17a). Then the sample undergoes lysis (Figure 9.17b) where DNA is broken into single strands and fragmented to form single-stranded DNA fragments. Next, hybridization with biotinylated detector probes and then capture probes is performed to form a sandwich structure. Then, an enzyme such as HRP is added, which conjugates to biotin. Finally, a substrate such as TMB is added and the electrochemical readout is performed using an appropriate voltage or voltage sweep. The electrical signal is monotonically related to the number of captured target analytes, thus an increased analyte concentration will lead to a higher electrical signal.

9.6.1 UTI – Standard of Care Diagnosis and Treatment

UTI diagnosis is currently performed using a standard culture of a urine sample, which involves feeding the bacteria with nutrients and cell culture media for about 18–24 hours. Diagnosis is done by a combination of clinical symptoms and a positive urine culture, and the usual prescribed course of treatment is antibiotics. If necessary, an antimicrobial susceptibility test (AST) can be performed in 48–72 hours to determine whether the bacteria present are susceptible to certain antibiotics.

9.6.2 UTI – Biosensor Diagnostics

By using the appropriate set of biomarker capture probes, electrochemical biosensors can potentially be used to perform much faster UTI diagnosis within 1 hour and AST in less than 3.5 hours. With traditional electrodes, multiplexing becomes challenging as each electrical contact needs to be addressed individually in addition to reference and counter-electrodes. One potential solution that has been proposed is solution-based circuits. In this design, columns of electrodes are overlaid with rows of electrochemical solution. The result is an array of biosensors that can be analyzed individually but with shared contacts, which greatly reduces the burden of multiplexing without compromising the limit of detection (a limit of detection of 1 cfu μl^{-1} has been shown, which is clinically significant). An example chip with nine probes is shown in Figure 9.18a. Figure 9.18b–d shows the response of the chip when spiked with three different bacteria. In particular, multiple probes can be addressed simultaneously. Using the same technology, a chip capable of testing 30 different probes for UTI diagnosis and assessment of antibiotic resistance was developed.

Generally speaking, the goal of biosensor diagnostics is to provide better, faster, and cheaper diagnostics using biomarkers for different diseases. Biosensors enable diagnostics with improved sensitivity and specificity depending on the molecular probe design of capture and detection probes. Biosensors also enable multiplex capability, or integration of several assays onto a single platform, commercialized electrochemical, optical, electrical, and magnetic biosensor chips can integrate up to thousands of assays on a single platform. The small size of biosensor chips also makes point-of-care applications easy to implement, while retaining the precision and multiplexity of lab-based methods.

9.6.3 Amperometric Readout

Alternative to cyclic voltammetry, one can conduct an amperometric measurement to detect analyte species. For this method, the potential is not scanned, but held constant at the point where background (parasitic) electrochemical reactions are minimized, so the output current is close to zero.

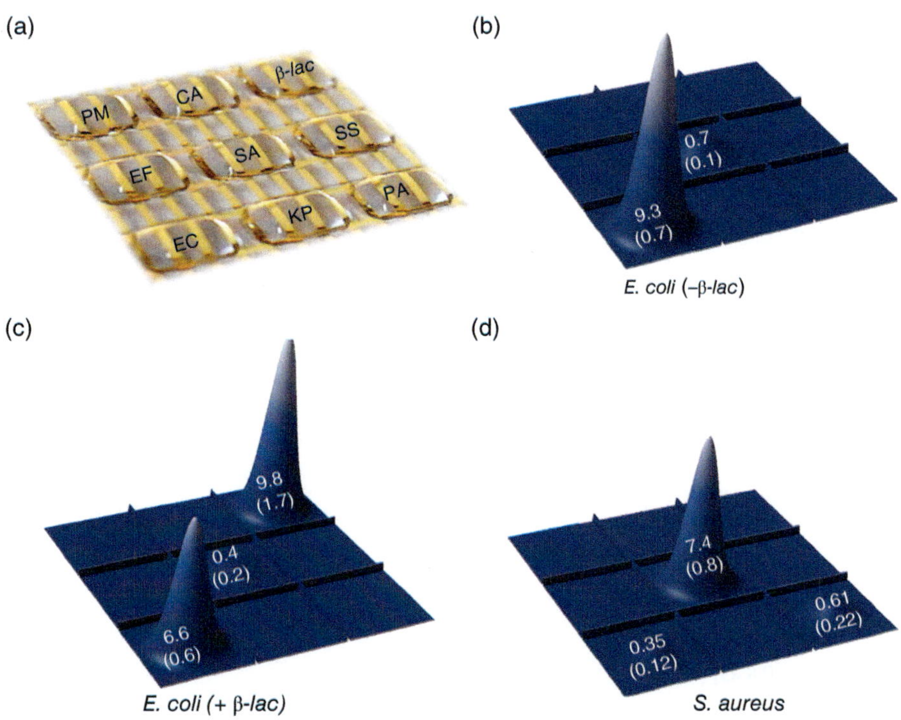

Figure 9.18 (a) Biosensor chip made of solution-based circuits and nine probes. (b–d) Chip results from three different bacteria. *Source:* Lam et al. [10]. Reprinted by permission from Springer Nature. Copyright © 2013 by Springer Nature.

However, if the detection sandwiches (capture antibody + target + labeled detector antibody) are present at the electrode surface, then the enzyme-substrate biochemical reaction generates product molecules that can interact with the electrode, which is held at the appropriate potential and, consequently, can generate detectable currents. Hence, this detectable current originated from the product can then be translated to the amount of analyte species through calibration of the detected current (signal). For example, the reactions are:

$$\text{Oxidation}: \quad HRP + 2 \cdot H_2O_2 + TMB \rightarrow HRP + TMBR^{+} + 2 \cdot H_2O + O_2$$

$$\text{Reduction}: \quad TMB^{2+} + 2 \cdot e^{-} \rightarrow TMB$$

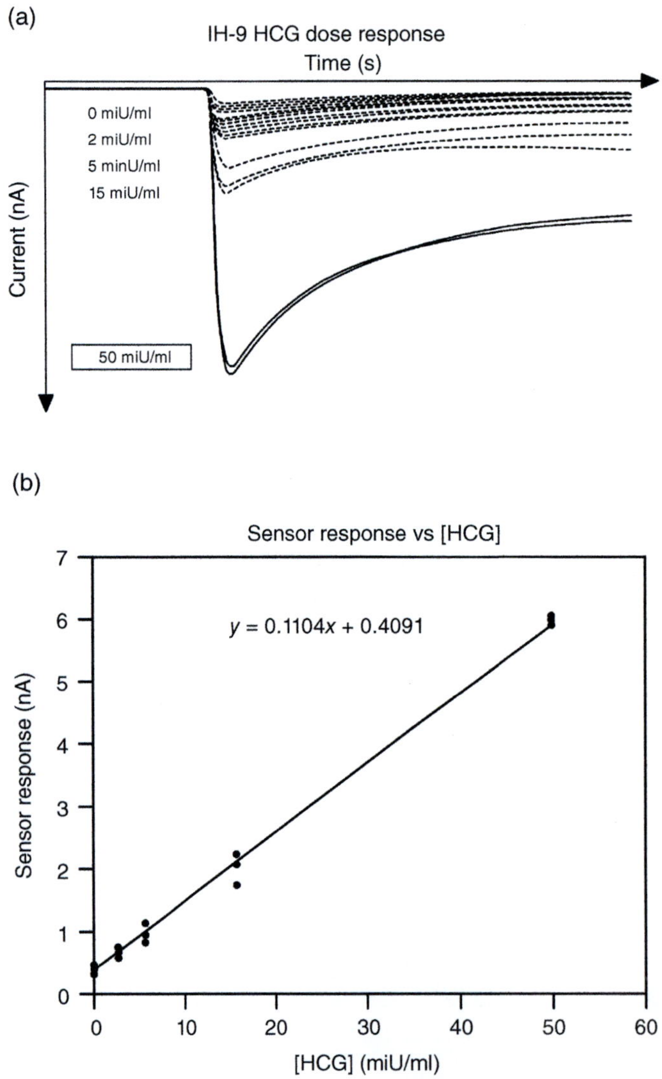

Figure 9.19 (a) An example of amperometric readout data: time courses of current signals. (b) Standard curve of hCG assays by electrochemical sensing. *Source:* Figures adapted from US patent US7723099B2 [11].

TMB^{2+} is being reduced back to TMB by the electrode (under a negative voltage). For certain commercial products, an alkaline phosphatase (ALP) + p-APP substrate system is used. ("Sodium Aminophenyl Phosphate" is full name for p-APP substrate.) Example systems are Abbott's i-Stat Troponin I and BNP cartridges for cardiovascular disease diagnosis.

Figure 9.19 shows an example of amperometric readout data. Figure 9.19a shows the current versus time plot for various concentrations of an analyte (HCG in this example). When the concentration is 0, there is still a signal present. This is called the background signal. Since the sensor detects redox reactions near the gold surface, it is possible to get signal from the reactions that occur naturally in the environment. When the concentration is increased to 50 mIU ml^{-1} (IU = International Unit), the signal level is significantly higher compared to the background level. The red dotted line specifies the time point used for detection. The signal level (current in nA) at this time point is recorded for all of the concentrations and shown in a current versus concentration plot in Figure 9.19b. Using this plot, which is the standard curve of the HCG electrochemical assay, one can easily determine the concentration of the analyte in an unknown sample by measuring the peak current.

9.7 Conclusion

Four major types of affinity-based biosensors including electrochemical, SPR, nanowire, and cantilever biosensors are presented in this chapter. All of them use a recognition element with ligands to capture the target analyte with high sensitivity and specificity. Once the target analyte is captured, different transduction mechanisms are used for detection measurements. The SPR, nanowire, and cantilever biosensors also have the advantage of being *label-free*, compared to other sensors that require an added label for target detection.

Problems

9.1 In an SPR biosensor, the incident wavelength (in air) is 633 nm, the refractive index of the gold layer is 0.40, and the refractive index of the prism next to the gold layer is 1.50.

A What is the critical incidence angle for total internal reflection?

B What is the range of the surface plasmon wave vectors that corresponds to the range of the incident angles?

9.2 Surface Plasmon Resonance (SPR) occurs when the incident light wave vector k_i (which is parallel to the conductor surface) is equal to the surface plasmon wave vector k_p. These wave vectors are defined as

$$k_i = \frac{2\pi}{\lambda} n_1 \sin\theta$$

$$k_p = \frac{2\pi}{\lambda} \cdot \frac{n_2 \cdot n_3}{\sqrt{n_2^2 + n_3^2}},$$

where λ is the wavelength of the incident light, n_1 is the refractive index of the prism, n_2 is the refractive index of the conductor (i.e. the gold layer), and n_3 is the refractive index of the sample medium.

A What is the incident angle for exciting SPR?

B What is the expression for the sensitivity of SPR measurement at the SPR angle, where sensitivity is defined as the ratio of the change in incident angle θ_p over the change in the refractive index of the sample medium?

Hint: You may need the following formula:

$$\frac{d}{dx}\left(\frac{ax}{\sqrt{a^2+x^2}}\right)=\frac{a^3}{\left(a^2+x^2\right)^{3/2}}$$

C The refractive indices of the prism, the gold layer, and the sample medium before binding to analytes are 1.7, 0.4, and 1.5, respectively. What is the SPR angle? If this SPR has the limit of detection (LOD) of 0.0001°, how much change in the refractive index of the sample medium can be detected at the SPR angle?

9.3 The equilibrium condition for ligand-analyte reaction is as follows:

$$L + A \leftrightarrow LA,$$

where L = ligand, A = analyte, $\theta = [LA]/[LA]_{max}$,

$$K_d = \frac{[L][A]}{[LA]}.$$

Derive the Langmuir isotherm formula, where $[LA]_{max\_}$ is a constant.

9.4 The kinetics equation was discussed in the chapter:

$$L + A \leftrightarrow LA,$$

where L = ligand, A = analyte, $\theta = [LA]/[LA]_{max}$,

$$K_d = \frac{[L][A]}{[LA]}.$$

A Derive the time dependence of coverage θ, i.e. the equation of the association curve, if $[A]$ is a constant, and initially all the ligands are unoccupied.

B If coverage $\theta = 0.5$ and $[A]$ turns zero at time $t = 0$, i.e. the biochip is washed with phosphate buffered saline (PBS) solution continuously at $t > 0$, derive the time course of θ, i.e. the equation of the dissociation curve.

C The on and off rates for binding between streptavidin (ligand) and biotinylated DNA (analyte) vary widely in the literature. If $k_{on} = 5 \times 10^6\ M^{-1}\ s^{-1}$, and $k_{off} = 10^7\ s^{-1}$, for the situation in (b), calculate the time required for the coverage to drop from 0.5 to 0.25.

D If your experiment time is limited to two hours, estimate the range of the off rate values you can measure reliably in (c).

E Now consider the situation in (a). If $[A] = 1$ nM, 1 pM, and 1 fM, respectively, calculate the time required for the coverage to increase from 0 to 0.5.

Hint: It may not be possible to reach coverage of 0.5 in certain situations.

9.5 The kinetics equation was discussed in the chapter:

$$\mathrm{Ab} + \mathrm{Ag} \leftrightarrow \mathrm{Ab}\cdot\mathrm{Ag}$$

$$\frac{\mathrm{d}\left[\mathrm{Ab}\cdot\mathrm{Ag}\right]}{\mathrm{d}t} = k_{\mathrm{on}}\left[\mathrm{Ab}\right]\left[\mathrm{Ag}\right] - k_{\mathrm{off}}\left[\mathrm{Ab}\cdot\mathrm{Ag}\right]$$

$$\theta \equiv \frac{\left[\mathrm{Ab}\cdot\mathrm{Ag}\right]}{\left[\mathrm{Ab}\cdot\mathrm{Ag}\right]_{\mathrm{max}}},$$

where Ab = antibody and Ag = antigen.

A Derive the time dependence of coverage $\theta(t)$, i.e. the equation of the association curve, if the concentration of antigen, [Ag], is constant and initially all the antibodies are unoccupied.

B If the coverage $\theta = 0.5$ and [Ag] turns to be zero at time $t = 0$, i.e. the biochip is washed with phosphate buffered saline (PBS) solution continuously at $t > 0$, derive the time course of coverage $\theta(t)$, i.e. the equation of the dissociation curve.

C The on and off rates of interaction between Carcinoembryonic Antigen (CEA) and antibody against it vary in the literature. If $k_{\mathrm{on}} = 2\times10^{5}\mathrm{M}^{-1}\mathrm{s}^{-1}$, and $k_{\mathrm{off}} = 10^{-5}\mathrm{s}^{-1}$, for the situation in part (b), calculate the time required for the coverage to drop from 0.5 to 0.25.

If you use an Si nanowire-based FET sensor with this antibody to detect CEA in a sample, how long does it take to obtain 90% of the fully saturated coverage? The concentration of CEA is 100 pM, and you flow the sample continuously at proper speed to maintain the constant concentration near the nanowire.

9.6 Some macromolecules exhibit cooperative binding in which multiple ligands can bind to the same macromolecule, such that we have:

$$A + nL \leftrightarrow AL_n \quad \text{where } n > 1$$

For example, hemoglobin exhibits cooperative binding with n = 2.8–3.0. In this case, the expression for the dissociation constant K_{d} for this cooperative binding reaction can be written as:

$$K_{\mathrm{d}} = \frac{\left[L\right]^{n}\left[A\right]}{\left[AL_n\right]}.$$

A Let θ be the fraction of binding sites that are occupied on the macromolecule. Derive the expression for θ in terms of L, n, and K_{d}.

B Describe an experimental plan to find the values of n and K_{d}.

9.7 In your own words, describe similarity and difference between the sensing mechanisms of SPR and Nanowire biosensors.

9.8 Estimate the zero-analyte level of the electrochemical sensor for hCG discussed in the chapter and explain why this value is nonzero

References

1 Mach, K.E., Wong, P.K., and Liao, J.C. (June 2011). Biosensor diagnosis of urinary tract infections: a path to better treatment? *Pharmacological Sciences* 32 (6): 330–336.

2 Patching, S.G. (January 2014). Surface plasmon resonance spectroscopy for characterization of membrane protein–ligand interactions and its potential for drug discovery. *Biochimica et Biophysica Acta (BBA) - Biomembranes* 1838 (1): 43–55.

3 Pol, E., Roos, H., Markey, F. et al. (October 2016). Evaluation of calibration-free concentration analysis provided by Biacore™ systems. *Analytical Biochemistry* 510: 88–97.

4 Patolsky, F. and Lieber, C.M. (April 2005). Nanowire nanosensors. *Materials Today* 8: 330–336.

5 Carrascosa, L.G., Moreno, M., Álvarez, M., and Lechuga, L.M. (March 2006). Nanomechanical biosensors: a new sensing tool. *TrAC Trends in Analytical Chemistry* 25: 196–206.

6 Gau, V., Ma, S.-C., Wang, H. et al. (May 2005). Electrochemical molecular analysis without nucleic acid amplification. *Methods* 37: 73–83.

7 Mohan, R., Mach, K.E., Bercovici, M. et al. (2011). Clinical validation of integrated nucleic acid and protein detection on an electrochemical biosensor array for urinary tract infection diagnosis. *PLoS ONE* 6 (10): e26846.

8 Berman, H.M., Westbrook, J., Feng, Z. et al. (2000). The protein data bank. *Nucleic Acids Research* 28: 235–242.

9 Liao, J.C. Yanbao Ma, Vincent Gau et al. (2006). A point-of-care micro-laboratory for direct pathogen identification in body fluids. 2006 1st IEEE International Conference on Nano/Micro Engineered and Molecular Systems, Zhuhai, pp. 1109–1112.

10 Lam, B., Das, J., Holmes, R.D. et al. (2001). Solution-based circuits enable rapid and multiplexed pathogen detection. *Nature Communications* 4. https://www-nature-com.stanford.idm.oclc.org/articles/ncomms3001.

11 Cary, M. et al. (2003) Immunoassay device with immune-reference electrode. US Patent US7723099B2.

Further Reading

BiaCore/GE; Vikram Joshi, Proxim Dx

Dill, L. and Grodzinski (2009). *Microarrays: Preparation, Microfluidics, Detection Methods, and Biological Applications*. New York, NY: Springer Science+Business Media, LLC.

Joe Liao, Yi Cui, Stanford University

Shena, M. (ed.) (2005). *Protein Microarrays*. Jones and Bartlett Publishers.

Patolsky, F., Timko, B., Zheng, G., and Lieber, C. (2007). Nanowire – based nanoelectronic devices in the life sciences. *MRS Bulletin* 32: 142–149. https://doi.org/10.1557/mrs2007.47.

Myszka, D.G., He, X., and Dembo, M. (1998). Extending the range of rate constants available from BIACORE: interpreting mass transport-influenced binding data. *Biophysical Journal* 75: 583–594.

10

Magneto-Nanosensor Biochips

10.1 Magnetism Overview

Most materials can be categorized into three different groups based on their magnetic properties: diamagnetic, paramagnetic, and ferromagnetic materials. These categories are summarized in Figure 10.1.

The vast majority of materials are diamagnetic; diamagnetic materials have closed electron shells (i.e. all of the orbitals have a pair of opposite spin electrons). The details of how orbitals are filled will not be covered in these course notes, but further information can be provided by learning about Aufbau Principle and Pauli Exclusion Principle. Since electrons in each orbital have opposing spins (i.e. spin angular momentums are opposite to each other), electrons in diamagnetic materials cancel out each other's magnetic effect and the atoms will have no net magnetic moments. Some examples of diamagnetic materials are air, wood, and glass. When an external magnetic field is applied to diamagnetic materials, the electron spins respond to the external field by creating an opposing magnetic field. When the external field is removed, the electrons return to their original states and the induced weak magnetic moments disappear.

Paramagnetic materials have atoms with unfilled valence shells and therefore have a magnetic moment even in the absence of an external magnetic field. The magnetic moments of these individual atoms are randomly oriented in different directions due to the thermal energy, and as a result, there is no net magnetization in the bulk material (macroscopic scale). When an external magnetic field is applied, each atom's magnetic moment rotates to align with the applied magnetic field because the aligned orientation is the lowest energy state. Even though the magnetic moments are aligned with the field, the thermal energy is still present. There is a balance between thermal energy (which favors random distribution of moments) and the magnetostatic energy (which favors alignment with the external field). For paramagnetic materials, the thermal energy (at room temperature) is still dominant and there is only slight alignment with the field. The result is a net magnetization along the external field; however, this magnetization is still weak due to the dominance of thermal energy.

Ferromagnetic materials are made of atoms with identical magnetic moments all with open shells. Ferrimagnetic materials (not covered in the chapter) contain at least two kinds of atoms with open shells and they have different magnetic moments. In the absence of an applied field, the magnetic moments of the atoms in these materials have spontaneous alignment. This means that even without an applied field, ferromagnetic/ferrimagnetic materials generate strong magnetic fields.

Biochips and Medical Imaging, First Edition. Adam de la Zerda and Shan Xiang Wang.

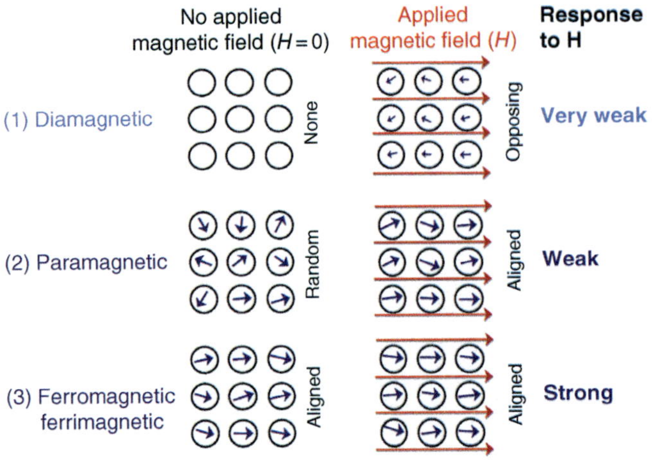

Figure 10.1 Classification of magnetic materials. The blue arrows denote atomic magnetic moments originated from spin and/or orbital angular momentum of electrons. *Source:* Callister [1]. Adapted with permission of John Wiley and Sons, Inc. Copyright © 2007; permission conveyed through Copyright Clearance Center, Inc.

Although paramagnetic materials have much weaker responses to external fields compared to ferromagnetic materials, paramagnetic materials can behave like ferromagnetic materials under certain conditions. For example, if the temperature of the material is lowered (i.e. thermal energy is removed), the magnetic moments of individual atoms align much better. Similarly, if the temperature of the ferromagnetic materials is raised high enough, thermal energy will overcome the alignment and they will behave like paramagnetic materials. These observations indicate that there is a phase transition point between paramagnetism and ferromagnetism for the same material.

10.2 GMR Magneto-Nanosensor Biochips

The magneto-nanosensor biochip is a type of biosensor that uses the principle of giant magnetoresistance (GMR) as a transduction mechanism to detect a change in resistance due to the capture of target analyte molecules. It can be used to detect the presence of analytes such as protein or DNA at higher sensitivity than ELISA, which could potentially be used in either benchtop or point-of-care applications.

Magneto-nanosensor biochips use materials that exhibit the phenomenon of giant magnetoresistance (GMR), which is characterized by a changing resistance in response to an applied magnetic field. GMR materials are typically made of several magnetic layers (e.g. iron) grown by molecular beam epitaxy (MBE) or sputtering, with alternating layers of different magnetizations separated by a nonmagnetic material such as chromium (Cr). Each of these magnetic layers are ferromagnetic, thus they contain ordered spins (magnetic dipoles) that align in the same direction if a sufficient magnetic field is applied (some spontaneous ferromagnetic materials don't require any applied field). Ferromagnetic materials such as pure iron and nickel-iron alloys exhibit up to a few percent of magnetoresistance ratio, defined as the relative change of its resistivity.

GMR materials can be in either the antiparallel state or parallel state, each with a different resistance R_{ap} and R_p. In the absence of an applied field, a GMR material is in the antiparallel state, thus travelling electrons with a particular spin direction will be scattered by the magnetic layers pointing in one direction, while electrons with the opposite spin will be scattered by the magnetic layers pointing in the other direction. Thus, alternating magnetization in a superlattice results in electron scattering at multiple interfaces and a high resistance (R_{ap}). When sufficient magnetic field is applied, the GMR material will be in the parallel state, such that the magnetization in each layer points in the same direction, allowing electrons of a certain spin to go through the material without scattering (or scattering much less than those in the antiparallel state). Thus, GMR material in the parallel state has a much lower resistance (R_p) compared to the antiparallel state (R_{ap}) (Figure 10.2). GMR materials have a high GMR ratio, which is defined as:

$$\text{GMR ratio} \equiv \frac{R_{ap} - R_p}{R_p} = \frac{G_p - G_{ap}}{G_{ap}}$$

$$G \equiv 1/R.$$

GMR materials are used in hard disk drives to read information in the magnetization direction of the ferromagnetic nanoparticles coated on disk platters, and greater GMR ratios enable reliable readout of smaller and fewer nanoparticles per binary bit, which translates into more information stored per disk. When a GMR sensor is near the disk with nanoparticles that are magnetized in one direction or another, the disk can generate a field with differing amplitude and direction that can affect the resistance of the GMR sensor. Albert Fert and Peter Grunberg shared the Nobel Prize in Physics in 2007 for the discovery of the GMR effect. GMR sensors have also been commercialized as magnetic field sensors to be used in automotives and appliances.

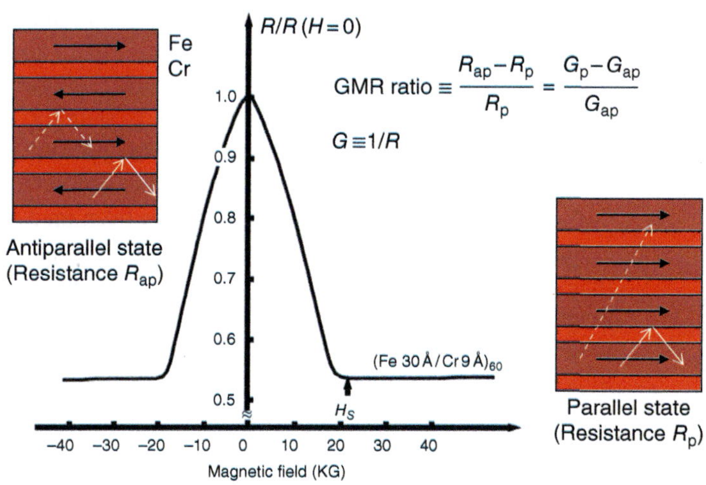

Figure 10.2 Giant magnetoresistance effect. Vertical axis shows the normalized resistance across the layers of GMR material. Horizontal axis shows the applied external magnetic field. When there is no applied magnetic field, the layers align themselves in antiparallel state and the resistance is maximum due to the scattering of both types of electrons. When applied field reaches about 20 KG Gauss or more, all of the layers align with the external field and form the parallel state configuration. In parallel state, the resistance is minimum because electrons with one type of spin don't get scattered. When the external field is −20 KG or less, again all the layers align with the magnetic field but this time they all point to the left instead of right. This state is also a low-resistance state. *Source:* Adapted from Baibich et al. [2]. Copyright © 1988 by The American Physical Society.

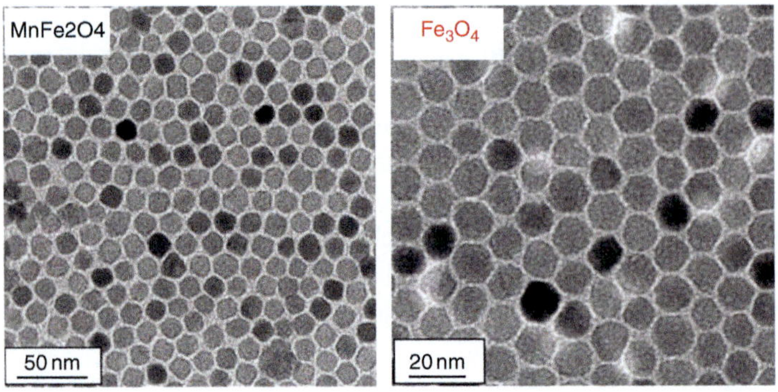

Figure 10.3 TEM images of ferrite nanoparticles. *Source:* Sun et al. [3]. Adapted with permission from Journal of the American Chemical Society. Copyright © 2004 by American Chemical Society.

10.2.1 Synthesis of Ferromagnetic Nanoparticles

Ferrite nanoparticles (Figure 10.3) can be synthesized using the bottom-up approach: the chemical route. A typical chemical synthesis for iron oxide nanoparticles would yield a mixture of magnetite (Fe_3O_4), which has the highest magnetization, along with γ-Fe_2O_3, and nonmagnetic phase α-Fe_2O_3. Monodisperse ferrite nanoparticles such as $MnFe_2O_4$ and Fe_3O_4 are suitable for single molecule detection since the magnetic moment is consistent across nanoparticles. When ferromagnetic nanoparticles are small enough (less than tens of nanometers), its magnetic moment will be pointing randomly due to thermal energy, similar to paramagnetic atoms. Such ferromagnetic nanoparticles are called superparamagnetic nanoparticles, which are ideal for biological applications because they would not agglomerate due to magnetic attraction. Superparamagnetic iron oxide (SPIO) nanoparticles are widely used in biomedicine, and will be used as molecular labels in magneto-nano biochips. In many cases, clusters of SPIO nanoparticles are also utilized because of their ready availability and colloidal stability.

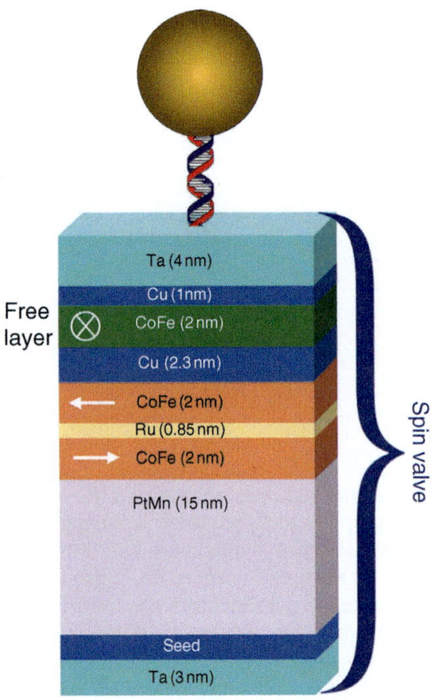

Figure 10.4 Spin valve DNA sensor.

Another synthesis method is the top-down approach: the physical fabrication route. For example, synthetic antiferromagnetic (SAF) nanoparticles have been made at Stanford by physical fabrication. These SAF nanoparticles consist of multiple layers of physically fabricated magnetic and nonmagnetic materials, in which the neighboring magnetizations are antiparallel, as in GMR materials. A field is then applied to orient the magnetizations toward the minimum energy direction to obtain a magnetic response.

Both superparamagnetic nanoparticles and SAF nanoparticles will generate a substantial dipole magnetic field only in the presence of an applied magnetic field.

10.2.2 Spin Valve (GMR) DNA Sensor

The spin valve DNA sensor is a special type of nanoengineered GMR material with a specific layered structure as shown in Figure 10.4. The key layers are the free layer (marked with ⊗) and the reference layer (marked with the left arrow), with a spacer layer of copper between the two. The reference layer (along with the underlying synthetic antiferromagnet) is engineered such that their magnetization does not change with applied field, while the free layer can respond to applied field and cause spin rotation in either direction (to the left or to the right). This spin rotation results in a minimum resistance when the free layer and reference layer are parallel to each other, and a maximum resistance when the free and reference layers are antiparallel to each other. In the absence of applied field (often called quiescent state), the free layer and the reference layer are perpendicular to each other, and the sensor resistance is at the midpoint between the minimum and maximum resistance. Thus, the spin valve DNA sensor is a nearly linear analog sensor. Note it is not the case for the $(Fe/Cr)_{60}$ GMR superlattice shown in Figure 10.4 where the sensor resistance is at the maximum value in the absence of applied field. When a tickling AC field is applied to the spin valve DNA sensor in a direction perpendicular to the quiescent magnetization of the free layer, the magnetization of the free layer will follow the tickling field to rock back and forth, giving a resistance variation nearly proportional to the tickling field. If the nanoparticle is captured at the surface of the spin valve sensor, its dipole field will cause a net shift of the sensor resistance signal due to the tickling field alone, and this shift is the biosensor signal that we detect to count the number of the nanoparticles captured. If the nanoparticles are further away from the free layer, the influence of the dipole field at the free layer drops very quickly, thus the spin valve sensor is a proximity sensor (only sensitive to nanoparticles bound to the local sensor surface).

10.2.3 Magneto-Nanosensor Chip Technology versus ELISA

Magneto-nanosensor biochips are similar to ELISA in that both types of sensors are coated with capture ligands (typically antibodies to detect target antigens) and then incubated with a sample and detection antibodies to form a sandwich structure (Figure 10.5). The difference between the two sensors lies in the transduction mechanism. For ELISA, the detection antibody is labeled by an HRP enzyme, which causes a substrate reaction signal that is optically detected. For magneto-nanosensor chips, the detection antibody is labeled by a magnetic nanoparticle and an applied tickling field induces a small dipole field from each magnetic nanoparticle, which causes a small resistance change in the spin valve sensor. The resistance change is then measured by either sending a bias current through the sensor and measuring the voltage or applying a bias voltage to the sensor and measuring the current. Note that the bias current or voltage can be AC or DC.

10.2.4 Magnetic Nanoparticle Tag

The magnetic nanoparticle tag produces a precise real-time signal since it is colloidally stable with no settling or precipitation, preventing detection of unbound tags. The structure consists of about 10 iron oxide nanoparticles inside a dextran polymer matrix, which has a surface conjugated with streptavidin (a binding agent). The streptavidin enables the nanoparticle to be conjugated with biotinylated detection antibodies (Figure 10.6). The 50-nm diameter magnetic nanoparticle tag features a detection range of a few hundred nm, and prevents magnetic cross talk between neighboring sensors.

10.2.5 Double Modulation Sensing (AC Bias Current and AC Applied Field)

Magneto-nano chips exhibit a large peak in the frequency spectrum analysis due to electromagnetic interference (EMI), often at the frequency of the AC applied field (e.g. tickling field). Since the tickling

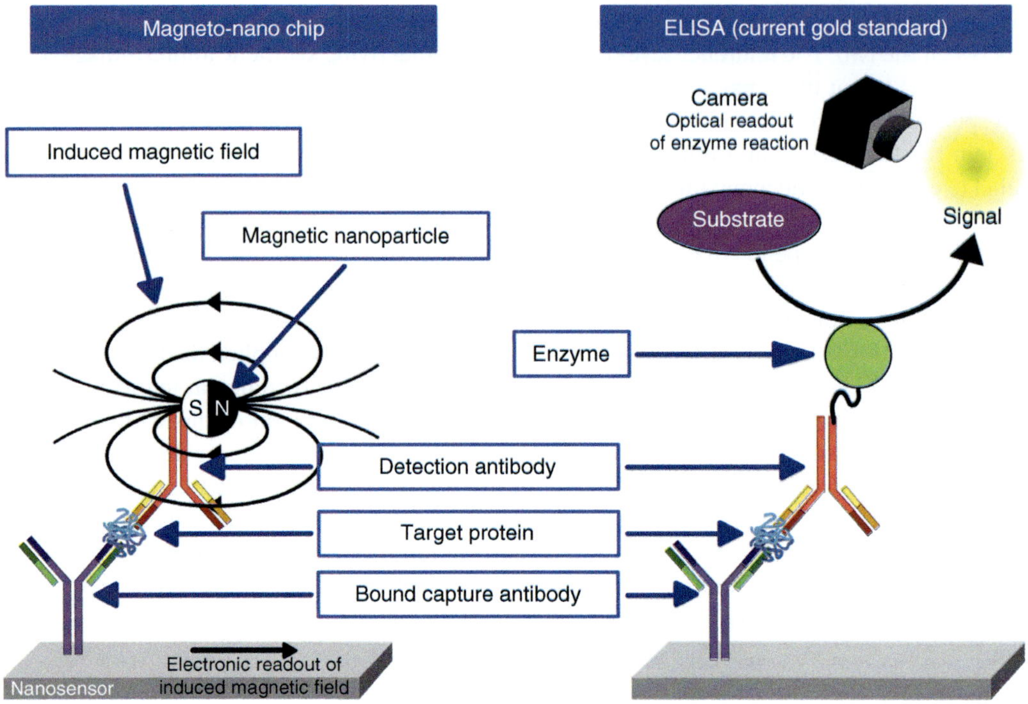

Figure 10.5 Magneto-nanosensor chip versus ELISA.

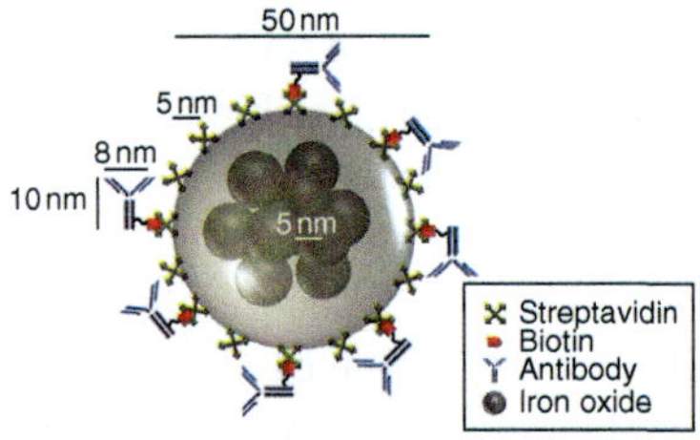

Figure 10.6 Magnetic nanoparticle tag. Source: Gaster et al. [4]. Reprinted by permission from Springer Nature: Nature Nanotechnology. Copyright © 2011 by Springer Nature.

field is much larger than the small field generated by individual nanoparticles captured by the sensor, a technique involving double modulation of the current and applied field is used to measure the signal from the nanoparticle alone, which is analogous to heterodyne radio reception. An AC-modulated current is passed through the sensor at frequency f_c, and the tickling field is modulated at a frequency f_f, which generates a resistance change in the sensor with the same frequency as the field. The voltage readout is the product of the current and resistance, which can be separated into three different frequency peaks: the carrier signal (at frequency f_c), the difference signal (at a frequency $f_c - f_f$), and the sum signal (at a frequency $f_c + f_f$) (Figure 10.7). The latter two are related to the resistance change due to the nanoparticles. If a nanoparticle is captured right at the top of the spin valve sensor center, the difference and sum peaks will decrease slightly, which is taken as the biosensor signal:

$$V_{\mathrm{GMR}}(t) = I_0 R_0 \cos(2\pi f_c t) + \frac{I_0 \Delta R_0}{2}\cos\left(2\pi\left(f_c - f_f\right)t\right) + \frac{I_0 \Delta R_0}{2}\cos\left(2\pi\left(f_c + f_f\right)t\right).$$

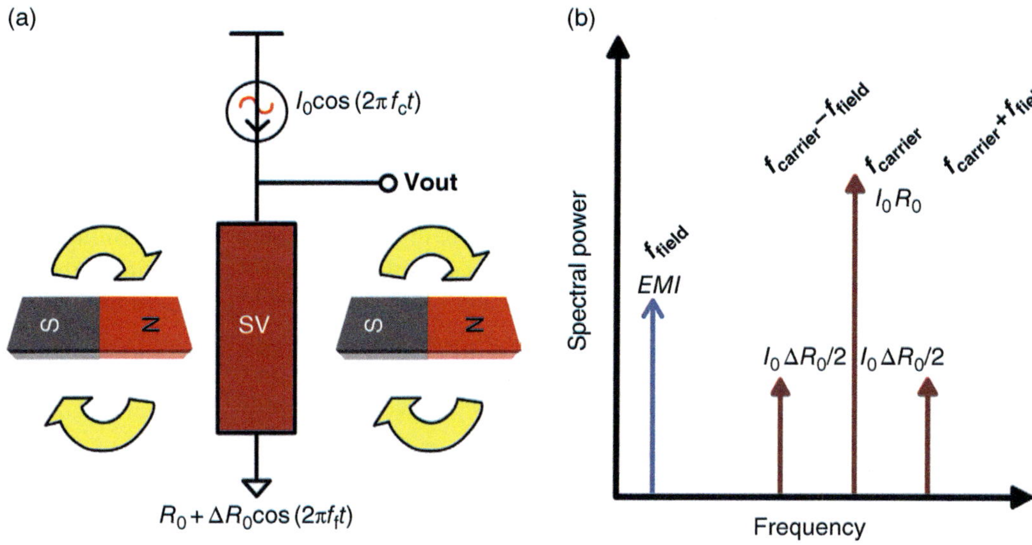

Figure 10.7 (a) Double modulation sensing and (b) spectral power of sensor signal.

10.2.6 Multiplex Readout Electronics

In order to read the sensors in a very short time, frequency-division or time-division multiplexing can be used, so that readout occurs while the biological processes are evolving on the chip. By passing the frequency-division or time-division multiplexed signals through shared replica paths, and subtracting the signal of two blocks, the net signal can be obtained (Figure 10.8). For example, by turning on the sensors at different time and frequency, four sensors can be read almost simultaneously, and the readout time can be reduced by a factor of 4 without compromising performance.

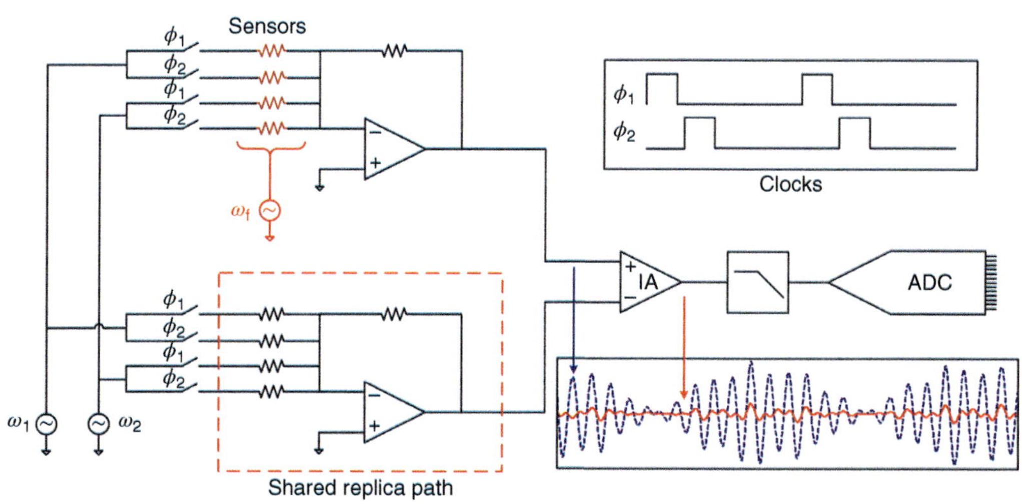

Figure 10.8 Multiplex readout electronics. *Source:* Hall et al. [5]. Reprinted from Biosensors and Bioelectronics. Copyright © 2010, with permission from Elsevier.

10.2.7 Sensitivity and Multiplexing of Magneto-Nanosensor Chip

A magneto-nanosensor chip can be multiplexed for different biomarker detection with high sensitivity. The graph in Figure 10.9 shows the sensor signal obtained for a chip that is functionalized with seven biomarkers (with 2–4 replicates per biomarker), along with positive and negative control sensors. Bovine serum albumin (BSA) protein is used for negative control to set the noise level in SNR calculations since it is very difficult for proteins to attach to, and thus should give zero signal theoretically. This chip is incubated with a sample containing seven different analytes in a reaction well and the resulting sensor signals are shown (each biomarker signal is represented by a different color). The magneto-nanosensor chip was able to process a seven-plex assay in about one hour, with all the seven biomarkers spiked at $1\,pg\,ml^{-1}$.

10.2.8 Dynamic Range of Magneto-Nanosensor Chip Compared to ELISA

Standard curves for both a magneto-nanosensor chip (with no magnetic signal amplification) and ELISA are shown in Figure 10.10. In this case, for the biomarker carcinoembryonic antigen (CEA), the magneto-nanosensor chip is about a thousand times more sensitive than ELISA, with six logs of linear dynamic range in log–log scale. Also, magneto-nanosensor chips can potentially detect even lower concentrations (50 attomolar) with magnetic signal amplification, which is done by adding linkers to nanoparticles so that they will conjugate and act as nucleation sites to attract more nanoparticles.

10.2.9 Matrix Effect Neutralized

A well-designed magneto-nanosensor chip will give similar concentration measurements for the same biomarker spiked into different matrix samples, such as serum, saliva, urine, cell lysate, phosphate buffer solution (PBS), etc. In other words, the matrix effect due to different samples should be neutralized, as seen in Figure 10.11.

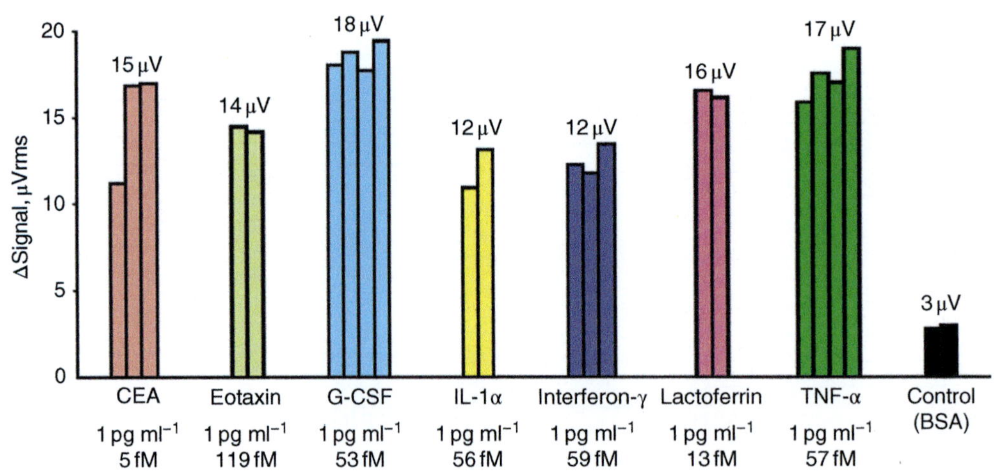

Figure 10.9 Magneto-nano chip signal level for seven different biomarkers and one control. *Source:* Osterfeld et al. [6]. Reprinted with permission from National Academy of Sciences. Copyright (2008) National Academy of Sciences, USA.

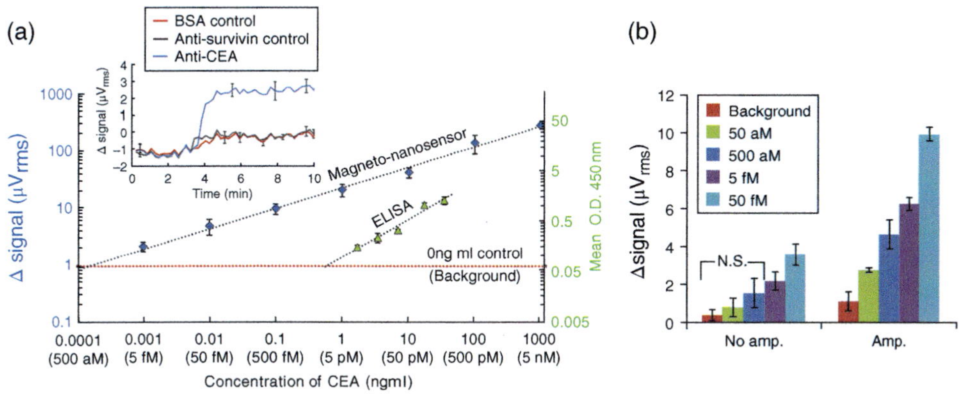

Figure 10.10 (a) Dynamic range comparison between magneto-nanosensor chip and ELISA. (b) Signal level comparison of magneto-nanosensor chip with and without amplification. *Source:* Gaster et al. [7]. Reprinted by permission from Springer Nature: Nature Medicine. Copyright © 2009 by Springer Nature.

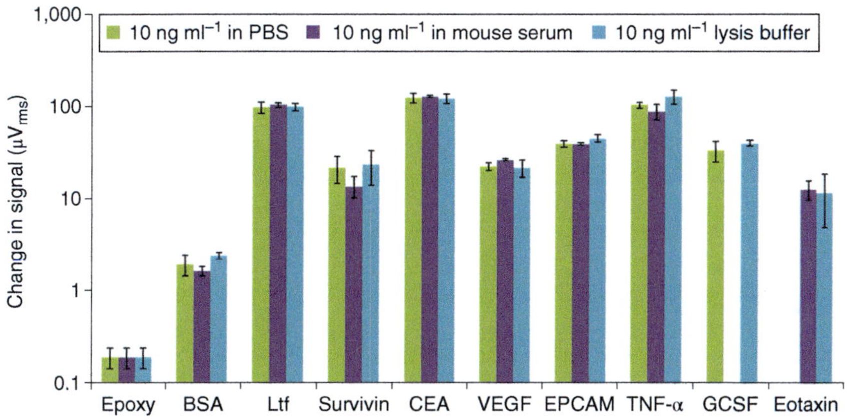

Figure 10.11 Signal level from 10 different biomarkers in three different matrices. Notice that there is very low variation between different media. *Source:* Gaster et al. [7]. Reprinted by permission from Springer Nature: Nature Medicine. Copyright © 2009 by Springer Nature.

10.2.10 Summary of Magneto-Nanosensor Chip

The magneto-nanosensor chip is a promising platform for in-vitro diagnostics for complex diseases that can be represented by multiple biomarkers, such as cancer and heart disease. Magneto-nanosensor chips typically have excellent sensitivity, detection time, and dynamic range (which depend on the specific biomarker and reagents used). For example, magneto-nanoprotein chips were shown to detect seven different tumor markers spiked at 10fM level, with an assay time of less than one hour and a dynamic range of six logs, which shows great promise for cancer diagnosis.

10.3 Point-of-Care Testing

Point-of-care (POC) testing refers to diagnostics done at the point of care, such as testing that can be performed at home without going to a doctor (e.g. a home pregnancy test). HIV/AIDS continues

Table 10.1 Summary of POC testing versus conventional lab testing.

POC testing versus conventional lab testing	
Advantages	**Disadvantages**
Quality of care can be improved by immediate results in some settings	Non-laboratorians may have difficulty with required QC, etc.
POC test can provide more efficient care, thus lowering costs	Typically higher unit cost of testing compared to central lab method
POC can save labor in following up results with patients (e.g. telephone)	Usually more personnel time per test compared to central lab testing
Patients can learn results immediately and not be "lost" to follow-up	Test unavailable at POC may require multiple collections
POC tests can improve patient flow through busy clinics and emergency departments	Testing workload may be difficult to add to existing staff responsibilities

to be a serious disease worldwide, with 39 million people afflicted with the disease, 2.7 million new cases, and 2.9 million deaths per year from the disease. To help fight this disease, China, India, and Thailand have each announced ambitious national programs to provide free anti-HIV drugs to people who need them most. An especially pressing need in POC testing is the large-scale rapid detection of diseases such as HIV/AIDS. Advantages and disadvantages of POC testing are summarized in Table 10.1.

10.3.1 Existing Divide with Diagnostics

Current methods of diagnostics are divided between central laboratory tests and existing POC tests. In general, central laboratory tests have high sensitivity and are customizable to each patient's needs; however, these tests are expensive and have a long turnaround time. In comparison, existing POC diagnostics are fast and low cost, but have relatively low sensitivity and can only measure one biomarker (single-plex detection).

10.3.2 Lateral Flow Immunochromatographic Assay

The lateral flow immunochromatographic assay (a.k.a. "strip test") is a common form of POC testing that can be done at home (e.g. a home pregnancy test). An example strip test is shown in Figure 10.12. There are two small lines of capture ligands embedded in the strip. The blood or urine sample is first dropped onto the left end of the strip, which then flows to the right due to capillary force. The sample picks up labeled detection antibodies and continues to move to the right. Once the sample reaches the test line with capture antibodies, a positive result will be displayed if the target analyte is present in the sample and is captured to form a sandwich structure. A negative result will be displayed if the target analyte is absent. In either case, some surplus detection antibodies pass through the test line and reach the control line at the far right end of the strip. Another set of capture antibodies at the control line will retain the labeled detection antibodies, which indicates that the test was valid. An absence of control line would indicate the reagents (antibodies, labels, etc.) are not working normally.

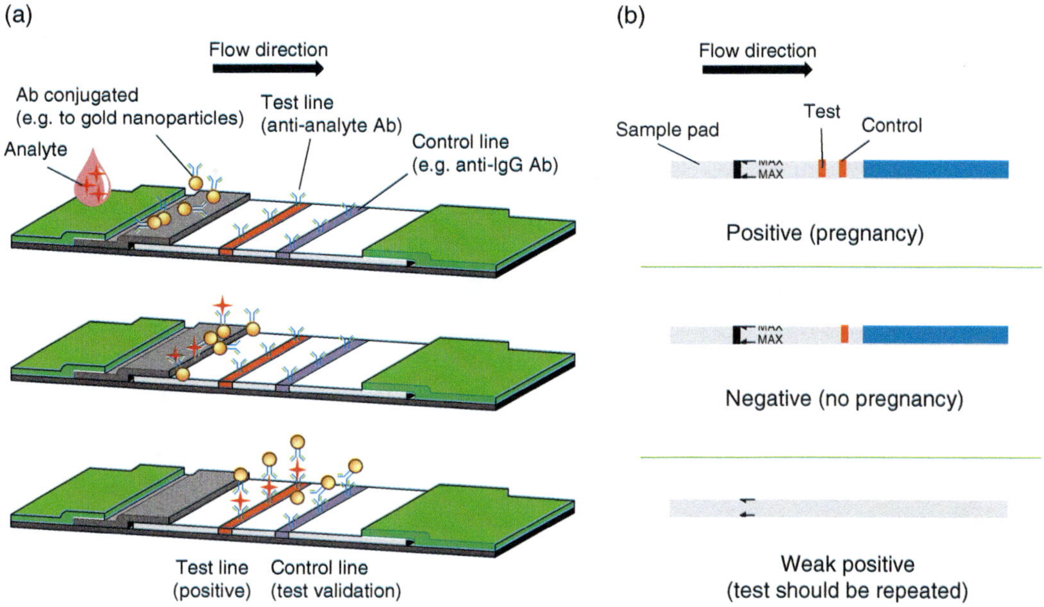

Figure 10.12 Lateral flow immunochromatographic assay: (a) 3-dimensional view of the assay process, (b) cross-sectional view of the assay process. *Source:* Koczuła and Gallotta [8]. Republished with permission of Portland Press, Ltd. Copyright © 2018; permission conveyed through Copyright Clearance Center, Inc.

10.3.3 NanoLab Handheld Diagnostic Lab

One goal of POC testing is to achieve a system that can combine the high sensitivity and customizability of lab tests with the low cost and high speed of current POC testing. For example, a device called the NanoLab (Figure 10.13) promises to provide affordable POC testing that is portable (about the size of a calculator), rapid and easy to use (within 15 minutes), and highly sensitive (more than 20 times more sensitive than existing POC tests).

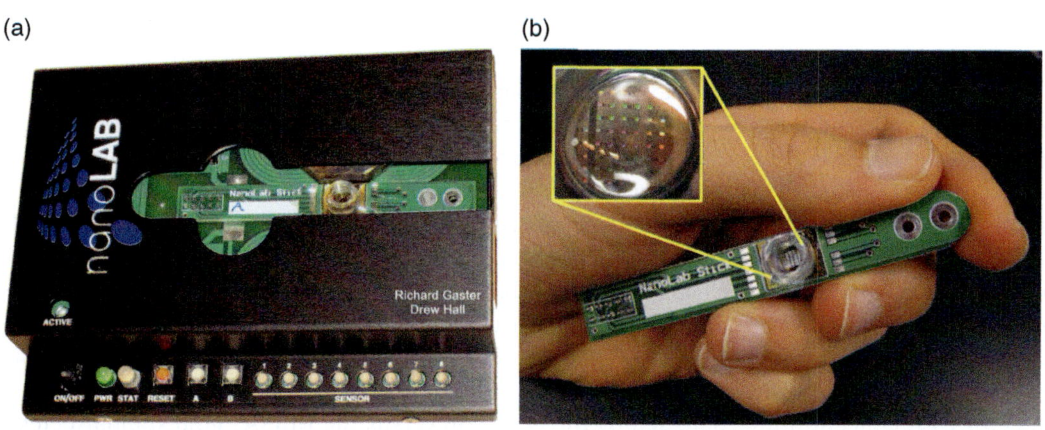

Figure 10.13 (a) NanoLab Station and (b) NanoLab Stick. *Source:* Reproduced from Gaster et al. [9], with permission of The Royal Society of Chemistry.

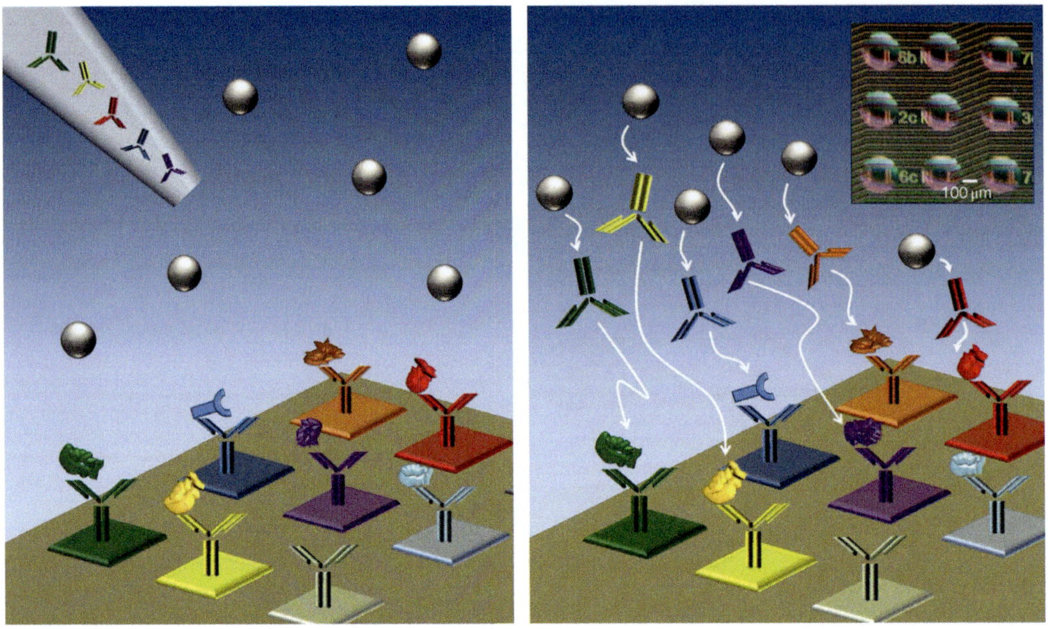

Figure 10.14 Auto-assembly immunoassay. *Source:* Gaster et al. [10]. Reprinted with permission from NanoLetters: American Chemical Society. Copyright © 2011 American Chemical Society.

10.3.3.1 Auto-Assembly Immunoassay

The auto-assembly immunoassay (Figure 10.14) consists of an array of GMR nanosensors, all functionalized with appropriate surface chemistry. After immobilizing unique capture antibodies over a unique, individually addressable sensor, and incubating with the protein of interest, the magnetic nanotags are added in solution above the sensor. Since there is no chemistry to link the magnetic nanotags to the captured antigen, no signal is detected by the underlying sensor. Once the detection antibody in solution is added, the detection antibody, which is labeled with biotin, is capable of linking the streptavidin-labeled magnetic nanotag to the captured analyte. In the presence of captured analyte and detection antibody complexes, the magnetic nanotags will congregate over the corresponding GMR sensors in high-enough concentration to be detected.

10.3.3.2 Real-Time Binding Data

The real-time binding data of the auto-assembly immunoassay (Figure 10.15) shows that the addition of the sample and magnetic nanotags contribute negligible signal (upon addition of the magnetic nanotags, there is a very small signal rise due to detection of unbound magnetic nanotags in solution above the sensor). However, once the detection antibody is introduced, the magnetic nanotags are clearly measurable on sensors functionalized with the appropriate capture antibody and antigen. The negative control sensors, coated with a noncomplementary antibody, anti-insulin antibody, remain flat, indicating negligible nonspecific binding. The *y*-axis units are the change in magnetoresistance normalized to the initial magnetoresistance presented in parts per million (ppm).

10.3.3.3 NanoLab Sensitivity

Data for CEA concentrations detected by the NanoLab versus the ELISA "gold standard" test show that NanoLab is 20 times more sensitive than ELISA (50 fM versus 1 pM, see Figure 10.16). Further, the NanoLab eliminates the need for any washing steps, which are a cumbersome

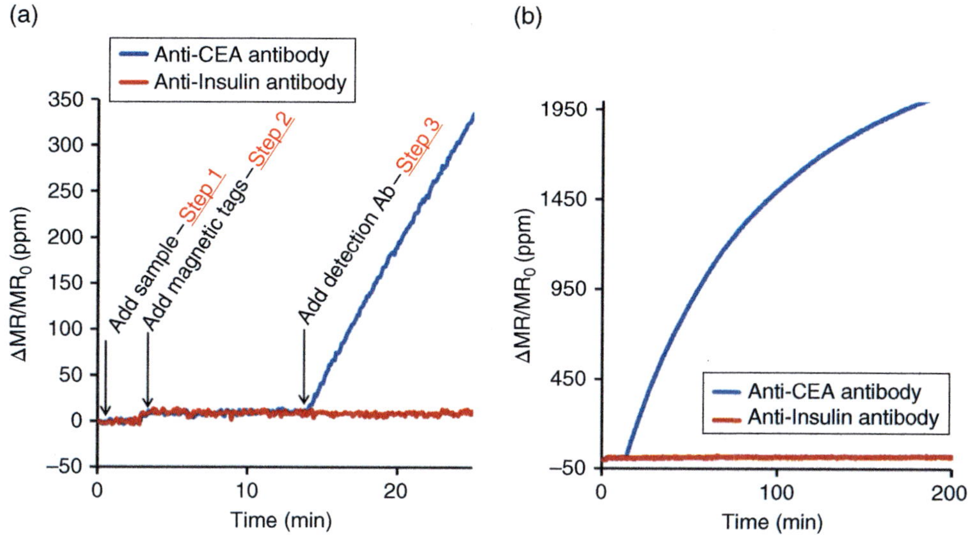

Figure 10.15 Real-time signal detection of the auto-assembly immunoassay (a) shows the initial signal detection while (b) shows the concentration detection over time. *Source:* Gaster et al. [10]. Reprinted with permission from NanoLetters: American Chemical Society. Copyright © 2011 American Chemical Society.

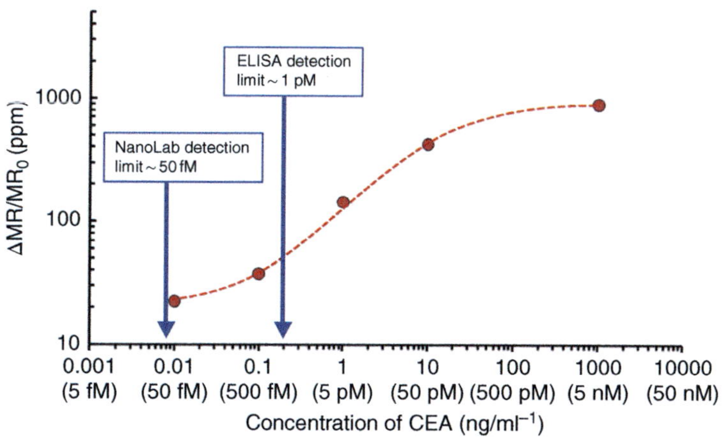

Figure 10.16 NanoLab sensitivity. *Source:* Gaster et al. [10]. Reprinted with permission from NanoLetters: American Chemical Society. Copyright © 2011 American Chemical Society.

and time-consuming part of fluorescent-based detection. This allows NanoLab testing to be faster and cheaper, and most importantly, to be used without training, even by patients themselves.

10.3.3.4 NanoLab and Point-of-Care Summary

If the NanoLab technology is widely commercialized, it would represent a technological advance that will hopefully be able to not only change the way medicine is practiced in the developing world, but also provide the developed world with a new medical infrastructure where everyone has the ability to literally take health care into their own hands.

10.4 Non-GMR Magnetic Nanobiosensors

10.4.1 Optomagnetic Biosensor (Lab on a Chip)

The optomagnetic biosensor, manufactured by Philips as a lab on a chip (Figure 10.17), features a microfluidic channel with magnetic nanoparticles that form a complex with analyte and capture ligands on the surface. The sensor signal is measured by the reflected light intensity, which depends on the concentration of nanoparticles at the sensor surface, by the mechanism of frustrated total internal reflection (f-TIR or FTIR). By modulating the force amplitude of an applied electromagnetic field, nanoparticles can be pulled closer to or away from surface, which corresponds to each ripple on the readout. The more the magnetic nanoparticles are bound to the surface, the less light is reflected (i.e. the more total internal reflection is frustrated). The net signal is the difference between the initial reflected light intensity when activating magnetic attraction and the final reflected light intensity after a stringency wash step, which removes the nonspecifically bound magnetic nanoparticles. The optomagnetic biosensor exhibits a limit of detection of 1 pM for the analyte cardiac troponin (cTn).

10.4.1.1 What is f-TIR?

f-TIR or FTIR stands for "frustrated total internal reflection," and this phenomenon has been used in the biometrics community to image fingerprint ridges since at least the 1960s. In 2005, Jeff Han popularized the use of f-TIR for touch screen sensing. When the user comes into contact with the surface, the light rays are frustrated since they can now pass through into the contact material (usually skin layer on top of the glass or acrylic plane), and the reflection is no longer total at that point (Figure 10.18). This frustrated light is scattered downward toward a photodetector or camera.

10.4.2 Magnetic Resonance Biosensor (Resonance Relaxation Shift Sensor)

The magnetic resonance biosensor, made by T2 Biosystems (Figure 10.19), features magnetic nanoparticles in solution, which can conjugate to target analyte molecules to create clusters and cause a change in resonance relaxation time (the time required to relax back to the equilibrium spin state after being oriented in certain spin state away from equilibrium; in this case, only spin–spin relaxation time T2 is measured). Before analyte is added, the nanoparticles in solution interact with water molecules and cause the water's hydrogen atoms to have a certain nuclear spin relaxation. If nanoparticles start to cluster due to the presence of analyte, there is now less nanoparticle–water spin–spin interaction, which results in a slower nuclear spin relaxation that can be measured as sensor signal. The magnetic resonance biosensor is miniaturized for POC application, but is singleplex with only two logs of dynamic range.

10.4.3 Immuno-PCR-Type Assays

There is at least one type of immuno-PCR assay that is being commercialized: the barcode assay (Figure 10.20a). The barcode assay uses magnetic particles with capture ligands, which capture target molecules, such as PSA, to form a sandwich assay with detector antibodies that are labeled with gold nanoparticles with barcode DNA. After the sandwich assay is formed, the magnetic nanoparticles with barcode DNA are magnetically separated, then the DNA strands are released from the gold nanoparticles, and, finally, the DNA strands are amplified by PCR methods. A slight variation of the assay utilizes antibody-DNA conjugates instead of coated gold nanoparticles (Figure 10.20b). These are some of the most sensitive tests available, but are also very complex.

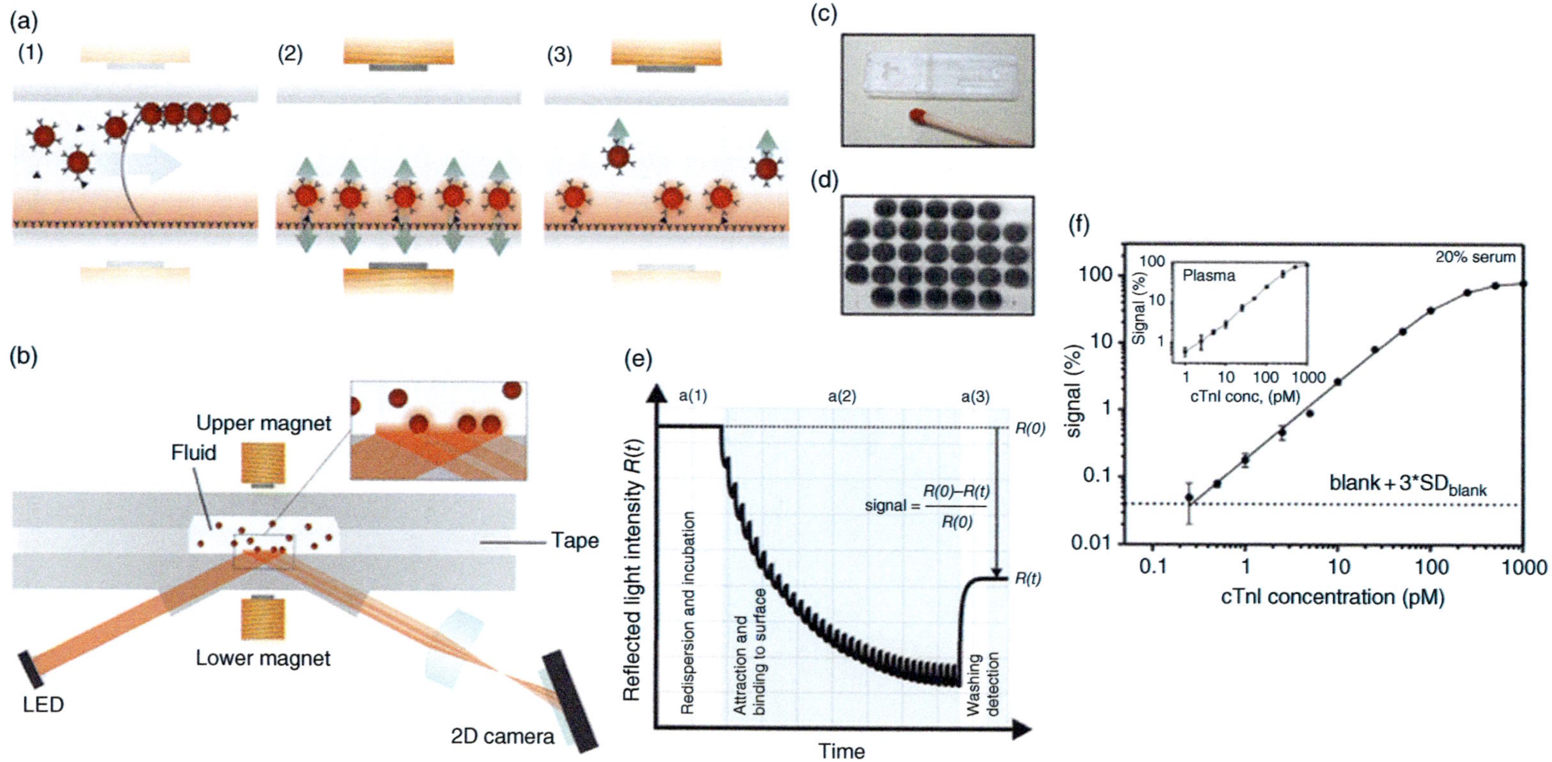

Figure 10.17 Optomagnetic biosensor based on actuated magnetic nanoparticles. (a) Schematic representation of the reaction microchamber showing successively the assay processes: (a1) filling of the microchamber, nanoparticle redispersion, and capturing of analyte; (a2) actuation of the particles during the process of binding to the surface; and (a3) removal of free and weakly bound nanoparticles from the sensing surface by magnetic forces. (b) The fluid microchamber placed in the optomagnetic system with electromagnets and detection optics. Light reflects from the sensor surface with an intensity that depends on the concentration of nanoparticles at the sensor surface, by the mechanism of frustrated total internal reflection (f-TIR). (c) Picture of an assembled disposable cartridge consisting of two structured plastic parts connected by double-sided adhesive tape. The cartridge has outer dimensions of 1 cm × 4 cm. The cartridge contains a sample inlet, a channel, a reaction microchamber, and a vent. A total sample volume of 10 μL is supplied, of which 1 μL is analyzed in the reaction microchamber. (d) f-TIR image of magnetic nanoparticles bound to the sensor surface via an immunoassay on 31 capture spots of 125 μm diameter each. (e) Schematic real-time curve of the measured optical signal for a single capture spot. The assay phases a1–a3 are indicated. The signal modulation in phase a2 is caused by switched actuation of the magnetic nanoparticles. (f) Calibration curve of the optical signal as a function of cTnI concentration in 20% human serum. Nanoparticles were mixed with the sample prior to injection into the cartridge. Signals were determined after the magnetic removal step. The inset shows a calibration curve of the integrated magnetic nanoparticle assay for cTnI in 100% plasma, with dry reagents inside the microchamber. Lines are guides to the eye. Data represent averages and standard deviations of 3 repetitions on different cartridges. *Source:* Reproduced from Bruls et al. [11], with permission of The Royal Society of Chemistry.

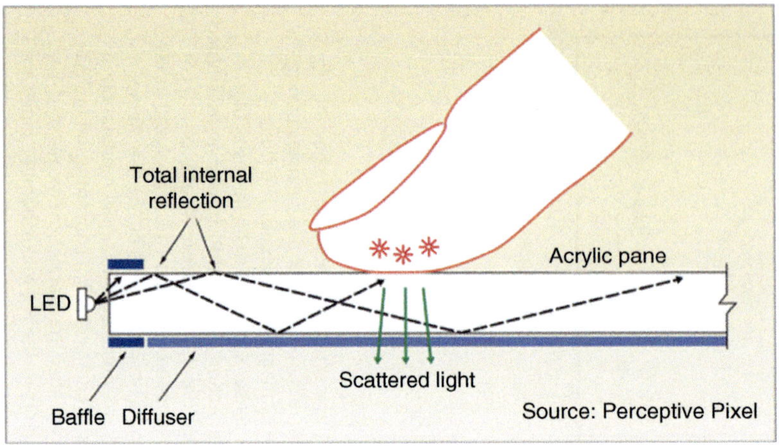

Figure 10.18 FTIR-based touch screen. *Source:* Copyright © 2007 IEEE. Reprinted with permission from Vaughan Nichols [12].

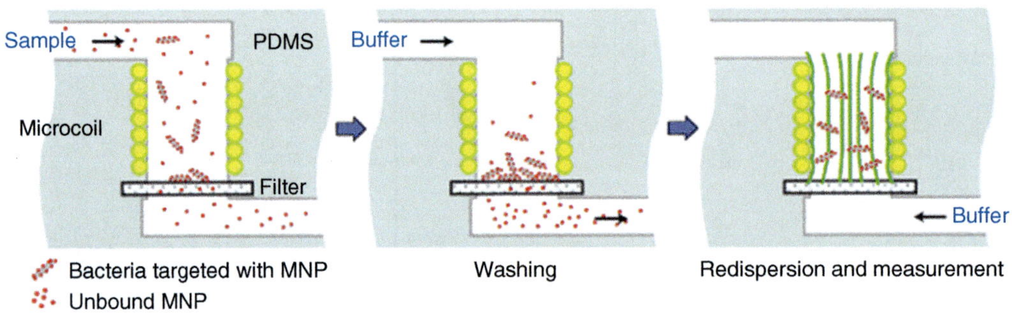

Figure 10.19 Magnetic resonance biosensor. *Source:* Lee et al. [13]. Republished with permission of John Wiley and Sons, Inc. Copyright © 2009 Wiley-VCH Verlag GmbH & Co. KGaA, Weinheim.

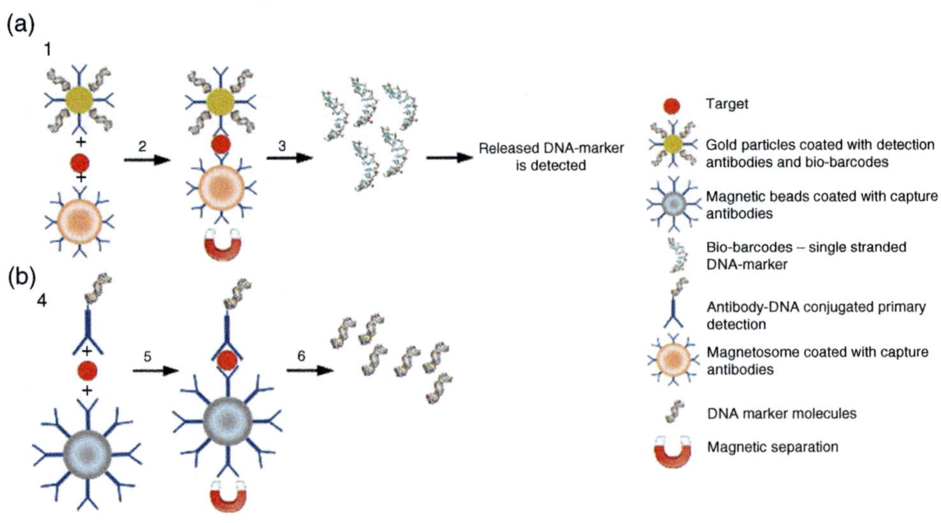

Figure 10.20 Barcode assays. The DNA markers are conjugated to either (a) gold nanoparticles or (b) detection antibodies. *Source:* Adler et al. [14]. Adapted by Taylor and Francis Ltd., with permission of The Royal Society of Chemistry.

10.5 Conclusion

The GMR magneto-nanosensor chip is a promising platform for in-vitro diagnostics for complex diseases that can be represented by multiple biomarkers, such as cancer and heart disease. Magneto-nanosensor chips typically have excellent sensitivity, detection time, and dynamic range. There are also several different non-GMR magneto-nanosensors that use magnetic nanoparticles in their transduction mechanism to achieve high sensitivity. Magneto-nanosensor chips can potentially be used in miniaturized POC platforms, such as the NanoLab, for rapid diagnosis of diseases including HIV/AIDS and malaria. If this NanoLab technology is widely commercialized, it would represent a technological advance that would hopefully be able to not only change the way medicine is practiced in the developing world, but also provide the developed world with a new medical infrastructure where everyone has the ability to literally take health care into their own hands.

Problems

10.1 One may use the original multilayer GMR superlattice discovered in 1988 for a magnetic biosensor in double modulation.

A Explain why the sensor resistance under an AC tickling field at a frequency of f_f can be approximately expressed as:

$$R = R_0 + \Delta R_0 \cos\left(4\pi f_f t\right)$$

B Derive an expression for the sensor voltage if the sense current is:

$$I = I_0 \cos\left(2\pi f_c t\right)$$

C Plot the frequency spectrum of the sensor voltage, and denote the nominal resistance (carrier) peak, the nanoparticle ΔR peaks, the EMI (electromagnetic interference) peak, and their respective frequencies.

10.2 Consider the GMR spin valve sensor discussed in the chapter (Figure 10.21):

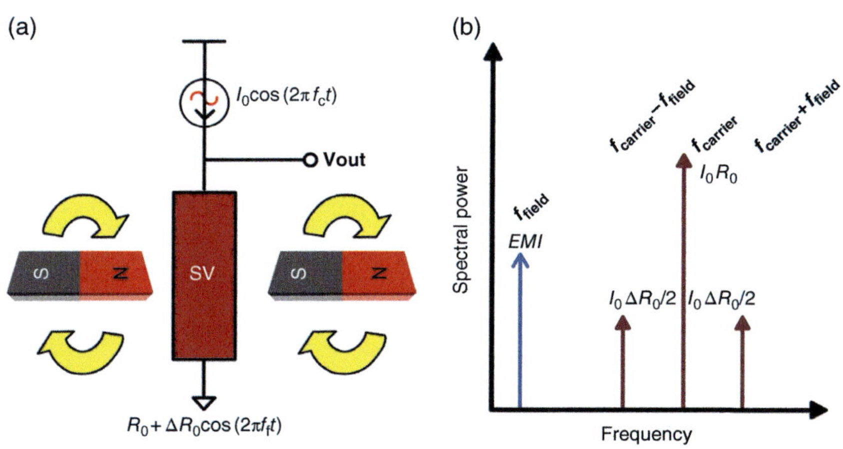

Figure 10.21 (a) Double modulation sensing and (b) spectral power of sensor signal.

If the sensor current is now changed to a square wave with a fundamental frequency of f_c, sketch the spectral power of the new sensor signal. The applied field is still sinusoidal with a frequency of f_f.
(Hint: You do not need to plot all spectral peaks, only those peaks that you think are the most important in this context.)

10.3 A GMR biosensor chip is typically used to detect multiple biomarkers from a single patient with a single chip and a single type of magnetic nanoparticle (MNP) labels. In this experiment, the GMR biosensor chip is extended to detect the same protein biomarker from both tumor and normal tissues on a single chip. To accomplish this, we label the protein biomarker from tumor tissue with MNP1, which will emit a magnetic field at a frequency of $f1$ under a DC bias magnetic field; we label the protein biomarker from the normal tissue with MNP2, which will emit a magnetic field at a frequency of $f2$ under the same DC bias field. The normal tissue and tumor tissue are then mixed to be interrogated with the GMR biosensor chip, on which all the sensors are immobilized with capture reagents which will bind to the said protein biomarker. The GMR sensor is sensitive enough to detect the magnetic signals from the MNPs. **Assume that the linear superposition principle applies to the GMR sensor in sensing magnetic fields, and that $f0 >> f1 > f2$.**

A If the GMR biosensors are passed with an AC current with a frequency of $f0$, and subject to the same DC bias magnetic field, how would the readout voltage in frequency domain look like after a blank sample (w/o normal or tumor tissues) are incubated with the chip?

B Keep the readout configuration the same for the subsequent questions. If only the normal tissue produces the protein marker, how would the readout voltage in frequency domain look like?

C If only the tumor tissue produces the protein marker, how would the readout voltage in frequency domain look like?

D If both tissues produce the protein marker, how would the readout voltage in frequency domain look like?

10.4 The binding kinetics equation is:

$$L + A \leftrightarrow LA,$$

where L = ligand, A = analyte, $\theta = [LA]/[LA]_{max}$,

$$K_d = \frac{[L][LA]}{[LA]}.$$

The time dependence of coverage q, i.e. the equation of the association curve, if $[A]$ is a constant, and initially all the ligands are unoccupied, is given by:

$$\theta = \frac{[A]}{[A]+K_d}(1 - e^{-(k_{on}[A]+k_{off})t}$$

The on and off rates for binding between an antibody immobilized on Magneto-Nanosensor and the specific target analyte are $k_{on} = 10^5\ M^{-1}\ s^{-1}$ and $k_{off} = 10^{-4}\ s^{-1}$.

A If the analyte concentration is 10 nM, calculate the incubation time needed for the sensor coverage to reach 0.5.

B If some amount of inhibitor molecules that can bind to the analyte and block the antibody-antigen-binding sites are accidently added to the sample, such that the effective analyte concentration is halved, calculate the incubation time needed to reach the same sensor coverage.

C If you were developing a portable magneto-nanosensor for point-of-care applications and the device would display readout results in five minutes after sample insertion, calculate the maximum and minimum sensor coverage if the analyte concentration ranges from 10 nM to 1 μM. For simplicity, assume the binding between the immobilized capture antibody and the target analyte is the only rate-limiting step (any other steps happen instantaneously).

D Based on what you know about magneto-nanosensor and binding kinetics, what can you do to increase the sensitivity of the portable device? Explain your answer.

10.5 Sofia purchased magnetic nanoparticles from a vendor to conduct her biochip assays, but somehow the vendor only provided her with the anisotropy constant ($K_u = 2 \times 10^4$ Jm^{-3}) and diameter of the particles ($d = 15$ nm). Thus, she decided to wait until more information was available because she thought that she could not figure out whether the particles would agglomerate or not.

A What is the blocking temperature T_B of the particle?

B Would you recommend that she start her experiment? Explain your rationale.

10.6 Choose a proper recognition element and transduction mechanism for each technique in the table below:

Recognition elements: antibody, DNA strand, antigen, and RNA.
Transduction mechanisms: Electrical, optical, mechanical, and magnetic.

Sensing technique	**Recognition element**	**Transduction mechanism**
Two-color cDNA microarray for mRNA detection		
Lateral flow pregnancy test for hCG (human chorionic gonadotropin)		
Cantilever sensor for measuring TNF-α (tumor necrosis factor-alpha)		
Luminex for detecting IL-6 (Interleukin-6)		
Magneto-nano-biochip for CEA (carcinoembryonic antigen) detection		
Antigen arrays for autoimmune diseases (using fluorophore-conjugated detection antibodies)		
DNA detection with Si nanowire-based FET sensors		
Mesoscale Discovery (MSD) electrochemiluminescence assay for monitoring VEGF (vascular endothelial growth factor)		

10.7 In your own words, describe similarity and difference between the sensing mechanisms of electrochemical, magnetic nanoparticle-based, and ELISA protein assays.

10.8 Explain how magnetic nanoparticle-based sensors are able to achieve a much lower limit of detection than ELISA.

10.9 POC versus Central Lab Testing: You have an idea to develop either (a) a POC device or (b) benchtop laboratory equipment for either lung cancer diagnostics or Influenza screening. Explain which footprint (a or b) you will choose for each disease diagnosis and why.

10.10 What is the main difference between SPR and optomagnetic biosensor?

References

1 Callister, W.D. (2006). *Materials Science and Engineering: An Introduction*, 7e. Wiley.
2 Baibich, M.N., Broto, M., Fert, A. et al. (1988). Giant magnetoresistance of (001)Fe/(001)Cr magnetic superlattices. *Physical Review Letters* 61: 2472.
3 Sun, S., Zeng, H., Robinson, D.B. et al. (2004). Monodisperse MFe2O4 (M = Fe, Co, Mn) Nanoparticles. *Journal of the American Chemical Society* 126 (1): 273–279.
4 Gaster, R.S., Xu, L., Han, S.-J. et al. (2011). Quantification of protein interactions and solution transport using high-density GMR sensor arrays. *Nature Nanotechnology* 6 (5): 314–320.
5 Hall, D.A., Gaster, R.S., Lin, T. et al. (2010). GMR biosensor arrays: A system perspective. *Biosensors and Bioelectronics* 25: 2051–2057.
6 Osterfeld, S.J., Yu, H., Gaster, R.S. et al. (2008). Multiplex protein assays based on real-time magnetic nanotag sensing. *PNAS* 105 (52): 20637–20640. doi: 10.1073/pnas.0810822105.
7 Gaster, R.S., Hall, D.A., Nielsen, C.H. et al. (2009). Matrix-insensitive protein assays push the limits of biosensors in medicine. *Nature Medicine* 15: 11.
8 Koczuła, K. and Gallotta, A. (2016). Lateral flow assays. *Essays in Biochemistry* 60: 111–120.
9 Gaster, R.S., Hall, D.A., and Wang, S.X. (2011). nanoLAB: An ultraportable, handheld diagnostic laboratory for global health. *Lab Chip* 11: 950.
10 Gaster, R.S., Hall, D.A., and Wang, S.X. (2011). Autoassembly Protein Arrays for Analyzing Antibody Cross-Reactivity. *NanoLetters: American Chemical Society* 11 (7): 3047.
11 Bruls, D.M., Evers, T.H., Kahlman, J.A. et al. (2009). Rapid integrated biosensor for multiplexed immunoassays based on actuated magnetic nanoparticles. *Lab Chip* 9 (24): 3504–3510. http://dx.doi.org/10.1039/B913960E.
12 Nichols, S.J.V. (2007). New interfaces at the touch of fingertip. *Computer Magazine* 40 (8): 12–15.
13 Lee, H., Yoon, T., and Weissleder, R. (2009). Ultrasensitive detection of bacteria using core–shell nanoparticles and an NMR-filter system. *Angewandte Chemie International Edition* 48: 5657–5660.
14 Adler, M., Wacker, R., and Niemeyer, C.M. (2008). Sensitivity by combination: immuno-PCR and related technologies. *Analyst* 133: 702–718, http://dx.doi.org/10.1039/B718587C.

11

Microfluidic Chips for Capturing Circulating Tumor Cells

11.1 Circulating Tumor Cells

Circulating Tumor Cells (CTCs) are tumor cells that break away from their original tumor and circulate throughout the body during metastasis, which is usually the final cause of death instead of the original tumor (Figure 11.1). Successful CTC enrichment can lead to early detection and treatment of metastatic cancer, as well as increase the understanding of CTC biology. A liquid biopsy would also provide feedback for therapeutic response. However, CTC enrichment is a challenge because CTCs are present in most cancer patients' blood at concentrations of around 1–100 CTC per ml of blood, compared to 5 billion red blood cells and 7 million white blood cells per ml of blood. Further, CTCs are delicate and short-lived, requiring rapid, gentle capture and elution. Finding just 1 CTC per ml of blood is clinically significant.

CTCs can be differentiated from other blood cells by size. They typically fall in the range of 12–25 μm in diameter, while erythrocytes (red blood cells) are 5–7 μm in diameter and **leukocytes** (white blood cells) are 7–15 μm in diameter. There is a clear size separation between CTCs and red blood cells. However, the size range of CTCs can overlap with some subtypes of leukocytes, such as monocytes which are 15–25 μm in diameter. Thus, size selection alone cannot detect and capture CTCs accurately.

11.2 Identifying CTC and WBC by 3-Color Staining

CTCs are often identified by immunostaining in which the cells are fluorescently labeled with antigen–antibody binding. Epithelial Cell Adhesion Molecule (EpCAM) bound to a capture antibody is often used for CTC capture, since EpCAM is expressed by nearly all carcinomas (85% of all solid tumors) and normal epithelial cells, but it not expressed by white blood cells (WBCs). A typical set of immunostaining antibodies may include DAPI for staining nuclei of CTCs and WBCs (with blue color), anti-Cytokeratin (CK)-FITC for staining epithelial cells (with green color), and anti-CD45-PE for staining WBCs (with red color). WBCs have a surface protein called CD45, which is not expressed in epithelial cells. Unlike WBCs, epithelial cells also express EpCAM on their surface and CK inside the cell but outside the nucleus. Thus, in this three-color staining scheme, CTCs would be stained blue and green (with no red), and WBCs would be stained blue and red (no green), as illustrated in Figure 11.2.

Biochips and Medical Imaging, First Edition. Adam de la Zerda and Shan Xiang Wang.

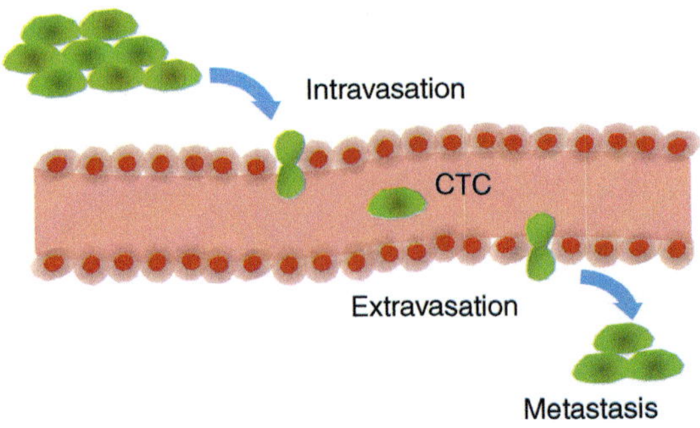

Figure 11.1 Circulating tumor cells.

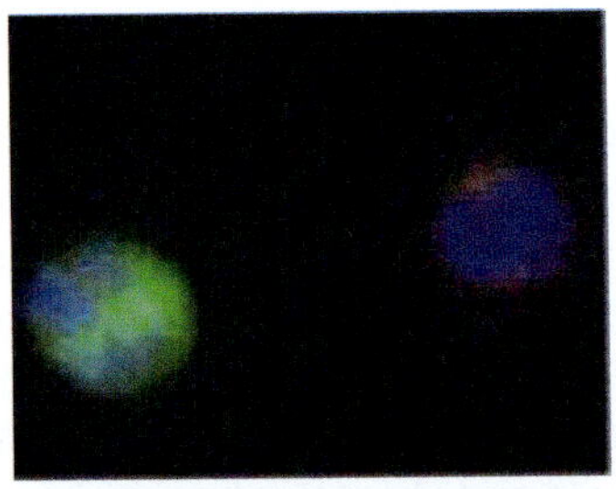

3 color imaging:

Marker	Tumor cell	White blood cell	Color
Anti-cytokeratin-FITC	+	–	Green
Anti-CD45-PE	–	+	Red
DAPI	+	+	Blue

PE: phycoerythrin, DAPI: 4′,6-diamidino-2-phenylindole, FITC: fluorescein isothiocyanate

Figure 11.2 3-color staining to distinguish cell types.

11.3 Fluorescence-Activated Cell Sorting (FACS)

One common method of cell sorting is Fluorescence-Activated Cell Sorting (FACS). This is similar to the flow cytometer used in the Luminex readout. Suppose three types of cells are to be sorted with FACS: those expressing GFP, those expressing CFP, and those expressing neither (Figure 11.3).

The mixture of cells expressing GFP and CFP is flowed through a channel, which eventually forms them into a single file. A laser connected to a photomultiplier tube forms the interrogation point, where each cell is excited with the laser and green or cyan color can be detected, depending on the GFP or CFP expression, respectively. An attached electrical wire can then charge the cells individually based on the color – for example, negatively charged for cyan and positively charged for green. Finally, a separation plate similar to a capacitor can sort the charged cells into three buckets: with the positively charged side attracting cyan, the negatively charged side attracting green, and noncolored cells in the middle. In this example, 3-plex FACS sorting is achieved with a throughput of up to 10^4 cells per second. Thus, FACS is not well suited for rare cells such as CTCs.

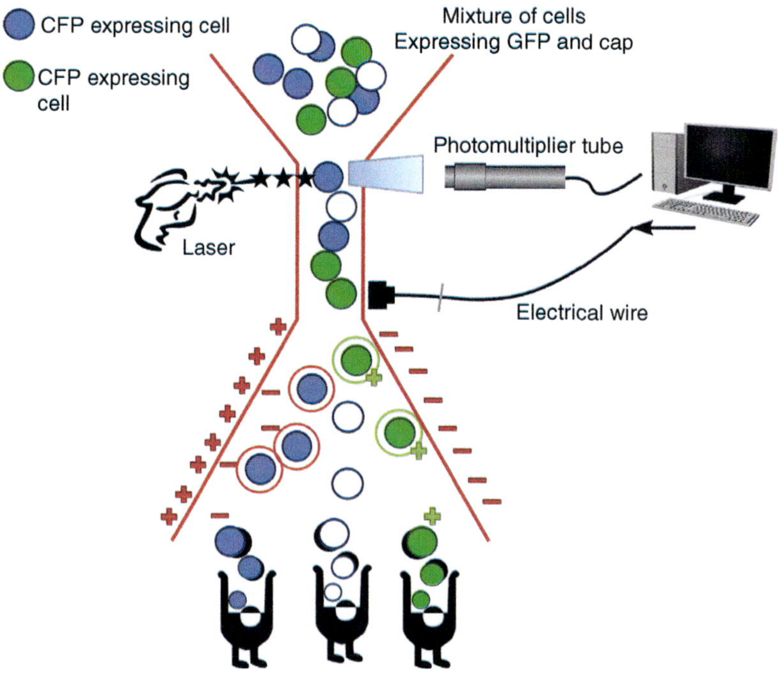

Figure 11.3 Fluorescence-Activated Cell Sorting (FACS). *Source:* University of Aberdeen – aye Switch [1]. Used under CC-BY 3.0 http://creativecommons.org/licenses/by/3.0.

11.4 Magnetically Activated Cell Sorting (MACS)

Another cell sorting technique is Magnetically Activated Cell Sorting (MACS) in which magnetically susceptible materials are extracted from a mixture using magnetic forces. In particular, rare cell enrichment has been performed with antibody-conjugated magnetic particles since the 1990s. Magnetic nanoparticles are first conjugated to antibodies and then added to the cell suspension, which will selectively bind to the target cells (Figure 11.4). Magnetic separation is then achieved by adding a permanent magnet to the sides of the flow column and then flowing buffer to wash away the unbound cells.

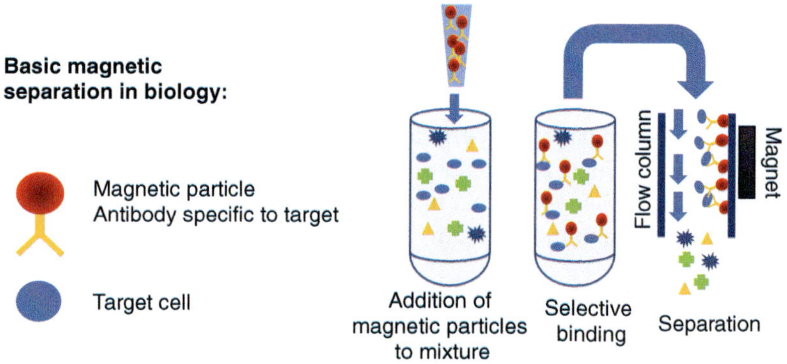

Figure 11.4 Magnetically Activated Cell Sorting (MACS).

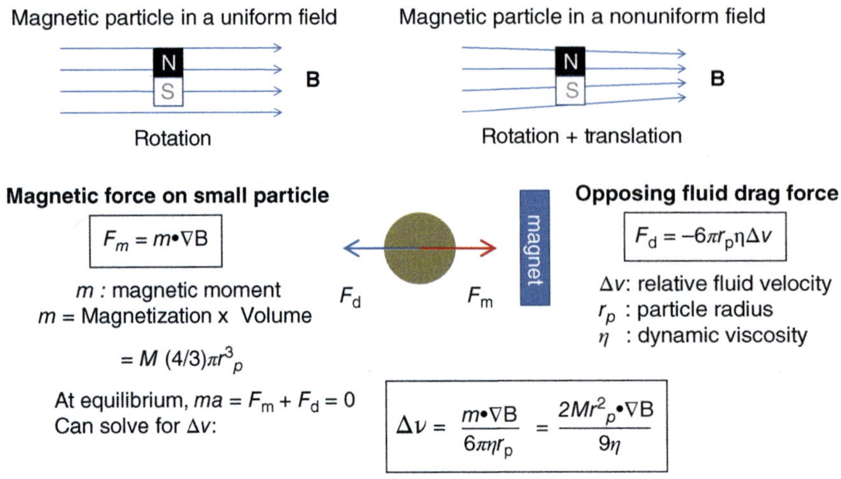

Figure 11.5 Theoretical basis of MACS.

The basic theory of MACS (Figure 11.5) relies on the fact that magnetic particles must have an applied nonuniform field in order to experience rotation and translation; otherwise, a uniform applied field will cause only rotation to the magnetic particle. In order for MACS to work effectively and efficiently, the magnetic force of the permanent magnet on the magnetic particles must balance out the opposing fluid drag force to reach steady state separation in equilibrium. The relative fluid velocity, given by the equation at the bottom of Figure 11.5, must fall into a reasonable range for efficient separation. Small particles typically require large M (magnetic dipole moment per volume) and field gradient to achieve reasonable capture time, while larger particles work better if the field gradient is limited.

11.5 Magnetic Separation Devices

Examples of typical magnetic separation devices are columnar flow devices (three-dimensional flow) and microfluidic devices (two-dimensional flow), each shown in Figure 11.6. The columnar flow devices consist of a vertical tube lined with soft magnetic material mesh, which can become magnetized with a permanent magnet to produce strong gradients in gaps. The magnetic mesh can capture magnetically labeled cells, after which the magnets can be removed and the column washed with washing buffer to elute and harvest the magnetically labeled cells or other biomolecules. Columnar flow devices have the advantage of high throughput in the ml h^{-1} range, but suffer from low field gradients ($<100\,\text{T m}^{-1}$) or retention in the nonuniform magnetic mesh. One example of a microfluidic device consists of patterned permanent magnets that create a field gradient as fluid flows through a channel, which again captures magnetically labeled cells. These devices have high field gradients due to closely spaced bar magnets and allow for optical inspection of separation, but suffer from low throughput in the $\mu\text{l min}^{-1}$ range.

11.5.1 CellSearch Platform

The CellSearch platform (from Immunicon/Veridex/Johnson & Johnson) is a system that can capture magnetically and fluorescently labeled CTCs from a blood sample for accurate measurement

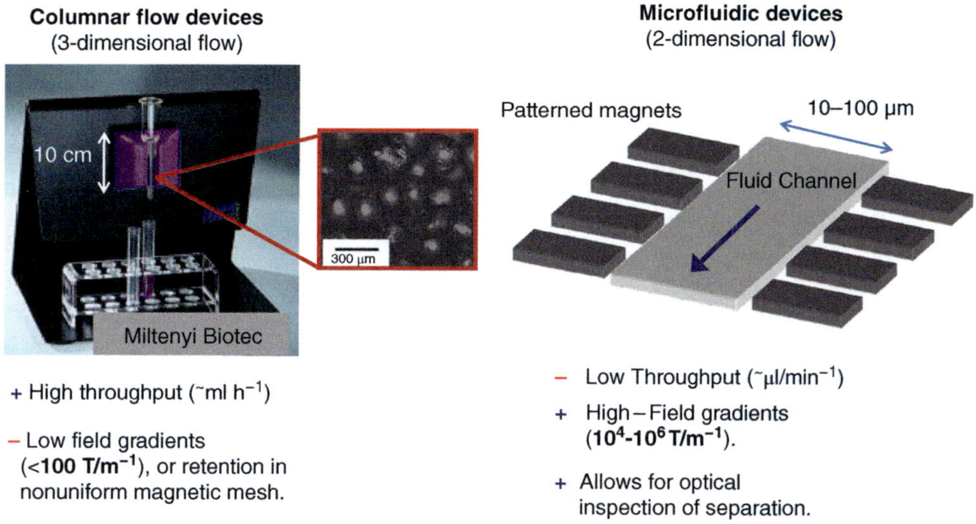

Figure 11.6 Columnar and microfluidic devices for magnetic separation.

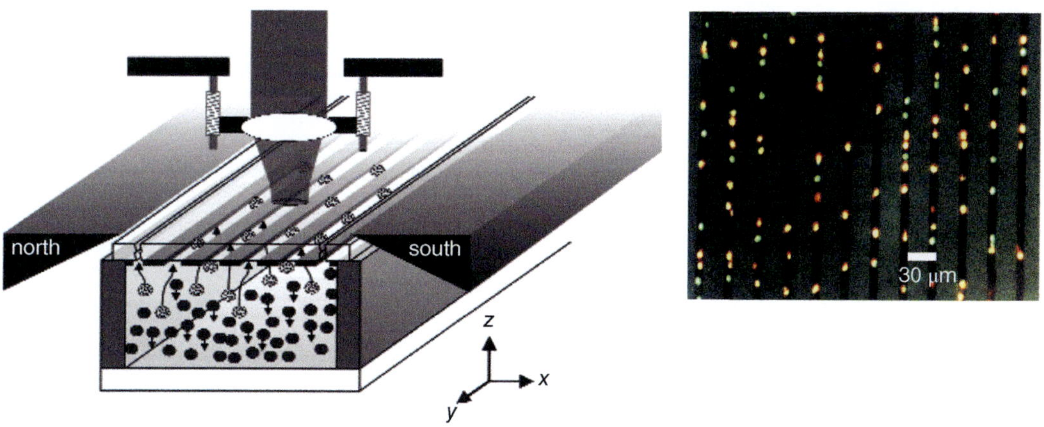

Figure 11.7 CellSearch platform. *Source:* Tibbe et al. [2]. Reprinted by permission from Springer Nature: Nature Biotechnology. Copyright © 1999 by Springer Nature.

(Figure 11.7). It is the only FDA-approved CTC enrichment technology platform. First, a whole blood sample is labeled with magnetic particle/anti-EpCAM complex and then loaded into the fluidic chamber. Permanent magnets and Ni lines on either side of the fluidic channel will attract CTCs to the top by creating a large field gradient (across a small gap). The cells are then stained with a three-color scheme, and a microscope can then observe their stained colors and count the captured cells as CTCs (or not) based on their color, size, shape, etc. (right image in Figure 11.7).

Figure 11.8 illustrates the criteria for identification of a CTC which includes a round to oval morphology, a visible nucleus (DAPI positive, DAPI is a dye that stains nuclei), positive staining for cytokeratin (CK) in the cytoplasm (CK-PE is a dye that stains CK), and negative staining for CD45 (expressed by many normal white blood cells, which CD45-APC stains). Row A shows a

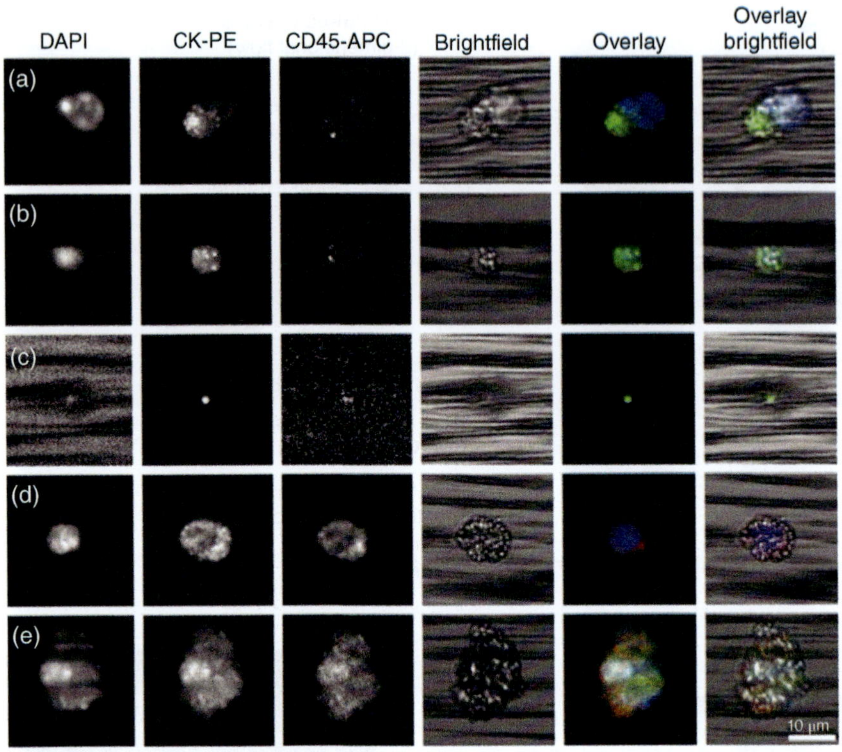

Figure 11.8 Identification of CTCs using CellSearch system. Row (a) shows an intact CTC; row (b) shows an apoptotic CTC; row (c) shows CTC debris; row (d) shows a leukocyte; and row (e) shows debris. *Source:* From Scholtens et al. [3]. Reprinted by permission from John Wiley and Sons, Inc. Copyright © 2011 International Society for Advancement of Cytometry.

definitively identified CTC while row B shows an apoptotic CTC and row C shows CTC debris. Row D shows a leukocyte (DAPI and CD45-APC positive, CK-PE negative). Row E shows debris (no clear stain results).

11.5.2 MagSifter for Cancer Cells

There are many emerging technologies being developed for CTC capture and enrichment. An example is the magnetic sifter (MagSifter) invented in Prof. Shan Wang's lab at Stanford. The MagSifter is a microfluidic device, about 7 mm × 7 mm in size, that is fabricated by first placing a silicon nitride membrane in a silicon backbone using reactive ion etch (RIE), then coating with NiFe film. The MagSifter contains about 38 000 pores in the soft magnetic NiFe film. The operating principle of the MagSifter is similar to MACS in that magnetic nanoparticles conjugated to EpCAM-antibody are used to label CTCs, and a permanent magnet is applied to capture the CTCs. The release of captured cells is enabled by removal of the magnetic field, which then demagnetizes the magnetic material. However, unlike MACS, the MagSifter enables both high capture efficiency due to the high field gradients at the small pore edges, as well as high throughput (sample volume processing in the $ml\,h^{-1}$ range) due to the dense pore arrays.

The MagSifter uses a three-color staining method of CTC identification, including DAPI for staining nuclei of CTCs and WBCs (with blue color), anti-Cytokeratin (CK)-FITC for staining epithelial cells (with green color), and anti-CD45-PE for staining WBCs (with red color). CTCs

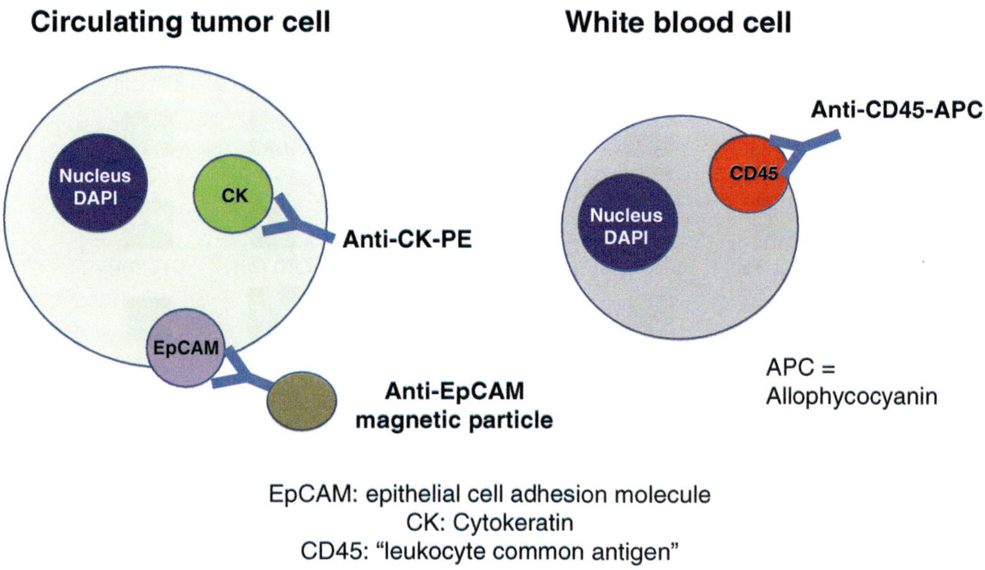

Figure 11.9 Staining scheme for capturing CTCs.

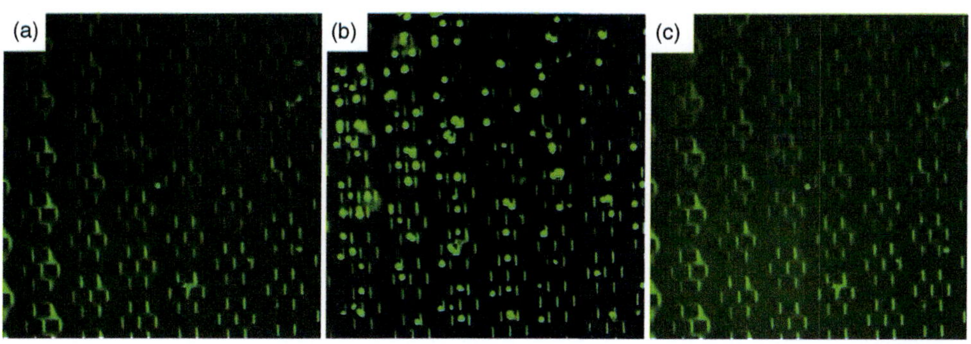

Figure 11.10 Fluorescent images of MagSifter (a) before capture, (b) after capture, and (c) after release steps. The cells are magnetically and fluorescently labeled.

would be stained blue and green (with no red), and WBCs would be stained blue and red (no green) (Figure 11.9). Figures 11.10 and 11.11 illustrate some captured CTCs from a lung cancer patient's blood sample using the MagSifter.

11.5.3 μ-Hall Detector

While anti-EpCAM complexes represent one of the most promising isolation schemes for CTCs, it may miss an important subclass of CTCs. As part of the process that allows CTCs to detach from the primary tumor (i.e. epithelial-mesenchymal transition), the CTCs may also reduce their expression of EpCAM. Additionally, CTCs are extremely heterogeneous, with different subclasses expressing different cell surface receptors (Figure 11.12a). Surface receptors (e.g. EpCAM, EGFR) are not only possible probes for CTC isolation, but their profiles on a patient's CTCs can also provide information about prognosis, treatment efficacy, and likelihood or recurrence. Issadore et al. [5] developed a μ-Hall detector (named because the detector is based on the Hall effect) that utilizes different sized

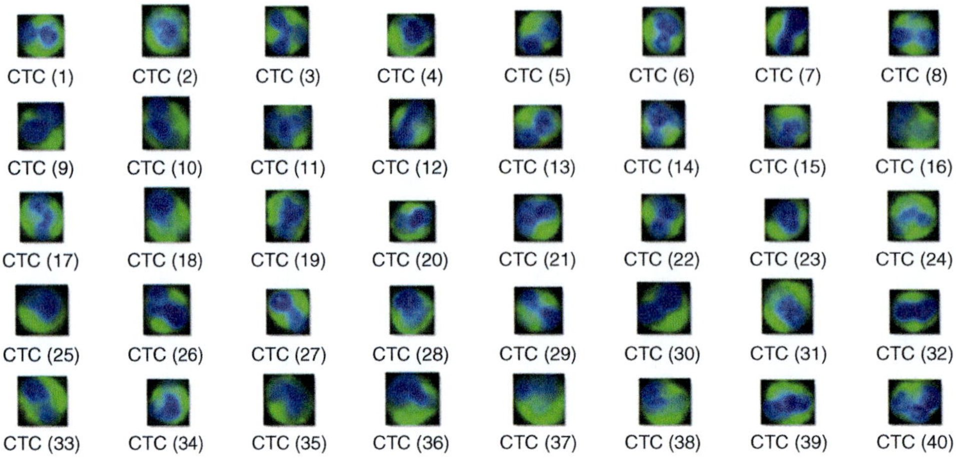

Figure 11.11 CTCs captured from a patient blood sample using MagSifter.

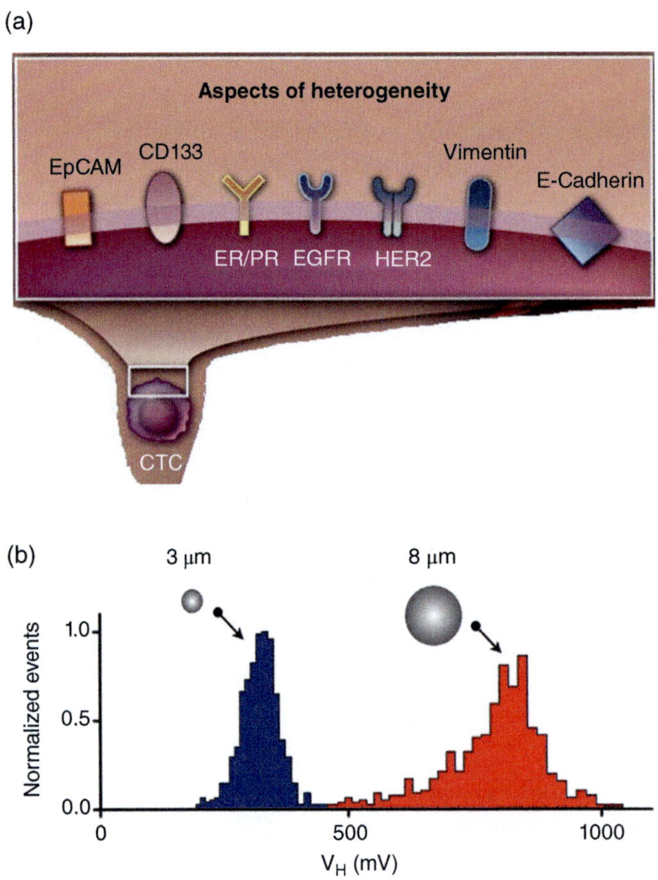

Figure 11.12 (a) Various surface biomarkers that can be present on CTCs. *Source:* From Lang et al. [4]. Copyright © 2012 American Association for the Advancement of Science. (b) Signal from μ-hall detector for two different sized magnetic nanoparticles. *Source:* From Issadore et al. [5]. Copyright © 2012 American Association for the Advancement of Science.

magnetic nanoparticles to isolate and profile CTCs based on three biomarkers: EpCAM, HER2/neu receptor, and EGFR. The measured signal is proportional to the volume of the nanoparticle (Figure 11.12b), which allows for quantification of each type of nanoparticle.

11.6 CTC Enrichment By Size Filtering

As previously mentioned, CTCs can be filtered by size separation rather than relying on antibody capture. Hosokawa developed a microcavity array (MCA) system integrated with a miniaturized device for CTC isolation without relying on EpCAM expression. The microcavity array consists of many small pores of 8–9 μm in diameter in a PDMS structure, which will effectively sort CTCs based on their larger size compared to typical RBC and most WBCs. After capture, a tricolor staining method with DAPI, CK-FITC, and CD45-PE is employed to distinguish CTCs from leukocytes. An alternative approach to pores for size filtration is to use centrifugal forces in a microfluidic channel. Hou et al. [6] demonstrated such an approach in a spiral microfluidic channel capable of separating CTCs from WBCs and RBCs (Figure 11.13).

11.7 CTC-CHIP (HARVARD UNIVERSITY)

Nagrath et al. [7] at Harvard University have developed a microfluidic platform called the CTC-chip (Figure 11.14), which is capable of efficient and selective separation of CTCs from blood samples. The CTC-chip is made of Si microposts coated with anti-EpCAM and attached to a Si substrate. The whole blood sample is then flowed through the CTC-chip, where the microposts slow down the flow and increase kinetic binding chance. The CTCs will be captured on these microposts and then interrogated and enumerated with 3-color staining from the top.

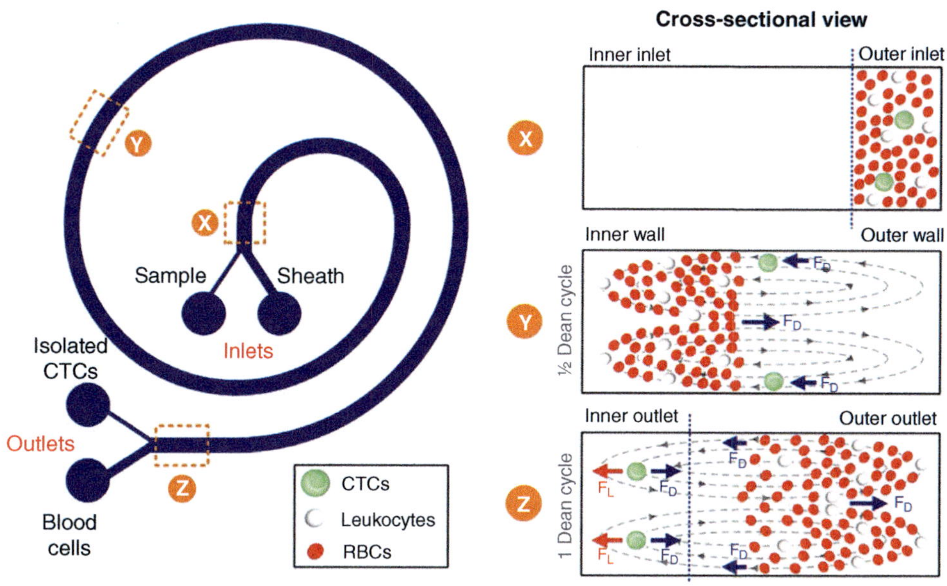

Figure 11.13 Spiral microfluidic chip for CTC isolation. *Source:* Hou et al. [6]. Adapted by permission from Springer Nature: Scientific Reports. Copyright © 2013 by Springer Nature.

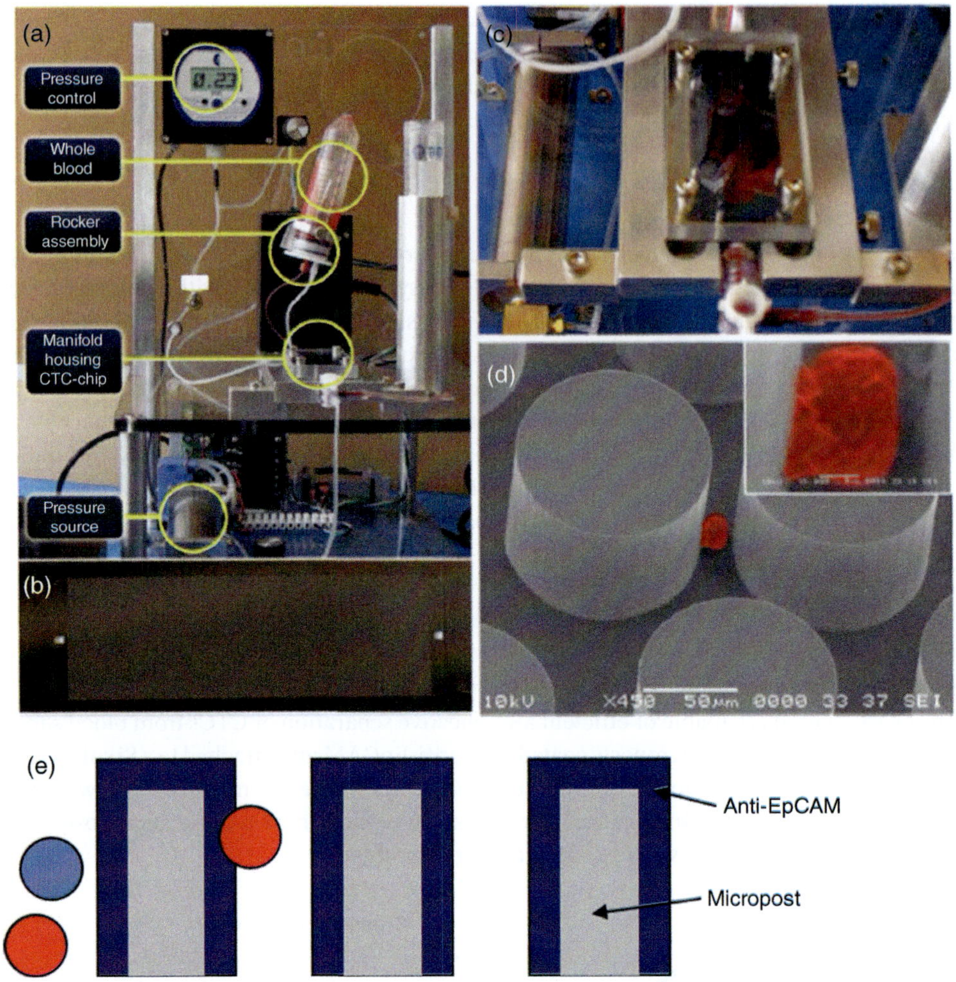

Figure 11.14 Harvard CTC-chip design and workstation. (a) The workstation setup for CTC separation. The sample is continually mixed on a rocker, and pumped through the chip using a pneumatic-pressure-regulated pump. (b) The CTC-chip with microposts etched in silicon. (c) Whole blood flowing through the microfluidic device. (d) Scanning electron microscope image of a captured NCI-H1650 lung cancer cell spiked into blood (pseudo coloured red). The inset shows a high magnification view of the cell. (e) Cross-sectional schematic showing three silicon microposts coated with anti-EpCAM capture antibodies which can capture EpCAM expressing CTCs in a blood sample. Source: Nagrath et al. [7]. Reprinted by permission from Springer Nature: Nature. Copyright © 2007 by Springer Nature.

11.7.1 The Third-Generation CTC Chip (CTC-iChip)

The third-generation CTC-iChip platform is an improvement upon the CTC-Chip. The CTC-iChip platform consists of three stages through which CTCs labeled with magnetic beads are flowed (Figure 11.15). The first stage is size-based sorting with microposts, which scatter the larger CTCs and WBCs downward to the second stage while allowing RBCs, platelets, and other small blood components to flow through and be flushed away. The second stage aligns the CTCs and WBCs into a single-file alignment due to inertial focusing. The final stage is magnetic separation which can be either positive-selection separation of anti-EpCAM-labeled CTCs away from WBCs, or alternatively, negative-selection separation of anti-CD45-labeled WBCs away from CTCs.

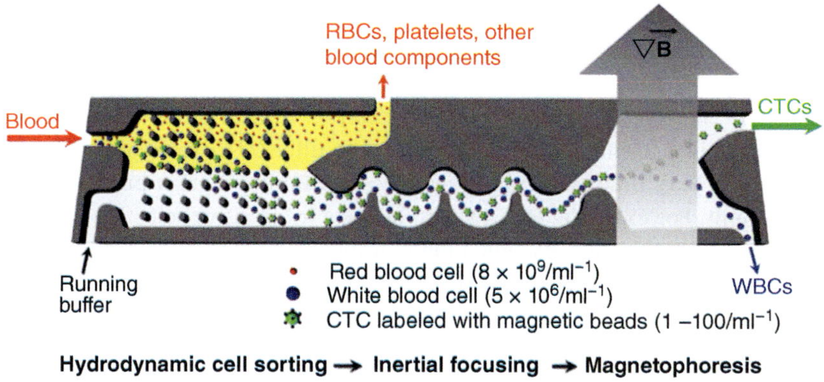

Figure 11.15 CTC-iChip design. *Source:* From Ozkumur et al. [8]. Copyright © 2013 American Association for the Advancement of Science.

After CTCs were collected by the CTC-iChip, they were stained in the typical DAPI/CK/CD45 tricolor scheme. CTCs/mL of whole blood were measured for samples from healthy donors compared to castrate-resistant prostate cancer (CRPC) patients, which demonstrated a clear separation between the two groups based on CTC identification.

11.8 Clinical Utility From CTCs

CTCs have the potential to enable liquid biopsy in the future, which is a biopsy done with a blood sample instead of a solid tissue. Currently, a biopsy is performed to screen for or diagnose a cancer tumor by using a needle to extract a small tissue sample, called a fine needle aspirate, from the suspected site. A biopsy may be painful, pose side effects or risks to the patient, or not be possible depending on the site. CTCs may also enable personalized medicine in which medical treatment for a cancer patient can be tailored based on the patient's personal genomic or proteomic data.

11.8.1 Liquid Biopsy

Research studies of CTCs have revealed insights that can potentially enable patient stratification or monitoring for personalized therapies. It has been found that the genotype and phenotype characteristics of CTCs can be different from the primary tumor due to the rapidly mutating nature of cancer cells. Thus, CTC analysis can enable patients to be stratified, i.e. placed into different diagnosis groups with targeted therapies, as well as be used to monitor the efficacy of a patient's therapy. During treatment, patients will typically develop drug resistance due to mutations. Physicians could measure this drug resistance from the CTCs, and thus monitor the efficacy of the therapy. In addition, the presence or absence of DNA mutations in a patient's collected CTCs could predict whether certain targeted therapies may be appropriate treatment options for that patient. One example is the Her2/neu gene, present in 20% of breast cancer patients, which attracts growth factors to allow tumor cells to grow. For these Her2/neu positive breast cancer patients, Trastuzumab (Herceptin) is an effective drug. Herceptin is a monoclonal antibody which latches onto growth factor receptors so that tumor cells will stop growing or go into remission. Advances in sequencing technology have made it possible to identify thousands of mutations in a single cancer sample and create mutation signatures (combinations of mutations). Looking at mutation signatures as opposed to individual mutations will allow for higher fidelity stratification, treatment evaluation, and drug resistance evaluation.

As a liquid biopsy, CTCs can be collected in many different ways. Physical properties such as size/deformability, density, and electric charges could be utilized to filter CTCs from other blood cells and components (Figure 11.16a). Biological properties such as different marker proteins can also be used for CTC enrichment. For example, EpCAM can be used for positive selection, either in vivo (inside the blood vessel) or ex vivo (e.g. a whole blood sample on a chip), and CD45 can be used for negative selection by depleting WBCs from the blood sample (Figure 11.16b).

After CTCs are collected from patient blood, there are many potential downstream analysis techniques for CTCs, including immunostaining for identification, fluorescence in-situ hybridization (FISH) for detection of the presence or absence of specific DNA sequences, DNA sequencing, qRT-PCR for mRNA quantification, expression analysis, or culture.

11.8.2 CTC Counts and Prognosis of Metastatic Breast Cancer

The survival plot (Kaplan–Meier plot) of metastatic breast cancer patients in Figure 11.17 indicates that patients with 5 or fewer CTCs per 7.5 ml of blood have a high survival rate past 18 months (over 70%), while patients with more than 5 CTCs per 7.5 ml of blood have a much lower survival rate past 18 months (about 30%). Thus, CTC count is indeed a very good prognosis biomarker, which can be used to decide whether to continue with the original therapy or to choose a different course of therapy. For example, a decreasing CTC count indicates that therapy

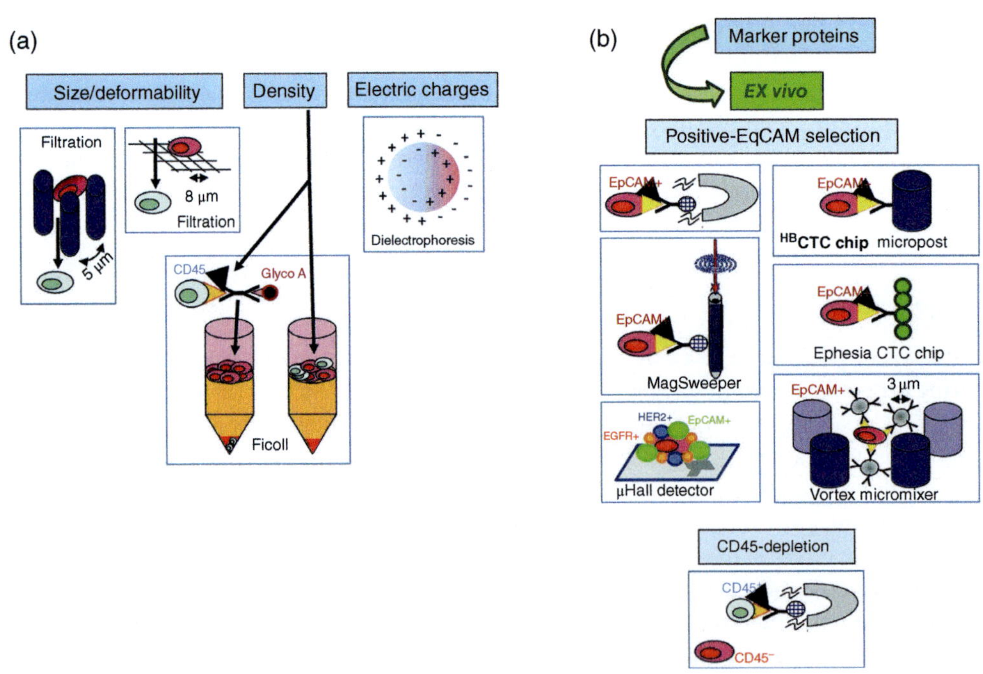

Figure 11.16 (a) Physical properties and (b) biological properties for CTC enrichment (liquid biopsy). *Source:* Alix-Panabieres et al. [9]. Republished with permission of Royal Society of Chemistry. Copyright © 2014 The Royal Society of Chemistry; permission conveyed through Copyright Clearance Center, Inc.

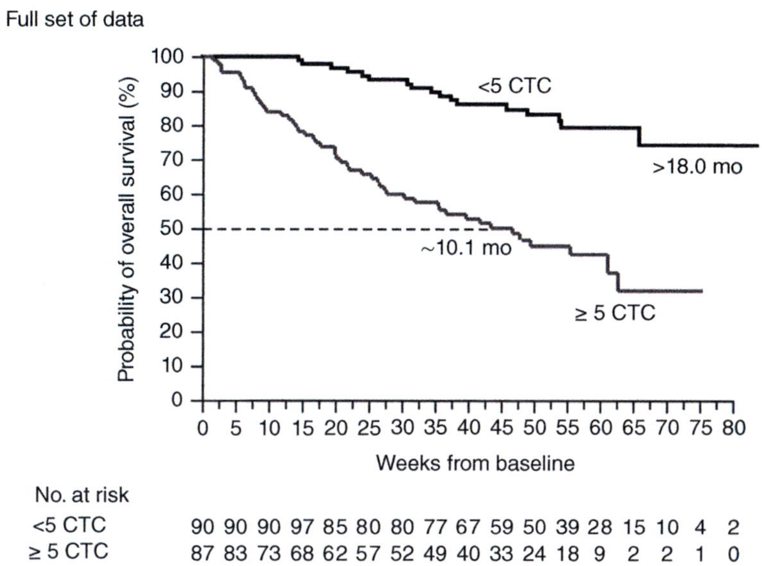

Figure 11.17 Prognosis of metastatic breast cancer based on CTC counts. *Source:* From Cristofanilli et al. [10]. Copyright © 2004 Massachusetts Medical Society. Reprinted with permission from Massachusetts Medical Society.

is working, while an increasing CTC count indicates that the patient's prognosis is deteriorating. It could be a powerful tool for serial monitoring of patients to provide continual care. A CTC test can predict patient prognosis for breast, colorectal, or prostate cancer, and CellSearch®-based CTC tests for these cancers have been approved by the FDA and are currently being marketed by Johnson & Johnson.

11.9 Conclusion

CTCs, although rare in blood circulation, are presumed to play a key role in cancer metastasis. FACS and MACS are two common approaches for cell sorting and have distinct pros and cons. Numerous microfluidic chips have been developed for capturing and enriching CTCs, including CellSearch, MagSifter, Size Filter, CTC-iChip, and many more. In the future, CTC enumeration and downstream analysis hold great promises for personalized medicine, especially in prognosis and early-stage cancer diagnosis.

Problems

11.1 You received a blood sample from a patient, and the sample was pretreated with EDTA (Ethylenediaminetetraacetic acid) to avoid clotting. To count the number of CTCs, you immunostained the cells with several cell markers, and observed them under a fluorescence microscope. You found that there were two different types of cells (Table 11.1):

A Based on the staining result, identify the cell type of A and B.

B If you want to confirm whether a cell is a CTC, what other criteria do you need to look out for?

Table 11.1 FITC, Cy3 and Cy5 are dye conjugates.

Cell ID	DAPI	Anti-Cytokeratin-Cy3	Anti-CD45-FITC	Anti-EpCAM-Cy5
A	+	+	−	+
B	+	−	+	−

C If you replace the dye (Cy5) of Anti-EpCAM-Cy5 with GFP (green fluorescent protein), what might be a possible problem?

D If you were to flow the sample through MagSifter to capture and enrich CTCs, what would you do differently from the above table during the immunostaining?

11.2 In your own words, describe pros and cons of Fluorescence-Activated Cell Sorting (FACS) and Magnetically Activated Cell Sorting (MACS).

11.3 One of the factors that determine the throughput of MACS is the speed at which the sample flows through it. Assuming speed is the only factor, we need to increase the speed to maximize the throughput while still ensuring that the magnetically labeled cells are captured. That means we need to increase the speed up to a certain point where the drag force on the cell becomes comparable to the magnetic force on the magnetic particles that bind to the cell. On average, you can label a cell with 100 magnetic nanoparticles, which have a magnetic moment of $m = 2\times10^{-16}\ \mathrm{A\cdot m^2}$. The diameter of the cell is about 15 μm. Using a unique design of magnets, a gradient of magnetic field of $10^5\ \mathrm{T\,m^{-1}}$ can be generated. You may assume that the fluid that contains the cells is water at 20 °C.

A What is the theoretical maximum speed of sample injection through the MACS column?

B How could you increase the throughput if you were to redesign the experiment?

11.4 Consider CTC counts-based molecular Dx test for metastatic breast cancer. If the number of CTCs per 7.5 ml is 5 for a particular patient, and the blood volume sampled randomly is 7.5 ml, then the mean of the CTC counts in a given sample is expected to be 5, and the standard deviation of the CTC counts is the squared root of 5.

A What is the chance that you will misclassify the patient as having a good prognosis (CTC counts = 4 or less)?

B Would your answer change if the volume of blood available for CTC counts is increased to 75 ml? The good prognosis criterion remains the same (CTC counts per 7.5 ml < 5, i.e. for 75 ml of blood, the CTC count is 44 or less).

Hint: You can assume the sample numbers of CTC counts in both situations obey a normal distribution. The mean in the second case is 50, while the standard deviation is its squared root.

References

1 University of Aberdeen (2010). *Flow cytometry Analysis of fluorescence Proteins*, iGEM 2010 Website. University of Aberdeen http://2010.igem.org/FACS_analysis_of_fluorescent_proteins.

2 Tibbe, A.G.J., de Grooth, B.G., Greve, J. et al. (1999). Optical tracking and detection of immunomagnetically selected and aligned cells. *Nature Biotechnology* 17: 12.

3 Scholtens, T.M., Schreuder, F., Ligthart, S.T. et al. (2012). Automated identification of circulating tumor cells by image cytometry. *Cytometry Part A* 81A: 138–148.

4 Lang, J.M., Casavant, B.P., and Beebe, D.J. (2012). Circulating tumor cells: getting more from less. *Science Translational Medicine* 4 (141): 141ps13. http://dx.doi.org/10.1126/scitranslmed.3004261.

5 Issadore, D., Chung, J., Shao, H. et al. (2012). Ultrasensitive clinical enumeration of rare cells ex vivo using a micro-hall detector. *Science Translational Medicine* 4 (141): 141ra92. DOI: 10.1126/scitranslmed.3003747.

6 Hou, H.W., Warkiani, M.E., Khoo, B.L. et al. (2013). Isolation and retrieval of circulating tumor cells using centrifugal forces. *Scientific Reports* 3: 1259.

7 Nagrath, S., Sequist, L.V., Maheswaran, S. et al. (2007). Isolation of rare circulating tumour cells in cancer patients by microchip technology. *Nature* 450: 7173.

8 Ozkumur, E., Shah, A.M., Ciciliano, J.C. et al. (2013). Inertial focusing for tumor antigen–dependent and –independent sorting of rare circulating tumor cells. *Science Translational Medicine* 5 (179): 179ra47. http://dx.doi.org/10.1126/scitranslmed.3005616.

9 Alix-Panabieres, C. and Pantel, K. (2014). Technologies for detection of circulating tumor cells: facts and vision. *Lab Chip* 14: 57–62.

10 Cristofanilli, M., Budd, G.T., Ellis, M.J. et al. Circulating tumor cells, disease progression, and survival in metastatic breast cancer. *New England Journal of Medicine* 351: 781–791.

Further Reading

http://scitation.aip.org/content/aip/magazine/physicstoday/article/67/2/10.1063/PT.3.2275
http://www.nature.com/articles/srep01259?WT.ec_id=SREP-631-20130301
http://stm.sciencemag.org/content/4/141/141ps13.full-text.pdf+html
http://www.nature.com/nature/journal/v500/n7463/pdf/nature12477.pdf

12

Molecular Diagnostics

12.1 Molecular Diagnostics (Dx)

Diagnosis (Dx) is both the process of attempting to determine a possible disease and the opinion reached by this process, which includes screening and early diagnosis. This chapter will introduce molecular diagnostics, a new discipline that distinguishes between normal and disease states at the molecular level, by examining molecules such as proteins and mRNA. Prognosis is the term that describes the expected course of a disease after diagnosis of the disease is made. Therapeutics (Rx) is the treatment and care of a patient with a disease. Molecular diagnosis may also help with therapy selection and monitoring through the development of personalized medicine.

12.1.1 Molecular Dx versus Traditional Dx

Before molecular diagnostics, clinicians categorized cancer cells obtained from a biopsy of a patient with clinical symptoms according to their pathology, i.e. according to their appearance (shape, color, etc.) under a microscope (Figure 12.1a). Borrowing from two new disciplines, genomics and proteomics, molecular diagnostics categorizes cancers using technology such as mass spectrometry and gene chips. Genomics is the study of all the genes in a cell or organism, while proteomics is the study of all of the organism's proteins. Molecular diagnostics determines gene and protein activity patterns – in different types of cancerous or precancerous cells, and captures this information as expression patterns (Figure 12.1b). Also called "molecular signatures," these expression patterns are improving clinicians' ability to diagnose cancer. Soon all cancers may be diagnosed this way.

12.2 Molecular Diagnostics for Cancer

12.2.1 Subtyping Cancer

Researchers also use microarrays to detect differences in patterns of gene activity even within the same tumor type. In many cases, researchers have discovered that what had been considered a single type of cancer – based on how the cells looked under a microscope – was really two, three, or even more subtypes, each with a distinct gene expression pattern. For example, using microarrays, researchers have identified new types of leukemia. They also discovered that the most common type of lung cancer, lung adenocarcinoma, has actually four distinct subtypes, each with its

Biochips and Medical Imaging, First Edition. Adam de la Zerda and Shan Xiang Wang.

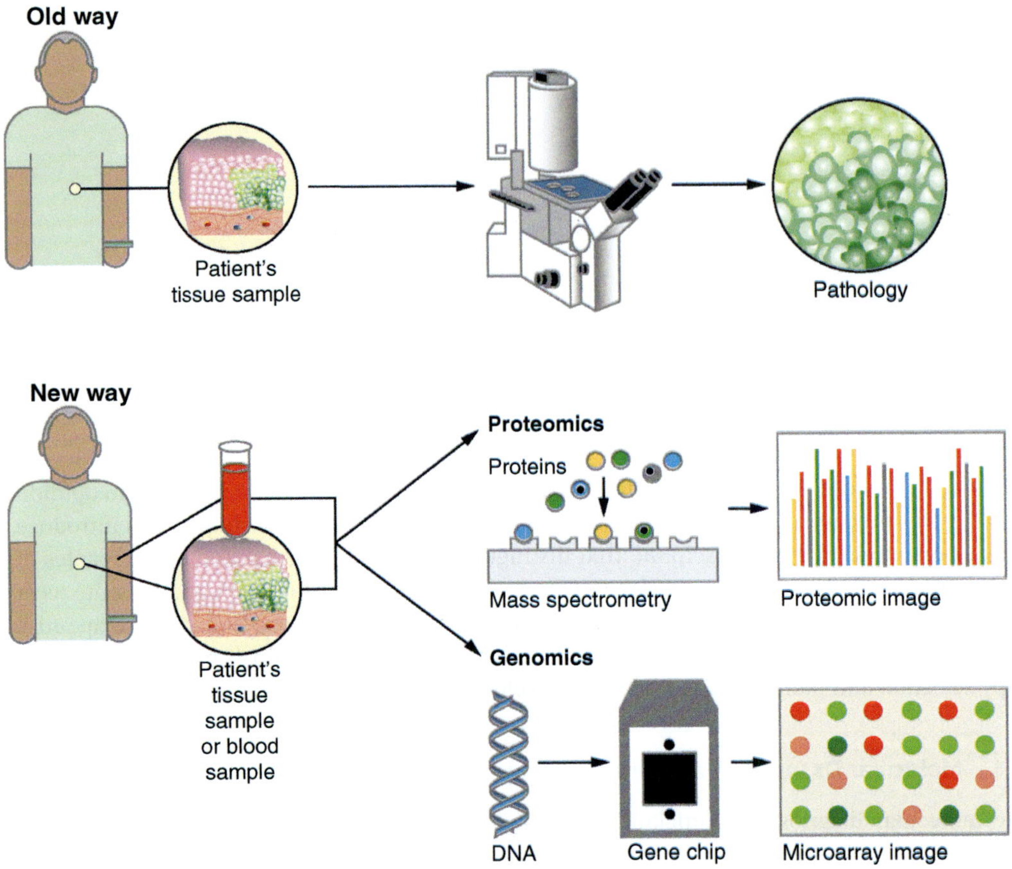

Figure 12.1 Molecular diagnostics versus traditional diagnostics. *Source:* From the Website of the National Cancer Institute (https://www.cancer.gov). Artwork by Jeanne Kelly.

own gene expression pattern (Figure 12.2). Given four patients with different subtypes of lung cancer, samples of tissue can be taken by biopsy and fed into a "lung-o-chip" microarray, which will detect the subtype of lung cancer present in each patient.

12.2.2 Protein Patterns and Diagnosis

To accomplish a molecular diagnosis based on active proteins in cancer, it is not necessary to identify every protein active in cancer; all that may be needed is to separate and preserve a unique subset, a pattern of proteins shared by all patients with the same cancer type. For example, researchers collected blood samples from a group of patients with diagnosed ovarian cancer and used mass spectrometry or protein assays (e.g. ELISA) to collect all the protein profiles that appeared in the patients' serum samples (Figure 12.3). Mass spectroscopy is done by first breaking the protein into peptides, then ionizing them and letting the samples pass through a mass spectrometer, which applies a magnetic field to charged particles that are measured as distinct lines due to different trajectories based on mass. While there was some variation from patient to patient, pooling enough samples of confirmed ovarian cancer enabled clinicians to use cluster analysis to determine what subset of proteins consistently served as markers for the presence of cancer. Identification of this subset was successful and today researchers are on their way to completing a method of molecular diagnosis for ovarian cancer.

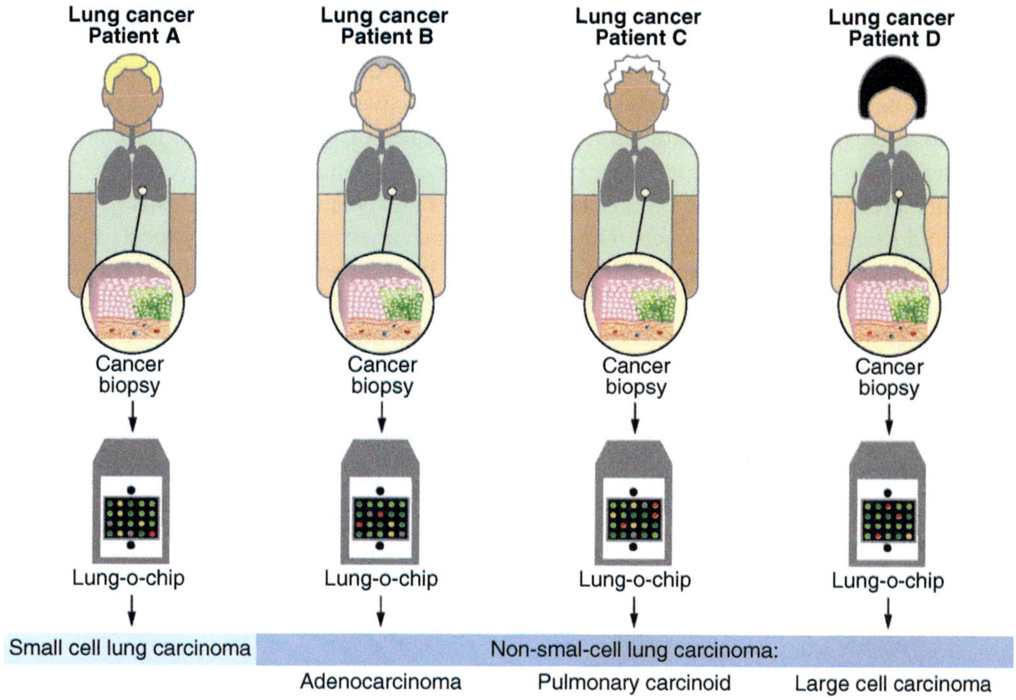

Figure 12.2 Subtyping lung cancer. *Source:* From the Website of the National Cancer Institute (https://www.cancer.gov). Artwork by Jeanne Kelly.

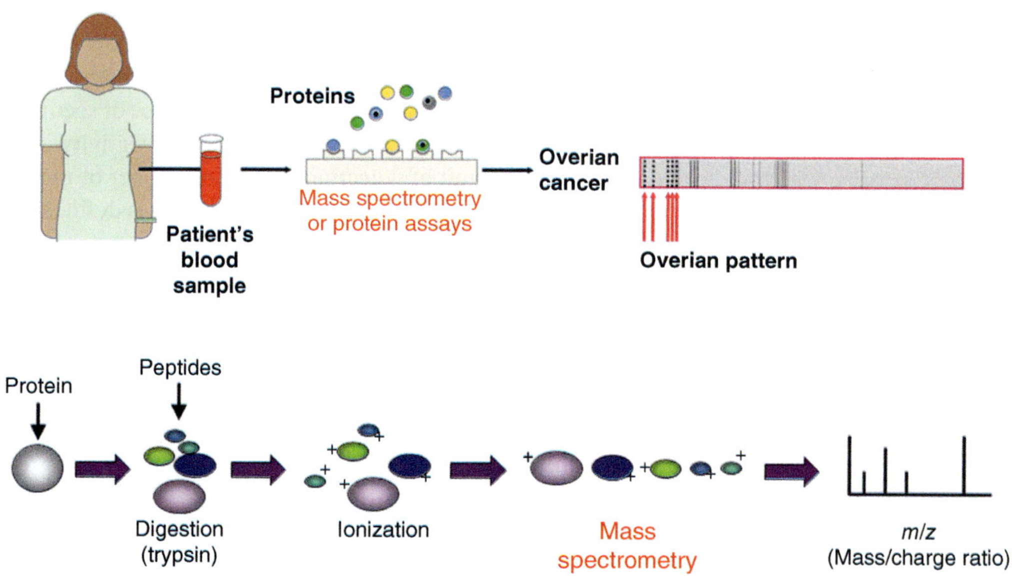

Figure 12.3 Protein-based diagnostics. *Source:* From the Website of the National Cancer Institute (https://www.cancer.gov). Artwork by Jeanne Kelly.

12.2.3 Protein Tumor Markers

For all forms of cancer, the importance of early detection is well documented. For lung cancer, the leading cause of cancer death, early detection leads to a five-year survival rate of over 50%, compared to a five-year survival rate without early detection of ~5%. Similarly, for colorectal cancer, survival rate is five times higher for patients with early detection. However, early detection through screening also comes at a cost because of false positives, which leads to wasted treatment and unnecessary side effects. The most effective cancer screening is expected to be a simultaneous assay of a panel of biomarkers, which can be used with a multivariate algorithm to produce an index-based diagnosis. As Table 12.1 shows, prostate-specific antigen (PSA) is a good biomarker for early prostate cancer screening. In prostate cancer screening, a PSA concentration greater than $4\,\text{ng ml}^{-1}$ indicates possible prostate cancer. CA-125 cannot be used for early screening of ovarian cancer yet, but it is used for diagnosis and treatment selection. Similarly, Her-2/neu is a biomarker used for diagnosis and treatment selection of breast cancer. It is important to note that each biomarker is not always useful and may be used only for certain subpopulations of certain cancers. Table 12.1 indicates the protein tumor markers recommended by the National Comprehensive Cancer Network (NCCN) and shows that diagnosis/prognosis and treatment monitoring are less challenging than screening.

12.3 Important Concepts in Diagnostics

12.3.1 Diagnostic Sensitivity

Molecular diagnostics (e.g. for ovarian cancer) must correctly detect all women who have the particular subtype of cancer, without incorrectly identifying people who do not have the disease. The first hurdle toward this goal is to develop a clinical diagnostic test with high sensitivity. Sensitivity answers this question: what percentage of people with a given type of cancer will have their cancer detected when a given screening test is used? If a test is not very sensitive, there will be many "false negative" results and individuals with cancer will go undetected. A test that yields many false negatives will obviously not be very good at reducing cancer deaths, giving a false sense of security to people who actually have the disease. Note the difference between diagnostic sensitivity and sensitivity of sensors, which indicates the minimum limit of detection (LOD) in number of molecules or their concentrations in biological media. Diagnostic sensitivity (Figure 12.4) is defined as the fraction of disease states that are detected:

$$\text{Sensitivity} = \frac{\text{TP}}{\text{TP} + \text{FN}},$$

where TP is the number of true positives and FN is the number of false negatives. Molecular tests based on IVDMIA (in vitro Diagnostic Multivariate Assay) produce a single index from multiple analytes and an index above or below a certain cutoff is reported as a positive or negative result, respectively.

12.3.2 Diagnostic Specificity

Another hurdle toward developing a clinical diagnostic test is the test's specificity. Specificity answers this question: what percentage of the people who do not have cancer are correctly identified as being free of disease? If a cancer test is not very specific, it will yield many "false positive"

Table 12.1 Biomarkers and their link with common malignancies.

NCCN recommendations on the use of tumor markers in common malignancies					
Site	**Analytes**	**Screening**	**Diagnosis and prognosis**	**Treatment selection and monitoring**	**Surveillance**
Acute myelogenous leukemia	Immunophenotyping markers		• (green)		
Bladder	NMP-22, BTA, M344		• (red)	• (red)	
Breast	Her-2/neu		• (green)	• (green)	
Colorectal	CEA		• (green)	• (green)	• (green)
Esophagus					
NSCLC					
Ovarian	CA-125		• (green)	• (green)	• (green)
Pancreas	CA-19-9		• (red)	• (red)	• (red)
Prostate	PSA	• (green)	• (green)	• (green)	• (green)
SCLC					
Stomach					

• Recommended in NCCN practice guidelines • Marker in development (no current consensus on utility) or used in investigational settings.

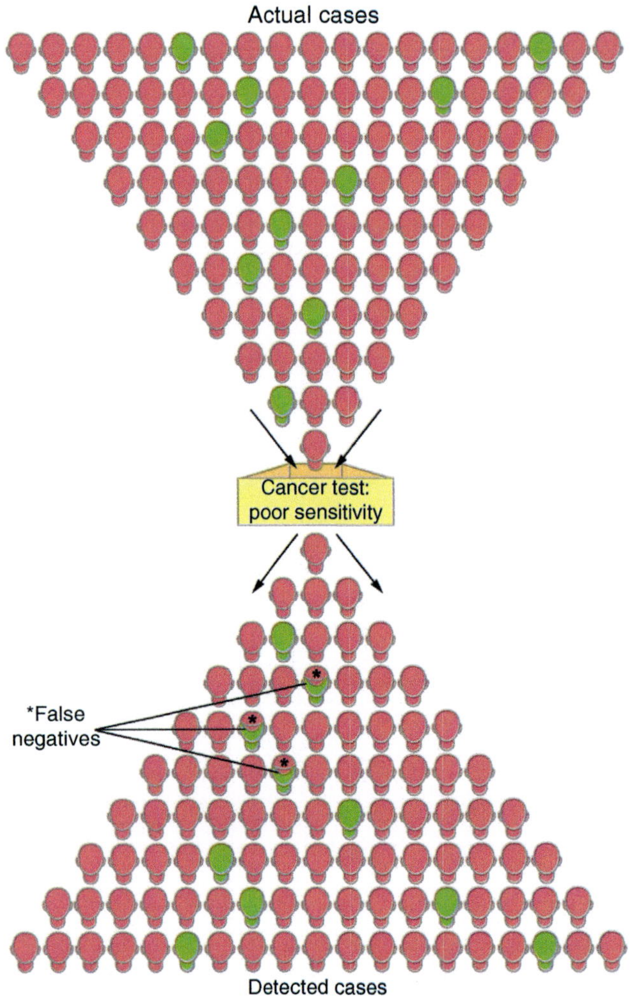

Figure 12.4 Diagnostic sensitivity. TP = 7, FN = 3, TP + FN = 10. *Source:* From the Website of the National Cancer Institute (https://www.cancer.gov). Artwork by Jeanne Kelly.

results; that is, a person will test positive even though they are cancer-free. Such error can lead to unnecessary and costly follow-up procedures and cause anxiety in the person misdiagnosed. Diagnostic specificity (Figure 12.5) is defined as the fraction of healthy states (negatives) that are diagnosed correctly as healthy states (true negatives):

$$\text{Specificity} = \frac{\text{TN}}{\text{TN} + \text{FP}},$$

where TN is the number of true negatives and FP is the number of false positives. The false positive rate is 1 – specificity.

High specificity is important for an ovarian cancer test because this cancer is a relatively rare disease occurring only in about 1 of 2500 postmenopausal women. The ovarian cancer diagnostic test is being developed and tested with women at risk of recurrence for ovarian cancer. If this use is successful, the test will next be extended to women at high risk for developing the disease.

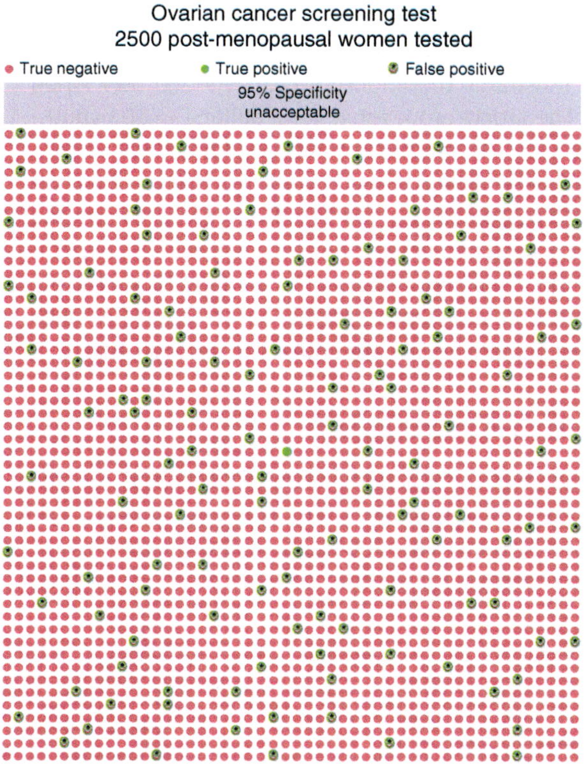

Figure 12.5 Diagnostic specificity. *Source:* From the Website of the National Cancer Institute (https://www.cancer.gov). Artwork by Jeanne Kelly.

12.3.3 Positive and Negative Predictive Values (PPV and NPV)

PPV is the probability of tested positives being correct while NPV is the probability of tested negatives being correct. They are given by the following equations:

$$\text{PPV} = \text{TP}/(\text{TP} + \text{FP})$$

$$\text{NPV} = \text{TN}/(\text{TN} + \text{FN}),$$

where TP is the number of true positives, FP is the number of false positives, TN is the number of true negatives, and FN is the number of false negatives.

12.3.4 If You Are an MD

Imagine a scenario in which you are given a new molecular diagnostic test to screen new patients from a general population with possible ovarian cancer, who have no prior history of cancer. Assume this molecular diagnostic test has a specificity of 95% and ovarian cancer has a prevalence of about 0.04%. If a female patient tests positive on this new test, what would you tell your "distressed" patient? It turns out that the probability of actually having ovarian cancer given a positive test result, the PPV, is only about $0.04\%/5\% = 0.8\%$. In general, PPV is usually low for low-prevalence diseases such as ovarian cancer since the majority of positive results are actually false positives.

PPV and NPV in Scientific Publishing

A 2013 article published in *The Economist* illustrates the importance of PPV and NPV when interpreting published results (Figure 12.6). The article argues that since about 1 in 10 hypotheses tested will be true, this implies that out of 1000 hypotheses, only 100 of them will be true. Assuming that the tests have a false positive rate of 5% and a sensitivity of 0.8, that would result in a total of 45 false positives (5% of 900), 80 true positives, and 20 false negatives. From the researcher's point of view, not knowing what is false and what is not, they will see 125 hypotheses as true, when, in reality, 45 of them are not. This gives values of PPV = 80/125 = 64% and NPV = 855/875 = 98%. Thus, the negative results are much more reliable based on an NPV much closer to 100% compared to PPV – but these negative results are unlikely to be published.

12.3.5 Cutoff Values in Molecular Dx: Myocardial Infarction (MI)

In molecular diagnosis of myocardial infarction (MI), those patients with NSTE (non-ST elevation in ECG) MIs are diagnosed with a blood test of cardiac troponin (cTn) as follows: a cutoff value (threshold) is set at the 99th percentile of a healthy reference population, or at the lowest measurable concentration with a CV (Coefficient of Variation) of 10% (functional sensitivity of an assay).

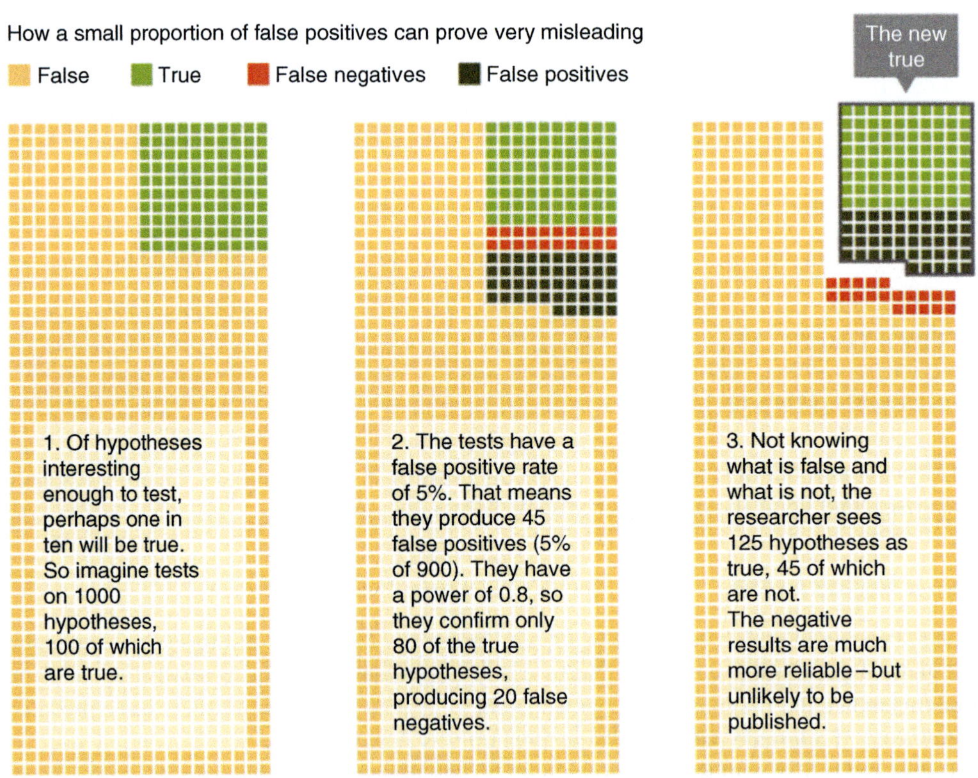

Figure 12.6 PPV and NPV in scientific publishing (adapted from The Economist). PPV = 80/125 = 64%. NPV = 855/875 = 98%. *Source:* From The Economist, "How Science Goes Wrong." © Copyright by The Economist Group Limited, London 2013.

For example, the Mayo clinic cutoff is 0.03 ng ml^{-1}. For cTn concentrations above the threshold, a positive result for heart attack is given. Lowering the threshold will increase false positives (i.e. a more sensitive but less specific test), while raising threshold will increase false negatives (i.e. a more specific but less sensitive test).

In more recent years, the 99th percentile of a healthy reference population is recommended as the cutoff for a positive MI indication. The probability that a single measured cTn result exceeds the estimated 99th percentile is equal to 1% for a person randomly selected from the general (reference) population. This criterion is irrespective of the imprecision profile of the analytical method as well as the lack of standardization of cTn assays.

12.3.6 Receiver Operating Characteristic (ROC) Curve

Figure 12.7 shows an example ROC curve, in which P(TP) is the true positive portion, a.k.a the True Positive Rate, and P(FP) is the false positive portion, a.k.a. the False Positive Rate (c.f. Section 12.3.7). If you have a large population and if you measure certain biomarkers to determine the state of the patients (i.e. healthy versus diseased), you'll get two Gaussian distributions for each state (shown as the left and right curves, respectively). If you choose your biomarkers wisely, these two Gaussians will sit farther apart. For example, a test to determine whether or not a subject has suffered from MI can measure the subject's cTn concentration. Subjects who have suffered from MI will have a higher concentration of cTn and their distribution would appear on the right. Healthy subjects will have lower cTn concentrations and their distribution curve will appear on the left. If you choose a biomarker that is useless for diagnosis, you would not get any separation between the healthy and diseased distributions. An example would be trying to detect MI but looking for a biomarker associated with ovarian cancer. In this case, you would get identical distributions of ovarian cancer biomarker in both healthy and diseased (MI) groups (unless there is a correlation between MI and ovarian cancer), and the test would be useless. The separation between two distributions depends on the quality of the test itself and does not depend on the choice of a threshold. This quality determines the ROC curve.

Using a threshold value allows your test to give a specific result. In the example above, the threshold moves the vertical bar in the distribution curves. Similarly, the threshold determines the operating point on the ROC curve. In both diagrams, green arrows represent the effect of threshold change. For example, you can set the threshold extremely low (i.e. left of the blue distribution curve) and your test will always give a positive result no matter what the actual state of the patient is. In this case, you will have 100% sensitivity but 0% specificity and your operating point on the ROC curve will shift all the way to the right (and intersect with the diagonal ROC because this kind of positive assignment is as useless as randomly distributing positives). Similarly, you can set the threshold extremely high (i.e. right of the red distribution curve) and your test will always give a negative result no matter what

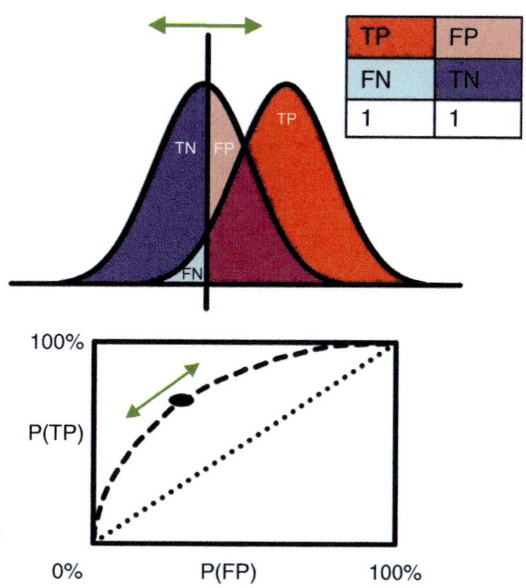

Figure 12.7 Example ROC curve.

the actual state of the patient is. In this case, you will have 0% sensitivity but 100% specificity and your operating point on the ROC curve will shift all the way to the left (and still intersect with the diagonal ROC). Ideally, you will want to set the threshold such that the operating point on the ROC curve is far away from the diagonal (i.e. pure chance ROC). Again it is important to note that changing threshold does not improve the ROC curve, it just defines what part of the ROC curve your test is operating. On the other hand, finding a better biomarker, which does a better job at differentiating diseased from healthy cases, will improve the ROC curve.

12.3.7 Additional Concepts in Diagnostics

Some rigorous definitions of important concepts are as follows. The True Positive Rate (TPR), a.k.a. sensitivity, is the probability of disease cases (TP + FN) that tested positive (TP). Thus, sensitivity = TP/(TP + FN) = TP/ "Disease Cases." FNs are disease cases that tested negative. The False Positive Rate (FPR), also known as (1 − specificity), is the probability of no-disease cases (TN + FP) being falsely reported as positive (FP). Thus, FPR = FP/(TN + FP) = FP/ "No − Disease Cases." FPs are no-disease cases that tested positive. Positive and Negative Predictive Values (PPV and NPV) are the probability of having the disease if given a positive test result, and probability of having no disease if given a negative test result, respectively. Accuracy is the percent of cases that are correctly classified, accuracy = (TP + TN)/all cases = (TP + TN)/(TP + TN + FP + FN). The receiver operating characteristic (ROC) curve is TPR versus FPR, i.e. the probability of a true positive (sensitivity) versus the probability of a false positive (1 − specificity), for all possible threshold values. The ROC curve reveals the trade-off between TPR (benefits) and FPR (costs). FP results in increased costs to treat individuals who are actually not diseased, while TPR results in a benefit of actual patients detected. The area under the curve (AUC) can be calculated for the ROC curve, which typically gives a value between 0.5 and 1. The closer the value of AUC is to 1, the better the diagnosis will be. A test with an AUC of 0.5 gives predictions that are as accurate as a coin flip (Figure 12.8).

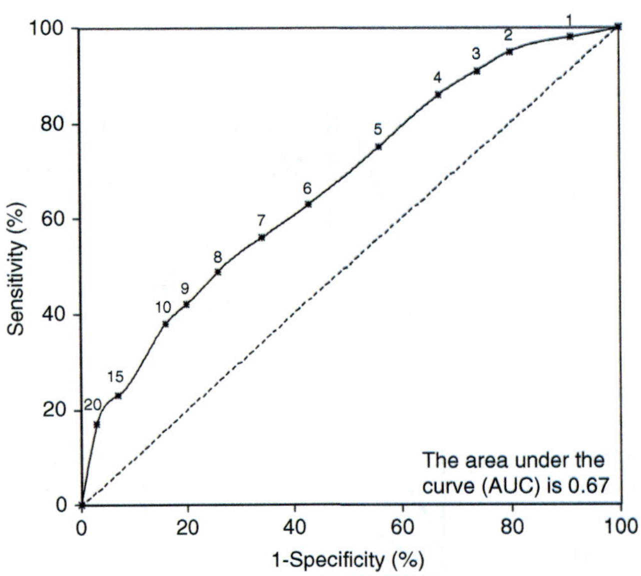

Figure 12.8 Example ROC curve and calculated AUC. *Source:* From Hoffman et al. [1]. © Copyright by Hoffman et al; licensee BioMed Central Ltd. 2002. Used under CC-BY license.

12.4 Conclusion

Molecular diagnostics is a new discipline that distinguishes between normal and disease states at the molecular level by examining molecules such as proteins and mRNA. Molecular diagnostics determine gene and protein activity patterns in different types of cancerous or precancerous cells. These "molecular signatures" are improving clinicians' ability to diagnose cancer. Molecular diagnosis may also help with therapy selection and monitoring through the development of personalized medicine, as well as provide prognosis for patients through methods such as genomic health breast cancer assay and CTC measurement.

Biochips could play a major role in disease diagnosis and prognosis, as well as personalized medicine. Sensitivity, specificity, PPV, NPV, and ROC curves need to be carefully considered for any biochip (or bioassay) to be used effectively.

12.5 Additional Information

Table 12.2 illustrates the concepts used in determining sensitivity and specificity. The fecal occult blood (FOB) screen test was used in 2030 people to look for bowel cancer:

12.5.1 ROC Curve Example for 2-Class Comparison (Healthy versus Disease State)

An example of an ROC curve for 2-class comparison (healthy versus disease state) is given in Figure 12.9. An appropriate threshold must be chosen to give the best tradeoff between sensitivity and specificity. If the threshold is set too low, the test will have high sensitivity but low specificity. As the threshold value is increased, the test's sensitivity remains high and specificity increases. The choice of a threshold cutoff can be subjective, depending on the social cost of the particular disease.

The area under the ROC curve (AUC) is commonly used as a summary measure of diagnostic accuracy. It can take values from 0.0 to 1.0. The AUC can be interpreted as the probability that a

Table 12.2 Example of how to determine sensitivity and specificity.

		Patients with bowel cancer (confirmed by endoscopy)		
		Condition positive	**Condition negative**	
Fecal occult blood Screen test outcome	Test outcome positive	**True positive** (TP) = 20	**False positive** (FP) = 180	Positive predictive value =TP/(TP + FP) =20/(20 + 180) **=10%**
	Test outcome negative	**False negative** (FN) = 10	**True negative** (TN) = 1820	Negative predictive value =TN/(FN + TN) =1820/(10 + 1820) **≈ 99.5%**
		Sensitivity =TP/(TP + FN) =20/(20 + 10) **≈67%**	**Specificity** =TN/(FP + TN) =1820/(180 + 1820) **=91%**	

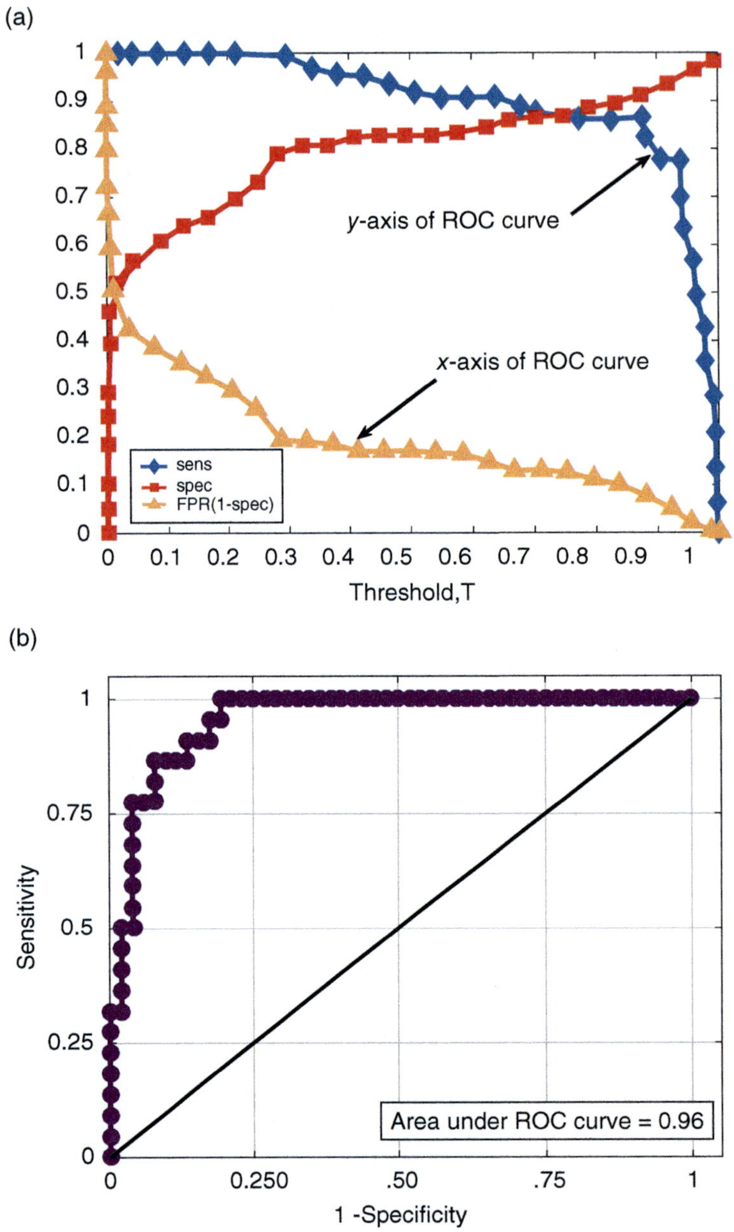

Figure 12.9 (a) Sensitivity, specificity, and false positive rate (FPR) as a function of threshold for 2-class comparison (healthy versus diseased state). (b) Receiver operating characteristic (ROC) curve built from (a).

randomly selected diseased case (or "event") will be regarded with greater suspicion (in terms of its rating or continuous measurement) than a randomly selected non-diseased case (or "non-event"). So, for example, in a study involving rating data, an AUC of 0.84 implies that there is an 84% likelihood that a randomly selected diseased case will receive a more suspicious (higher) rating than a randomly selected non-diseased case. Note that an AUC of 0.50 means that the diagnostic accuracy in question is equivalent to that which would be obtained by flipping a coin (i.e. random chance). It is possible but not common to run into AUCs less than 0.50. It is often informative to report a 95% confidence interval for a single AUC in order to determine whether the lower endpoint is > 0.50 (i.e. whether the diagnostic accuracy in question is, with some certainty, any better than random chance).

$$\text{AUC} = \text{integral}\left[\text{TPR} \times d(\text{FPR})\right] = \text{integral}\left[\text{TPR} \times d(\text{TNR})\right] \text{ for all threshold values.}$$

12.5.2 Personalized Medicine

12.5.2.1 Breast Cancer Treatment #1

Herceptin is a good example of a pharmacogenomics success story. In the 1980s, researchers discovered that some women who had particularly fast-growing breast cancers expressed extra copies of a gene called *Her-2/neu*. The genes were producing many copies of a protein that appeared to be driving the growth of the cancer cells. In the early 1990s, an antibody was developed that latches onto the Her-2/neu proteins on the surface of a cancer cell. Herceptin binds to Her-2/neu receptors and stops them from binding to growth factors and spurring on cancer-cell growth, and through this "stop signal" can also stop propagation of survival signals within the cancer cell (Figure 12.10). Some women who were given the experimental antibody saw their cancer growth slow or stop altogether when their Herceptin treatment was combined with cytotoxic chemotherapy. The Food and Drug Administration approved Herceptin in late 1998 as a therapy for a subcategory of women who test positive for high levels of the Her-2/neu protein (about 25–30% of all breast cancer patients).

To test for high levels of Her-2/neu protein, breast cancer patients are first screened with an immunohistochemistry assay for Her-2/neu overexpression before treating with Herceptin. Immunohistochemistry is the localization of antigens or proteins in tissue sections using labeled antibodies as specific reagents through antigen–antibody interactions that are visualized by a marker such as fluorescent dye, enzyme, or colloidal gold. Herceptin treatment for a subset of breast cancer patients represents the dawn of personalized medicine, in which treatment options are tailored for the specific patient's molecular state.

12.5.2.2 Finding New Drugs and Selecting Therapy

Another important use of microarrays occurs in pharmacogenomics, an area of research that studies why certain drugs work in combination with particular genetic expression patterns, but not with others. This information is being used to design new drugs that target cancer cells without

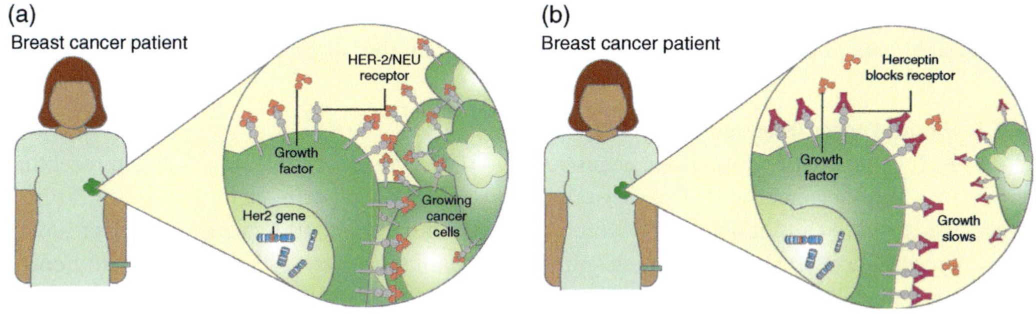

Figure 12.10 (a) Growth factor binds to Her-2/neu receptors. (b) Herceptin blocks Her-2/neu receptors. *Source:* From the Website of the National Cancer Institute (https://www.cancer.gov). Artwork by Jeanne Kelly.

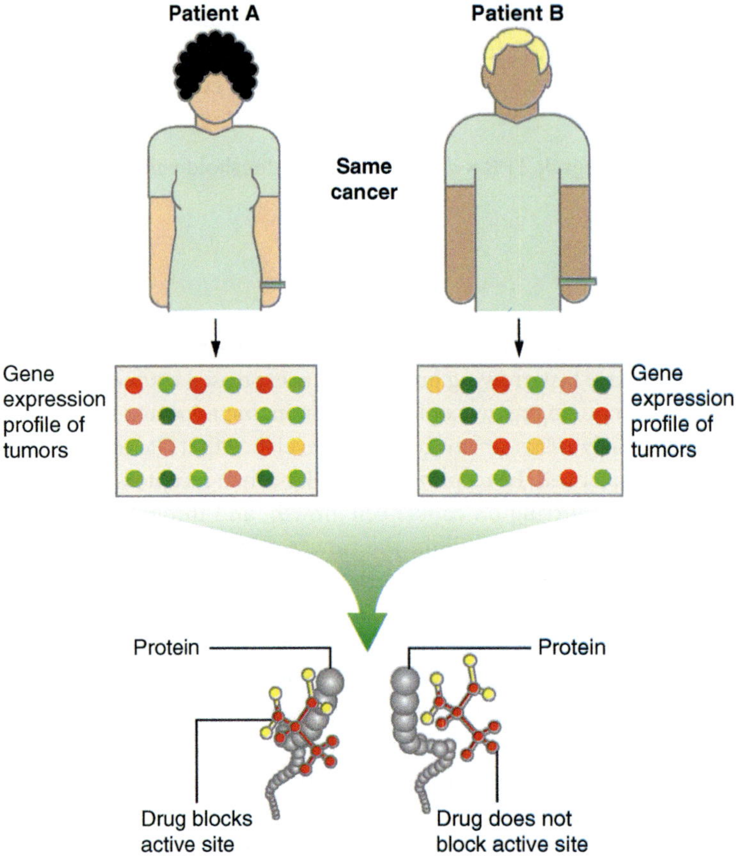

Figure 12.11 Determination of the effectiveness of cancer drugs based on protein blocking. *Source:* From the Website of the National Cancer Institute (https://www.cancer.gov). Artwork by Jeanne Kelly.

affecting normal ones. Given patients A and B with the same type of cancer, a microarray assay can be performed to determine the gene or protein expression profiles of tumors, as shown in Figure 12.11. Then protein samples can be taken from the patient to test if a proposed drug is able to block the protein's active sites and render them ineffective. If so, then the proposed drug is effective for that particular patient. Once such a drug is adopted, the microarray assay can be used to select the right patient population who will benefit from such therapy.

12.5.2.3 Breast Cancer Treatment #2

About 15% of women with lymph node negative (LN−) (i.e, cancer is still local), estrogen receptor positive (ER+) breast cancer will have a distant recurrence, i.e. a recurrence in the distant future. However, because we cannot determine which women will have distant recurrence, 50% of LN−, ER+ women will receive chemotherapy, despite its attendant morbidity (ill health), mortality, cost, and the knowledge that the majority of treated women will receive no benefit from the treatment. Therefore, a goal to improve prognosis is to develop a test that can identify those women who will not benefit from and don't need chemotherapy.

12.5.2.4 Genomic Health Breast Cancer Assay (This Section is Optional and for Advanced Readers Only)

By conducting a genomic health breast cancer assay, 16 cancer and 5 reference genes are selected that are related to different aspects of breast cancer, such as proliferation (metastasis), invasion, Her-2, estrogen (hormone expression), and reference genes to make the test more accurate (Figure 12.12). These 21 genes are selected for the best RT-PCR performance and robust predictions. By combining the readings of all 21 gene expressions into a recurrence score (RS) algorithm, we can calculate a recurrence score index that predicts the risk of recurrence. An RS below 18 indicates low risk, an RS above 31 indicates high risk (usually the 15% previously mentioned fall here), and RS scores between those extremes indicate an intermediate risk. One drawback is the high cost of this test, currently about $2000–$3000 per test.

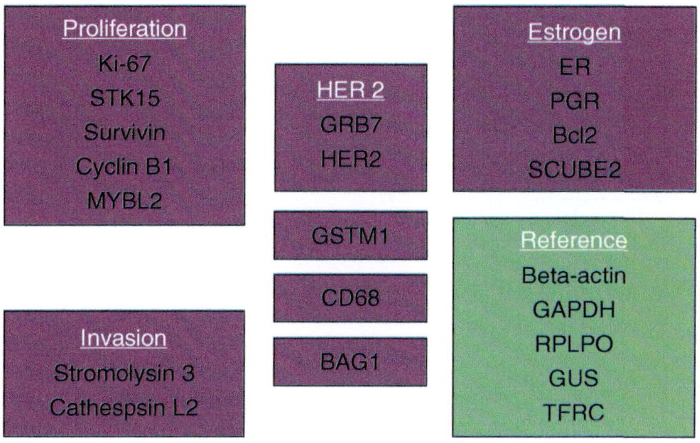

Figure 12.12 16 cancer and 5 reference genes used for Genomic Health Breast Cancer Assay.

Problems

12.1 Analytical specificity is defined as:

A The minimum number of copies reliably detected by the assay
B The intended purpose of the assay
C Agreement between sample replicates, both within an assay run and between independent assay runs, when tested by the same laboratory
D The degree to which the assay does not detect (amplify) other pathogens

12.2 The following is paraphrased from a news release in GenomeWeb, 26 February 2016: Researchers at University of Pennsylvania and Veracyte Inc. are developing a genomic diagnostic test, called Percepta, to stratify lung cancer and benign cases (no cancer) after an indeterminate result from a bronchoscopy (an endoscopic procedure to inspect lung area optically). The researchers used the Percepta test to evaluate samples from the 77 patients who underwent additional invasive procedures including surgical lung biopsy and transthoracic needle biopsy. Of these 77 patients, 42 were ultimately diagnosed as benign cases (no cancer). If the Percepta were used to guide decision making, invasive biopsy procedures could have been avoided in 50% of benign cases. Further, among 35 patients that were diagnosed with lung cancer by biopsy, four patients were missed by the Percepta test.

A What are the numbers of TP, FP, TN, and FN of the Percepta test in this study of lung cancer?

B What are the diagnostic sensitivity, diagnostic specificity, PPV, and NPV of the Percepta test for lung cancer in this study?

C Is it reasonable for this test to be used for rule out of lung cancer? Why or why not?

12.3 Prevalence of a given disease, normalized by the relevant population, can be expressed as the number of existing cases of the disease divided by the total population at a given point in time:

$$p = \frac{\text{TP} + \text{FN}}{\text{TP} + \text{FN} + \text{TN} + \text{FP}},$$

where $\text{TP} + \text{FN} + \text{TN} + \text{FP} = C$ is the total population. Prove the following:

A Diagnostic sensitivity and specificity can be expressed as:

$$\text{Sensitivity} = \frac{\text{TP}}{p \times C}, \quad \text{Specificity} = \frac{\text{TN}}{(1-p) \times C}.$$

B Positive predictive value and negative predictive value can be expressed as:

$$\text{PPV} = \frac{p \times \text{Sensitivity}}{p \times \text{Sensitivity} + (1-p) \times (1 - \text{Specificity})},$$

$$\text{NPV} = \frac{(1-p) \times \text{Specificity}}{p \times (1 - \text{Sensitivity}) + (1-p) \times \text{Specificity}}.$$

C The accuracy of a diagnostic test is defined as the percentage of correctly classified cases out of all cases tested. Express the accuracy in terms of sensitivity, specificity, and prevalence (p).

D For a given diagnostic test with nearly perfect sensitivity and specificity (~95% or higher), and a disease with very low prevalence ($p \ll 1\%$), show that the PPV is proportional to the prevalence.

12.4 You are given a new molecular diagnostic test for ovarian cancer to screen patients from a general population with no prior history of cancer. The sensitivity and specificity of the test are known to be 100 and 95%, respectively, and the prevalence of ovarian cancer in the general population is ~0.1% (all cases of ovarian cancer at one time).

A If a female patient tests positive, what is her probability of actually having ovarian cancer? Would you say this test is predictive or not?

B The accuracy of a diagnostic test is defined as the percentage of correctly classified cases out of all cases tested. What is the accuracy of the new molecular diagnostic test?

C A diagnostic test with a sensitivity and specificity of 100 and 95%, respectively, is generally regarded as very accurate. How can such an accurate test be not so predictive?

D How useful is such an "accurate" test in real practice?

12.5 Consider a molecular Dx test for metastatic breast cancer that counts CTCs. If the number of CTCs per 7.5 ml is 5 for a particular patient, and the blood volume sampled randomly is 7.5 ml, then the mean of the CTC counts in a given sample is expected to be 5, and the standard deviation of the CTC counts is the square root of 5.

A What is the chance that you will misclassify the patient as having a good prognosis (CTC counts = 4 or less)?

B Would your answer change if the volume of blood available for CTC counts is increased to 75 ml? The good prognosis criterion remains the same (CTC counts per 7.5 ml $<$ 5, i.e. for 75 ml of blood, the CTC count is 44 or less).

Hint: You can assume the CTC count in both situations obeys a normal distribution. The mean in the second case is 50, while the standard deviation is the square root of 50.

12.6 Troponin I is the most commonly used protein biomarker for detecting heart attack, and its 99 percentile concentration of the healthy population is chosen as the cutoff, meaning that anyone above that concentration will be tested as "positive." Assume that the prevalence of heart attack is about 0.1% in a population of 1 million people, and all of them at the time of testing have a troponin I concentration above 15 $pg\,ml^{-1}$. The newly FDA-approved Roche's "next-generation" troponin I test is adopted here, whose 99th percentile concentration of the healthy population is 14 $ng\,l^{-1}$. (Its LOD is 5 ng/l.)

A What are the numbers of TP, FP, TN, and FN of the troponin test for heart attack?

B What are the diagnostic sensitivity, diagnostic specificity, PPV, and NPV of the test?

C Is it reasonable for this test to be used for rule in and rule out of heart attack? Why or why not?

12.7 A new serum test for advanced cancer is developed whose purpose is to differentiate the advanced cancer, having an effective targeted drug therapy, from early-stage cancer, for which the drug is not effective but not harmful. A study is done comparing the performance of the serum test in cancer patients and healthy individuals (i.e. no cancer). It is found that the serum test is positive in all patients with the advanced cancer, is positive in 25% of the subjects with early stage cancer, and in 10% of healthy individuals. It is known that one in five cancer patients are advanced stage. The prevalence of this cancer in the general population is 0.13%.

A What is the confusion matrix of this serum test?

B What are the specificity, sensitivity, NPV, and PPV of the serum test, which is designed to differentiate advanced cancer from early-stage cancer?

C Now a doctor wants to repurpose the serum test to screen the general population to detect both early and advanced stages of this cancer. What is the relevant confusion matrix in this case?

D What are the specificity, sensitivity, NPV, and PPV of the serum test which is designed to detect cancer in the general population?

E Do you think the original and repurposed serum tests are clinically useful? Why or why not?

12.8 If we were to rely on pure chance to distinguish those subjects with a disease versus those without a disease, prove that the ROC curve would fall along a straight diagonal line, which is referred to as the Chance Diagonal in diagnostics.

12.9 Your research team found that CA-1891 is upregulated in the bloodstream of stomach cancer patients. To confirm whether this biomarker is good enough for screening of stomach cancer, you obtained 10 serum samples from your collaborators for testing your recently developed biochips. Five of them are the samples from the patients in their early stages and the rest of them are from healthy donors. The measurement results of the concentrations of CA-1891 in the samples are shown in Table 12.3.

Table 12.3 Concentrations (pg ml^{-1}) of CA-1891 in five healthy donors and five patients with early-stage stomach cancer.

Unit: (pg/ml)	Healthy donors	Patients
1	37.1	55.1
2	55.2	54.3
3	48.6	50.0
4	34.8	49.6
5	16.2	37.6

A Using this small set of data, sketch the Receiver Operating Characteristic (ROC) curve.

B What cutoff value would you choose to screen stomach cancers for this device? Explain your rationale.

12.10 Considering the results of a particular biochip-based blood test in two populations: one population with a disease and one population without the disease. The distributions of the test results are shown in Figure 12.13 with two curves, where TP, FP, TN, and FN denote true positives, false positives, true negatives, and false negatives for a given criterion value of the test, which is the cutoff (threshold) value of the tests between people who test positive and those who test negative.

A Given the distributions in Figure 12.13 for the diseased and healthy populations, sketch how sensitivity and specificity will vary with the criterion value chosen for the test.

B Sketch the ROC curve for the test described above. If you could change the blood test and thus the distributions given earlier, what would you need to do (qualitatively speaking) to get an AUC = 0.999?

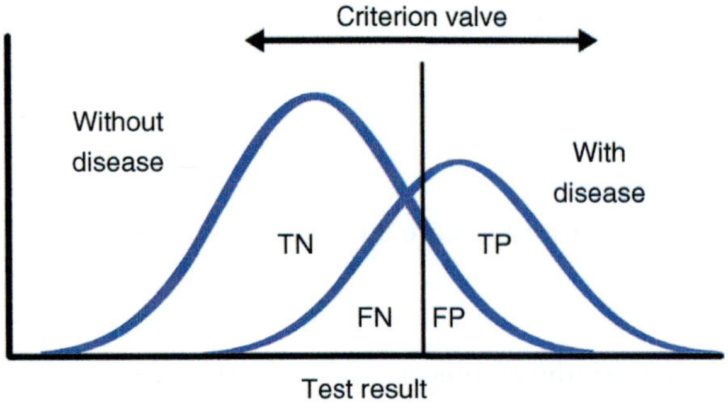

Figure 12.13 Distribution curves of a biochip-based blood test in two populations: with disease and without disease.

12.11 Solve the following problems related to molecular Dx with biochips.

A For a population of 800, the prevalence of a disease is 50%. If a biochip-based diagnostic test has a sensitivity of 76%, and a specificity of 88%, what are TP, FN, FP, and TN?

B Figure 12.14 shows three different ROC curves. If one wants to maximize the sum of sensitivity and specificity in choosing a particular point on an ROC curve, prove that the vertical distance from that point to the diagonal line should also be the maximum. Denote that point for each curve (A, B, C).

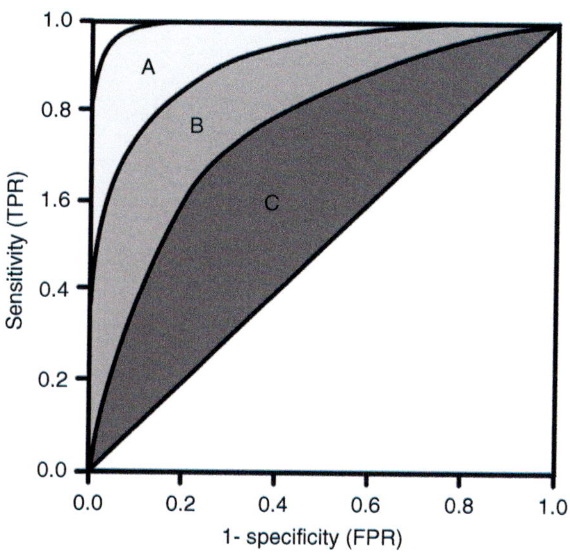

Figure 12.14 Three different theoretical ROC curves.

Reference

1 Hoffman, R.M., Gilliland, F.D., Adams-Cameron, M. et al. (2002). Prostate-specific antigen testing accuracy in community practice. *BMC Family Practice* 3 (19) https://doi.org/10.1186/1471-2296-3-19.

Further Reading

Cristofanilli, M., Budd, G.T., Ellis, M.J. et al. (2004). Circulating tumor cells, disease progression, and survival in metastatic breast cancer. *N. Engl. J. Med* 351 (8): 781–791.

The HER2 testing conundrum (2010). *Nature Biotech* 28 (2): 117.

13

Magnetic Resonance Imaging

13.1 Medical Imaging – Categorization

The clinical purpose of imaging is to perform diagnosis or monitor therapy for a patient. Medical imaging modalities can be categorized in similar ways as biochips. For example, where biochips are categorized based on what analyte is measured, imaging modalities can be categorized based on what molecule or structure is visualized. Further categorizations can be considered, including "what produces the imaging signal?" In imaging, the signal can come from either intrinsic molecules (i.e. a molecule that already exists in the body) or extrinsic agents (i.e. externally introduced contrast agents). A summary of biochip versus imaging categorizations is provided in Table 13.1.

13.1.1 Imaging is Synergistic to Biochips

Medical imaging is synergistic to biochips when used as a medical tool for the diagnosis and monitoring of diseases. The first line of defense is to use biochips for screening a disease by analyzing blood samples or other body liquids. Then, patients identified by the biochip test can proceed to the second line of defense, which is imaging to validate the biochips' findings and provide spatial localization and molecular information on the disease (e.g. localizing "hot spots" where a tumor has potentially metastasized).

13.2 Overview For Imaging Section

The imaging portion of the course will cover several imaging modalities including magnetic resonance imaging (MRI), positron emission tomography (PET), single photon emission computed tomography (SPECT), fluorescence imaging, Raman imaging, optical coherence tomography (OCT) and photoacoustic imaging. For each imaging modality, the physics behind the imaging modality, the physics of contrast agents, some examples of contrast agents, and some real-world applications will be covered. Imaging modalities cover the full range of the electromagnetic spectrum, ranging from low-energy radio waves for MRI to high-energy gamma rays for nuclear imaging (Figure 13.1).

Biochips and Medical Imaging, First Edition. Adam de la Zerda and Shan Xiang Wang.

Table 13.1 Biochip and imaging categorizations.

Biochip	Imaging
What is measured?	**What is visualized?**
DNA, RNA, proteins, cells	Bones, oxygen, receptors, genes
How is it captured?	**What produces the signal?**
Antibodies, single-stranded DNA	Endogenous or exogenous molecules
Signal amplification?	Signal amplification?
Many signaling molecules per analyte	**Many signaling events per target**
How is the signal measured?	**How is it imaged?**
Optics, electricity, etc. . .	MRI, Ultrasound, Optics
What is the clinical purpose?	**What is the clinical purpose?**
Screening cancer, etc. . .	Diagnosis, monitoring, therapy

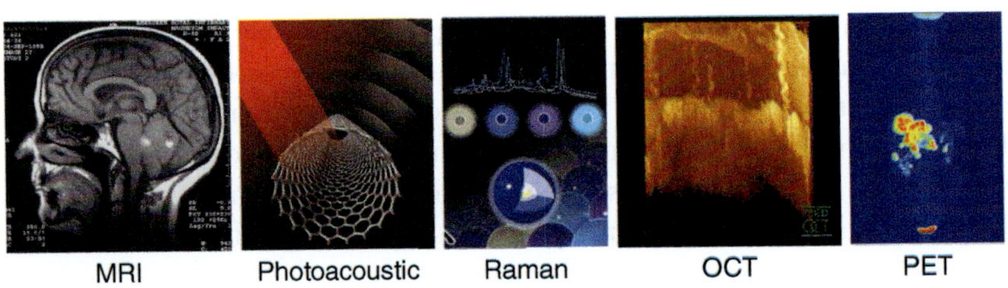

Figure 13.1 Various imaging modalities that rely on different regions of the electromagnetic spectrum. *Source:* Fastfission~commonswiki [2]. CC0-1.0 public domain https://creativecommons.org/publicdomain/zero/1.0/; Photoacoustic image courtesy of Jim Strommer. Raman image courtesy of Jim Strommer, Dr. Cristina Zavaleta, and Dr. Sanjiv Gambhir; Source of OCT image: BoP commonswiki [4], used under CC-BY-SA 2.0 AT https://creativecommons.org/licenses/by-sa/2.0/at/deed.en; Source of ultrasound image: Moroder [5], Used under CC-BY-SA 3.0 https://creativecommons.org/licenses/by-sa/3.0/; Source of PET image: Damato [6]. CC0-1.0 public domain https://creativecommons.org/publicdomain/zero/1.0/.

13.2.1 Imaging Terminology

Table 13.2 defines some important terms related to imaging. Imaging is the act of visualizing in the context of physical space. SNR is the signal-to-noise ratio. SBR is the signal-to-background ratio. Resolution describes the image's spatial resolution (in the physical domain) or temporal resolution (in the time domain). Time of acquisition is the time duration for capturing an image. Tomography is an imaging modality that shows depth, as opposed to imaging the surface of an object. in vivo (i.e. in living) indicates imaging done on a live animal, while ex vivo imaging is done outside the animal, and in vitro imaging is done in cells or bioliquids. A pixel (i.e. picture element) is one element in a 2-D image, while a voxel is one element in a 3-D image.

13.2.2 Contrast Agent Terminology

Table 13.3 defines some important terms related to contrast agents. A contrast agent is a molecule that gives off an imaging signal. An imaging agent is a type of contrast agent that is molecularly targeted to a biomarker (e.g. tumor receptor with a target antibody). A biomarker is a molecular target (e.g. a cancer-specific receptor). A molecular imaging agent is another term for an imaging agent. An agent is a shortcut for either contrast or imaging agent. A probe is either a contrast agent or an imaging agent. The signaling part refers to the part in the imaging agent that produces the imaging signal and the targeting part is the part in the imaging agent that targets the biomarker.

Table 13.2 Imaging terminology.

Term	Definition
Imaging	The act of visualizing in the context of physical space
SNR	Signal-to-noise ratio
SBR	Signal-to-background ratio
Spatial resolution	Resolution in the physical domain
Temporal resolution	Resolution in the time domain
Time of acquisition	Time duration for capturing an image
Tomography	Imaging modality that shows depth (as opposed to imaging the surface of an object)
in vivo/in living subject	In a live animal
ex vivo	Outside the animal
in vitro	In cells or bioliquids
Pixel	One element in a 2D image
Voxel	One element in a 3D image

Table 13.3 Contrast agent terminology.

Term	Definition
Contrast agent	A molecule that gives off an imaging signal
Imaging agent	A contrast agent that is molecularly targeted to a biomarker
Biomarker	A molecular target (e.g. cancer-specific receptor) *(this definition is very specific to imaging, not biochips!)*
Molecular imaging agent	Same as imaging agent
Agent	Shortcut for either contrast or imaging agent
Probe	Shortcut for either contrast or imaging agent
Signaling part	The part in the imaging agent that produces the imaging signal
Targeting part	The part in the imaging agent that targets the biomarker
Endogenous/intrinsic contrast	That already existed in the body
Exogenous contrast	That does not exist naturally in the body

13.3 MRI: Past, Present, and Future

Medical imaging has seen significant improvement in recent years: an early MRI image of the area just below the diaphragm from 1978 and a modern high-resolution MRI image of the brain from 2005 are shown in Figure 13.2a and b. In the future, MRI molecular imaging approaches will be able to generate images of not only a patient's anatomy and physiology, but also specific molecules associated with the occurrence and progression of disease, e.g. the distribution of angiogenic receptors (promoting tumor angiogenesis – the growth of new blood vessels) in cancer cells. For example, the red color on Figure 13.2 represents imaging agents (external particles that produce a signal and are molecularly targeted to certain molecules) that

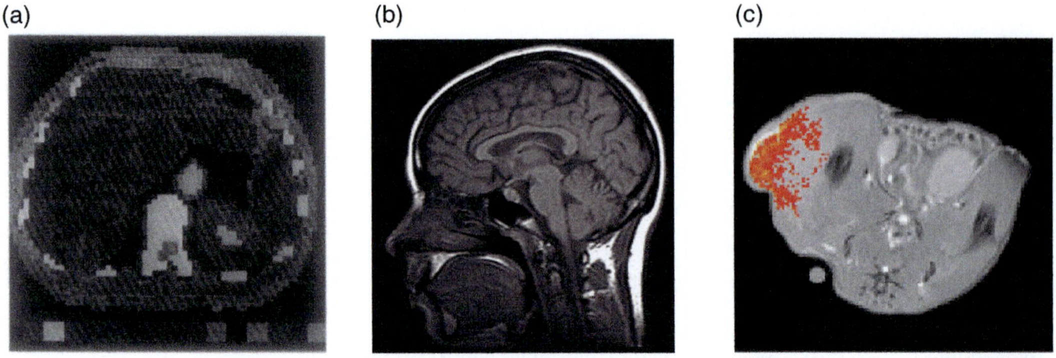

Figure 13.2 (a) MRI image from just below the diaphragm, 1978 (*Source:* Reprinted from Mansfield and Pykett [1], Copyright © 1978 Published by Elsevier, Inc. with permission from Elsevier), (b) MRI Image of the Brain, 2005 (*Source:* Fastfission commonswiki [2]. CC0-1.0 public domain https://creativecommons.org/publicdomain/zero/1.0/), and (c) MR Molecular Image of angiogenic receptors in a tumor (*Source:* Reprinted from Geralda et al. [3], Copyright © 2008, with permission from Elsevier).

were injected into an animal. Once injected, they bound to their target molecule and increased the MRI signal in regions where that molecule was present. MR molecular images are much more powerful in this way relative to traditional MR images because they provide information about the molecular composition of the tumor.

13.4 Physics of MRI Overview

MRI is a noninvasive imaging technique, which is done by nonionizing magnetic fields. MRI has many intrinsic contrasts (e.g. water and fat) and can produce images at any 2D plane or in 3D. MRI can generate many different types of images, including water content, fat content, flow, etc. There have been eight Nobel Prizes given for MRI to date (1943–2003).

As shown in Figure 13.3, an MR image is obtained by first putting the patient into a powerful magnet generating a static magnetic field of several Tesla. Next, a sequence of radio frequency (RF) pulses is produced by RF coils. Finally, the RF signal is switched off and the RF coils are used as antennas to measure any RF "echo" signals that are emitted from the patient. Using simple Fourier transform techniques, the "echo" signals are then used to reconstruct a 3D image of the patient.

13.5 Physics of MRI

A proton spins around its axis like a planet and its positive charge (i.e. a moving electric field) induces a **magnetic dipole** (Figure 13.4). When protons, such as the ones in hydrogen, are placed in a strong external magnetic field, they will align themselves, either parallel or antiparallel, with the magnetic field (with different energy levels). There is a slight net magnetization of hydrogen protons toward the magnetic field (about 7 out of 10 million protons). This is because parallel protons have lower energy, making the parallel state slightly more energetically favorable (Figure 13.5). However, this very low magnetization is balanced by the fact that there are many ^1H atoms in the body (e.g. H_2O – water), so a detectable MRI signal can be measured from the body.

The number of protons that align parallel with the field is slightly more than the number that align antiparallel. If the proton's magnetic field is tipped, the protons will also move like a spinning

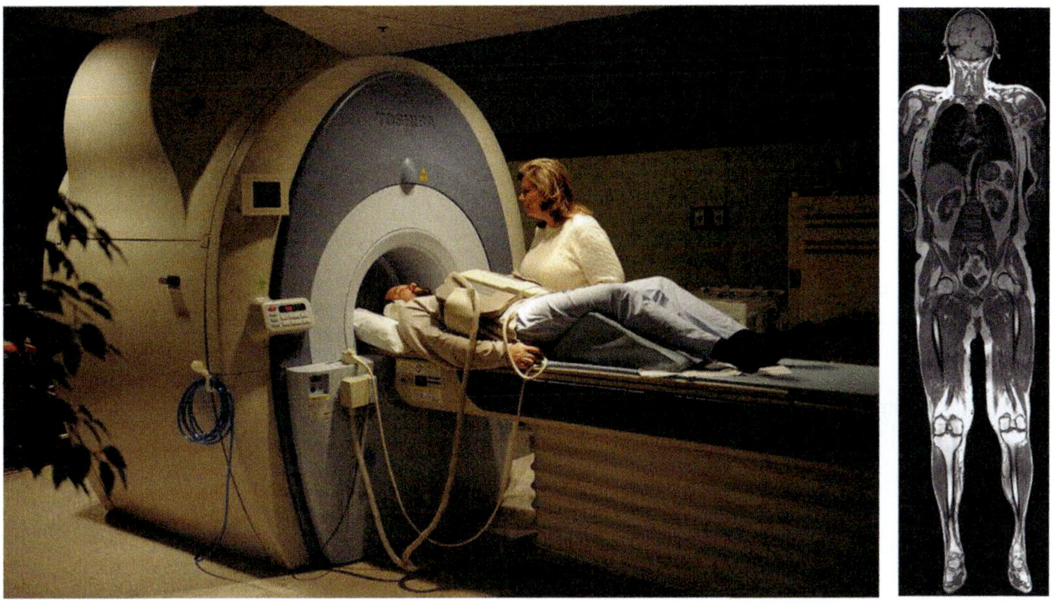

Figure 13.3 An MRI machine and a full-body MRI image. Source of left image: United States Air Force [7]. CC0-1.0 public domain https://creativecommons.org/publicdomain/zero/1.0/; Source of right image: Reprinted from Schmidt et al. [8], Copyright 2009, with permission from Elsevier.

top in a two-axis motion, called precession (Figure 13.6), about the direction of the magnetic field B_0 (z-axis). The precession angular frequency (ω) depends on the magnetic field strength (B_0) and the gyromagnetic ratio (γ) according to the Larmor equation: $\omega = \gamma B_0$.

In steady state, as there are more protons aligned parallel to the external magnetic field, there is a net magnetic moment (M_z) aligned along the $+z$ axis. To "tip" the protons' magnetic moment: a transverse RF field is applied at the Larmor frequency, tipping the magnetization vector away from the z-axis. With the proper strength and duration, M can be tipped as much as 180°.

Important Note: Tipping by RF pulse conserves the magnitude of the magnetic moment. For example, assume that initial magnetic moment is M_0 and it is pointing in $+z$ direction. After a 90-degree tip, the magnetic moment will be still M_0 but it will lie on the transverse plane (xy plane). If we apply a 180-degree pulse, the magnetic moment will be M_0 again, but this time, the vector will point to the $-z$ direction.

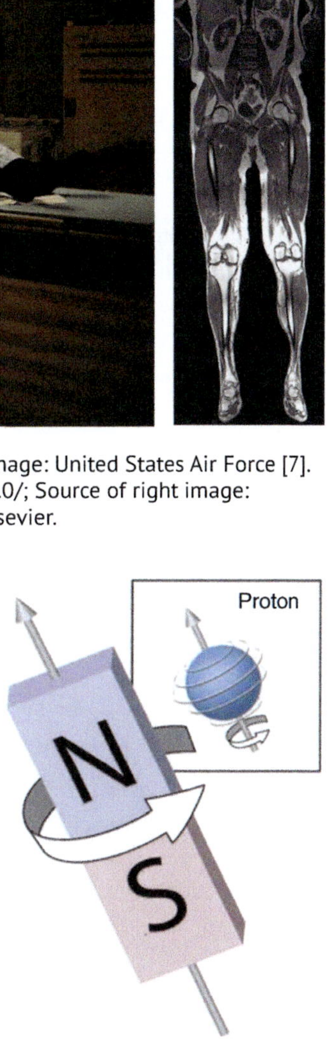

Figure 13.4 Spinning protons induce magnetic dipoles.

13.5.1 T_1 and T_2 Time Constants

Precessing protons will gradually return to equilibrium in the z-axis direction at an exponential rate: the magnetization vector on the z-axis (longitudinal magnetization) at a time constant T_1 (due to vibrational or translation energy to the lattice), and the magnetization vector on the xy-axes (transverse magnetization) at a time constant T_2 (due to energy transfer to neighboring nuclei), see

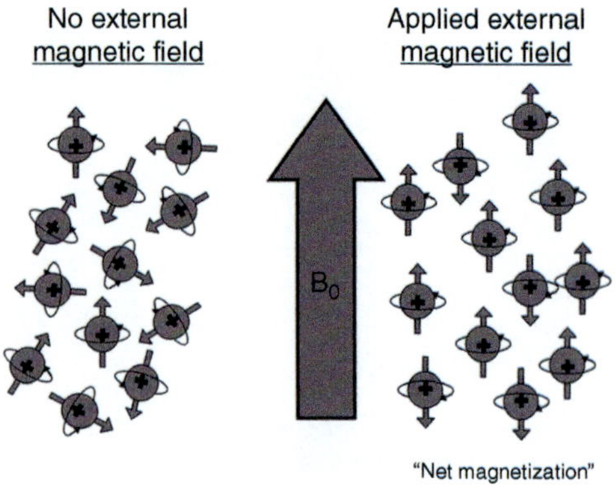

Figure 13.5 Protons align with magnetic fields. *Source:* Pooley [9], Copyright © 2005, RSNA.

Figure 13.7. The time constants are defined as the time required for the difference between the magnetization and its equilibrium value to decrease by a factor of e. The values of the T_1 and T_2 parameters depend on the type of matter (water, fat, brain matter, etc.) being imaged, which allows differentiation between tissues. For example, liquids have long T_1 and T_2 times compared to fats, which have short T_1 and T_2 times.

Important Note: The relaxation does not necessarily conserve the magnitude of the magnetic moment. The longitudinal (M_z) T_1 relaxation is **independent** of transverse (M_{xy}) T_2 relaxation. The detailed explanation below may help you understand this concept.

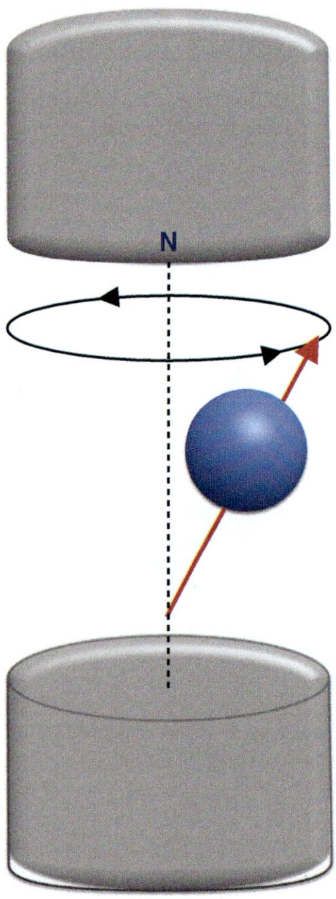

Figure 13.6 Proton precession.

13.5.2 Detailed Overview of MRI Physics

When we are talking about magnetic moments in MRI, we are usually talking about bulk magnetic moment. For example, in a voxel, the signal might arise from millions of protons each with a small magnetic dipole. The magnetic moment we measure in MRI is the vector sum of all these little magnetic moments. When we apply a tip to these moments, we actually apply a rotating external magnetic field. This field creates a torque on the magnetic moments in accordance to $\tau = m \times B$, where τ is the torque, m is magnetic moment, and B is the external magnetic field. This torque is the reason why magnetic dipoles precess and it is the same reason why magnetic moments tip with the RF pulse. Figure 13.6 shows how the main magnetic field (the strong B_0 field, typically around 3 T) causes precession.

The cross product of M and B is perpendicular to the planes created by the M and B vectors. You can find the direction of applied torque using the right-hand rule. Curl your fingers from M to B and your thumb points in the direction of the applied torque on M. As you can see here, the external magnetic field B causes the precession of magnetic dipole M.

We already know that these magnetic dipoles precess in the external magnetic field. Ideally, they all precess with the Larmor frequency, but they are not in phase. In a voxel with 1 million protons, you can assume that the phases of their dipoles are randomly distributed (i.e. they are rotating at the same speed but they don't start their rotations at the same time). In the end, the dipoles form a cone because of their random phase distribution. You will get net magnetization in the $+z$ direction because the transverse components of the dipoles cancel each other. Since the starting positions of their precessions are randomly distributed, dipoles are evenly spaced around a cone as they precess. This

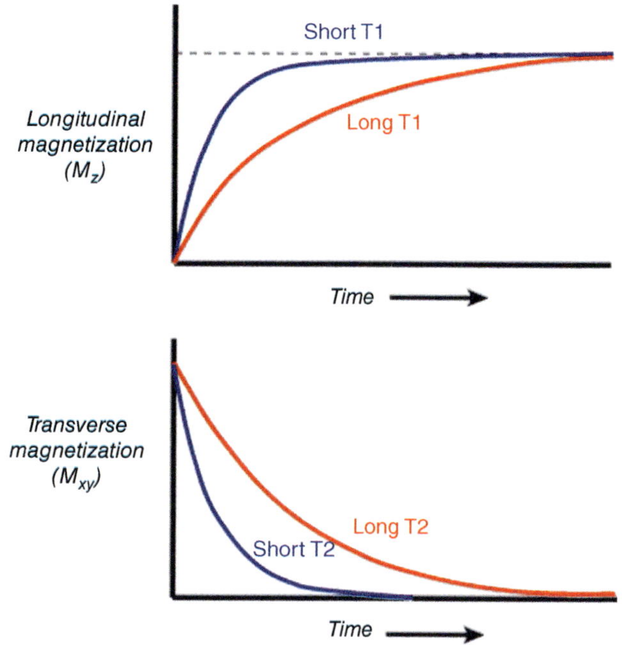

Figure 13.7 Longitudinal and transverse magnetizations versus time. *Source:* Image courtesy of Allen D. Elster, MRIQuestions.com.

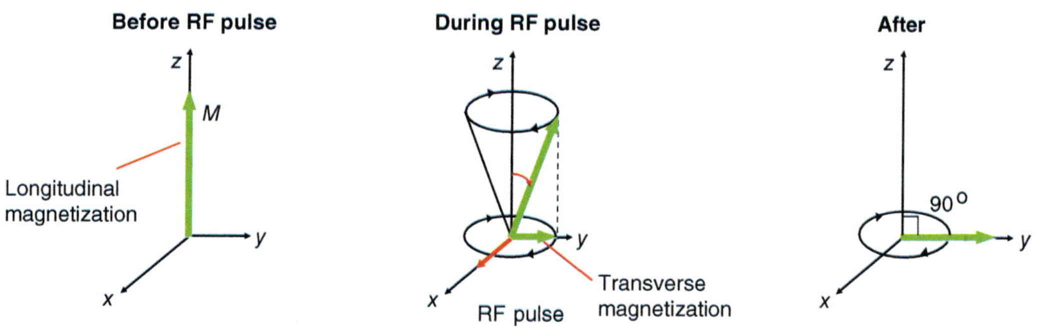

Figure 13.8 Tipping magnetic dipoles with RF pulse. The applied magnetic field (RF) is in the +*x* direction and the dipole tips 90° to the +*y* direction.

causes the transverse components to cancel each other and create a net magnetic moment (M_0) in the $+z$ direction.

Now let's see what happens when we apply the RF pulse. As we mentioned earlier, the RF pulse is basically a rotating magnetic field. For now, assume there is no precession. When we apply a second magnetic field in the $+x$ direction (the first one is the main magnetic field along $+z$), we would cause a torque on the magnetic dipoles. This is illustrated in Figure 13.8. We showed before that when the magnetic field is along the $+z$ axis, the dipole precesses about the $+z$ axis due to the torque created by the cross product. The exact same thing happens here. When we apply an external magnetic field in the $+x$ direction, the dipole wants to precess around $+x$ axis. We apply this magnetic field only for a short time so that we get partial rotation around $+x$ axis. In the example in Figure 13.8, the external magnetic field (RF pulse) is applied such that the dipoles only rotate ¼ cycle. This is equivalent to a 90-degree tip.

Now let's explain why we call this magnetic field an RF pulse. First of all, we call it a pulse because it is applied for a very short duration, just enough to tip the magnetic dipole 90 or 180°. Why do we call it an RF signal? Remember that the dipole is precessing about the $+z$ axis during the RF pulse. When you look at Figure 13.8, you will see that if we keep the RF magnetic field in the $+x$ direction and precess the magnetic dipole (green vector), it will first start tipping toward the $+y$ axis while precessing about the $+z$ axis. Eventually, the magnetic dipole will rotate 180° about $+z$ and the same RF pulse (that is still pointing in the $+x$) will tip it back to the $+z$ axis. Let's repeat it again. Assume that RF pulse (red vector) is constant and fixed. Also, assume that now we have precession (green vector). When the tipping starts, the green vector tips slightly toward the $+y$ axis and the vectors will look like the middle image in Figure 13.8. Now while doing this tip, the green vector is still precessing, and, as a result, it actually spirals down. Now imagine a scenario where the green vector rotates about the $+z$ axis and circles to the other side of the cone (similar to the middle image in Figure 13.8 but this time, the green vector is on the left side of the cone). Now the cross product of red vector and green vector still causes a torque toward the $+y$ axis, but this time, the torque pushes the green vector toward the $+z$ axis. As a result of this, after one cycle of precession, there would be no net tipping on the dipole. In order to cause actual tipping, we need to apply the RF magnetic field (the red vector) at the same frequency as the Larmor frequency. When we do that, both the red vector and green vector stay in the same frame of reference (i.e. since both of them rotate around $+z$ with Larmor frequency, they behave like there is no precession at all). Hence, when we apply the external magnetic field at the Larmor frequency, the whole cone of dipoles tip toward the $+y$ axis. Now the question is: how do you create a rotating magnetic field (the red vector in Figure 13.8)? One way of achieving is using coils. If you remember Faraday's Law, inducing current in a coil causes a magnetic field through the coil (right-hand rule). We can place two coils, one facing the x-axis and another facing the y-axis. The net magnetic field from these coils will be the vector sum of each coil's magnetic field. If we apply sine waves to these coils (one should be 90° out of phase), we can create a rotating magnetic field. Since we want the magnetic field to rotate at the Larmor frequency, we need to set the frequency of these sine waves to the Larmor frequency. This frequency for Hydrogen under 1 T is 42.5781 MHz and it turns out to be in the RF range. This is the reason why we call it an RF pulse. If you happen to use higher magnetic fields like 7 T, this frequency increases into microwave range.

Now that we have tipped the magnetic dipoles onto the $+y$ axis, we can look into the decay process. There is one more important concept that one has to understand the relaxation, called dephasing (Figure 13.9). The dipoles that are tipped interact with each other (spin–spin interaction) and change their precession speed. This is called dephasing and it is the main reason for T_2

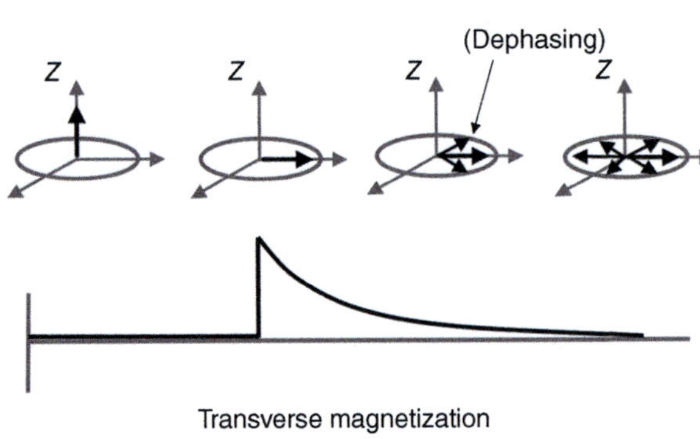

Figure 13.9 Dephasing and T2 relaxation. *Source:* Pooley [9], Copyright © 2005, RSNA.

decay. Initially, all of the dipoles were pointing in the $+y$ direction (more or less) and they were in phase. When some of them slow down, they lag behind the group and get out of phase slowly. Similarly, when some of the dipoles speed up, they lead the group and get out of phase too. This creates a uniform phase distribution over time and causes the signal to decay because the dipoles on the opposite angles cancel each other's transverse component. This is illustrated in Figure 13.9. This is the reason why the magnitude of the bulk magnetic moment is not conserved during relaxation. Individual dipoles observe the rules of physics but their cumulative behavior is different. Let's assume that T_2 time is extremely short compared to T_1. After a 90-degree tip, we have a vector of M_0 pointing at the $+y$ direction. Because of the short T_2, dipoles dephase really fast and we completely lose net transverse magnetization. After dephasing, the net magnetic moment will be zero and then it will start to rise in the $+z$ direction with T_1 decay. Again, if you think about the individual dipoles, this would be equivalent to creating a disk of dipoles (pointing in every direction on the xy-plane) and then as these dipoles slowly rise to the $+z$ axis the disk would turn into a cone (still cancelling xy-components but this time with a net $+z$ component). Eventually, as the dipoles return to their original orientation, this cone gets narrower and narrower until it returns to its starting size.

This section should make it clear that T_1 and T_2 relaxations are independent processes and the explanation is not really simple. This is a simplified explanation of why those two relaxations are different. Multiple other factors like T_2^* decay are not mentioned for simplicity.

13.6 Image Acquisition in MRI

In order to generate an image, spatial localization is achieved by adding a gradient field, which is a small magnetic field along the z-axis whose intensity changes linearly with x- and y-positions, e.g. $B = \left(B_0 + G_x x + G_y y\right)\hat{z}$. Therefore, the Larmor frequency is now dependent on the x- and y- positions: $\omega x, y = \gamma(B_0 + G_x x + G_y y)$, which enables the use of Fourier transform to retrieve the ^{1}H concentration in the x- and y-coordinates and generate an image. Localization in the z-axis is given by an additional transient gradient field $G_z(t)$ that selects for a specific z slice. This allows the MRI image to first focus on one plane and acquire an image of that plane, then move to the next plane to acquire an image, and so on.

When acquiring an image, an RF field is first applied, then after a wait time of TE, the echo signal coming out from the patient is measured, which generates one point in the Fourier domain. This process is then repeated many times for different acquisitions, waiting a time TR between each acquisition (Figure 13.10).

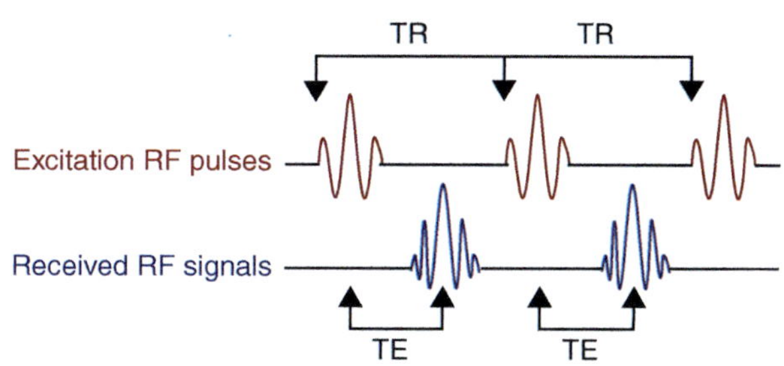

Figure 13.10 Excitation and received RF pulses.

13.6.1 T_1-Weighted Images

A T_1-weighted MRI image measures the change in magnetization in the z-axis, e.g. the time required to return to equilibrium in the z-axis, resulting in an image that highlights differences in T_1 of the tissues. The first applied RF pulse inverts M_0 by tipping it by 180°, which then relaxes with T_1 time coefficient. The second RF pulse, sent TE time after the first one, flips M_z by 90°, thereby turning the magnetization to points in the transverse plane (Figure 13.11). The magnetization in the z-axis can be described by the following equations:

$$\frac{dM_z}{dt} = \frac{M_0 - M_z}{T_1}, \qquad M_z\big|_{t=0} = -M_0$$

$$M_z\big|_{t=\mathrm{TE}} = M_0\left[1 - 2\exp\left(-\mathrm{TE}/T_1\right)\right]$$

The 90-degree pulse allows the pickup coil to measure transverse magnetization alone, even though the signal actually represents the magnetization in M_z.

Since the longitudinal magnetization changes over time, a value of TE is chosen such that the contrast between the longitudinal magnetization values for each different type of matter present in the sample is maximized. A shorter T_1 gives a more positive contrast (i.e. whiter color) on the MRI image. For example, a T_1-weighted MR image of the brain shows mostly white matter, which appears white on the image. However, gray matter would appear darker and cerebrospinal fluid (CSF) would appear even darker on the image (Figure 13.12).

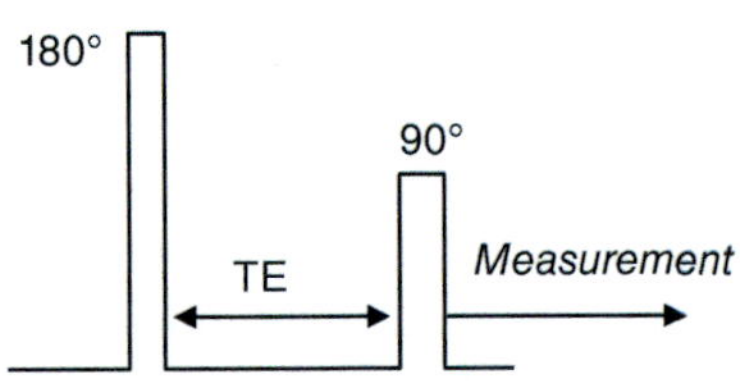

Figure 13.11 RF pulses and equations for a T1-weighted image.

13.6.2 T_2-Weighted Image

By applying a different sequence of RF pulses, T_2-weighted images can be produced (Figure 13.13), which measure the change in transverse magnetization over time. Typically, a

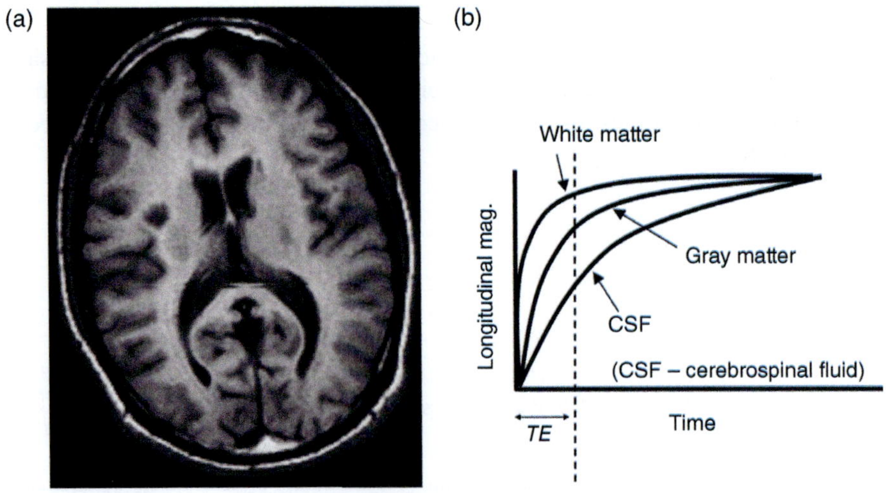

Figure 13.12 (a) T_1-weighted MRI image of the brain, (b) longitudinal magnetization versus time. *Source:* Pooley [9], Copyright © 2005, RSNA.

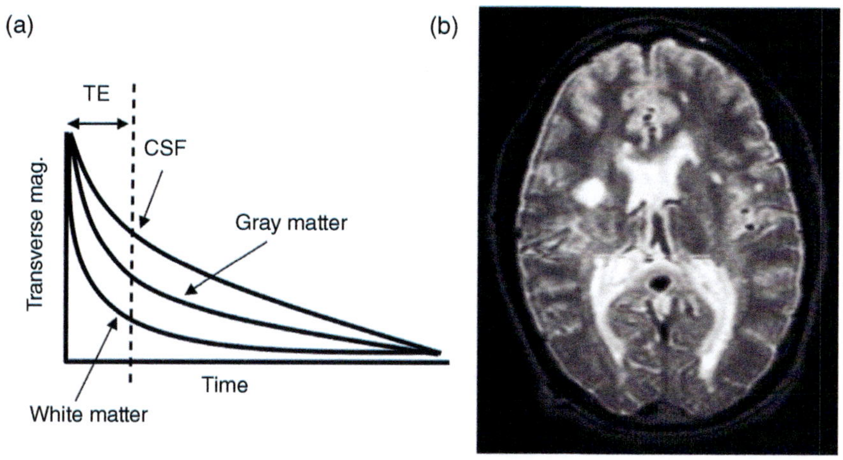

(c) $M = M_0[1 - \exp(-TR / T_1)] \exp(-TE / T_2)$

Figure 13.13 (a) Transverse magnetization versus time, (b) T2-weighted MRI image of the brain, and (c) equation for the T2-weighted image. *Source:* Pooley [9], Copyright © 2005, RSNA.

long value of TR is chosen (a few times T_1 so that differences in T_1 do not contribute to the image) and the TE value is chosen according to the desired contrast (typically long).

Finally, many other imaging sequences can be applied in an MRI scan, each of which measures physical parameters including: proton density, flow/velocity, fat, diffusion, temperature, blood oxygen levels, and more.

13.6.3 Calculation of T_1-Weighted and T_2-Weighted Magnetizations

Consider a system where the net magnetization of the system is M_{z0} and M_{xy0} on the $\hat{z}$-axis and the transverse plane, respectively, at time $t = 0$.

Find:

$$M_z(t) \text{ and } M_{xy}(t)$$

Answer:

M_z and M_{xy} go back to equilibrium exponentially with time constants T_1 and T_2, respectively. Therefore:

$$\begin{cases} M_z(t) = A * e^{-\frac{t}{T_1}} + B \\ M_{xy}(t) = C * e^{-\frac{t}{T_2}} + D \end{cases} \quad \text{where } A, B, C, \text{ and } D \text{ are constants we need to find.}$$

When $t \to \infty$: The magnetization returns to equilibrium, therefore $\begin{cases} M_z = M_0 \\ M_{xy} = 0 \end{cases}$

Therefore:

$$M_z(t \to \infty) = A * 0 + B = B = M_0 \quad \to B = M_0$$

$$M_{xy}(t \to \infty) = C * 0 + D = D = 0 \quad \to D = 0$$

At t = 0:

$$M_z(t=0) = M_{z0} = A*1 + B = A + B = A + M_0 \quad \rightarrow A = M_{z0} - M_0$$

$$M_{xy}(t=0) = M_{xy0} = C*1 + D = C + D = C \quad \rightarrow C = M_{xy0}$$

Therefore:

$$M_z(t) = (M_{z0} - M_0) * e^{-\frac{t}{T_1}} + M_0$$

$$M_{xy}(t) = M_{xy0} * e^{-\frac{t}{T_2}}$$

13.6.4 MRI Tradeoffs

An intrinsic tradeoff in MRI is that the SNR depends linearly on the resolution and on the square root of the readout time:

$$\text{SNR} \propto \Delta x \Delta y \Delta z \sqrt{\text{total readout time}}.$$

Therefore, in order to improve resolution by twofold on each axis (keeping the same SNR), the total readout time must be increased by a factor of 64. However, this is not realistic, as the cost of acquiring an MRI scan is proportional to the total readout time. Because of the relatively long readout time and high costs, MRI scans are typically used to image patients that are known to have a certain disease or highly suspected to have a disease, rather than as a screening tool for large numbers of patients.

13.7 MRI Contrast Agents

13.7.1 How Contrast Agents Work

Contrast agents for MRI typically create contrast by shortening the T_1 or T_2 coefficients of water molecules around them. Contrast agents are commonly administered to the patient in one of two ways: orally (when target organ is within the gastrointestinal tract) or intravenously (i.e. into the vein), when the target is accessible through the systemic circulation. Common contrast agents for MRI include gadolinium (Gd^{3+}, the most commonly used T_1 contrast agent), manganese (another T_1 contrast agent), and iron oxide (a T_2 contrast agent).

Contrast agents affect T_1 and/or T_2 of the molecules around them, due to resonant fields between the contrast agent and the proton that can flip the proton's spin, thereby shortening either T_1 or T_2 relaxation times, or both. Every contrast agent is characterized by two relaxivity coefficients, r_1 and r_2, which affect T_1 and T_2 as follows:

$$\frac{1}{T_{1(\text{observed})}} = \frac{1}{T_{1(\text{original})}} + Cr_1$$

$$\frac{1}{T_{2(\text{observed})}} = \frac{1}{T_{2(\text{observed})}} + Cr_2,$$

where C is the contrast agent concentration in units of mM, and r_1 and r_2 are the contrast agent relaxivities in units of $[(\text{mM s})]^{-1}$.

The ideal contrast agent would be injected into the circulatory system of the body, produce the desirable contrast at the desirable location, and shortly after, leave the body (usually through the urinary system). It should also be nontoxic and produce a high signal with low injection dose.

13.7.2 Gadolinium (Gd^{3+})

Gadolinium is the most common MRI contrast agent, with seven commercial Gd-based MRI contrast agents approved by the FDA. Since gadolinium is highly toxic, it must be cleared from the body quickly and be contained (a.k.a. chelated) within another molecule so it cannot interact much with the body. The chelation must be carefully designed such that water molecules will be able to interact with the Gd^{3+}, but not allow gadolinium to be free in the body and interact with other biomolecules. Some common Gd-containing contrast agents include Gadoteridol and Gadopentetic acid (Gd-DTPA), shown in Figure 13.14.

13.7.3 Gd^{3+} for Imaging Stroke and Brain Tumors

Stroke patients often incur a defect of the Blood–Brain Barrier (BBB), a protecting layer on the brain blood vessels that protects the vascular of the brain from foreign material leaking into it. T_1- weighted MRI images (shown in Figure 13.15) can indicate BBB defect with Gd^{3+} contrast agent. The image on the left shows a T_1-weighted MRI scan before the injection of the contrast agent, while the right image, which was taken after the injection of the contrast agent, shows the areas affected by the stroke. A higher signal appears in areas where a high concentration of contrast agent is present, where the T_1 value is reduced.

Similar to strokes, brain tumors can disrupt the BBB, allowing Gd-DPTA contrast agent to accumulate in the tumor (Figure 13.16). Eventually, molecular imaging may enable real-time imaging of a brain tumor during surgery so that the surgeon is able to resect (i.e. surgically remove) only the portion of the brain affected by the tumor and minimize healthy brain tissue removal.

13.7.4 Smart Contrast Agents (Imaging Agents)

Smart imaging agents, or activatable imaging agents, do not naturally give a signal. Only upon activation (typically by an enzyme) will the imaging agents produce an imaging signal. For

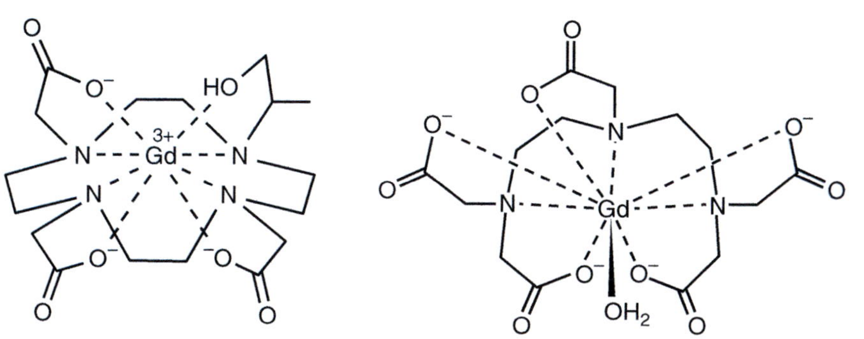

Figure 13.14 Common Gd-containing contrast agents (Gadoteridol on the left and Gd-DTPA on the right).

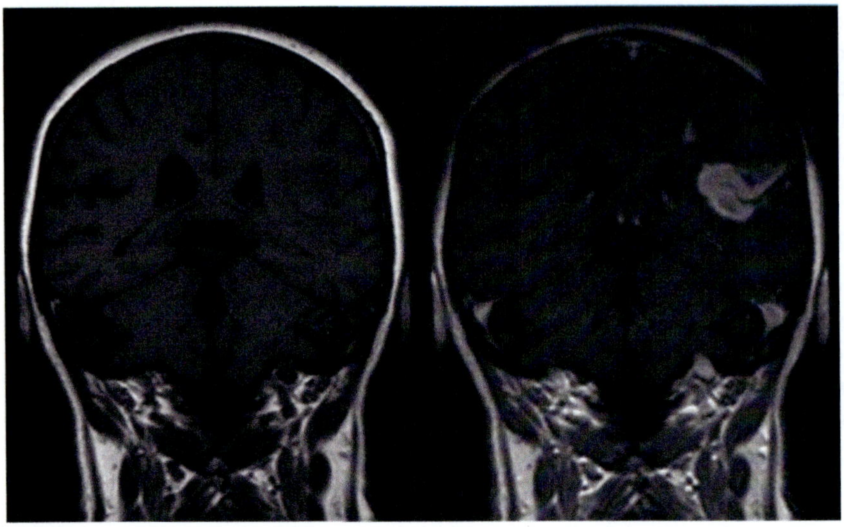

Figure 13.15 Image of stroke patient's brain (without and with contrast agent). *Source:* Hellerhoff, [10]. Used under CC-BY-SA 3.0 https://creativecommons.org/licenses/by-sa/3.0/.

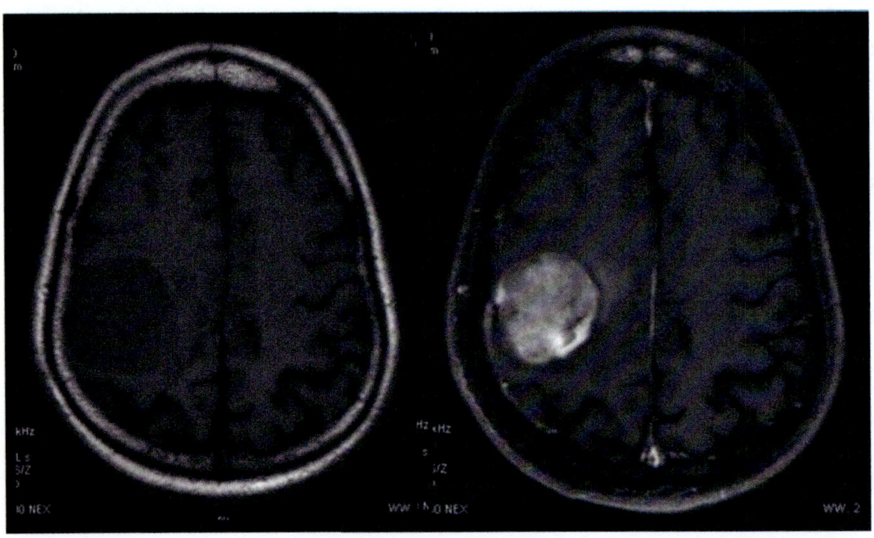

Figure 13.16 Image of a patient with brain tumor (without and with contrast agent). *Source:* Udare et al. [11]. Poster ECR 2014/C-1685. Figure 1. Courtesy of Dr. Amar Ramesh Udare.

example, an imaging agent can be created by chelating Gd^{3+} with a cap-like structure that does not give a signal. This cap can be cleaved off by the β-galactosidase enzyme, enabling the imaging agent to interact with water molecules, producing an imaging signal. Thus, only in cells that express LacZ (the gene that encodes for β-galactosidase enzyme) will the imaging agent be cleaved and produce a signal on a T_1-weighted image. For example, a fish that is genetically engineered to express the LacZ gene will produce a high imaging signal, while nongenetically engineered fish will display much lower signal due to small intrinsic levels of LacZ expression and natural intrinsic T_1-weighted MRI signal (Figure 13.17).

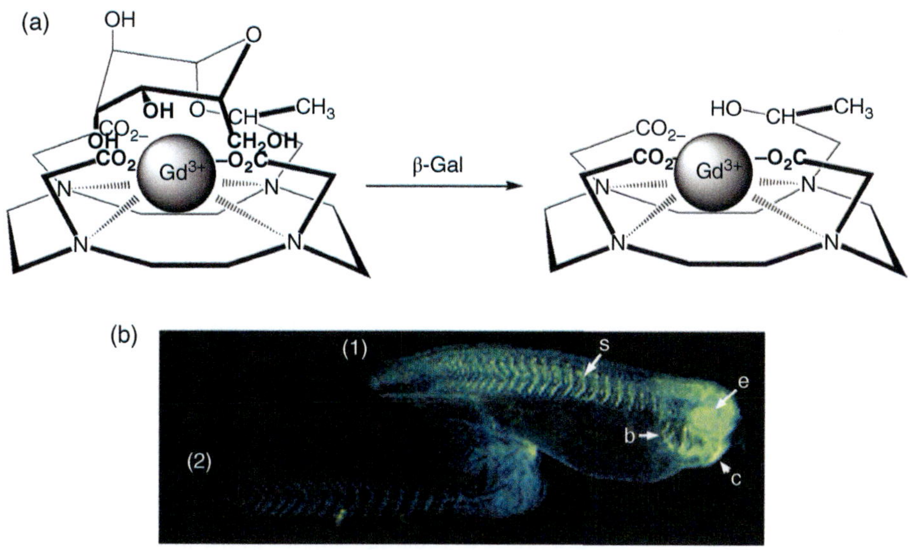

Figure 13.17 (a) Imaging agent cleaved by β-Gal (*Source:* Louie et al. [12]. Reprinted by permission from Springer Nature: Nature Biotechnology, Copyright © 2000 by Springer Nature), (b) Fish #1 (expressing LacZ) and Fish #2 (low LacZ). (*Source:* Louie et al. [12], Reprinted by permission from Springer Nature: Nature Biotechnology, Copyright © 2000 by Springer Nature).

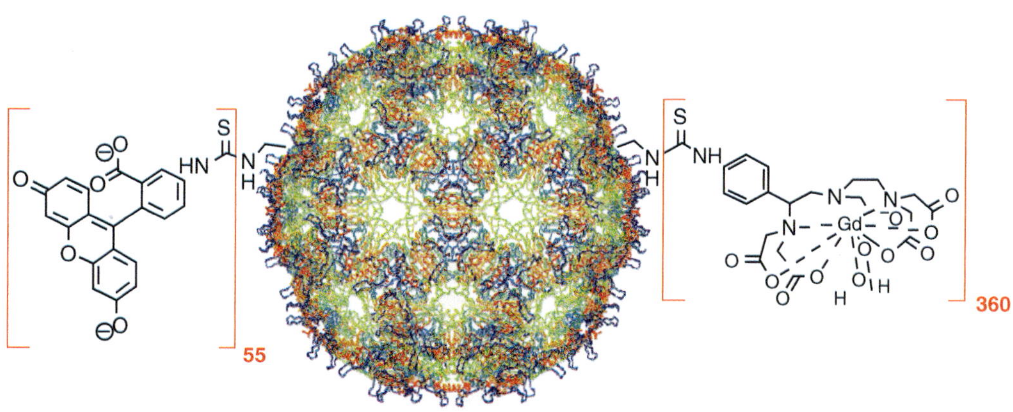

Figure 13.18 Gd-DPTA nanoparticle contrast agent. The molecule shown on the right is a fluorescent dye (FITC) and the molecule on the right is Gd-DTPA. *Source:* Anderson et al. [13]. Reprinted (adapted) with permission from Nano Letters: American Chemical Society, Copyright © 2006 American Chemical Society.

13.7.5 Gd-Nanoparticle Contrast Agent

One way to improve the performance of a contrast agent is to attach many Gd-DPTA molecules to a single nanoparticle (27 nm in diameter, shown in Figure 13.18). By placing many Gd^{3+} atoms in close proximity to each other, the imaging signal can be amplified synergistically by a factor higher than the actual increase in contrast agent. For example, a nanoparticle with 360 Gd-DPTA molecules attached to it will result in a 440-fold improvement in r_1 compared to a single Gd-DPTA.

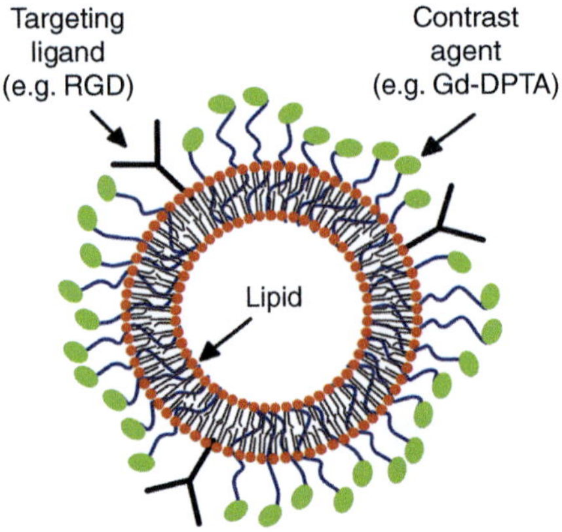

Figure 13.19 Gd-DPTA liposome-targeted contrast agent.

13.7.6 Targeted Contrast Agent

In addition to signal amplification, targeted contrast agents can also be designed to accumulate selectively in certain areas of the body. For example, a liposome (capsule made of lipid bilayer, like the cell membrane) can be coated with 90 000 Gd-DPTA molecules as well as RGD peptides that target to $\alpha_V\beta_3$ integrin (an integrin that is associated with angiogenesis in new blood vessels). Such a particle is shown schematically in Figure 13.19. This targeted contrast agent can then accumulate in areas of atherosclerosis, which were recently shown to undergo angiogenesis, much like cancer cells. Rather than a still image, targeted contrast agents can show where active angiogenesis is occurring, as well as which blood vessels are prone to causing embolus in the future.

13.7.7 Iron Oxide Nanoparticles

Iron oxide nanoparticles are used as T_2 contrast agents for MRI. The nanoparticles are made of several iron oxide cores about 10 nm in diameter, which have a dextran coating of about 100 nm in diameter. These iron oxide nanoparticles have the advantage of low toxicity so that they can be heavily loaded into cells and their effect on MRI is much larger than the cell volume (unlike Gd^{3+}). One use of iron oxide nanoparticles is to monitor the location of therapeutic stem cells in the body. Figure 13.20 shows an example in which mesenchymal stem cells (MSCs) were labeled with iron

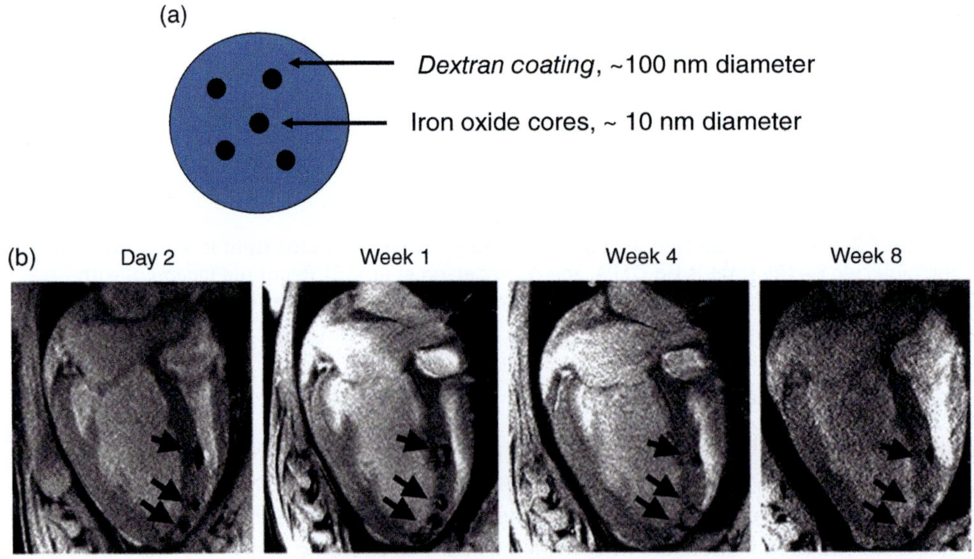

Figure 13.20 (a) Iron oxide nanoparticle, (b) application to stem cell therapy monitoring. *Source:* Amado et al. [14]. Copyright © (2005) National Academy of Sciences, USA.

oxide nanoparticles and injected into a pig's heart with myocardial infarction (MI). The labeled MSCs then travelled to the area of heart muscle death and caused regeneration and regrowth. The T_2-weighted MR image allowed monitoring of the location of the MSCs, which appear as dark drops on the image (Figure 13.20b).

13.8 Conclusion

MRI is a very common and powerful imaging technique that can provide images of many common tissues in the body, such as the brain, heart, and other organs. Future advances in molecular imaging would be revolutionary to imaging technology, allowing the imaging of not only the patient's anatomy and physiology, but also the molecular information, which are the underpinnings of disease initiation and progression (e.g. visualizing the distribution of angiogenic receptors in a tumor). Molecular imaging is an extremely powerful tool that can provide detailed real-time information about the molecular composition of body tissues such as tumors.

Problems

13.1 MRI physics typically involves an applied magnetic field: $\boldsymbol{B} = (B_x, B_y, B_z)$, relaxation times T_1 and T_2, and a gyromagnetic ratio, $\gamma > 0$. Generally, we are interested in understanding how these quantities affect the nuclear magnetization of the tissue of interest, $\boldsymbol{M} = (M_x, M_y, M_z)$. If the tissue has a steady state magnetization of $\boldsymbol{M_0} = (0, 0, M_0) = M_0\hat{z}$, then the magnetization can be related back to the other quantities through a set of differential equations known as the Bloch equations. Suppose the initial magnetization of a tissue has $M_x(t = 0) = m_x$, $M_y(t = 0) = 0$, and $M_z(t = 0) = m_z$.

A In the absence of any applied magnetic field (not even a constant large magnetic field in the z-axis), what would we expect the magnetization to be after an infinite amount of time has passed?

B Now, look at the Bloch equations:

$$\frac{dM_x(t)}{dt} = \gamma\left(M_y(t)B_z(t) - M_z(t)B_y(t)\right) - \frac{M_x(t)}{T_2}$$

$$\frac{dM_y(t)}{dt} = \gamma\left(M_z(t)B_x(t) - M_x(t)B_z(t)\right) - \frac{M_y(t)}{T_2}$$

$$\frac{dM_z(t)}{dt} = \gamma\left(M_x(t)B_y(t) - M_y(t)B_x(t)\right) - \frac{M_z(t)}{T_1} + \frac{M_0}{T_1}$$

We will consider what happens when we apply a constant magnetic field in the z direction. Thus, we set $B_x(t) = 0$, $B_y(t) = 0$, and let $B_z(t) = B_z$.

v) Write down the differential equations for $M_x(t)$, $M_y(t)$, and $M_z(t)$.

vi) Solve the differential equations for $M_z(t)$.
Hint: The solution to differential equations of the form, $\frac{dw(t)}{dt} = -aw(t) + d$, is $w(t) = ce^{-at} + \frac{d}{a}$ where c is some constant determined from the initial conditions.

vii) Solve the differential equations for $M_x(t)$, and $M_y(t)$.
Hint: The differential equations for $M_x(t)$ and $M_y(t)$ are linked as a system of differential equations. The general solutions of the following system of differential equations

$$\frac{dw(t)}{dt} = -aw(t) + bv(t)$$

$$\frac{dv(t)}{dt} = -bw(t) - av(t)$$

are given by

$$w(t) = e^{-at}\left(c_1 \cos(bt) + c_2 \sin(bt)\right)$$

$$v(t) = e^{-at}\left(-c_1 \sin(bt) + c_2 \cos(bt)\right)$$

Where c_1, c_2 are constants determined by the initial conditions. To be unnecessarily explicit: c_1, c_2 are constants used in both equations.
Additional hint: Let $w(t) = M_x(t)$, and $v(t) = M_y(t)$. What must a and b be in this case?

viii) Using either what you know about MRI or what you obtained from the previous part, determine the length of the magnetization in the xy plane: $|M_{xy}| = \sqrt{M_x(t)^2 + M_y(t)^2}$.

ix) Explain how changing B_z affects the behavior of $M_x(t)$ and $M_y(t)$.

13.2 We want to acquire MR images with ^{19}F being the contrast (as opposed to ^{1}H). The gyromagnetic ratio of ^{19}F is $\frac{\gamma}{2\pi} = 40.05 \frac{\text{MHz}}{\text{Tesla}}$. The polarizing field is known to be 1.5T.

A What is the new Larmor angular frequency?

B What may be the challenge in acquiring MRI images of ^{19}F?

13.3 For the following RF excitation pulses, find $M_z(t)$ and $M_{xy}(t)$.
You can assume $M_{t=0} = M_0\hat{z}$.

A RF pulse of 180°

B RF pulse of 90°

C A train of 90° pulses separated by time TR from each other. You can assume that $T_2 \ll TR$ (but you cannot assume anything on T_1). If it's easier for you, you can draw $M_z(t)$ and $M_{xy}(t)$ on a graph and give the explicit analytical expression for only one of the TR periods.

13.4 A common MR pulse sequence used to establish contrast is the saturation recovery sequence with spin echoes. As shown in Figure 13.21, the sequence consists of a 90-degree excitation followed by a 180-degree refocusing pulse that is TE/2 after the 90-degree pulse.

A If the tissue has a steady state magnetization of $\boldsymbol{M_0} = (0,\ 0,\ M_0) = M_0\hat{z}$ and the repetition time $TR \gg T_2$, draw M_z and M_{xy} on Figure 13.21.

B Derive analytical expressions for M_z and $|M_{xy}|$ for the time points in the table below where $(t)^-$ indicates immediately before a pulse and $(t)^+$ indicates immediately after the pulse.

Figure 13.21 Saturation recovery sequence with spin echoes.

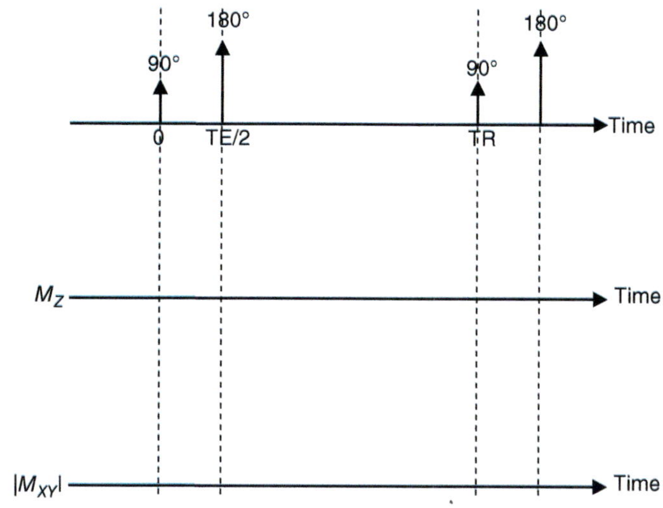

Time	M_z	$\|M_{xy}\|$
$(TE/2)^-$		
$(TE/2)^+$		
$(TR)^-$		
$(TR)^+$		

Time	M_z	$\|M_{xy}\|$
$(TR)^-$		
$(TR)^+$		
TR + TE	X	

C If $\mathbf{TE/2 \gg T_1}$, derive analytical expressions for M_z and $|M_{xy}|$ for the time points in the table below where $(t)^-$ indicates immediately before a pulse and $(t)^+$ indicates immediately after the pulse.

D If an image of $|M_{xy}|$ was captured at $t = \text{TR} + \text{TE}$ using the equations derived in part (c), how would you set TR and/or TE to make it a T_1 weighted image?

E If an image of $|M_{xy}|$ was captured at $t = \text{TR} + \text{TE}$ using the equations derived in part (c), how would you set TR and/or TE to make it a T_2 weighted image?

13.5 Fill in the table below with either *brighter/darker* to denote whether white matter and gray matter would appear brighter or darker on either T_1-weighted or T_2-weighted images. Explain the reasoning for your decision.

Note: White matter and gray matter are two types of tissues in the brain. Their names do not necessarily refer to how they are visualized on an MR image.

	T_1-weighted image	T_2-weighted image
White matter		
Gray matter		

13.6 Assume that a voxel (small volume) of tissue has net magnetization of M_0 in $+z$ direction under 1 Tesla. We apply a 180^0 RF pulse, then wait for $t = 1000$ ms and apply a 90^0 pulse. Right after the 90^0 pulse, the amplitude of measured signal is $|M_{xy}| = (0.53)M_0$.
You may find Table 13.4 useful.

A What type of weighting is used in this measurement?

B What are the two possible values for the time constant? Using the provided tables, determine the type of tissue.

C If we were to image fat tissue using the same pulse sequence, would it look brighter or darker in the MRI image compared to the tissue in part (b)?

D We don't want to see the fat tissue in the MRI image, how would you suppress the signal coming from fat only (i.e. how would you time the pulses)? Hint: Use the same sequence used in this problem, and find the correct t value.

E What is the optimum value of t if we want to maximize the signal difference between white matter and gray matter?

13.7 A certain tissue has a $T_1 = 500$ ms. At a certain magnetic field B_0, Gd-DTPA was measured to have relaxivity $r_1 = 4\ (\text{mM s})^{-1}$.

A What is the minimal concentration of Gd-DTPA required in order to reduce T_1 by 50%?

B We attached 1000 Gd-DTPA on the surface of a liposome and measured the T_1 of decreasing concentrations of the new particle in water (results from the experiment are in Table 13.5). What is the relaxivity r_1 of the new particle?

(Hint: You may want to use Excel's linear curve fitting feature).

C What is the minimal concentration of the new particle that is required to reduce T_1 of the original tissue (the one with $T_1 = 500$ ms) by 50%?

Table 13.4 T1 and T2 values for various tissues.

Tissue	T1 (ms)*	T2 (ms)
Gray matter	810	100
White matter	690	92
Muscle	740	47
Fat	240	85
Kidney	590	58
Liver	430	43

Table 13.5 Concentrations of a new particle in water and the measured T_1 values.

Concentration (μM)	T_1 (sec)
1	0.1
0.5	0.2
0.25	0.33
0.125	0.75

D How many Gd-DTPA molecules (that are not bound to any nanoparticle) would be needed to create the same effect on T_1 as the effect that one nanoparticle has on T_1? (i.e. the nanoparticle being the same liposome with 1000 Gd-DTPA on its surface)?

13.8 We would like to take a T_1-weighted MRI image of an organ that is composed of two tissue types: Tissue-A and Tissue-B with T_1 values of $T_{1,A}$ and $T_{1,B}$, respectively. It is known that $T_{1,A} < T_{1,B}$. You can assume that M_0 of both tissues is the same.

A What should be the TE of the MR sequence to eliminate any signal from Tissue-B in the T_1-weighted image?

B The patient is injected with a Gd contrast agent that spreads homogeneously through the organ. The contrast agent has a T_1 relaxivity of r_1 and its concentration in the tissue is C. Does the value of TE that you calculated in (a) need to change because of the contrast agent? If so, what is the new value?

C The contrast between Tissue-A and Tissue-B is defined as: $C_{A,B} = |M_A - M_B|$. For the TE value you calculated in (b), did the contrast agent have an effect on the contrast between the tissues? If so, did it increase or decrease?

D Assuming the contrast agent is *not* homogeneously distributed in the tissue (i.e. its concentration C isn't constant), is it still possible to eliminate the signal of Tissue-B from the T_1-weighted image? Explain.

13.9 A certain healthy tissue has a T_1 of 1000 ms. A tumor that is growing within this tissue has a T_1 of 800 ms. Because of the difference in T_1, we decide to acquire a T_1-weighted image of the tissue to visualize the tumor. The contrast between tissue A and tissue B is defined as $C_{A,B} = |I_A - I_B|$, where I_A and I_B are the image intensities for tissues A and B, respectively. Throughout the question, you may assume that M_0 of the tumor and that of the healthy tissue are the same.

A What is the contrast between the tumor and the surrounding tissue, $C_{\text{tumor,tissue}}$, in the T_1-weighted image, if the time between the RF pulse and the received echo is chosen to be TE = 500 ms?

B An imaging agent with a relaxivity value of $r_1 = 3\,\text{mM}^{-1}\,\text{s}^{-1}$ is administered to the patient and is localizing in the tumor area, which now shows a $T_1 = 500$ ms. What is the concentration of the imaging agent in the tumor?

C With the new $T_1 = 500$ ms of the tumor, what TE should be used to achieve an image with maximized contrast between tumor and healthy tissue $C_{\text{tumor,tissue}}$? What is $C_{\text{tumor,tissue}}$ at this TE?

13.10 A tissue has a steady state magnetization of $M_0\,\hat{z}$ and decay times of T_1 and T_2. A 90° RF pulse is applied and the system is then allowed to decay back toward steady state.

A What are $M_z(t)$ and $M_{xy}(t)$? (Assume $t = 0$ is the time immediately after the 90° RF pulse.)

B A new MRI sequence for measuring the total length of M has been developed. Given that the magnitude of the vector is not conserved through the decay toward steady state, what is the magnitude of the magnetization vector $|M(t)|$?

C For the following cases, find what is the shortest length of the magnetization vector during its decay toward steady state:

i) $T_1 = T_2$

ii) $T_1 = \dfrac{T_2}{2}$

iii) $T_1 = \dfrac{3T_2}{2}$

D We now add a contrast agent to the tissue with relaxivity coefficients r_1 and r_2 and concentration c. With the contrast agent in the tissue, will the shortest length of the magnetization vector be longer or shorter in the following cases? Explain.

i) $r_1 > 0$ and $r_2 = 0$

ii) $r_1 = 0$ and $r_2 > 0$

References

1 Mansfield, P. and Pykett, I.L. (1969). Biological and medical imaging by NMR. *Journal of Magnetic Resonance* 29 (2): 355–373.

2 Fastfission commonswiki, https://commons.wikimedia.org/wiki/File:MRI_brain.jpg

3 van Tilborg, G.A.F., Mulder, W.J.M., van der Schaft, D.W.J. et al. (2008). Improved magnetic resonance molecular imaging of tumor angiogenesis by avidin-induced clearance of nonbound bimodal liposomes. *Neoplasia* 10 (12): 1459–1469.

4 User:BoP (28 August 2005). Supplied by the medOCT group, Center of biomedical Engineering and Physics, Medical University Vienna, Austria.

5 Moroder, https://commons.wikimedia.org/wiki/File:CRL_Crown_rump_lengh_12_weeks_ecografia_Dr._Wolfgang_Moroder.jpg.

6 Damato, https://commons.wikimedia.org/wiki/File:PET-MIPS-anim.gif.

7 United States Air Force, http://www.scott.af.mil/News/Art/igphoto/2000294961/

8 Schmidt, G.P., Reiser, M.F., and Baur-Melnyk, A. (2009). Whole-body MRI for the staging and follow-up of patients with metastasis. *European Journal of Radiology* 70: 393–400.

9 Pooley, R.A. (2005). Fundamental physics of MR imaging. *RadioGraphics* 25: 1087–1099.

10 Hellerhoff, https://commons.wikimedia.org/wiki/File:Bluthirnschranke_nach_Infarkt_nativ_und_KM.png

11 A.R. Udare, A. Mahajan, S. Juvekar, P. Shetty, M. Thakur, A. Moidayi. 2014. Role of functional MRI in evaluating intraaxial brain tumors – Advances and pitfalls. *European Society of Radiology*. https://posterng.netkey.at/esr/viewing/index.php?module=viewing_poster&task=viewsection&pi=119714&ti=405031&searchkey= doi: https://doi.org/10.1594/ecr2014/C-1685

12 Louie, A.Y., Huber, M.M., Ahrens, E.T. et al. (2000). in vivo visualization of gene expression using magnetic resonance imaging. *Nature Biotechnology* 18: 321–325.

13 Anderson, E.A., Isaacman, S., Peabody, D.S. et al. (2006). Viral nanoparticles Donning a paramagnetic coat: conjugation of MRI contrast agents to the MS2 capsid. *Nano Letters: American Chemical Society* 6 (6): 1160–1164.

14 Cardiac repair with intramyocardial injection of allogeneic mesenchymal stem cells after myocardial infarction", Luciano C. Amado, Anastasios P. Saliaris, Karl H. Schuleri, Marcus St. John, Jin-Sheng Xie, et al., Proceedings of the National Academy of Sciences 2005, 102 (32) 11474-11479; doi: https://doi.org/10.1073/pnas.0504388102.

Further Reading

http://abhijitpoddar.100webspace.net/researchpage/UGC_MRP_05_06_forweb/elearningnode27.html

Pooley, R.A. (2005). Fundamental physics of MR imaging. *Radiographics* 25: 1087–1099.

Shan Wang MSE347 course slides.

http://en.wikipedia.org/wiki/MRI_contrast_agent

14

Radionuclide Imaging

14.1 Radioactivity

A **radionuclide** is an atom with an unstable nucleus, which has excess energy that can be transferred to either a newly created radiation particle or an electron. During this process of radioactive decay, the radionuclide also emits gamma rays and/or subatomic particles. **Radionuclide imaging**, or nuclear imaging, uses radionuclides and their radioactive decay to produce images of tissues (Figure 14.1), using either positron emission tomography (PET) or single photon emission computed tomography (SPECT). Unlike MRI, for which the body naturally produces a good signal without administration of an external contrast agent, nuclear imaging requires the injection of contrast agents or imaging agents since the body naturally is not radioactive enough to produce a detectable and specific signal.

14.1.1 Gamma Decay

An atom or atom within a molecule that is in an unstable state (i.e. a radionuclide) can undergo three different types of radioactive decay: alpha, beta, or gamma. Beta and gamma decay are applicable for nuclear imaging. During **gamma decay** (Figure 14.2), nucleons rearrange themselves to a less energetic, more stable configuration, giving off electromagnetic energy in the form of high-energy (i.e. very short wavelength) gamma photons. For gamma imaging, a metastable parent atom is required, i.e. the atomic number (number of protons) Z does not change during decay:

$$^{A}X_{z} \rightarrow {}^{A}X_{z} + \gamma,$$

where X is an atom, A is the mass number (number of neutrons and protons), and Z is the atomic number (number of protons). When a metastable atom undergoes gamma decay, the mass number (i.e. total number of protons and neutrons) does not change, but one electron moves from one shell to another, and thus emits high-energy gamma rays on the order of several keV. Some examples of nuclei that can undergo gamma decay include ^{111}In, ^{123}I, ^{125}I, ^{99m}Tc, and ^{201}Tl.

Every different isotope will release gamma rays with different energies during gamma decay. Therefore, analysis of the energy spectrum can determine which atoms have undergone gamma decay (similar to fluorescent tags with different colors). As an example of gamma decay, ^{99m}Tc (where the m stands for metastable) can decay into regular ^{99}Tc and gamma rays, which is a more energetically favorable and stable state.

Biochips and Medical Imaging, First Edition. Adam de la Zerda and Shan Xiang Wang.

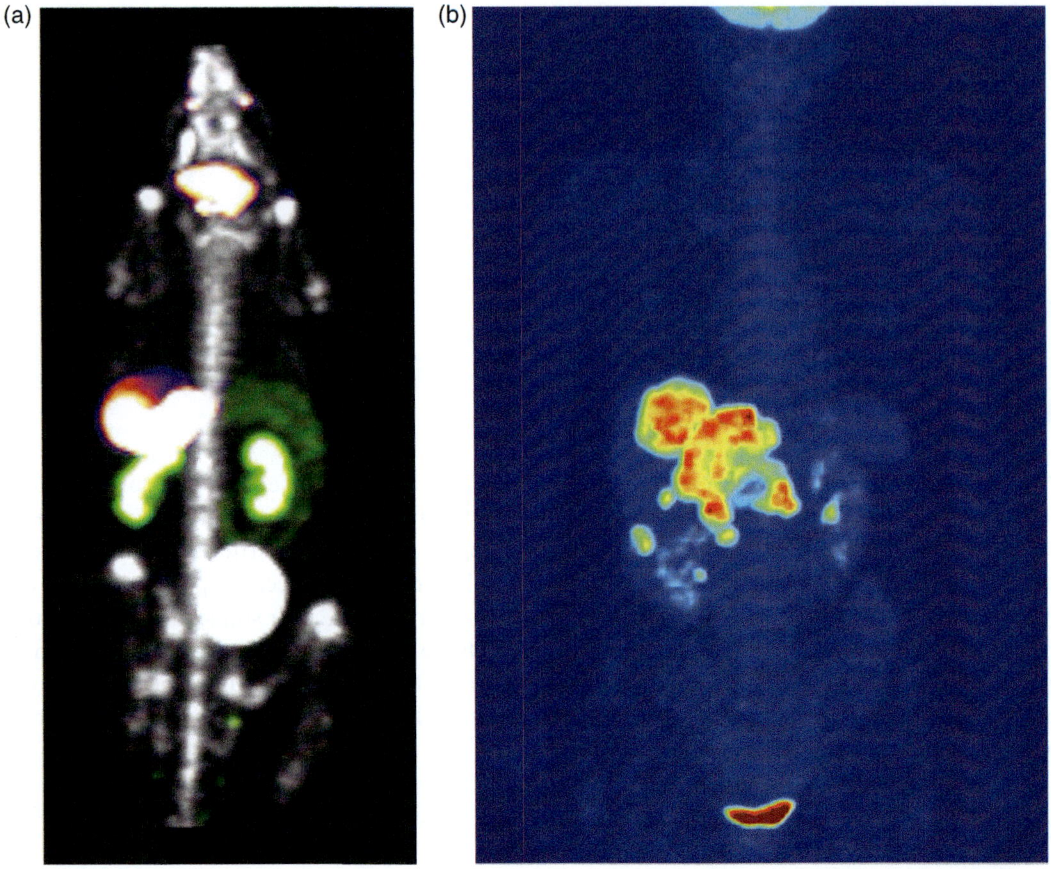

Figure 14.1 (a) PET (*Source:* Courtesy of JP Norenberg, Keck-UNM Small-Animal Imaging Resource [KUSAIR]), (b) SPECT (*Source:* Damato [1] CC0-1.0 public domain https://creativecommons.org/publicdomain/zero/1.0/).

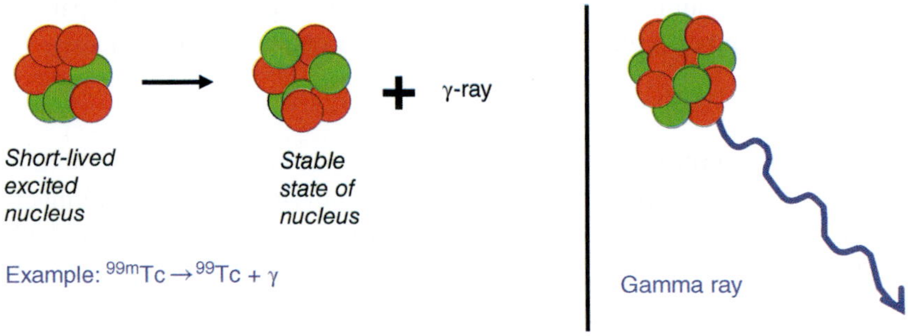

Figure 14.2 Gamma decay of ^{99m}Tc. *Source:* Image courtesy of Dr. Craig Levin.

14.1.2 Beta Decay

As with gamma decay, **beta decay** occurs when nucleons transform in order to obtain a more stable configuration. This involves the emission or absorption of a beta particle, which is a high-energy electron or positron. There are three subtypes of beta decay: electron emission, positron emission, and electron capture.

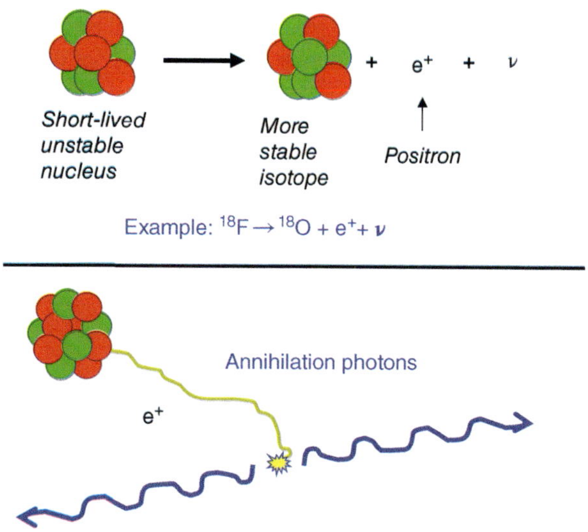

Figure 14.3 Positron emission. *Source:* Image courtesy of Dr. Craig Levin.

Electron emission: $n \rightarrow p + e^- + \gamma$ $\quad {}^{A}X_z \rightarrow {}^{A}Y_{Z+1} + e^- + \gamma$

Positron emission: $p \rightarrow n + e^+ + \gamma$ $\quad {}^{A}X_z \rightarrow {}^{A}Y_{Z-1} + e^+ + \gamma$

Electron capture: $e^- + p \rightarrow n + \gamma$ $\quad e^- + {}^{A}X_z \rightarrow {}^{A}Y_{Z-1} + \gamma$

In **electron emission**, one neutron decays to become a proton and an electron. In **positron emission** (Figure 14.3), one proton decays to become a neutron and a positron. The positron, which is the antimatter complement to an electron, will travel a short distance (1 mm on average) to find the nearest electron and disintegrate to release energy according to Einstein's $E = mc^2$ equation (which describes the conversion between mass and energy). In **electron capture**, a proton and an electron combine to form a neutron. An example of beta decay is positron emission of ^{18}F to produce ^{18}O and an emitted positron (e^+), which will annihilate with an electron and emit two photons of energy 511 keV, which travel in opposite directions due to conservation of momentum. Examples of β-decaying nuclei are ^{3}H, ^{14}C, ^{32}P, ^{11}C, ^{13}N, ^{15}O, and ^{18}F. Examples of electron capture decaying nuclei include ^{111}In and ^{201}TI.

14.1.3 Radioactivity Decay Kinetics

Radioactivity is a random process, i.e. if N_0 identical unstable parent nuclei were present initially, the most probable number N surviving after a time t is given by:

$$N(t) = N_0 e^{-\lambda t},$$

where λ is the **decay constant**. The decay constant is related to the **half-life** $\tau_{1/2}$ by:

$$\lambda = \frac{\ln(2)}{\tau_{1/2}},$$

which means that after a time $\tau_{1/2}\tau$, there will be half the number of unstable nuclei left that have not decayed. Activity is defined as the number of decays per unit time, and is given by:

$$\text{Activity}(t) = -\frac{dN}{dt} = \lambda N(t) = \lambda N_0 e^{-\lambda t}.$$

Activity is measured by Ci (Curies) or Bq (becquerels, or disintegrations per second), where 1 $Ci = 3.7 \times 10^{10}$ and is the activity of 1 g of ^{226}Ra.

14.1.4 Half-Life of Common Radionuclides

Each radioactive isotope has a different energy (keV) and half-life, typically ranging from 20 minutes to 8 days. Half-lives of some common radionuclides are given in Table 14.1. Two radionuclides often used in nuclear imaging are ^{99m}Tc and ^{18}F, which have half-life values of 6 hours and 110 minutes, respectively. These are good lifetimes for imaging as they allow sufficient time for the imaging agent to distribute in the body and bind to its target and still be able to produce radioactivity. Lifetimes that are too long are also unfavorable as they result in low activity, which imposes scanning over long periods of time. In contrast, ^{131}I has a half-life of eight days. Due to its very long lifetime, it is not used in imaging but is rather used in various nuclear medicine therapies where Iodine is targeted (e.g. thyroid gland). Similarly, ^{11}C is not suitable for imaging due to its short half-life of 20 minutes.

^{14}C has a very long half-life of 5730 years; thus, it is used in carbon dating of fossils and old organic artifacts. We can do this because naturally occurring ^{14}C constitutes about 1 part per trillion of atmospheric carbon. Since plants fix the atmospheric carbon into their bodies, in all living organisms, there is one radioactive ^{14}C for every 1 trillion carbon atoms. As long as the organism is alive, the ratio of ^{14}C stays constant because ^{14}C is replenished. After the organism dies, this replenishment stops and radioactive decay starts reducing the ^{14}C ratio. One can use carbon dating to determine the year of death by looking at the ratio of ^{14}C to ^{12}C.

Table 14.1 Half-life of common radionuclides.

Isotope	Energy (keV)	Half-life
^{67}Ga	93, 185, 300	78 h
^{111}In	172, 247	67 h
^{113m}In	392	100 min
^{123}I	159	13.2 h
^{131}I	364	8 d
^{99m}Tc	140	6 h
^{201}Tl	80, 167	73 h
^{133}Xe	80	5 d
^{18}F	511	110 min
^{11}C	511	20.4 min
^{4}C	156	5730 yr (!!)

14.2 Basics of Positron Emission Tomography (PET)

Positron Emission Tomography (PET) is a form of radionuclide imaging which relies on the detection of two photons traveling in opposite directions as the result of positron annihilation with an electron (Figure 14.4). The positron comes from positron emission of an injected radionuclide source.

During a PET scan, the patient is surrounded by a cylindrical array of **gamma detectors**, which will capture photons coming out of the body resulting from positron emission with a specific energy of 511 keV. Detectors opposite each other in the circle will click at nearly the same time and indicate that radioactivity from the same annihilation occurred somewhere along the line between them (Figure 14.5). PET is a nuclear medicine tomographic imaging technique that uses a tracer compound labeled with a radionuclide that is a positron emitter. A PET study yields cross sectional image slices representing uptake/biodistribution of the radioactively labeled chemical. PET provides quantitative information of rates of biological processes, such as metabolism, cell proliferation, etc.

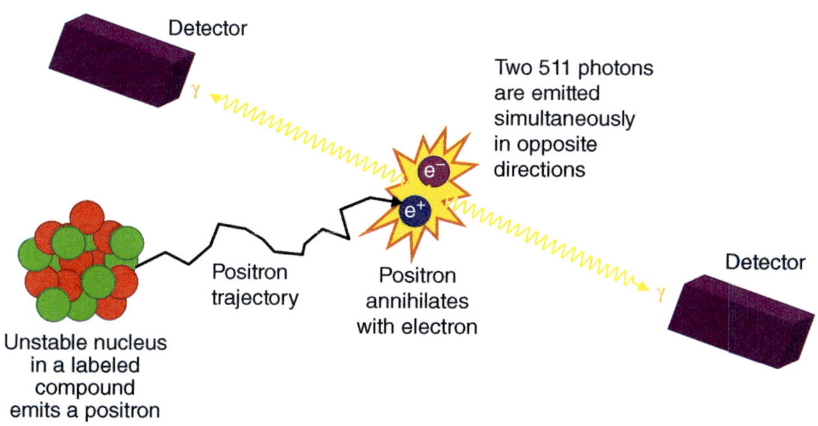

Figure 14.4 Positron annihilation with an electron. *Source:* Zereshk [2]. CC0-1.0 public domain https://creativecommons.org/publicdomain/zero/1.0/

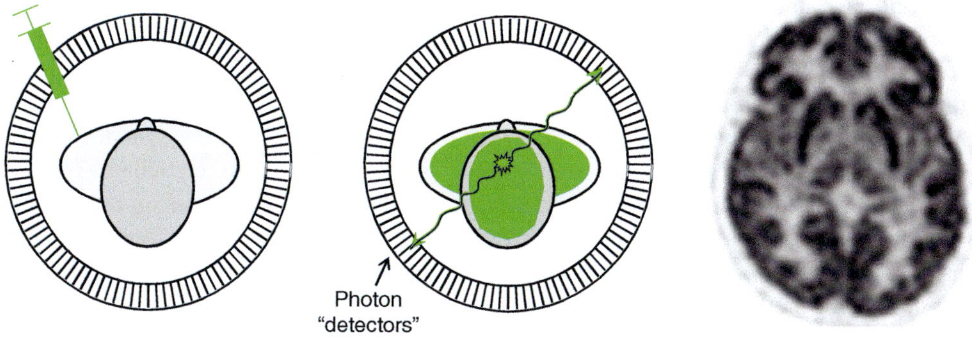

Figure 14.5 PET scan. *Source:* Image courtesy of Dr. Craig Levin.

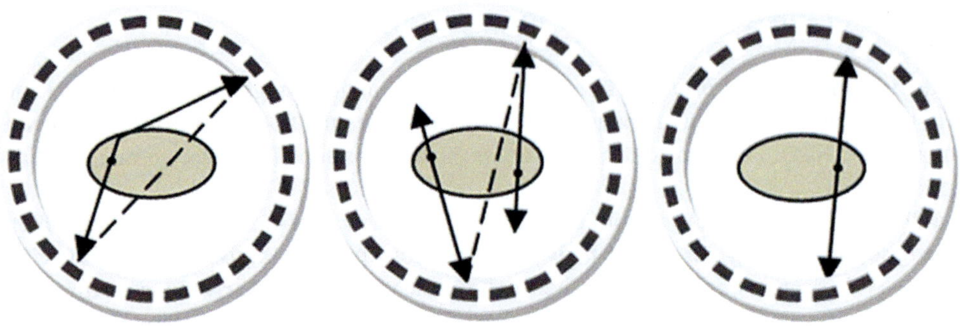

Figure 14.6 Coincidence types. *Source:* Than et al. [3].

14.2.1 Types of Coincidences

True coincidence is the simultaneous detection of the two emissions resulting from a single decay event, which indicates that the annihilation location occurred somewhere along a straight line between the two detectors. A **scatter coincidence** occurs when one or both photons from a single event are scattered and both are detected, resulting in an incorrectly drawn line (mistake). One way to counteract scatter coincidences is to use photodetectors that only respond to specific photon energies since photons change energy after scattering. A **random coincidence** is the simultaneous detection of emission from more than one decay event, which will also result in an incorrectly drawn line. Each of these three coincidence types is depicted in Figure 14.6.

14.2.2 Basics of PET – Detector

A PET detector consists of a **scintillation crystal** and a **photomultiplier tube (PMT)**, shown in Figure 14.7. The scintillation crystal converts an X-ray photon (gamma ray) to many (tens of thousands) visible photons. The PMT converts the photons into electrical signals (using the photoelectric effect) and further amplifies the signal by multiplying electrons inside a vacuum tube. The sensitivity of the detector is high enough to detect a single X-ray photon. Alternatively, some detectors use scintillation crystals and semiconductor-based detectors such as CCD cameras, CMOS cameras, Si photodetectors, or avalanche photodiodes. These detectors eliminate the need for a bulky photomultiplier and the detector size decreases significantly.

The internal structure of a PMT with a scintillator crystal is shown in Figure 14.8. An incident X-ray (gamma) photon is converted to thousands of visible photons in the scintillator crystal. These photons then hit the photocathode of the PMT and cause a release of electrons. A PMT is basically a vacuum tube and free electrons released by photocathode accelerate toward the dynodes. Each dynode in Figure 14.8 has more positive potential than the previous one. Accelerated electrons with high kinetic energy hit the dynodes and release more electrons. This causes an avalanche effect and the number of electrons increases significantly by the time they reach the anode.

The most important parameter of scintillation crystal materials is the **light yield**, which gives the number of photons emitted per unit energy of gamma ray accepted. Another desirable characteristic is a very short decay time so that only two detectors click at one time. This is important in determining the annihilation location, otherwise multiple detectors may click and we cannot tell

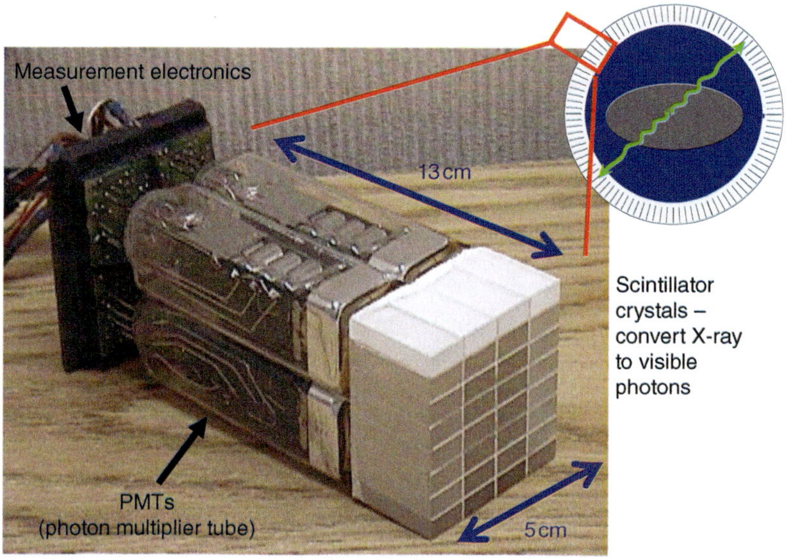

Figure 14.7 PET detector. *Source:* Image courtesy of Dr. Craig Levin.

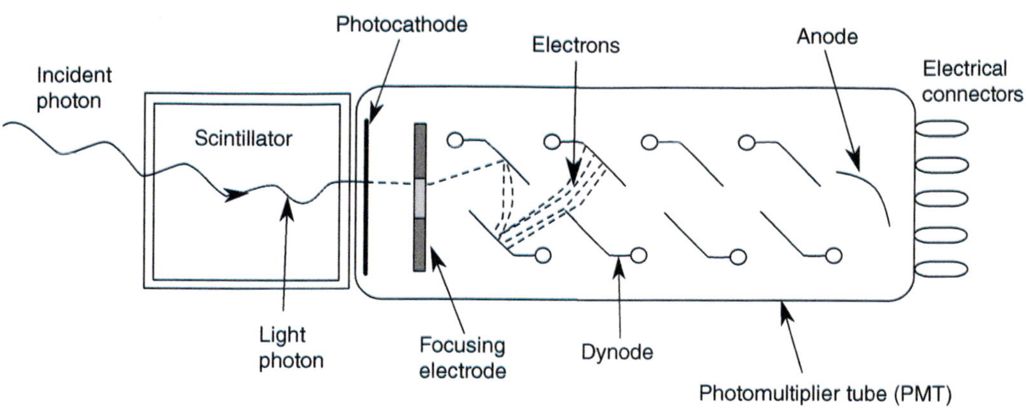

Figure 14.8 Internal structure of PMT with a scintillator crystal. *Source:* Mako098765 [4]. CC0-1.0 public domain https://creativecommons.org/publicdomain/zero/1.0/.

where the radioactivity came from. The characteristics of some scintillation crystal materials are given in Table 14.2.

14.2.3 Importance of Counts

As a higher number of counts are measured to form an image, the SNR is increased, resulting in better quality images (Figure 14.9). However, it may be difficult to get a high number of counts, which would require high radioactivity that can be harmful to the body. The alternative is to use a low amount of radioactivity and wait for a long time to accumulate a sufficient number of counts; however, imaging costs will increase with longer scan time, and patient movement can cause image blurring.

Table 14.2 Characteristics of various scintillation crystal materials.

Scintillation Crystal	Density (g/cm^3)	Effective Z	Peak Wavelength λ_{max} (nm)	Refractive Index at λ_{max}	Decay Time (ns)	Light Yield (Photons/MeV)
NaI(Tl)	3.67	51	410	1.85	230	38 000
$Bi_4(GeO_4)_3$	7.13	75	480	2.15	300	8200
CsI(Tl)	4.51	54	540	1.80	1000	39 000
$Lu_2(SiO_4)O$:Ce	7.40	66	420	1.82	40	28 500
$Gd_2(SiO_4)O$:Ce	6.71	59	440	1.85	60	9500
BaF_2	4.88	65	220	1.56	0.6	10 000

Source: Courtesy of Dr. Craig Levin.

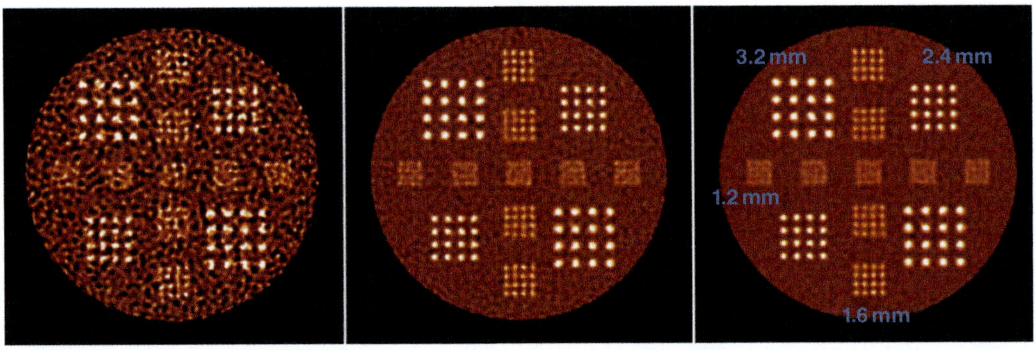

Figure 14.9 PET scans with varying counts. *Source:* Li et al. [5]. Used Under CC-BY 3.0 https://creativecommons.org/licenses/by/3.0/ © 2014 The Authors. Published by American Association of Physicists in Medicine and John Wiley & Sons Ltd.

14.2.4 PET Time of Flight

If the detectors are fast enough to localize in time the arrival of each photon, the photon origin may be narrowed down so that the distance x between the midpoint of the detectors and the annihilation location can be found (due to the difference in time of flight). This is described by the following two equations:

$$\Delta t = \left(d_2 - d_1\right) / c = 2x / c$$

$$x = \Delta t * \frac{c}{2},$$

where Δt is the difference in the time of flight and x is the distance between the detector midpoint and annihilation location (Figure 14.10). For example, if the detectors had infinite time resolution and two clicks are detected at exactly the same time, then the annihilation location was at exactly the center. Otherwise, difference in times can be used to determine the annihilation location along the line, down to a resolution of several cm. Faster detectors result in more accurate image resolution, which allows for a shorter scan time and lower cost.

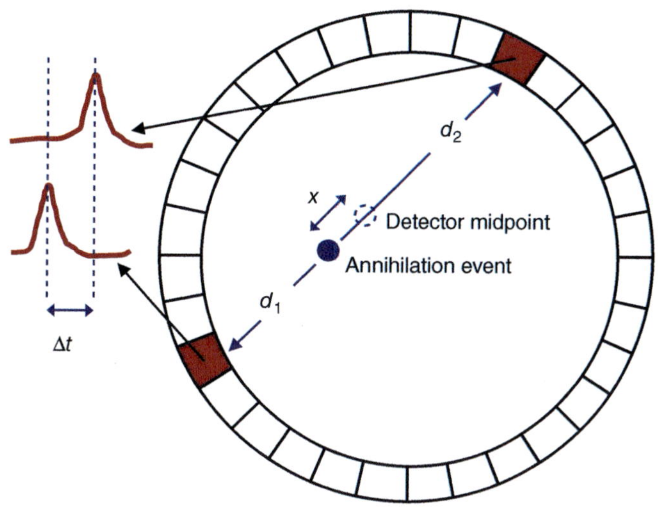

Figure 14.10 PET time of flight detection.

14.2.5 PET/CT

A **CT (computer tomography)** scan is a tomographic X-ray imaging system, which highlights anatomical features of tissues. PET and CT can be combined to form a new device that provides both anatomical information (from CT) as well as molecular information (from PET) on the same image. In general, it is difficult to interpret a PET scan without the context of what is being imaged. However, CT and PET scans can be performed at the same time and their images can be overlaid to obtain much higher quality images, where the CT scan provides some context for interpreting the PET spots (Figure 14.11). Nearly all commercial PET scanners currently in use also feature a CT scan as well.

14.3 Single-Photon Emission Computer Tomography (SPECT)

14.3.1 Basics of SPECT

Single-photon emission computer tomography (SPECT) is another radionuclide imaging modality that relies on the detection of radioactivity effects. Gamma-emitting radionuclides are administered to the patient. Unlike PET, where the 511 keV gamma photons are generated after the annihilation of the emitted positron, SPECT radionuclides emit gamma photons directly. The photons emitted in SPECT are not necessarily 511 keV; they can have different energy levels determined by the source being used. Single photons that are emitted from the patient are first passed through a **collimator**, which only allows perpendicular beams to go through and blocks the beams coming from other angles. As a result, collimators effectively produce parallel gamma beams that are incident on the detectors. Detectors with high-energy resolution will be able to differentiate two photons from different radionuclides, which enable multiplexing. The detectors only detect photons that arrive perpendicular to the camera plane; otherwise, the metal plates of the collimator absorb the photons. By rotating the detectors in a 360-degree circle around the body, a 3-D image can be reconstructed (Figure 14.12).

To allow only parallel photons to reach the detector, collimators made of metal plates with holes are built into SPECT systems. By choosing plates with the right length, thickness, and distance

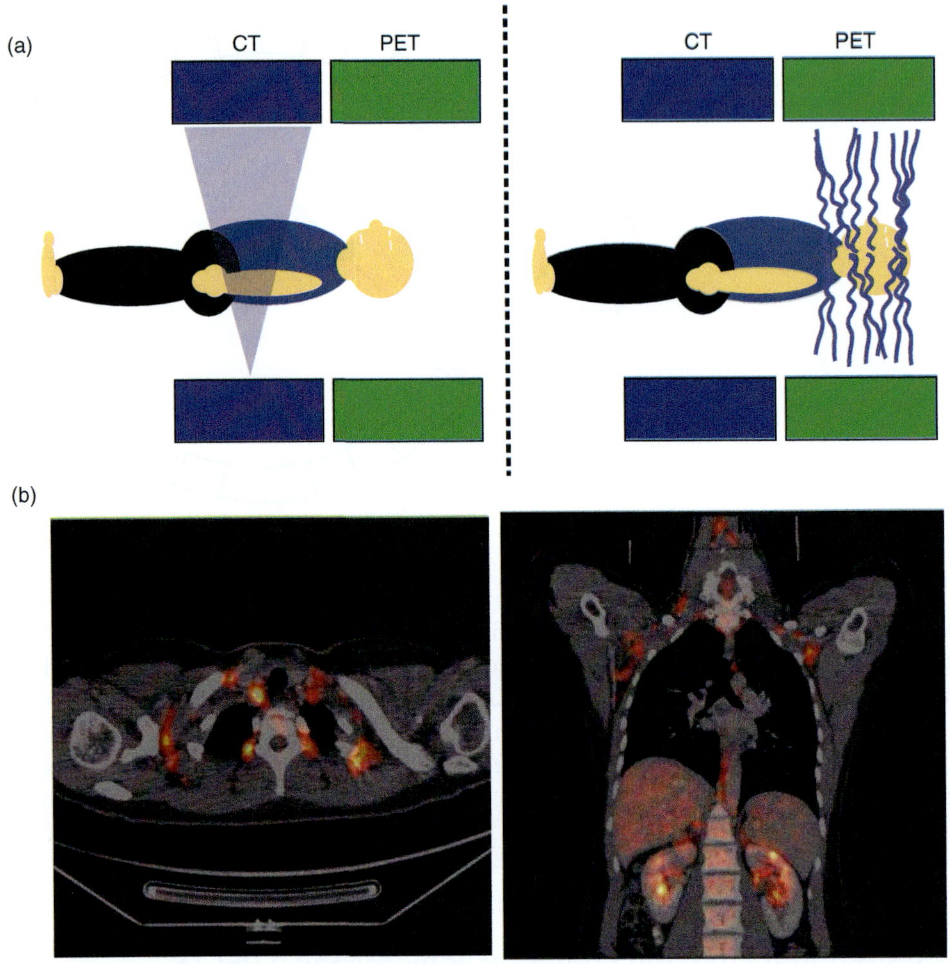

Figure 14.11 (a) PET/CT systems first scan with CT to get anatomical image and then with PET to get the functional image (*Source:* Courtesy of Dr. Craig Levin). (b) Overlapped PET/CT images. (*Source:* Hg6996 [6]. CC0-1.0 public domain https://creativecommons.org/publicdomain/zero/1.0/).

between holes, a SPECT system can be designed with a desired sensitivity. For a parallel-hole collimator with a gamma ray passing a distance w through one plate of length l, thickness t, and separation distance d, a collimator can be designed to allow a certain percentage of photons through (Figure 14.13). For example, the condition on the collimator thickness necessary for allowing a maximum of 5% of the original light intensity to pass through (for non-perpendicular rays) can be calculated as follows:

$$\text{want: } e^{-\mu w} \le 0.05$$

$$t \ge \frac{6d/\mu}{l - 3/\mu}.$$

For the parallel-hole collimator pictured in Figure 14.13, the plate thickness must be at least 0.13 mm to limit the transmission to 5%. Note that the physical parameters of the collimator can be

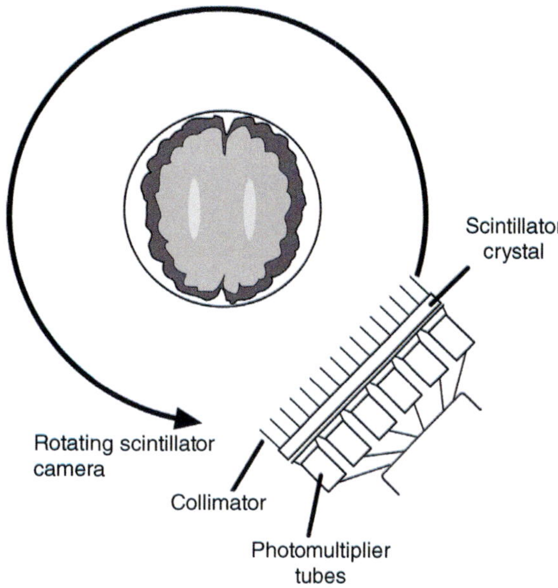

Figure 14.12 SPECT camera is rotated around the subject to create a 3D functional image.

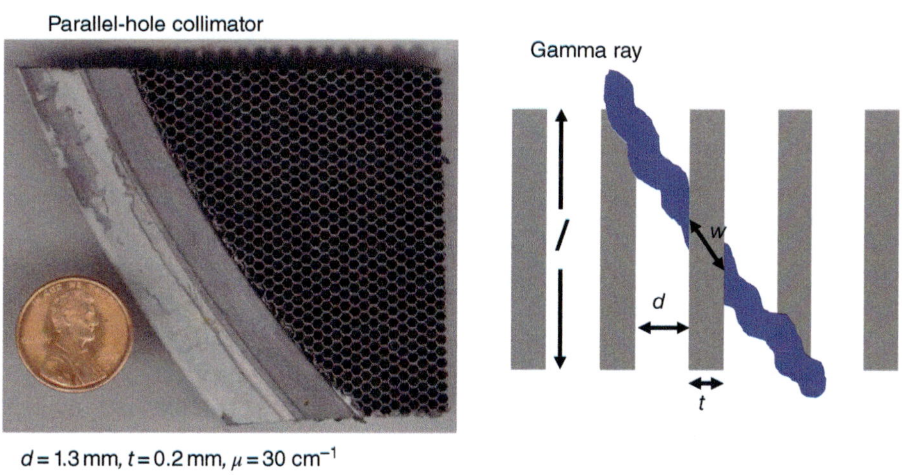

Figure 14.13 Image of an actual collimator and the metal plate thickness requirement for 95% attenuation of non-perpendicular beams. *Source:* Image courtesy of Dr. Craig Levin.

related by $t = 2\,dw/(l-w)$. If the gamma ray is perpendicular to the detector, the collimator does not cause any attenuation.

14.3.2 SPECT Configurations

For rapid imaging, multiple heads can be designed into a SPECT system, e.g. a triple-head system that only scans 120° instead of 360°. The SPECT industry has settled on a double head system to save costs since scintillating crystals are expensive. Modern SPECT systems can use tens or even hundreds of panels made from MEMS, so the rotation can be performed very quickly (Figure 14.14).

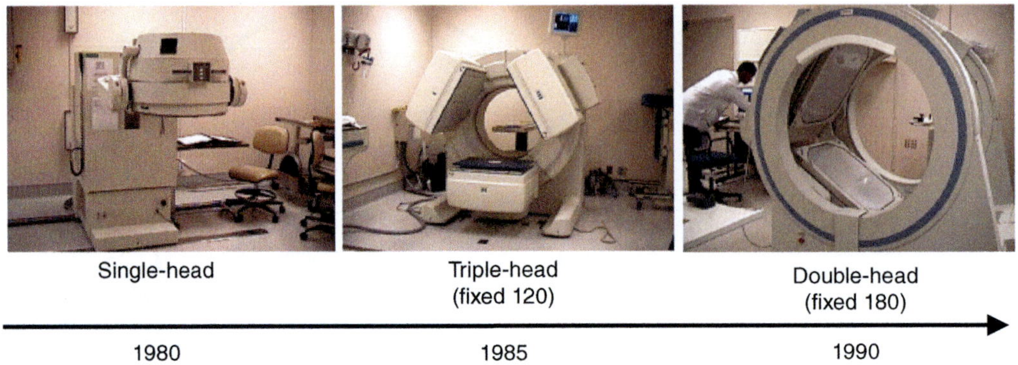

Figure 14.14 SPECT configurations over time. *Source:* Image courtesy of Dr. Craig Levin.

Table 14.3 SPECT versus PET

	SPECT	PET
Energy	Lower-energy γ rays	Higher-energy γ rays
Spatial resolution	5–7 mm	2–4 mm
Temporal resolution	Minutes	10 seconds – minutes
Depth	No limit	No limit
Sensitivity	10–100 pM	1–10 pM
Quantitative degree	++	+++
cost	$$$	$$$$
Multiplexing (imaging multiple probes simultaneously)	Yes (different isotopes result in different photon energies)	No (all photons are 511 keV)
Advantages	Many probes available, multiplexing	High sensitivity, isotope can substitute naturally occurring atoms, quantitative
Disadvantages	Low sensitivity, radioactivity	Costly synthesis, radioactivity

14.3.3 SPECT versus PET

SPECT and PET systems are similar in that they measure radioactivity to form an image, but they have many differences, which are summarized in Table 14.3. Most notably, SPECT has the advantage of multiplexing capability and the disadvantage of low sensitivity, while PET has the advantages of high sensitivity and quantitative detection and the disadvantage of costly synthesis. Both forms of radionuclide imaging have the disadvantage of radioactivity and its associated side effects on the patient.

14.4 Contrast and Imaging Agents

14.4.1 Contrast Agents

Contrast agents should ideally have several properties, including **good clearance**, **specific signal**, **non-toxicity**, and **amplification**. Good clearance through the patient's system is typically handled by the urinary system and is important for reducing toxicity and other side effects. An oral contrast agent may not efficiently reach the target in the gastrointestinal tract, so a contrast agent is usually administered through intravenous (IV) injection, allowing the kidneys clear it out. Getting a specific signal from the contrast agent is vital for image quality. A good contrast agent should rapidly find its target and accumulate in the targeted region to create a specific signal. It is also important for the contrast agent to clear out the circulation as fast as possible because the contrast agents in the blood circulation at the time of imaging may cause extra background noise. Amplification of the signal may be implemented by leveraging some biological mechanism that will allow many contrast agents accumulate in the target by interacting with only one target molecule (e.g. enzyme), thereby increasing specific signal from the target tissue or cell.

14.4.2 Imaging Agents

Contrast agents are non-targeted, i.e. they do not target a specific molecular event in a tissue. Imaging agents are targeted by either direct or indirect targeting. In direct targeting, the imaging agent can either bind to the target (e.g. radiolabeled antibody targeted to a receptor) or be "activated" or "captured" by the target (e.g. FGD and FLT). In indirect targeting, the imaging agent interacts with a protein that is expressed by the same promoter as the target protein so that a high level of that protein indicates a high level of the target protein.

14.4.3 Radioactive Glucose – FDG

A common imaging agent used in PET is **^{18}F-Fluorodeoxyglucose (FDG)**, shown in Figure 14.15. It is the most frequently used PET agent and has multiple uses in imaging cancer, heart disease, and neural diseases. It is created by replacing a hydroxyl (OH) group in glucose with radioactive fluorine (^{18}F), which is then administered to the patient.

FDG targets areas of high glucose metabolism, such as tumor cells, because both glucose and FDG are transported into cells as part of the glycolytic pathway. Hexokinase enzyme is essential for phosphorylation (i.e. adding a phosphate group) in glucose metabolism and is upregulated upon high metabolism by a cell (e.g. in a cancer cell). Upon interaction with either FDG or glucose, hexokinase phosphorylates the molecule (i.e. adds phosphorus to it), which traps it inside the cell (amplification). While phosphorylated glucose continues in the glycolytic pathway (i.e. metabolism of glucose), the phosphorylated FDG becomes trapped inside the cell and does not continue in the glycolytic pathway, which amplifies the image signal (Figure 14.16). Therefore, FDG is an imaging agent for glucose metabolism and FDG uptake is dependent on the number of glucose channels and hexokinase activity.

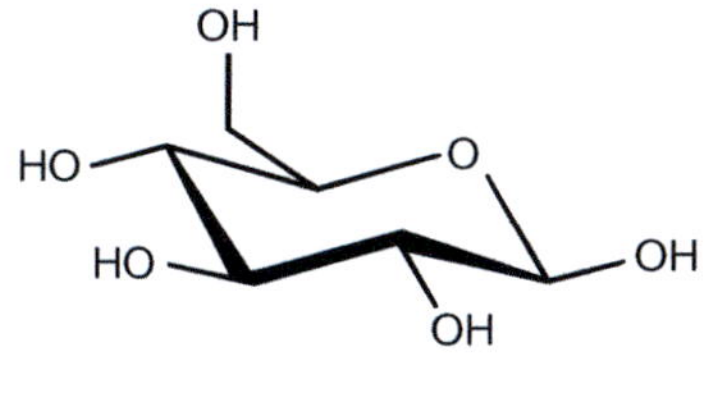

D-Glucose

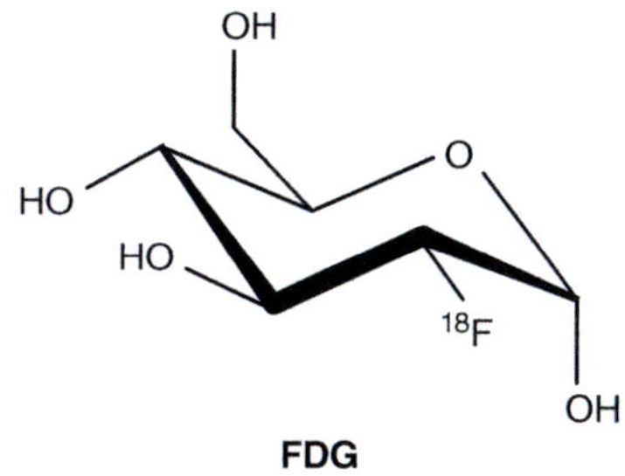

FDG

Figure 14.15 Regular glucose and FDG. *Source:* Yikrazuul [7]. CC0-1.0 public domain https://creativecommons.org/publicdomain/zero/1.0/; Anypodetos [8]. CC0-1.0 public domain https://creativecommons.org/publicdomain/zero/1.0/.

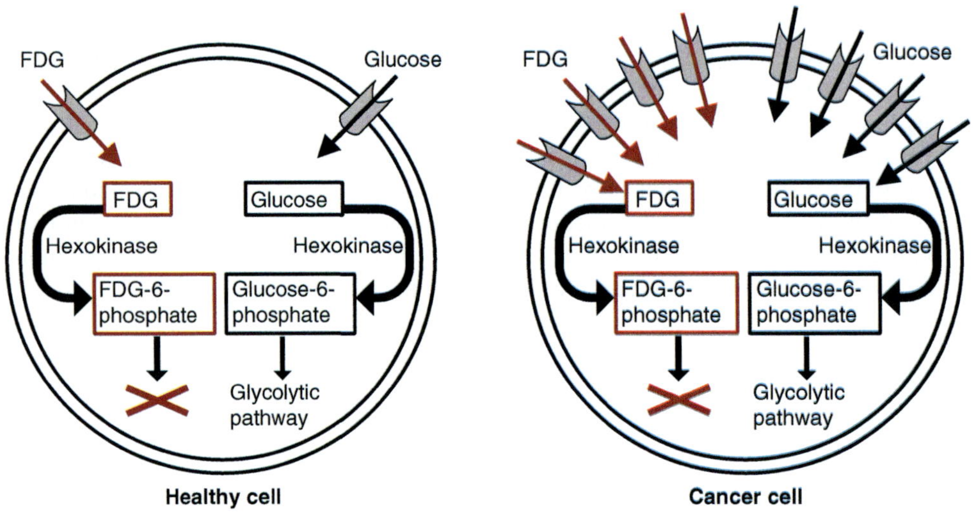

Figure 14.16 FDG accumulation in a cancer cell compared to a normal cell.

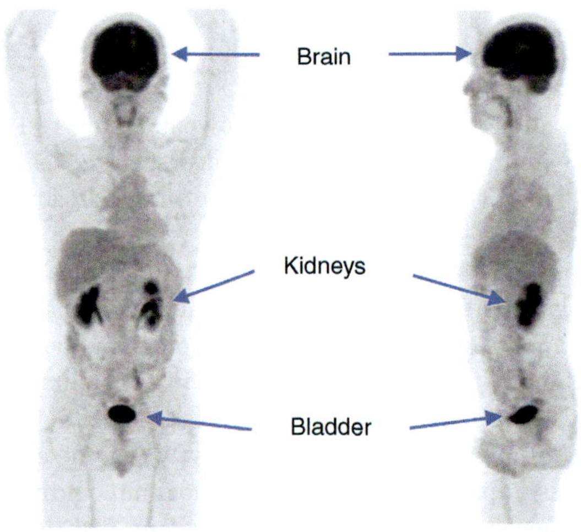

Figure 14.17 FDG-PET of a healthy person. *Source:* By courtesy of Hamamatsu Medical Imaging Center.

An FDG-PET scan of a healthy person (Figure 14.17) shows that there are no sites of especially high glucose metabolism occurring, other than the brain (which has high intrinsic metabolic activity and is therefore typically left out of FDG scans). The bladder shows a high signal as FDG is cleared from the body through the urinary system and therefore collected in the bladder.

14.4.4 FDG-PET in Monitoring Treatment

FDG-PET can be used to monitor cancer treatment. For example, an FDG-PET image of a 63-year-old patient with squamous cell carcinoma shows intense focal accumulation of FDG in the tumor before therapy (Figure 14.18a, the tumors are indicated by arrows). The tumor is also visualized in a T_1-weighted MRI. After four weeks of chemoradiotherapy treatment, the FDG-PET image reveals normalization of FDG uptake, i.e. the "hot spot" has disappeared and glucose metabolism activity is much lower, indicating that the treatment is working (Figure 14.18b). The MRI still

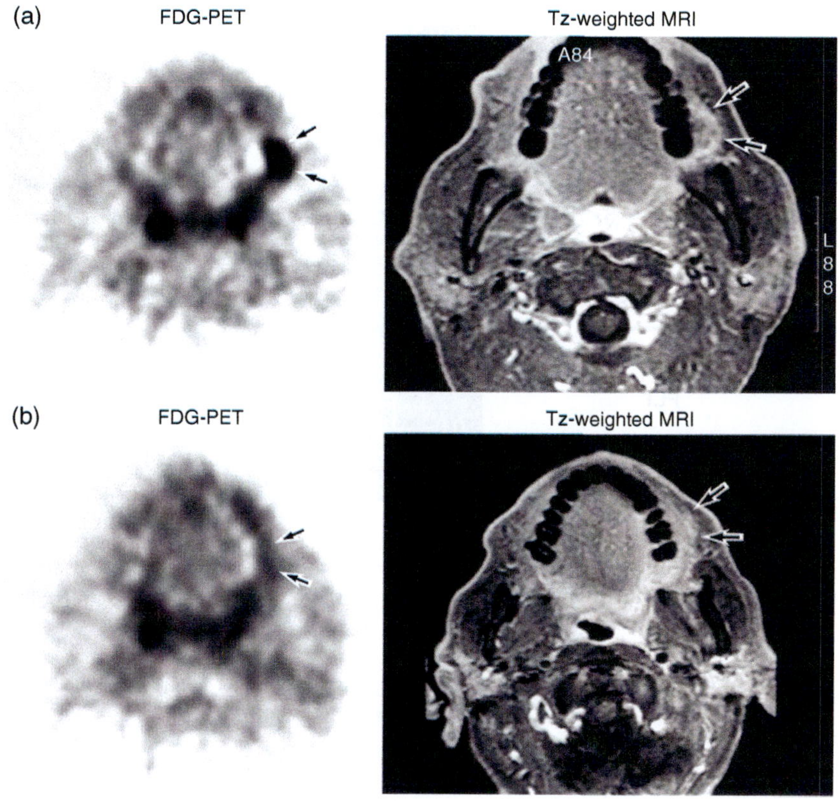

Figure 14.18 (a) Pretreatment and (b) post-treatment images. *Source:* Kitagawa et al. [9]. This research was originally published in JNM. Figure 1. © by the Society of Nuclear Medicine and Molecular Imaging, Inc.

shows contrast enhancement in the tumor, which falsely indicates residual tumor. Therefore, an FDG-PET image was more specific than the MRI image and the patient was able to avoid surgery.

14.4.5 ^{18}FLT Imaging Agent

FLT is **3′-Deoxy-3′-[^{18}F]fluorothymidine**, another imaging agent that is made by replacing a hydroxyl (OH) group in Thymidine by radioactive ^{18}F. Thymidine kinase-1 enzyme (TK-1), an enzyme that is expressed during the DNA synthesis phase of the cell cycle, is responsible for phosphorylating Thymidine and is upregulated in cells with high proliferation activity. TK-1 also phosphorylates FLT; however, since FLT cannot be used by cells to build DNA, it cannot exit the cell after phosphorylation and is trapped inside proliferating cells (just as FDG is trapped inside cells with high glucose metabolism). [^{18}F]FLT-PET is used to detect and monitor tumor proliferation, evaluate the stage of tumor, and detect metastasis. For example, [^{18}F]FLT-PET/CT scans of a patient with non-small-cell lung cancer show reduction of tumor "hot spots" that indicate cell proliferation activity (Figure 14.19).

14.4.6 FDG versus FLT

Due to their different targeting mechanisms, FDG-PET and FLT-PET can each detect certain tumors that the other may miss. For example, the brain does not produce as much signal with

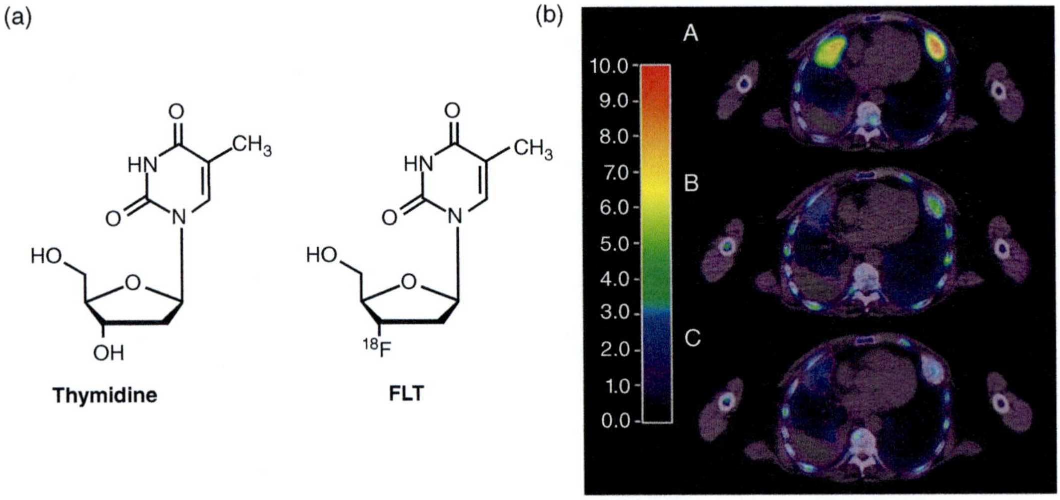

Figure 14.19 (a) Regular Thymidine and FLT. *Source:* Leung [10], (b) FLT-PET/CT scans of non-small-cell lung cancer patient before (top), after 7 days (middle), and 26 days (bottom) after start of tyrosine kinase inhibitor treatment. *Source:* Reprinted from Bollineni et al. [11], Copyright © 2018, with permission from Elsevier.

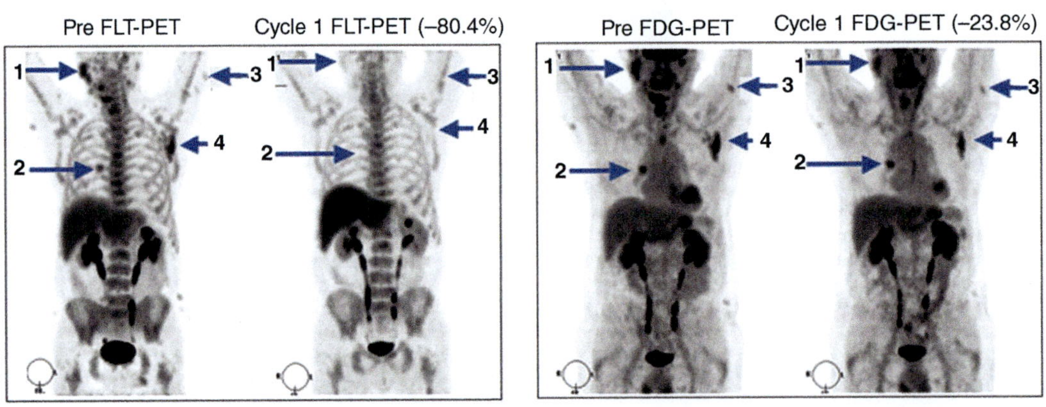

Figure 14.20 FLT (left images) and FDG (right images) of a patient before therapy ("Pre" images) and three weeks into treatment ("Cycle 1" images). *Source:* From Leonard, et al. [12], Republished with permission of American Society of Hematology: Blood. Copyright © 2012; permission conveyed through Copyright Clearance Center, Inc.

FLT-PET compared to FDG-PET since brain cells divide slowly. Both imaging agents show high signal in the bladder due to accumulation in the excretory system. Figure 14.20 shows comparison between FLT and FDG images of a patient both before and three weeks into treatment. Note that in the images taken during treatment, all the tumors are more easily detected using FDG as opposed to FLT.

14.4.7 ^{99m}Tc-MDP Bone Scan

^{99m}Tc-Methyl diphosphonate (^{99m}Tc-MDP) is a commonly used contrast agent for skeletal imaging, primarily for detection of neoplasm (cancer), infections, or trauma (Figure 14.21). Since

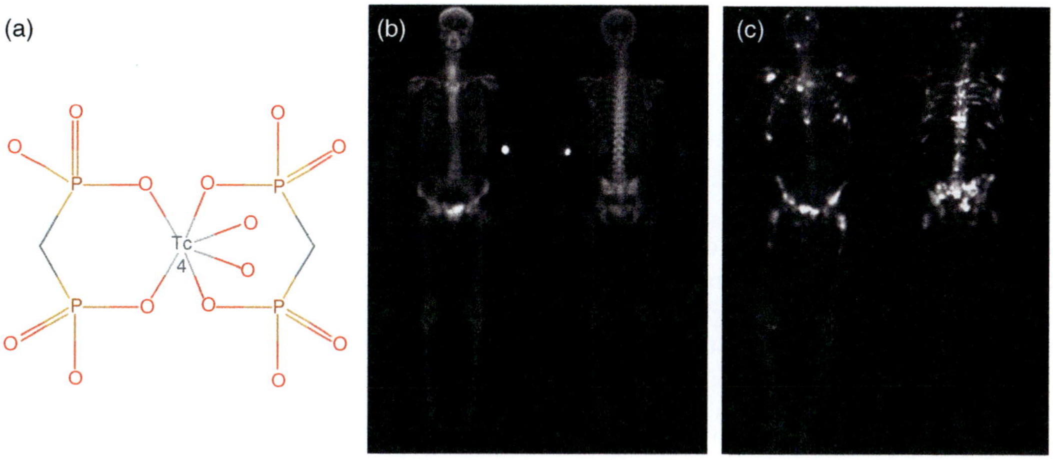

Figure 14.21 (a) ^{99m}Tc-MDP molecule (*Source:* Chopra [13]), (b) ^{99m}Tc-MDP scan of a healthy patient (*Source:* NMT Procedures 2011 [14]. Used under CC-BY-SA 3.0 https://creativecommons.org/licenses/by-sa/3.0/), and (c) ^{99m}Tc-MDP scan of a metastatic prostate cancer patient (*Source:* McAninch and Lue [15], Copyright © 2013 by The McGraw-Hill Companies, Inc.).

treatment of internal bone injuries requires very invasive procedures, proper diagnosis is critical. ^{99m}Tc-MDP-SPECT provides detailed information about the anatomy and physiological state of the bone. Bone ^{99m}Tc-MDP-SPECT is used to detect early bone death, to investigate internal derangement and stress fractures of the knee, and also to monitor bone metastasis in breast, gastric, and prostate cancers.

Bone SPECT imaging reveals changes in bone metabolism (bone turnover or blood flow) rather than changes in bone structure. It is very sensitive because it reveals the metabolism of the bone, but usually specificity is very low (i.e. many diseases will cause an abnormal bone scan). Bone SPECT imaging is useful for stress fractures (the result of repeated low-level impact) and confirmation of fracture when radiography is normal.

14.4.8 SPECT Multiplexing

SPECT has multiplexing capability to image multiple contrast or imaging agents. Since each radioactive isotope produces a different energy γ, SPECT detectors with sufficiently high-energy resolution can separate the SPECT to their components. For example, the image in Figure 14.22 shows

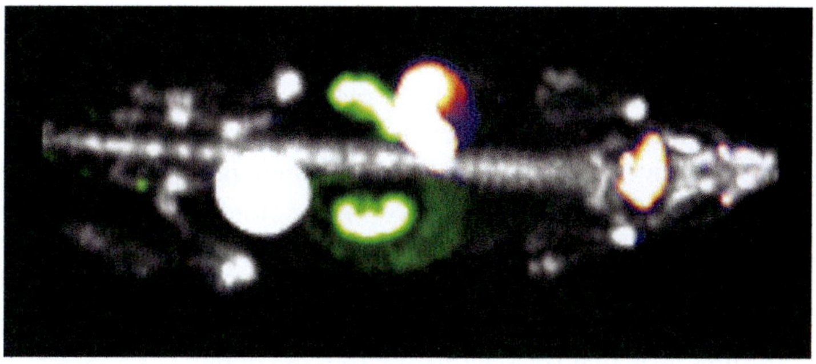

Figure 14.22 Multiplexed SPECT imaging with three different radioactive tracers. *Source:* Courtesy of JP Norenberg, Keck-UNM Small-Animal Imaging Resource (KUSAIR).

multiplexing with multiple imaging agents: ^{99m}Tc-MDP bone uptake is visualized in gray, ^{123}I uptake (red) is clearly visible in the thyroid, small intestine, and eyes, while ^{201}Tl (green) uptake is mostly evident in the kidneys.

14.5 Conclusion

PET and SPECT are two forms of radionuclide imaging, which use radioactive decay of injected contrast or imaging agents to produce images of tissues. Compared to MRI, nuclear imaging has some advantages, including higher resolution and sensitivity, and multiplexing capability with SPECT. Unlike MRI, for which our body will naturally give a good signal without injection, nuclear imaging requires the injection of contrast agents or imaging agents since the body naturally is not radioactive enough to produce a good signal. Therefore, nuclear imaging has the disadvantages of toxicity and side effects from radioactivity, in addition to higher cost.

Problems

14.1 At time $t = 0$, a batch of FDG was prepared and inserted into a syringe. One hour later, the activity from the syringe was measured to be 5 mCi and its content was injected in full to a patient.

A How many radioactive FDG molecules were in the syringe at the time of injection?

B How many radioactive FDG molecules were in the syringe at time $t = 0$?

14.2 Suppose we have a radionuclide X that decays with decay constant λ_X to form a daughter nucleus Y. This daughter nucleus then decays with decay constant λ_Y. Let N_X and N_Y be the number of X and Y nuclei, respectively, present at time t, and also let $N_{X0} = N_X(t = 0)$. Also, it is known that $\lambda_X > \lambda_Y$. The activity of Y is given by:

$$-\frac{dN_Y}{dt} = \lambda_Y N_Y - \lambda_X N_X = \lambda_Y N_Y - \lambda_X N_{X0} e^{-\lambda_X t},$$

to which the solution (assuming $N_Y(t = 0) = 0$) is:

$$N_Y(t) = \frac{\lambda_X}{\lambda_Y - \lambda_X} N_{X0}\left(e^{-\lambda_X t} - e^{-\lambda_Y t}\right).$$

A We would expect the shape of $N_Y(t)$ to look like (choose one and explain why).

i) Increasing with t

ii) Increasing with t up to a maximum value, then decreasing to zero

iii) Increasing with t up to a maximum value, then staying at a constant value

B Find the time at which the maximum value occurs.

C Find the time at which there is an equal amount of radionuclide X and radionuclide Y.

D Assuming $\lambda_X < \lambda_Y$, is there a maximal proportion between λ_Y and λ_X for which there is a time t_0 where $N_X(t_0) = N_Y(t_0)$? If so, find that maximal proportion. Otherwise, explain.

14.3 A patient with cancer walks into a clinic to get a PET scan. He is injected with the radioactive FDG molecules with an activity of 1 mCi at time $t = 0$. At time $t = 1$ hour, the doctor measures an activity of 3.7×10^6 Bq from the tumor.

Please assume:

1) Non-tumor cells capture a negligible amount of FDG molecules.
2) All FDG molecules not captured by tumor cells will be cleared out of the bloodstream after one hour of injection.
3) Once an FDG molecule is captured by a cell, it will stay in the cell for the next six hours.
   - **A** How many FDG molecules are captured by the tumor? What percentage of the original injected FDG molecules was captured by the tumor?
   - **B** At $t = 3$ hours, what will be the activity from the tumor? How many radioactive FDG molecules are now present in the tumor?

14.4 ^{22}Na, a positron-emitting isotope of sodium with a half-life of 2.6 years, is often used to create point-sources to test PET detectors and systems.

- **A** Sarah has recently purchased a ^{22}Na point source to test her newly developed PET detector. The source came with an information sheet stating that the activity of the source was measured to be 100 μCi at the time of preparation. How many parent nuclei were present at the time of preparation?
- **B** Sarah initially set the point source 2 cm away from her single detector as shown in Figure 14.23. Assuming each decay results in two 511 keV photons oriented at 0° and 180°, all the photons travel along a straight line, and she measures for 1 second, how many photons should reach the detector when using the point source 100 days after its preparation?
- **C** To model the annihilation photons passing through the body, Sarah placed the point source inside a container of water shown below with a linear attenuation coefficient of $\mu(511\,\text{keV}) = 0.096\,\text{cm}^{-1}$, as shown in Figure 14.24. Using the same assumptions as in part (b), how many photons should reach the detector when using the point source 100 days after its preparation? *Hint: Recall that the Beer–Lambert relates the attenuation of photons travelling through a medium as* $\frac{I}{I_0} = e^{-\mu l}$.
- **D** She is surprised to find that her detector is only detecting 30% of the calculated photons in part (c). Give three reasons why this may be occurring.

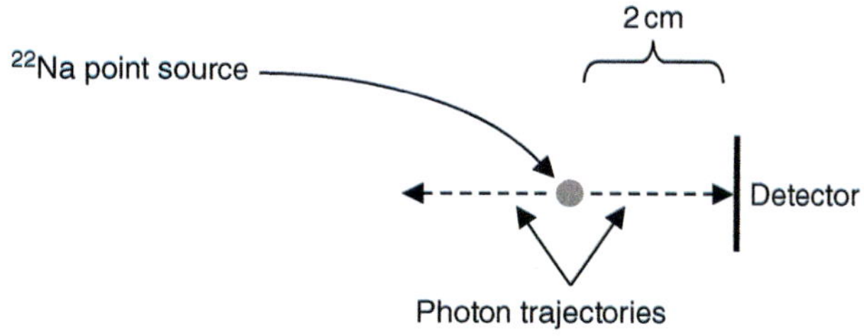

Figure 14.23 Schematic of experiment using a ^{22}Na point source.

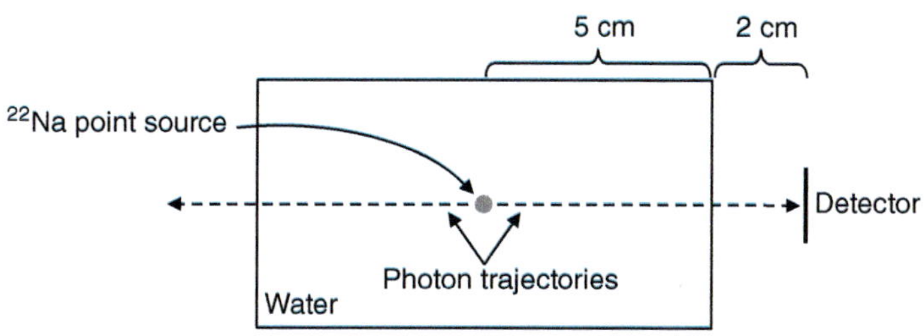

Figure 14.24 Schematic of experimental setup used for modeling annihilation photons.

14.5 A patient is injected with ^{18}FLT. A time-of-flight PET system is used to acquire an image of the patient. The PET system detectors can localize signals in time with an accuracy of ± 0.1 ns. During the scan, two opposite detectors have "clicked" 0.5 ns one after the other (the right detector clicked first, and the left detector clicked 0.5 ns later).

Where did the radioactive decay occur? With what accuracy can that be determined? (You may assume that both detectors lie on the x-axis and that $x = 0$ is exactly the midpoint between the detectors).

14.6 Explain why PET/CT imaging is more commonly used in hospitals than traditional PET imaging, despite the much higher cost of PET/CT systems.

14.7 A SPECT linear collimator was designed with septum thickness t, displacement between septa d, length of septa l, and septa absorbance μ. The designer would like to find the minimum required septa thickness t such that any beam that goes through the septa (i.e. a beam that the collimator is intended to remove and prevent from reaching the detectors, by hitting one of the sides of the collimator) would be attenuated to at least 0.05 of its original intensity. As linear collimators are intended to allow only γ rays that are nearly perpendicular to the detectors to go through, you may assume that $l >> 2d + t$. You may consider unwanted γ rays as rays that hit one of the sides of a septum (i.e. ignore rays which hit the front side of the septum).
Hint: The final solution is given in the chapter; you only need to find the way to it. . .

14.8 Explain why SPECT has a lower sensitivity and a lower spatial resolution compared to PET.

14.9 ^{18}FDG is a PET imaging agent that is based on a ^{18}F that is attached to a glucose molecule.
- **A** How many ^{18}FDG molecules are in a vial that measures 3 mCi of activity?
- **B** The ^{18}F in this ^{18}FDG is five hours old. What portion of the glucose-like molecules in the vial is still radioactive?
- **C** How would your answer to (a) and (b) change if instead of ^{18}FGD, we had ^{99m}Tc-MDP in the vial?

14.10 ^{18}FLT is a PET imaging agent that is based on a ^{18}F that is attached to a thymidine molecule.
- **A** What is the activity (in Ci) of 10^9 molecules of ^{18}FLT?
- **B** After three hours, how many radioactive molecules are left from the original 10^9?
- **C** How would your answers to (a) and (b) change if instead of ^{18}F, one attaches ^{99m}Tc to the thymidine?

14.11 Explain the mechanism of targeting and amplification for FDG and FLT and highlight the similarities and differences between the two radiotracers.

14.12 We created a new imaging agent ^{18}FLA (Deoxy-^{18}Fluoro-adenosine). As a reminder, deoxy-adenosine is the nucleobase "A" in the DNA. Similar to deoxy-thymidine ("T" in DNA), there is a kinase enzyme called "adenosine-kinase" (AS) which phosphorylates deoxy-adenosine.
- **A** Explain what kind of cells this new imaging agent will target.
- **B** Explain the amplification mechanism of ^{18}FLA.

References

1 Damato, https://commons.wikimedia.org/wiki/File:PET-MIPS-anim.gif
2 Zereshk, https://commons.wikimedia.org/wiki/File:Coincidence_detection_Persian.PNG
3 Than, T.D., Alici, G., Harvey, S. et al. (2014). Concept and simulation study of a novel localization method for robotic endoscopic capsules using multiple positron emission markers. *Med. Phys.* 41: 072501. doi:10.1118/1.4881316.
4 Mako098765, https://commons.wikimedia.org/wiki/File:Photomultipliertube.svg
5 Li, Y., Matej, S., and Metzler, S.D. (2014). Image reconstructions from super-sampled data sets with resolution modeling in PET imaging. *Med. Phys.* 41: 121912. doi:10.1118/1.4901552 https://aapm.onlinelibrary.wiley.com/doi/full/10.1118/1.4901552.
6 Hg6996, https://sv.wikipedia.org/wiki/Fil:Brownfat_PETCT.jpg
7 Yikrazuul, https://commons.wikimedia.org/wiki/File:Beta-D-Glucose.svg
8 Anypodetos, https://commons.wikimedia.org/wiki/File:Fluorodeoxyglucose_18-F_skeletal.svg
9 Kitagawa, Y., Nishizawa, S., Sano, K. et al. (2003). Prospective comparison of 18F-FDG PET with conventional imaging modalities (MRI, CT, and 67Ga scintigraphy) in assessment of combined intraarterial chemotherapy and radiotherapy for head and neck carcinoma. *J Nucl Med.* 44 (2): 198–206.
10 Leung, K. (2004). 3'-Deoxy-3'-[18F] fluorothymidine. In: *Molecular Imaging and Contrast Agent Database (MICAD) [Internet].* Bethesda, MD: National Center for Biotechnology Information (US); 2004–2013. https://www.ncbi.nlm.nih.gov/books/NBK23373/.
11 Bollineni, V.R., Kramer, G.M., Jansma, E.P. et al. (2016). A systematic review on [18F]FLT-PET uptake as a measure of treatment response in cancer patients. *European Journal of Cancer* 55: 81–97.
12 Leonard, J.P., LaCasce, A.S., Smith, M.R. et al. (2012). Selective CDK4/6 inhibition with tumor response by PD0332991 in patients with mantle cell lymphoma. *American Society of Hematology: Blood* 119 (20): 4597–4607.
13 Chopra, A. (2007). 99mTc-Methyl diphosphonate. In: *Molecular Imaging and Contrast Agent Database (MICAD) [Internet].* Bethesda (MD): National Center for Biotechnology Information (US); 2004–2013. https://www.ncbi.nlm.nih.gov/books/NBK24575/.
14 NMT Procedures 2011, https://nmt-procedures-2011.wikispaces.com/Whole+Body+Bone+Scan
15 McAninch, J.W. and Lue, T.F. *Smith & Tanagho's General Urology*, 18ee. McGraw Hill Professional.

Further Reading

Molecular Imaging and Contrast Agent Database (MICAD). Bethesda, MD: National Center for Biotechnology Information (US). http://www.ncbi.nlm.nih.gov/books/NBK5330/
Craig Levin BIOE 222A lectures
Sanjiv Sam Gambhir BIOE 222A lectures
http://en.wikipedia.org/wiki/Photomultiplier

15

Fluorescence and Raman Imaging

15.1 Introduction to Optical Imaging

Optical imaging is based on the detection of light that has interacted with tissue. It has advantages over other imaging modalities such as MRI, PET, and SPECT, which are expensive, require a long scan time, have low sensitivity (MRI), and use radioactivity (PET and SPECT). The advantages of optical imaging include high resolution, low cost, multiplexing ability, and ability to use during surgery (intraoperative).

Optical imaging is based on the **usable optical spectrum** range of 400–1300 nm wavelength, which includes the visible spectrum and part of the infrared spectrum. Unlike the ionizing radiation used in nuclear imaging, optical imaging uses nonionizing radiation. Light waves with different wavelengths and frequencies will have different energies of light. The energy of a photon is inversely proportional to its wavelength, and is given by:

$$E_{\text{photon}} = hf = \frac{hc}{\lambda},$$

where λ is the wavelength (m), f is the frequency (Hz), c is the speed of light (m/s), E_{photon} is the photon energy, and h is Planck's constant (6.6×10^{-34} J·s). Figure 15.1 shows the range of usage electromagnetic spectrum. Specifically, for optical imaging, wavelengths between 400 and 1300 nm are mostly used (and 650 and 1300 nm *in vivo*).

15.2 Photon/Tissue Interaction

Photons of light can interact with bodily tissue in multiple different ways, including transmission, reflection, refraction, scattering, absorption, and fluorescence (Figure 15.2). In **transmission**, a "ballistic photon" will pass through the tissue without any interaction. In **reflection**, a photon is reflected back 180° from the surface of the tissue, without a change in energy. In **refraction**, a photon changes its direction of propagation due to a change in speed of propagation (or a change in refractive index) according to Snell's Law. In **scattering**, a photon changes its propagation direction. Scattering is measured as μ_s (units of cm^{-1}), and is typically elastic (with no energy change), but sometimes (about 1 in 10 million events) its inelastic (with a change in energy). In **absorption**, which is measured as μ_a (units of cm^{-1}), a photon is absorbed by the material, and typically energy is converted into heat. **Fluorescence** is a subtype of absorption where the absorbed energy is released as a lower energy photon (e.g. blue light causes the emission of red light).

Biochips and Medical Imaging, First Edition. Adam de la Zerda and Shan Xiang Wang.

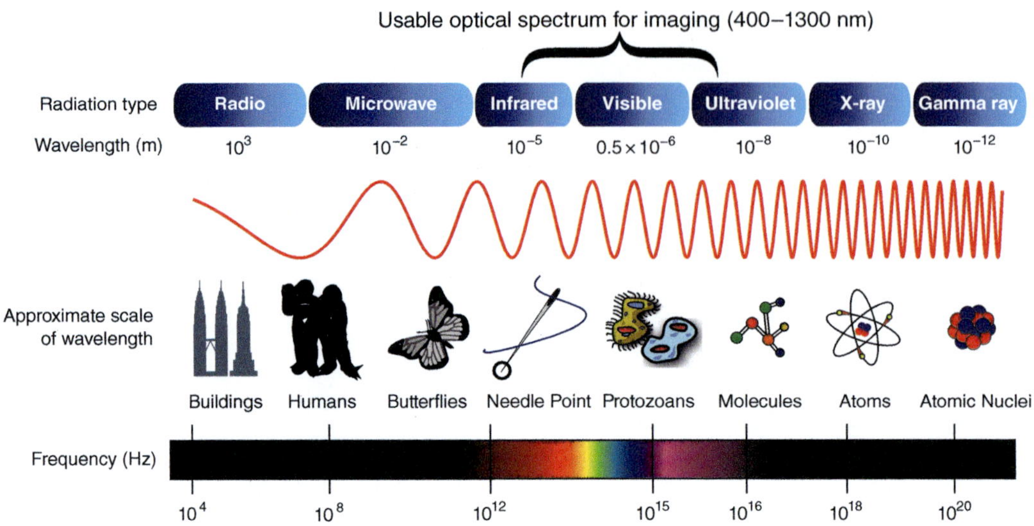

Figure 15.1 Spectrum of optical imaging. *Source:* Courtesy of NASA [1], CC0-1.0 public domain https://creativecommons.org/publicdomain/zero/1.0/

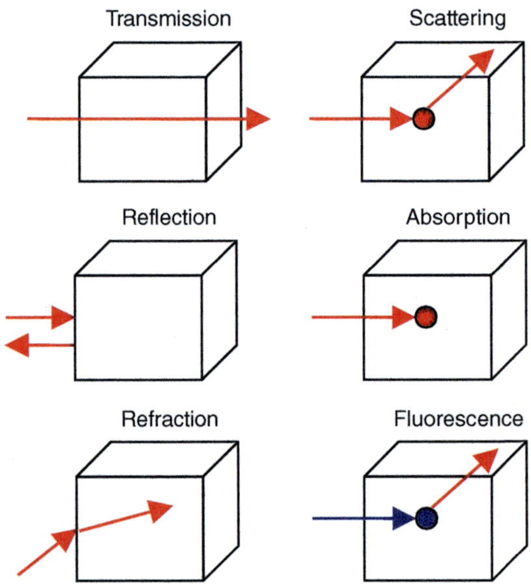

Figure 15.2 Photon/tissue interaction.

15.2.1 Tissue Penetration

Scattering and absorption coefficients will determine how deep a light ray will penetrate a tissue. The lower μ_s and μ_a are, the deeper the light will penetrate. $1/\mu_s$ is the mean scattering-free path (average distance between consecutive photon-scattering events), and $1/\mu_a$ is the "mean free path" for photon travel prior to absorption. The constants μ_s and μ_a depend on the wavelength and the

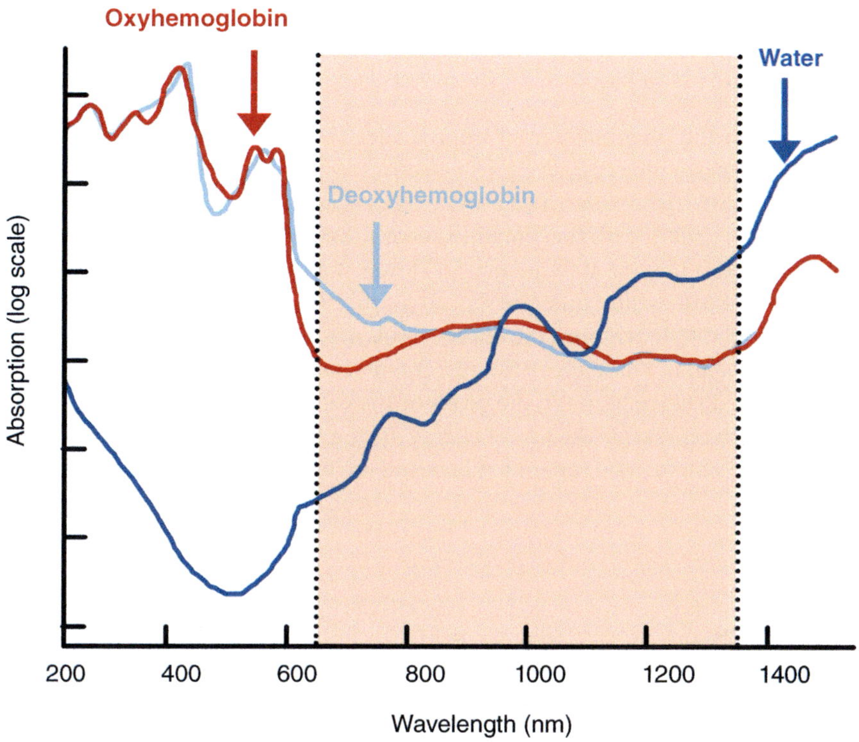

Figure 15.3 Absorption of water and hemoglobin. Notice that around 650–700 nm oxygenated hemoglobin (red) absorbs less light than deoxygenated hemoglobin (blue). Since this region corresponds to red light, oxyhemoglobin appears redder than deoxyhemoglobin.

type of tissue or material, e.g. water, melanin, oxygenated hemoglobin (HbO_2), and deoxygenated hemoglobin (Hb). Recall from Chapter 2 that the extinction coefficient depends on μ_s and μ_a. Hemoglobin (Hb) has high absorption at low wavelengths (less than 650 nm), while water is absorbing at high wavelengths beyond the visible spectrum (greater than 1300 nm). Hence, the "optical window" for optimal tissue penetration is $650 < \lambda < 1300$ nm (Figure 15.3). Typically, other absorbers in the body contribute less to the optical tissue penetration.

There are a number of numerical models to estimate light propagation in tissues, including the radiative transfer equation, the diffusion equation (a simplified version of the radiative transfer equation), and simulations such as finite element and Monte Carlo.

Radiative equation:

$$\frac{1}{c}\frac{\delta I(r,t,\hat{s})}{\delta t}+\hat{s}\cdot\Delta I(r,t,\hat{s})+(\mu_a(r,t))+\mu_s(r,t))I(r,t,\hat{s})=q(r,t,\hat{s})+\mu_s(r,t)\int_{4\pi}f(\hat{s},\hat{s}')I(r,t,\hat{s})\mathrm{d}^2\hat{s}'.$$

The diffusion equation (a simplified version of the radiative equation, valid for depths greater than ~1 mm):

$$-D(r)\Delta^2 I(r)+\mu_a(r)I(r)=q(r).$$

15.3 Fluorescence Imaging

15.3.1 Physics of Fluorescence Imaging

Fluorescence imaging relies on the phenomenon of fluorescence (Figure 15.4), which occurs as follows. First, a photon of light at frequency f_{ex} excites an electron to a higher energy state (from S_0 to S'_1) (**excitation**). Second, the electron moves to a lower energy state S_1 through a (nonradiative) vibrational **relaxation** ("Stokes shift"), with the remaining energy being lost mostly as heat. Third, as the electron moves back to S_0, a photon at frequency f_{em} (lower than f_{ex}) is emitted (**emission**). Different fluorescent molecules will exhibit different f_{ex} and f_{em} profiles.

In molecules, as opposed to individual atoms, the energy levels are bands (i.e. S_0, S'_1, and S_1 represent a continuum of energy bands). Therefore, a fluorescent molecule is characterized by excitation and emission spectra. The distance between the peaks of the excitation and emission spectra is called the **Stokes shift**, which represents the loss of energy during the relaxation step of fluorescence (Figure 15.5). Ideally, we want a good separation between the two spectra. So, having a large Stokes shift is desirable.

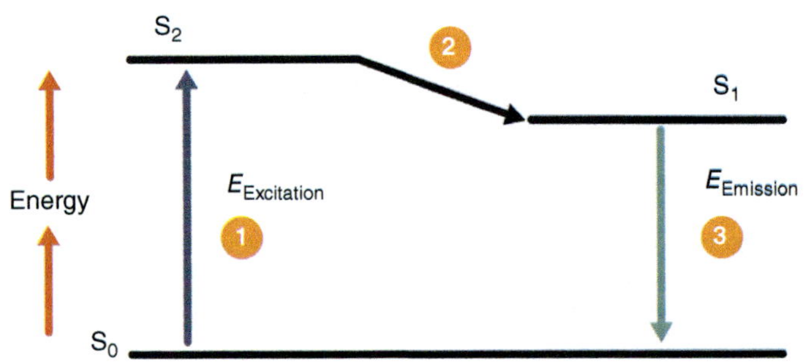

Figure 15.4 Fluorescence steps. *Source:* Courtesy of Bio-Rad.

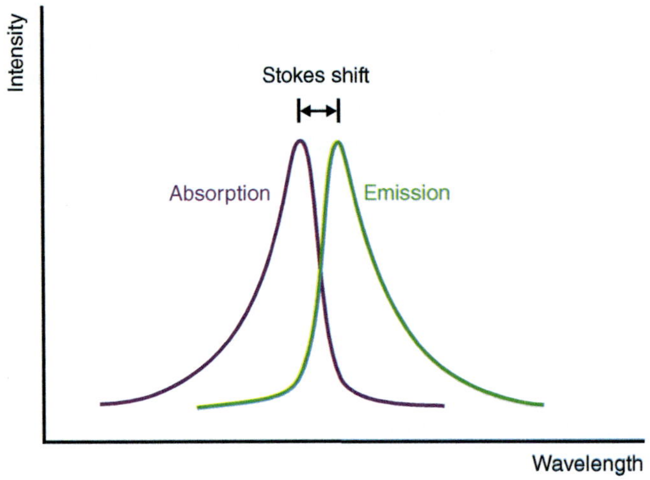

Figure 15.5 Excitation and emission spectra of a fluorescent dye. *Source:* Jacopo Werther [2], used under CC-BY-SA 3.0 https://creativecommons.org/licenses/by-sa/3.0/.

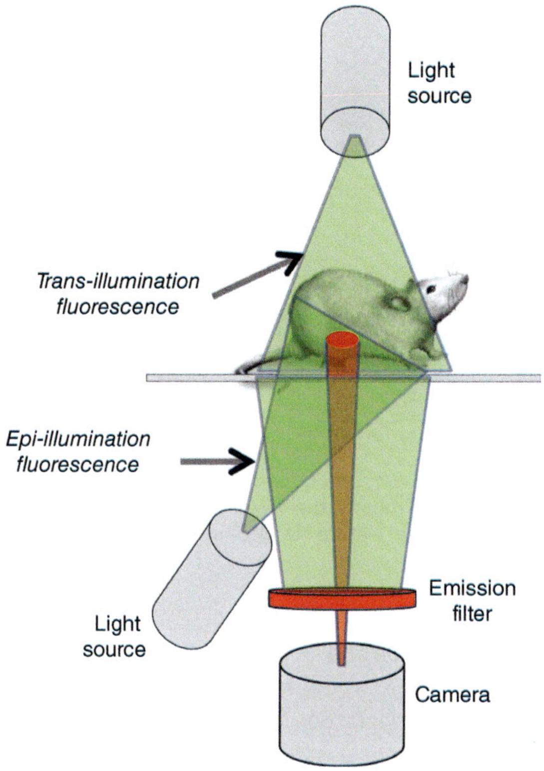

Figure 15.6 Fluorescence imaging setup.

Many implementations of fluorescence imaging systems exist. One common implementation is shown in Figure 15.6. A broad white light source is combined with an excitation filter to illuminate a narrow spectrum of wavelength onto an animal. The fluorescent light that is created within the object reaches the surface of the tissue and filtered by an emission filter (intended to filter out all the excitation light and only allow the fluorescent light through). Third, the fluorescent light is detected optically by a detection apparatus such as a CCD camera. Fluorescence can either be epi-illumination fluorescence (i.e. from the same side as the camera) or trans-illumination fluorescence (i.e. illumination on the opposite side of the camera), which is more challenging since the light needs to penetrate through the entire subject, such as a mouse.

As fluorescent light from the target is propagating through the tissue, it is scattered. This leads to a rapid decrease in spatial resolution as the depth of the target increases, which is one of the biggest disadvantages of fluorescence imaging. For example, epi-fluorescence imaging of a tissue-mimicking phantom with a 4.2 mm-wide inclusion filled with fluorescent quantum dots (QDs) emitting at 800 nm (Figure 15.7a) shows a full-width half-max (FWHM) of 11.5 mm for at a depth of 4.5 mm (Figure 15.7b).

Figure 15.7 actually represents a bigger problem than just blurring of the image. Since the purpose is to determine the actual structure (the cylinder) by looking at the image acquired (on the right), the blurring due to scattering leads to an ill-posed problem. For example, by looking at the image alone, there is no way of knowing if the object is small but located deep in the tissue, or large but located near the surface. As the object goes deeper into the tissue, the image on the

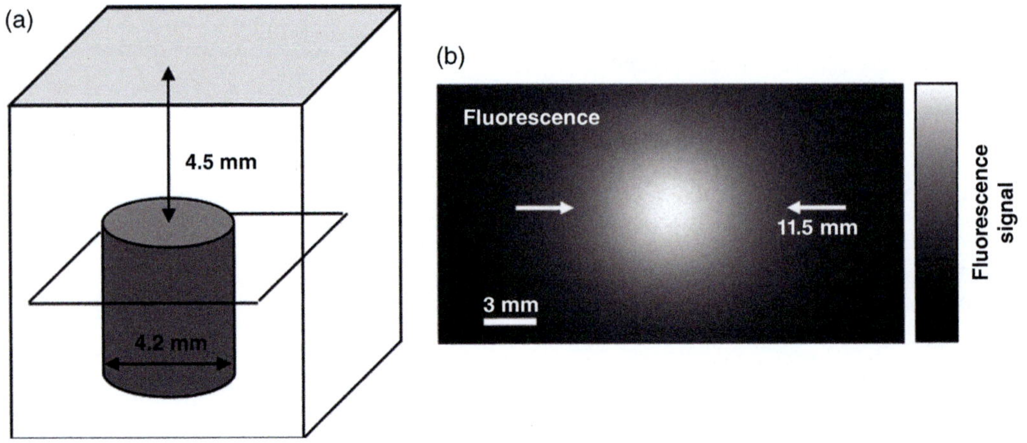

Figure 15.7 (a) Tissue-mimicking phantom with an inclusion of fluorescent quantum dots emitting at 800 nm.(b) Epi-fluorescence of the phantom showing FWHM of 11.5 mm for the 4.2 mm wide inclusion. *Source:* Zerda et al. [3]. Reprinted by permission from Springer Nature: Nature Nanotechnology, Copyright © 2008 by Springer Nature..

surface becomes larger. In Figure 15.7, the object is 4.2 mm wide and located at a depth of 4.5 mm, but the image is 11.5 mm wide. However, a very similar image would have been obtained if the object was 11.5 mm wide and located just below the surface. So, these two scenarios are indistinguishable.

15.3.2 Contrast Agents for Fluorescence Imaging

Fluorescence signal sources can either be **endogenous** (i.e. naturally occurring in the subject) or **exogenous** (i.e. contrast or imaging agents administered to the subject). An endogenous fluorescence signal, or **autofluorescence**, is created by tissue molecules that are fluorescent (e.g. NADH, collagen, riboflavin, folic acid, and melanin). Their excitation and emission spectra are mostly in the range less than 600 nm. In animal imaging, autofluorescence imposes a major hurdle as a "background signal" from sources such as skin and food (Figure 15.8). One of the nicest advancements in the field was the development of nonfluorescent food because it reduces the background fluorescence caused by food autofluorescence.

15.3.3 Contrast Agents – Small Molecules

An exogenous fluorescence signal can be obtained by administering contrast agents to the subject in the form of small molecules or nanoparticles. There are several small-molecule fluorescent contrast agents that are currently used in humans, such as fluorescein and indocyanine green (ICG) (Figure 15.9). They feature the advantage of good urinary clearance. In addition, these fluorophores can be attached to a targeting agent to become an imaging agent and bind to a molecular target. However, small-molecule contrast agents typically have disadvantages of low signal (which results in low sensitivity) and photobleaching of the fluorescence signal, which occurs in response to long laser irradiation. **Photobleaching** is the loss of fluorescence ability in the fluorophores. When fluorophores are exposed to large amounts of light, they change their molecular conformation and lose their ability to fluoresce. Under standard conditions, fluorophores can last several

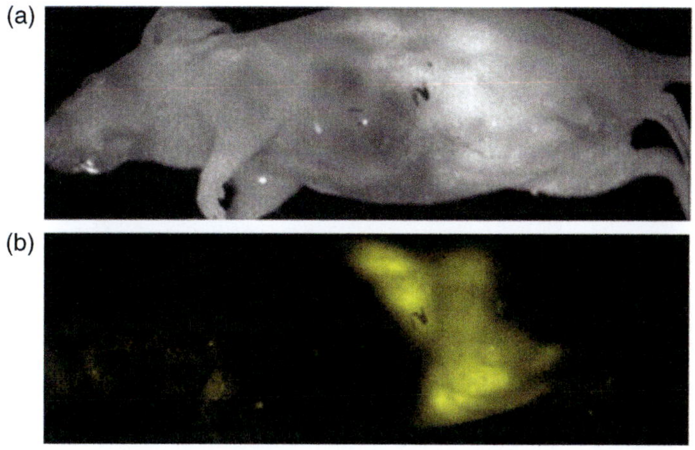

Figure 15.8 (a) Autofluorescence of skin, (b) food. Source: Levenson and Mansfield [4].

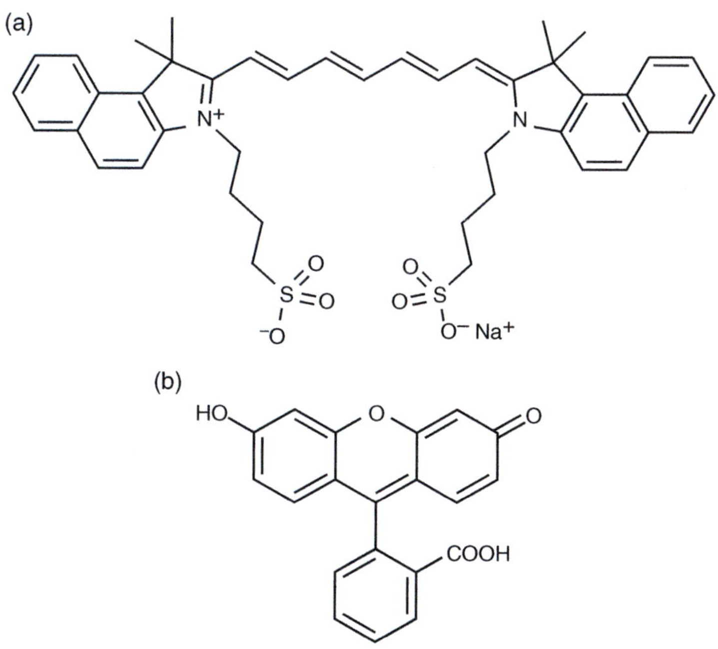

Figure 15.9 (a) Molecular structure of ICG, and (b) Fluorescein.

minutes, hours, or even several days. An example of small-molecule fluorescence imaging is fluorescein angiography (FA) for scanning of the retina (the posterior part of the eye where photodetectors convert light into an electrical signal and send it to the brain) to detect age-related macular degeneration (Figure 15.10). A few minutes after injecting the patient with a fluorescein contrast agent, most of the fluorophores will clear from the blood except for a small portion, which leaks out of the blood vessels in the diseased area.

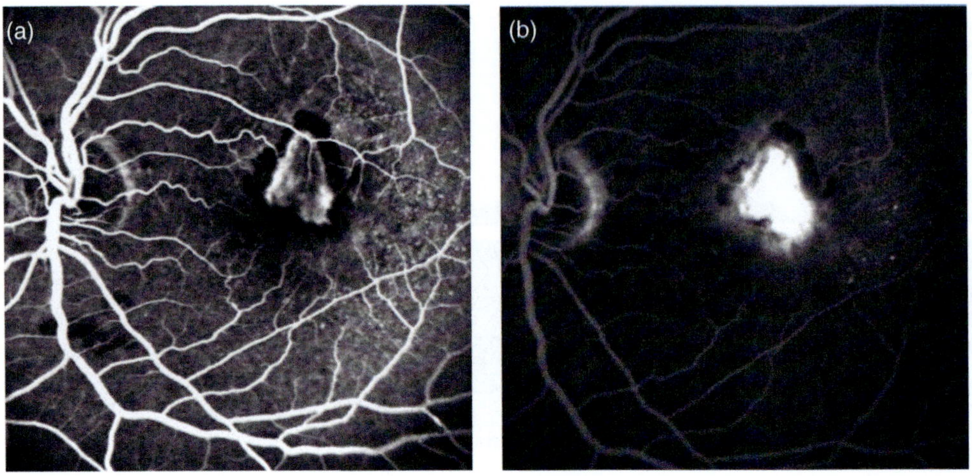

Figure 15.10 Fluorescein angiography (FA). (a) Imaging shortly after injection. (b) Image showing the leakage area. *Source:* Michels et al. [5]. Republished with permission of Association for Research in Vision and Ophthalmology: Investigative ophthalmology & Visual Science, Copyright © 2006; permission conveyed through Copyright Clearance Center, Inc.

15.3.4 Contrast Agents – Nanoparticles

Nanoparticles such as quantum dots are another class of exogenous contrast agents that can be used for fluorescence imaging. **Quantum dots (QDs)** are nanoparticles that are 15–20 nm in diameter. Because they are larger in size than small molecule contrast agents, QDs get more exposure to light and therefore exhibit increased sensitivity. Although QD contrast agents have the advantages of high brightness and no photobleaching, they are potentially toxic. Quantum dots are typically composed of a CdSe core and a ZnS shell. By increasing the size of the QDs, their emission wavelength can be increased. Therefore, QDs of various sizes can be mixed to cover a wide spectrum of fluorescence (Figure 15.11). Since QDs have a very broad excitation spectrum, they can all be excited by the same wavelength of light, but respond by emitting fluorescent light at different wavelengths, which enables multispectral imaging.

15.3.4.1 Applications of QDs

Multispectral imaging can be performed by injecting different-sized QDs into different locations. An example is shown in Figure 15.12, where different-sized QDs were used to image a mouse's lymphatic system operation. Algorithms such as least squares (spectral deconvolution) can then be used to isolate overlapping spectral components.

Another application of QD fluorescence imaging is the use of QDs targeted to $\alpha_v\beta_3$ integrins. RGD is a peptide (fraction of a protein) with a sequence of three key amino acids: arginine (R), glycine (G), and aspartic acid (D). This RGD peptide has been shown to selectively bind to the angiogenic receptor – $\alpha_v\beta_3$ integrin. Hence, QDs with RGD peptides can be used to identify areas of angiogenesis (via direct targeting), such as tumor cells. In one experiment, two identical mice were injected with human glioblastoma (a rapidly growing brain cancer) cells, which formed a tumor on their shoulders. A mouse was then injected intravenously with the QD-RGD (left mouse in Figure 15.13) and a control mouse was injected with QD without the RGD peptide (right mouse). This control experiment is very important as it provides evidence that QD-RGD targeted the $\alpha_v\beta_3$ integrin in the tumor as opposed to nonspecifically accumulating in the tumor. The liver, for

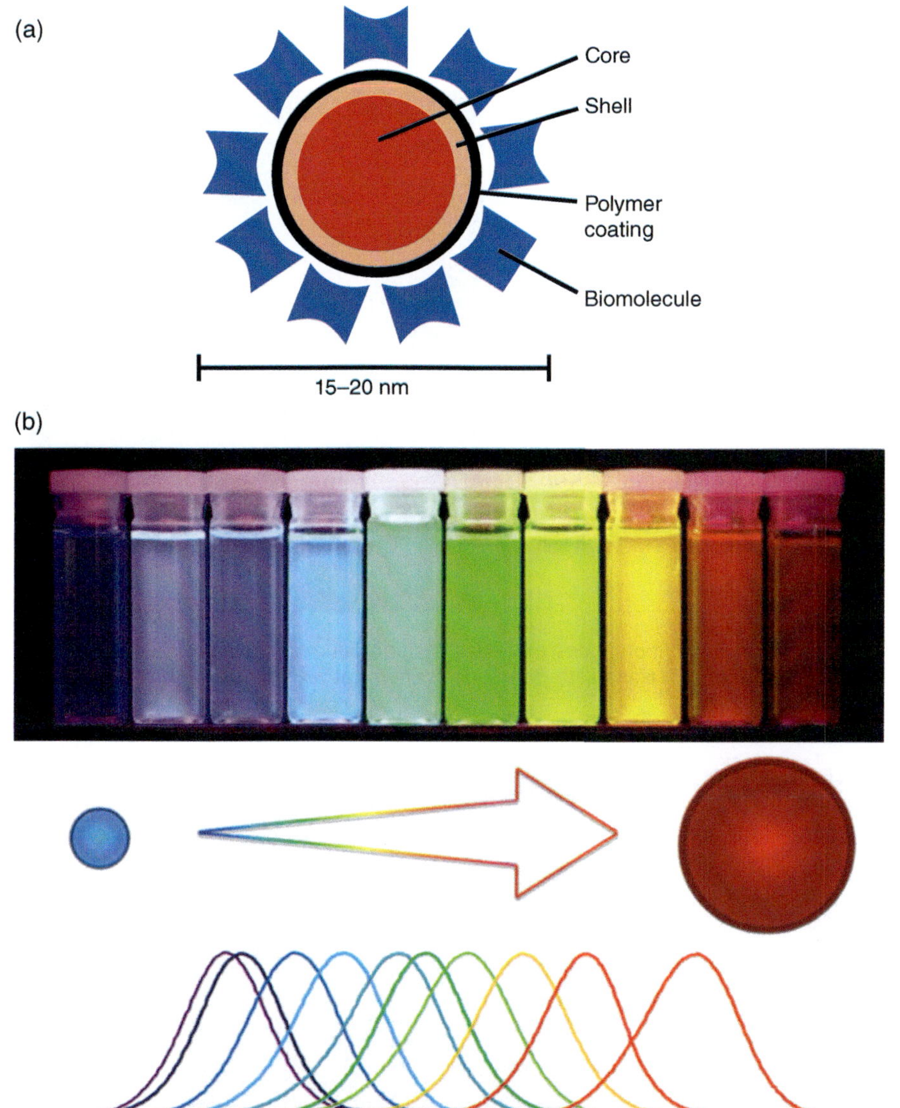

Figure 15.11 (a) The QD structure, (b) size vs. color and fluorescence spectrum. *Source:* Reproduced ("Adapted" or "in part") from Zrazhevskiy et al. [6], with permission of The Royal Society of Chemistry.

example, is nonspecifically taking up the QD-RGD (strong red signal at the mid-right level of the images) in both mice.

15.3.5 Fluorescence Resonance Energy Transfer (FRET)

Fluorescence Resonance Energy Transfer (FRET) is a special case of fluorescence imaging that allows the use of "activatable imaging agents." When a fluorophore is in close proximity with a quencher molecule, an excited donor fluorophore may transfer energy to the acceptor quencher

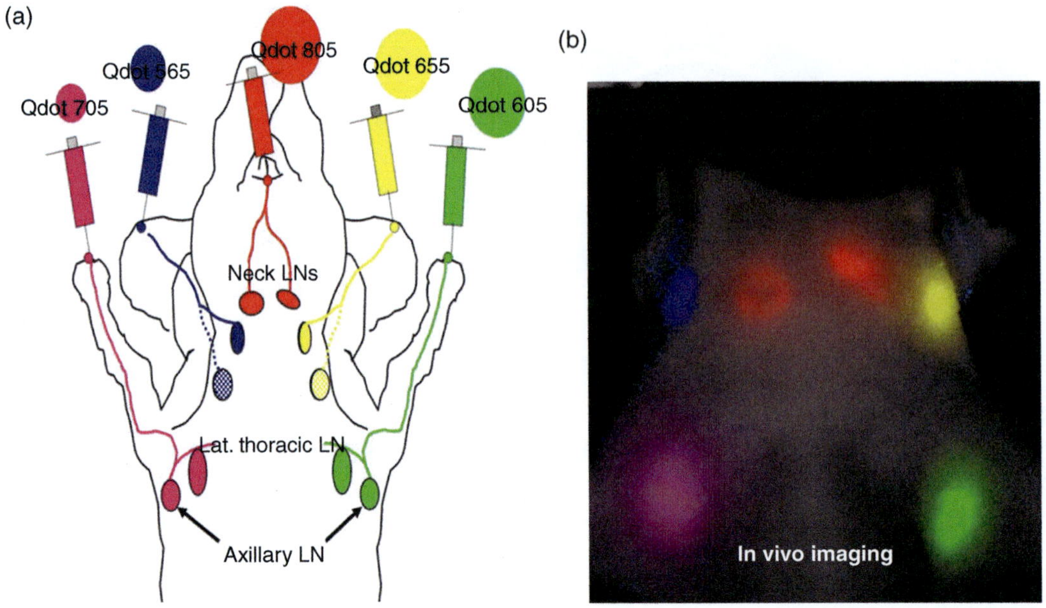

Figure 15.12 (a) Injection of QDs into lymph nodes, (b) *in vivo* imaging. *Source:* Kobayashi et al. [7]. Reprinted (adapted) with permission from Nano Letters: American Chemical Society, Copyright © 2007 American Chemical Society.

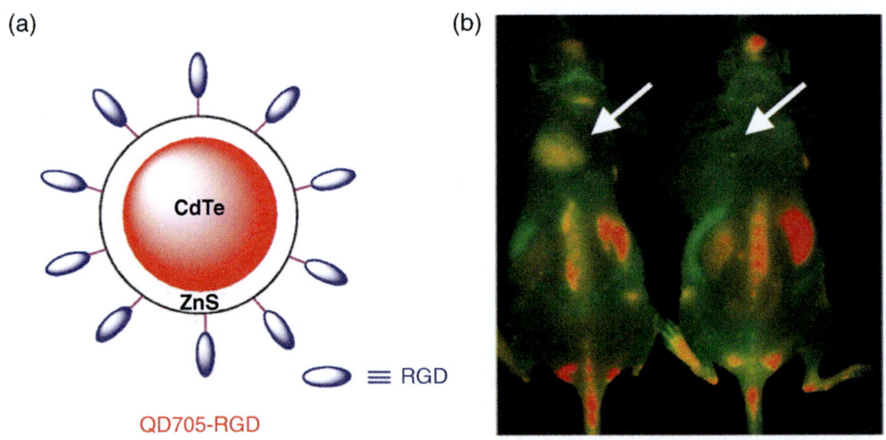

Figure 15.13 (a) QD with RGD peptides. (b) The mouse on the left is injected with QD-RGD. The mouse on the right (control) is injected with QDs only (no RGD). Arrows indicate tumor locations. *Source:* Cai et al. [8]. Reprinted (adapted) with permission from Nano Letters: American Chemical Society, Copyright © 2006, American Chemical Society.

through non-radiative dipole-dipole coupling, rather than fluorescence (Figure 15.14). The efficiency of FRET depends on $1/R_0^6$ (where R_0 is the distance between the two molecules). Hence, fluorescence typically occurs when R_0 is greater than 10 nm, and FRET occurs when R_0 is less than 10 nm (i.e. when most fluorescence is quenched). By controlling the interaction of fluorophores and quencher molecules, FRET can be activated in certain targeted areas. The acceptor can also be a fluorophore and fluoresce instead of a quench.

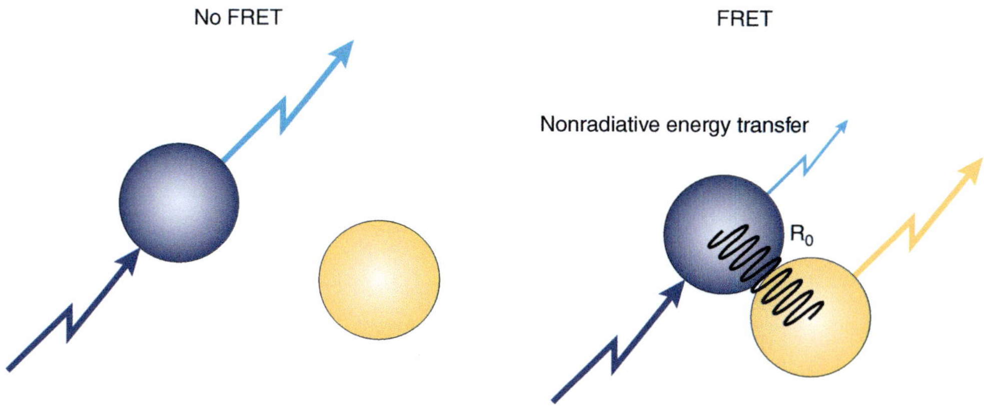

Figure 15.14 Fluorophore (blue) and quencher (yellow). *Source:* Rudolf et al. [9]. Reprinted by permission from Springer Nature: Nature Reviews Molecular Cell Biology, Copyright © 2003 by Springer Nature.

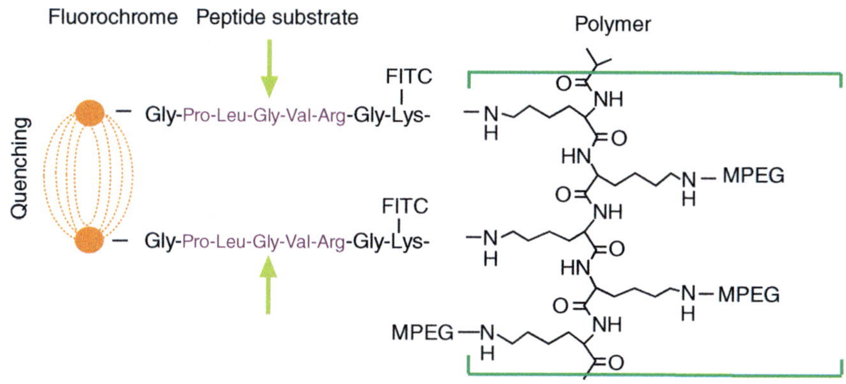

Figure 15.15 Cleavage of fluorophore and quencher by MMP-2. *Source:* Bremer et al. [10]. Reprinted by permission from Springer Nature: Nature Medicine, Copyright © 2001 by Springer Nature.

15.3.5.1 Application of FRET

One example of the application of FRET is the imaging of areas of tumor metastasis. A contrast agent contains a fluorophore and a quencher molecule. Each of the molecules has a small amino acid sequence that is recognized and cleaved by MMP-2 (matrix metalloproteinase-2, an enzyme responsible for tumor metastasis). Hence, in the presence of MMP-2, the fluorophores and quenchers separate and fluorescence occurs (Figure 15.15). This type of imaging can be used to determine if drugs targeting metastasis are effective (e.g. prinomastat which tries to deactivate metastasis), and the effectiveness of many different drug versions can be easily quantified, saving a significant effort in the research and development of new drugs. This is demonstrated in Figure 15.16 when mice-bearing HT1080 tumors (human fibrosarcoma) that express MMP-2 were treated with the antimetastatic drug prinomastat and imaged using FRET. As can be seen, the presence of MMP-2 decreased in the treated mouse compared to the untreated mouse, suggesting a decrease in tumor metastasis.

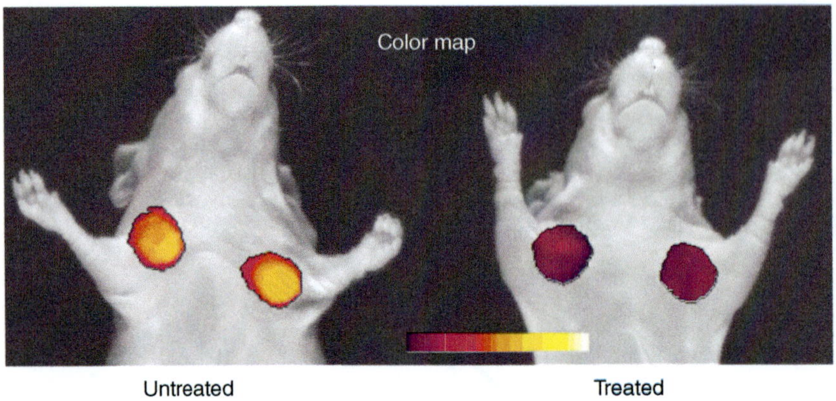

Figure 15.16 Comparison of untreated (left) and treated (right) tumors in mice using FRET imaging *Source:* Bremer et al. [10]. Reprinted by permission from Springer Nature: Nature Medicine, Copyright © 2001 by Springer Nature.

15.4 Raman Imaging

15.4.1 Physics of Raman Imaging

Raman imaging relies on the physics of light scattering in tissue. As previously mentioned, scattering is one possible form of light-tissue interaction, which occurs either elastically or inelastically (Figure 15.17). Scattering almost always occurs elastically, but about one in 10 million scattering events is inelastic, in which the photon loses some energy and is scattered with a higher wavelength ($\lambda_s > \lambda_i\lambda$). Different materials will exhibit different Raman scattering "signatures" (i.e. Raman shift), which is defined as:

$$\text{Raman shift} = \frac{1}{\lambda_i} - \frac{1}{\lambda_s}, \left(\text{in units of cm}^{-1}\right)$$

and describes the Raman effect, for which Sir Chandrasekhara Venkata Raman won the Nobel Prize in 1930.

15.4.2 Contrast Agents for Raman Imaging

Endogenous (i.e. intrinsic) contrast is typically very weak, but also very specific in some organisms such as bacteria. For example, Figure 15.18a shows the unique Raman shift signatures for eight different bacteria species.

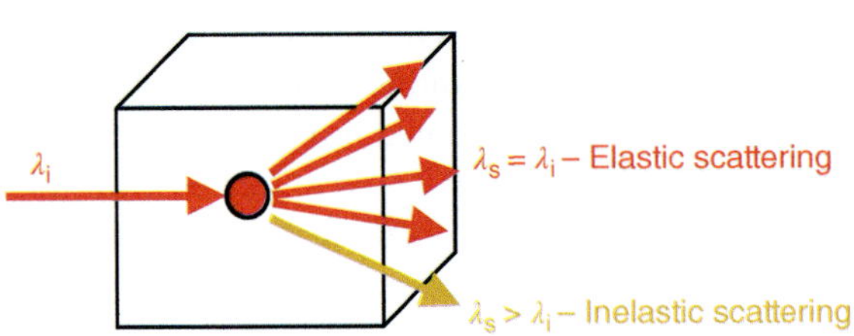

Figure 15.17 Raman scattering.

Exogenous contrast agents for Raman imaging include **single-walled carbon nanotubes (SWNTs)** and **surface-enhanced Raman scattering (SERS)** agents. **SWNTs** are single-layered carbon sheets rolled into a tube-like shape (Figure 15.18b), which exhibit a characteristic peak (a.k.a. G-band) at 1600 cm^{-1} (Figure 15.18c).

SERS agents typically consist of a spherical gold core surrounded by an organic reporter and silica coating, which can be attached with biological recognition molecules (such as antibodies)

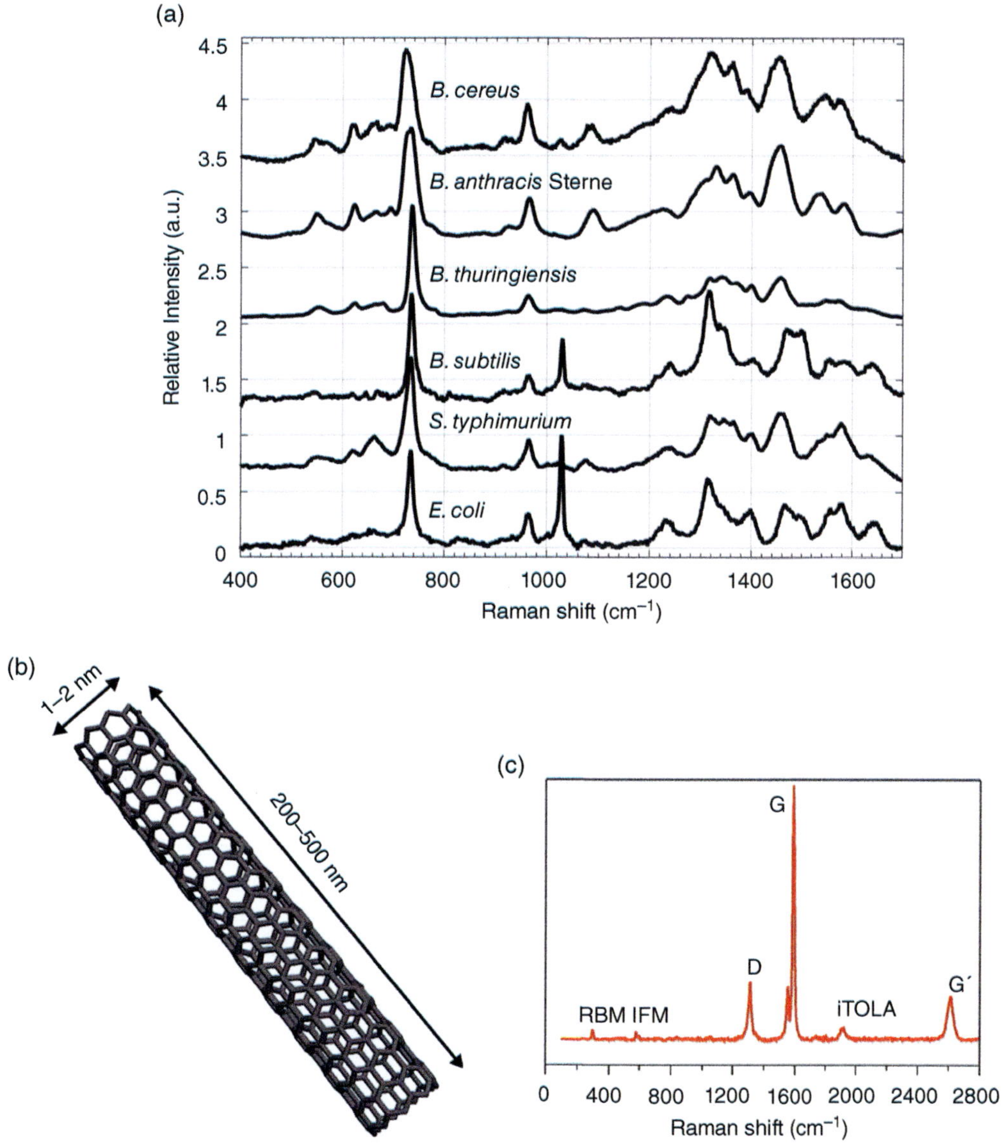

Figure 15.18 (a) Raman shift signatures of six different bacteria species. *Source:* Premasiri et al. [11]. Reprinted (adapted) with permission from The Journal of Physical Chemistry B: American Chemical Society, Copyright © 2005, American Chemical Society. (b) SWNTs shape (*Source:* Courtesy of Professor Guosong Hong), and (c) characteristic peak of Raman shift (peak indicated by G). *Source:* Dresselhaus et al. [12]. Reprinted (adapted) with permission from Nano Letters: American Chemical Society, Copyright © 2010, American Chemical Society.

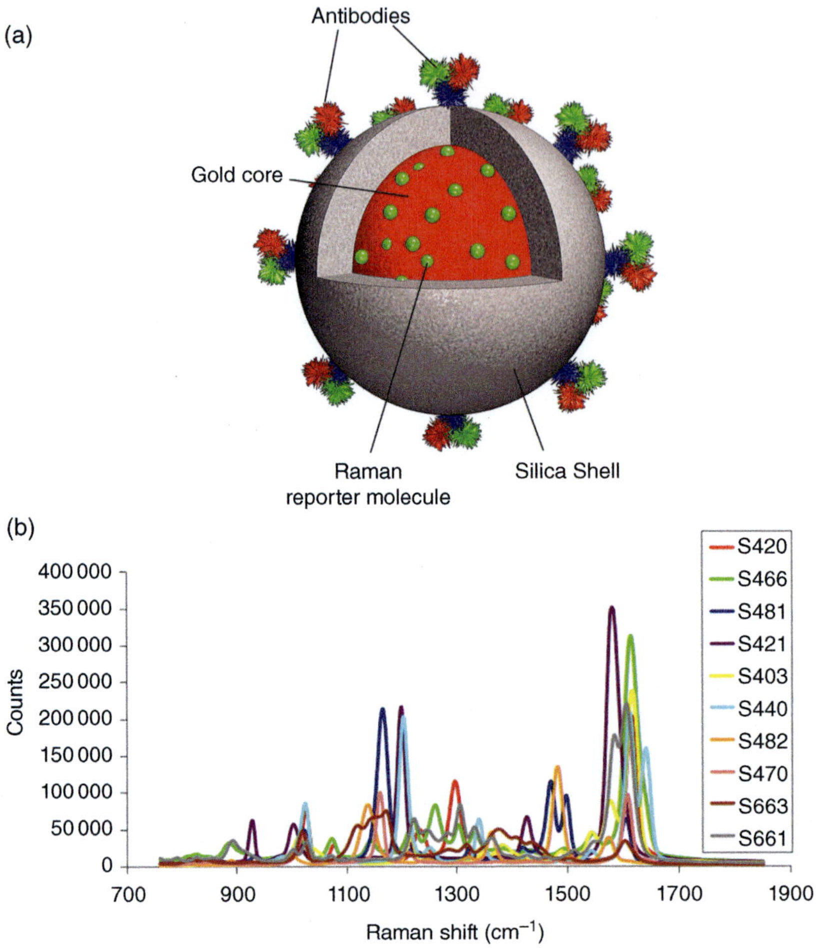

Figure 15.19 (a) SERS structure. *Source:* Paxon et al. [13]. (b) Raman shift spectrum of ten different contrast agents. *Source:* Zavaleta et al. [14]. Copyright © (2009) National Academy of Sciences, USA.

that bind to certain proteins (Figure 15.19a). Metals enhance the Raman scattering of molecules as they come in close proximity to the molecule, by a factor of up to 10^{11}, enabling a very high sensitivity with a limit of detection of about 10 pM. SERS agents have high multiplexing capability; Figure 15.19b shows the Raman signature of 10 different Raman contrast agents, which were constructed using ten different organic reporters.

15.4.3 Raman Spectroscopy Imaging Instrument

Raman imaging can be performed using the apparatus shown in Figure 15.20. In this system, a sample is illuminated by a laser and moved by a robotic arm. For every point (x, y) on the image plane, the whole Raman spectrum is acquired simultaneously, and the robotic arm moves the sample in the x–y plane to acquire an entire image. This setup uses grating filters to separate wavelengths from each other like a prism, such that each CCD pixel detects a different wavelength. A least-squares algorithm (deconvolution) then unmixes the spectra from each other to find the entire Raman spectrum for each point. Because of its ability to resolve and separate signals from

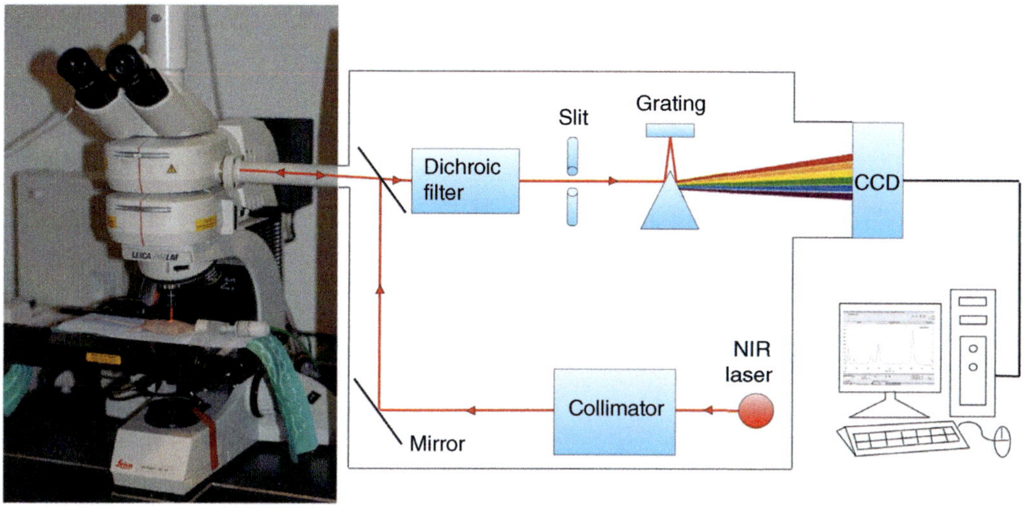

Figure 15.20 Raman spectroscopy imaging instrument. *Source:* Image courtesy of Dr. Cristina Zavaleta.

different sources, the background signal in Raman imaging is negligible, rendering the technique much more sensitive than fluorescence imaging.

15.4.4 Application – Raman Imaging

As an example of Raman imaging, a mouse was implanted with human glioblastoma (invasive brain cancer) in the shoulder and then injected intravenously with SWNT-PEG_{5000}-RGD to target $\alpha_v\beta_3$ integrin. For the mouse not to reject the human tumor, its immune system was genetically compromised, which also led to hair loss (Figure 15.21a). The PEG (polyethylene glycol) reduces the toxicity of the contrast agent by minimizing the direct SWNT interaction with the body immune system, as well as rendering it water-soluble. The RGD peptides cause the Raman contrast agent to accumulate in the tumor, which can be seen by comparison to the control image with plain SWNTs without RGD (Figure 15.21b). The control image shows a much smaller signal, with some artifacts due to random circulation and image reconstruction artifacts.

Raman imaging has high multiplexing capability, i.e. the ability to uniquely resolve multiple contrast agents in the same image. As an example, a mouse was injected with ten different types of SERS contrast agents, each of which was independently resolved into different images by a least-squares algorithm. Due to the different and unique Raman shifts of each contrast agents, one can multiplex many such contrast agents, despite the significant overlap of their spectra. In the example shown in Figure 15.22, different contrast agents are injected into different locations but in actual application, they will circulate in the bloodstream and bind to their targets. Using deconvolution, it is still possible to detect each agent's signal level, even if they are located in the same position.

15.5 Fluorescence Imaging vs. Raman Imaging

Table 15.1 compares the characteristics of fluorescence imaging, multispectral fluorescence imaging, FRET imaging, and Raman spectroscopy imaging.

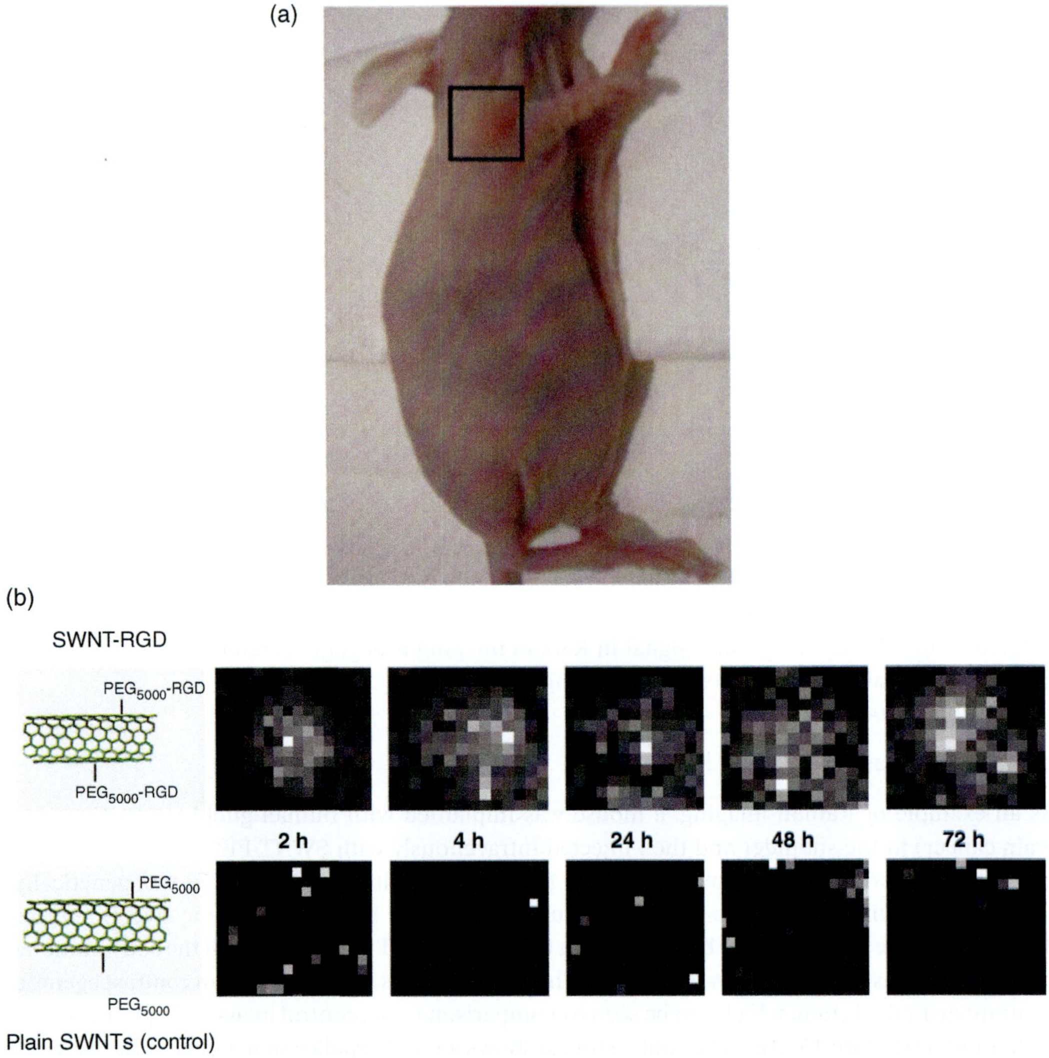

Figure 15.21 (a) Nude mouse with human glioblastoma in the shoulder. (b) Raman imaging with SWNT-RGD and the control (plain SWNTs). *Source:* Zavaleta et al. [15]. Reprinted (adapted) with permission from Nano Letters: American Chemical Society, Copyright © 2008, American Chemical Society.

Other optical imaging techniques include intravital microscopy, confocal microscopy, two-photon microscopy, optical coherence tomography (OCT), bioluminescence, diffuse optical spectroscopy, time-domain and frequency domain fluorescence imaging, and many others.

15.6 Conclusion

Fluorescence imaging and Raman spectroscopy imaging are two forms of optical imaging, which are based on the detection of light that has interacted with tissue. Optical imaging has advantages over other imaging modalities such as MRI, PET, and SPECT, which are expensive, require a long

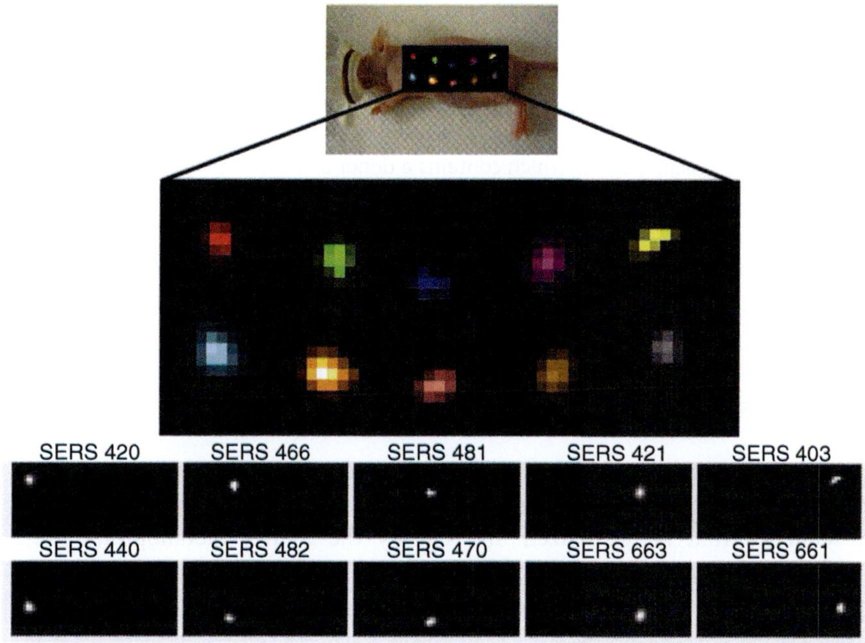

Figure 15.22 Multiplexed Raman imaging. *Source:* Zavaleta et al. [14]. Copyright © (2009) National Academy of Sciences, USA.

Table 15.1 Comparison of various optical imaging modalities.

Differences	Fluorescence	Multi-spectral fluorescence	FRET	Raman spectroscopy imaging
Temporal resolution	<1 s	Seconds	Seconds	Minutes
Sensitivity	1 nM	100 pM	1 nM	10 pM
Background level	High	Medium	High	Low
Cost/system complexity	Low	Medium	Medium	High
Multiplexing ability	Low	Medium	Low	High
Intrinsic signal		Autofluorescence		Very low
Contrast agents	Many	Many	Many	Few

scan time, have low sensitivity (MRI), and use radioactivity (PET and SPECT). The advantages of optical imaging include high resolution, low cost, high sensitivity, multiplexing ability, and ability to use during surgery (intraoperative).

Problems

15.1 Oximetry is a noninvasive method for monitoring a patient's oxygen saturation. A light source and a photodetector are placed on opposite sides of the patient's fingertip, and the light is passed through the fingertip to the detector to measure the absorbance. The final readout of the device is the percentage of oxygenated hemoglobin.

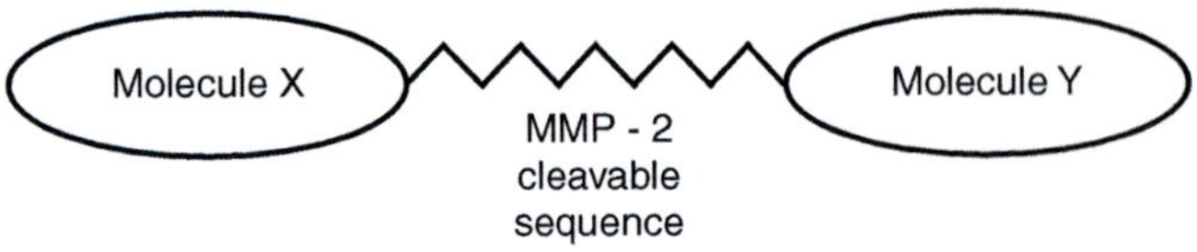

Figure 15.23. Schematic of a new imaging agent, which contains a donor and acceptor held together by a cleavable sequence.

A Based on the plot of molar coefficient vs. wavelength (Figure 15.3), what is the optimal wavelength for the oximetry to maximize the signal?
B Single wavelength measurement might be problematic. What do you think are possible problems with it? How would you improve this technique?

15.2 An imaging agent is represented in Figure 15.23. Molecules X and Y represent the donor and acceptor of the fluorophore, respectively. The MMP-2 cleavable sequence is a short amino acid sequence that is recognized and cut by the matrix metalloproteinase-2 (MMP-2).
What does the imaging agent target? Briefly explain the targeting mechanism.

15.3 Explain the following in your own words:
A In fluorescence imaging, what are the advantages of using nanoparticles as contrast agents compared to small-molecule fluorescent contrast agents?
B What is the advantage of Raman imaging compared to fluorescent imaging?

References

1 NASA. http://mynasadata.larc.nasa.gov/images/EM_Spectrum3-new.jpg
2 Jacopo Werther, https://commons.wikimedia.org/wiki/File:Stokes_shift.png
3 de la Zerda, A., Zavaleta, C., Keren, S. et al. (2008). Carbon nanotubes as photoacoustic molecular imaging agents in living mice. *Nature Nanotechnology* 3: 557–562.
4 Levenson, R. M. and Mansfield, J. R. (2006), Multispectral imaging in biology and medicine: slices of life. *Cytometry*, 69A: 748-758. doi:https://doi.org/10.1002/cyto.a.20319
5 Michels, S., Hansmann, F., Geitzenauer, W., and Schmidt-Erfurth, U. Influence of treatment parameters on selectivity of Verteporfin therapy. *Investigative Ophthalmology & Visual Science* 47 (1).
6 Zrazhevskiy, P., Sena, M., and Gao, X. (2010). Designing multifunctional quantum dots for bioimaging, detection, and drug delivery. *Chem. Soc. Rev.* 39: 4326–4354.
7 Kobayashi, H., Hama, Y., Koyama, Y. et al. Simultaneous multicolor imaging of five different lymphatic basins using quantum dots. *American Chemical Society* 7 (6): 1711–1716.
8 Cai, W., Shin, D.-W., Chen, K. et al. Peptide-labeled near-infrared quantum dots for imaging tumor vasculature in living subjects. *American Chemical Society* 6 (4): 669–676.
9 Rudolf, R., Mongillo, M., Rizzuto, R., and Pozzan, T. (2003). Looking forward to seeing calcium. *Nature Reviews Molecular Cell Biology* 4: 579–586.
10 Bremer, C., Tung, C.-H., and Weissleder, R. (2001). in vivo molecular target assessment of matrix metalloproteinase. *Nature Medicine* 7: 743–748.

11 Premasiri, W.R., Moir, D.T., Klempner, M.S. et al. Characterization of the surface enhanced raman scattering (SERS) of bacteria. *The Journal of Physical Chemistry B: American Chemical Society* 109 (1): 312–320.
12 Dresselhaus, M.S., Jorio, A., Hofmann, M. et al. Perspectives on carbon nanotubes and graphene raman spectroscopy. *Nano Letters: American Chemical Society* 10 (3): 751–758.
13 Tracy L. Paxon, R. Scott Duthie, Casey Renko, Andrew Burns, Frank J. Mondello and Marie Lesaicherre, “Identifying biological agents with surface-enhanced Raman scattering”, *SPIE Newsroom*, 18 April 2011, doi: https://doi.org/10.1117/2.120113.003645
14 “Multiplexed imaging of surface enhanced Raman scattering nanotags in living mice using noninvasive Raman spectroscopy”, Cristina L. Zavaleta, Bryan R. Smith, Ian Walton, William Doering, Glenn Davis, Borzoyeh Shojaei, Michael J. Natan & Sanjiv S. Gambhir, *Proceedings of the National Academy of Sciences* Aug 2009, 106 (2) 13511–135116. doi: https://doi.org/10.1073/pnas.0813327106.
15 Zavaleta, C., De la Zerda, A., Liu, Z. et al. Noninvasive Raman spectroscopy in living mice for evaluation of tumor targeting with carbon nanotubes. *Nano Letters: American Chemical Society* 8 (9): 2800–2805.

Further Reading

http://www.piercenet.com – Dyelight680
http://en.wikipedia.org/wiki/Autofluorescence
Rowe, A. (2009). Top Raman, ACS Meeting News: surface-enhanced spectroscopic tool could yield health care, global security applications. *Science and Technology* 87 (38): 36–38.
Cristina Zavaleta, PhD

16

Optical Coherence Tomography

16.1 Introduction

Optical Coherence Tomography (OCT) is a high-resolution, three-dimensional, subsurface imaging modality. Similar to Raman spectroscopy and fluorescence imaging, which were discussed in Chapter 15, OCT consists of sending light into the sample and measuring the light that returns. While fluorescence and Raman spectroscopy capture light that has been altered (i.e. wavelength shifted), OCT measures the unaltered back reflected light. In essence, light is sent into a sample and the back reflected light from each surface within the sample is detected and measured. Figure 16.1 shows this basic operating principle overlaid on a cross sectional OCT image of a tadpole. A cross sectional image shows what would be seen if the tadpole were cut in half lengthwise and then imaged from the side. As demonstrated in the figure, depth information is collected along a line (dictated by the spot size of the light source), which is termed an A-scan. To build a cross sectional image, termed a B-scan, the light is scanned in a single direction along the sample. Finally, combining many B-scans acquired along an orthogonal direction produces a 3D volume of the sample.

OCT is a relatively new imaging modality; it was first demonstrated in 1990. For comparison, MRI was invented in 1971, CT in 1972, and ultrasound in 1941. OCT has quickly become a standard practice in ophthalmology and optometry clinics, and is gaining popularity in various other medical fields. OCT works with wavelengths inside the near-IR optical window (discussed in Chapter 15) and therefore achieves very high image resolution (micrometers) but is limited to a shallow imaging depth (a few millimeters). This chapter will cover the basic physics, applications, and contrast enhancement mechanisms for OCT. Two implementations of OCT will be discussed: Time-Domain OCT and Spectral-Domain OCT.

16.1.1 Mirrors and Photodiodes

Before explaining the physics of OCT, a few basic optical components need to be understood: mirrors and photodiodes. Fully reflective mirrors (Figure 16.2a) completely reflect any incoming light rays. That is, the intensity of the reflected light is equal to that of the incoming light. Semi-reflective mirrors (Figure 16.2b) reflect a portion of the light; the remaining light is transmitted

Biochips and Medical Imaging, First Edition. Adam de la Zerda and Shan Xiang Wang.

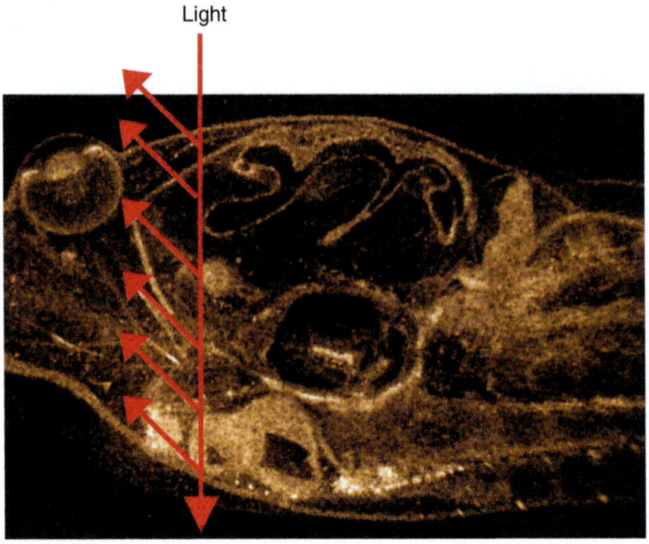

Figure 16.1 Basic operating principle of OCT overlaid on a cross sectional image of a tadpole. *Source:* Photo courtesy of Thorlabs; https://www.thorlabs.com/images/TabImages/OCT_PW11.pdf

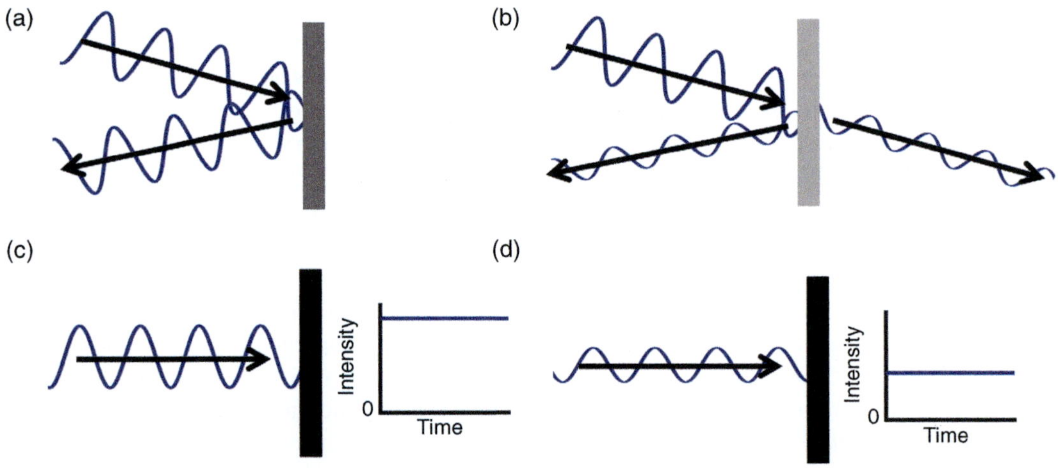

Figure 16.2 Basic optical components. (a) Fully reflective mirror. (b) Semi-reflective mirror. (c) and (d) Photodiodes with associated intensity readings for various incoming light waves.

through the mirror. The relative intensities of the transmitted and the reflected light are described by the reflection coefficient of the mirror. If a mirror has a large reflection coefficient, then the mirror reflects a large portion of the incoming light; a fully reflective mirror has a reflection coefficient of one.

Photodiodes are a type of optical detector; they measure the time-averaged intensity of a light wave (Figure 16.2c and d). The time over which the signal is averaged is called the integration time. The integration time of a photodiode can be large compared to time-varying fluctuations in the light intensity. If this is the case, the photodiode would not be sensitive to these changes. It should also be noted that if the light source is composed of many wavelengths, then the photodiode measures the time-averaged intensity of the sum of all wavelengths.

16.1.2 Time of Flight

A biological sample (e.g. tissue) can be modeled of as a series of semi-reflective mirrors; at each depth in the sample, some of the light is reflected back and the rest is transmitted through. To construct an image of the sample, two sets of information are required: (a) the location (depth) of each sample mirror, and (b) the reflection coefficient of each sample mirror. Performing time of flight measurements would be the simplest method of obtaining this information (Figure 16.3). That is, to send light into the sample and measure both the time at which the light returns and the intensity of the returning light.

The depth and reflection coefficient of each mirror could be calculated from the return times and intensities, respectively. Unfortunately, current optical detectors can only achieve resolutions on the order of centimeters. That is, the light travels too fast for the detectors to differentiate the return times from within a biological sample. Therefore, trying to perform time of flight measurements would not yield useful depth information about the sample. Fortunately, this information can be measured through other mechanisms, such as interferometry.

16.1.3 Interferometry (Monochromatic)

A key optical component for interferometry is the beam splitter. A beam splitter is a semi-reflective mirror, positioned at an angle to the incoming light, which splits incoming light into two orthogonal paths as shown in Figure 16.4. Beam splitters can also be made of other components

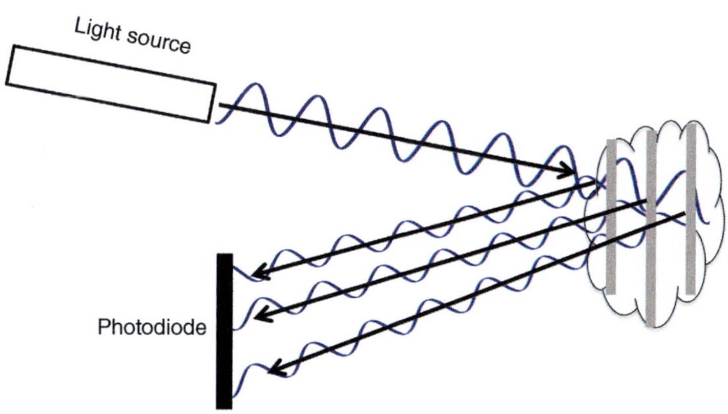

Figure 16.3 Theoretical setup for time of flight measurements using light.

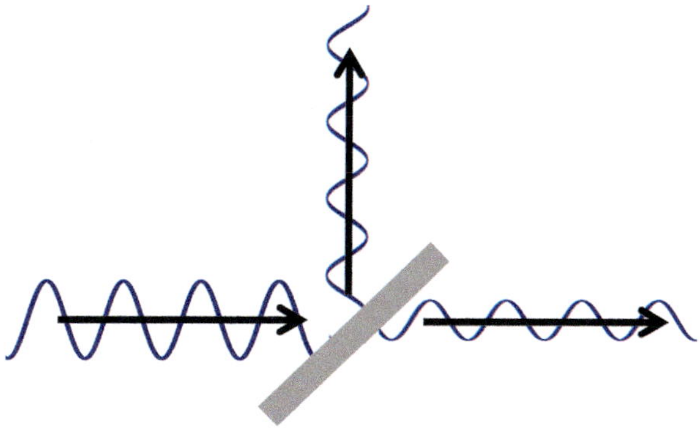

Figure 16.4 Schematic of a beam splitter, which splits an incoming light wave into two orthogonal paths.

(e.g. two triangular glass prisms). A basic interferometer consists of a light source, a beam splitter, mirrors in each path, and a detector (Figure 16.5). The light from each path (called an arm) is reflected back toward the beam splitter where the photons reflected from both paths interfere (i.e. are summed together). The resultant wave is then measured using a photodiode. The intensity measured by the photodiode is a function of the path length difference between the two arms. Examples of interference patterns are shown in Figure 16.6. The top two rows show light waves from the two arms of the interferometer. If the light travels the same distance in each arm, then the waves arrive at the beam splitter in phase. That is, the peaks of one wave align with the peaks of the other, as shown in the center column. When these two waves interfere, the result is a wave with

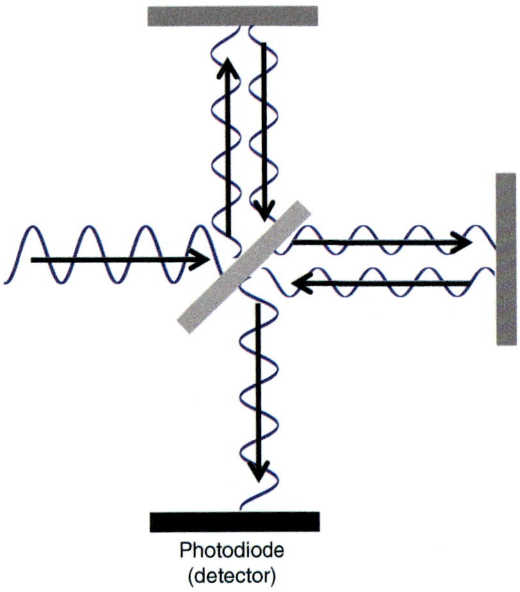

Figure 16.5 Basic interferometer setup.

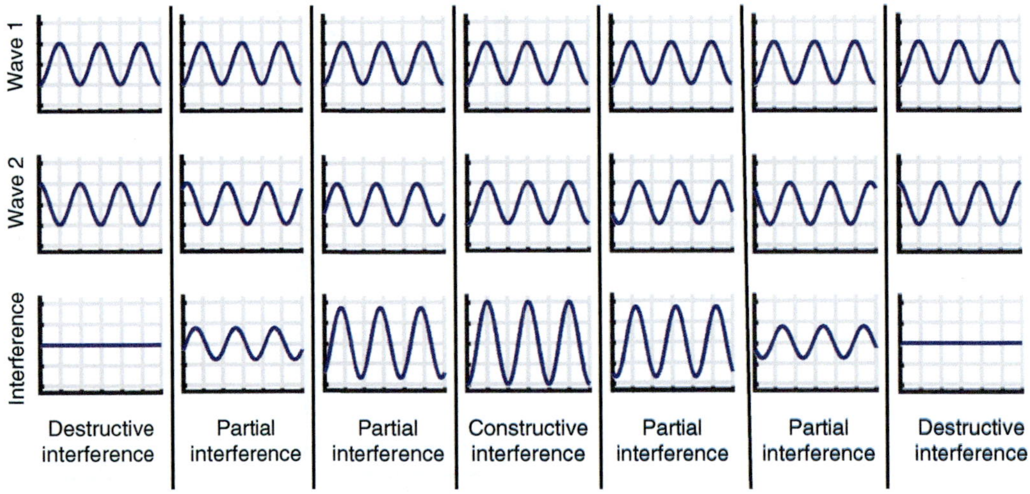

Figure 16.6 Types of interference. The bottom row is the resultant wave after interfering the light waves from the top two rows.

twice the amplitude (note that, in practice, the resultant amplitude will be less than twice because some of the returning light can travel back toward the source through the beam splitter; however, this concept is beyond the scope of this book). This situation is called constructive interference. Note that constructive interference occurs when the difference in path lengths is zero or a whole-integer multiple of the wavelength of light. Destructive interference (shown in first and last columns of Figure 16.6) occurs when the path length difference is an odd multiple of half the wavelength. In this scenario, the waves arrive at the beam splitter completely out of phase (i.e. the peaks from one wave align with the troughs of the other). The amplitude of the summed waves is zero. When the waves arrive partially out of phase, the result is partial interference, and the amplitude of the resultant wave is between twice that of the original waves and zero. Therefore, the intensity of the resultant wave provides information about the path length difference between the two mirrors. Note that the interference patterns shown assume monochromatic light (i.e. light of just a single wavelength).

If a biological sample is modeled as just a single mirror, then the basic interferometer of Figure 16.5 can be used to measure the distance to the sample by replacing one of the mirrors with the sample (Figure 16.7). The path containing the sample is termed the sample arm and the other arm is termed the reference arm. The graph shown is the result of mechanically moving the reference mirror (to change the reference path length) and measuring the intensity for each position. When the path lengths are matched, the light from the sample and reference mirror constructively interferes giving a maximum reading at the detector. The waves destructively interfere when the path lengths differ by half a wavelength, which results in an intensity of zero at the detector. This pattern repeats when the path lengths differ by a full wavelength because constructive interference occurs again. Therefore, the interferometric signal provides information about the distance to the sample, but the exact distance cannot be calculated due to ambiguity in the signal. If the sample is modeled as two semi-reflective mirrors (Figure 16.8), it becomes apparent that this ambiguity prevents the usability of such a system for biological imaging. The intensity measured by the photodiode is now a function of the distance between the reference mirror and each sample mirror. The location and value of the maximum intensity are a function of the distance between the two sample mirrors. However, the change in these parameters is also a repeating function; the distance between the mirrors can only be calculated within a multiple of the wavelength. That is, the exact distance between the sample mirrors cannot be determined. Therefore, performing interferometry with a monochromatic source does not provide any useful depth information about the sample.

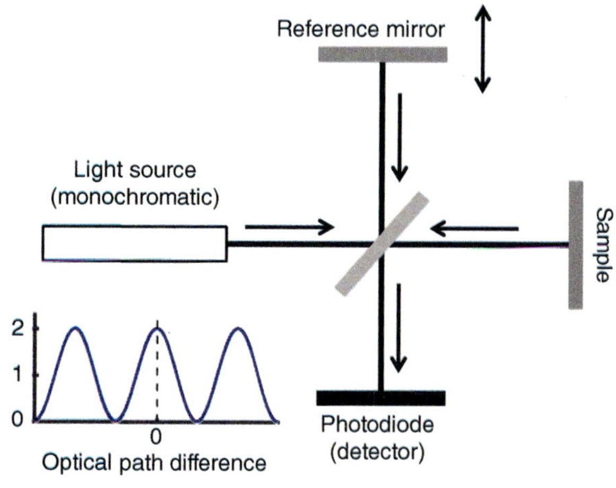

Figure 16.7 Interferometer with a monochromatic source and a single sample mirror. The detected signal as a function of reference mirror position is shown.

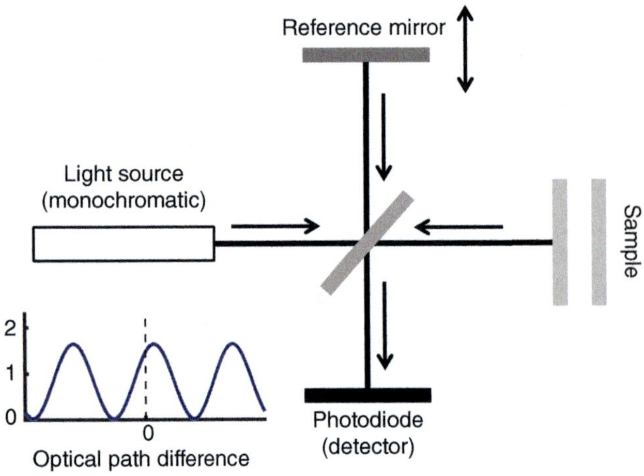

Figure 16.8 Interferometer with a monochromatic source and sample composed of two semitransparent mirrors. The detected signal as a function of reference mirror position is shown.

16.1.4 Time-Domain OCT (TD-OCT)

OCT overcomes the ambiguity discussed earlier by replacing the monochromatic source with a broadband source. While the emission from a broadband source contains many wavelengths, it can be modeled by a single effective waveform. When all the wavelengths have a fixed-phase relationship, the effective waveform is a pulse (Figure 16.9a). The coherence length, τ_C, describes the width of the pulse. In practice, the wavelengths emitted from a broadband source do not have a fixed-phase relationship. In this case, the main frequency and amplitude of the waveform vary (Figure 16.9b); here, the coherence length describes the distance over which the wave has a predictable phase and amplitude. The coherence length is often described as the length over which the wave is nicely sinusoidal. The coherence length is a function of the source spectrum; the

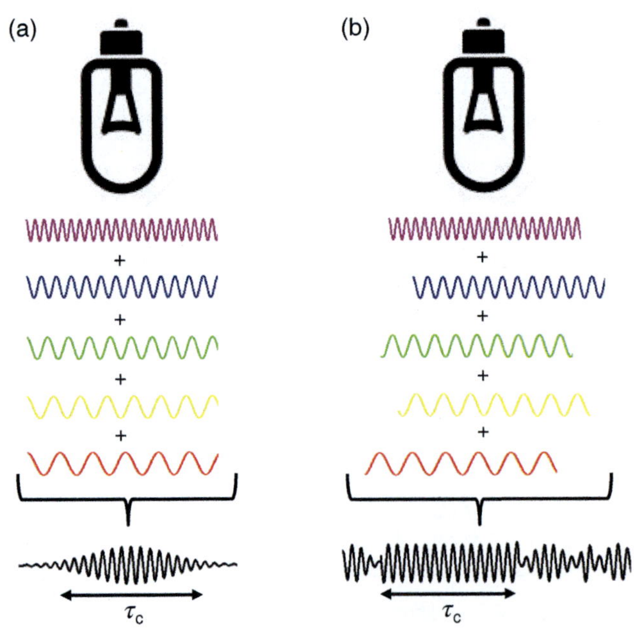

Figure 16.9 Effective waveforms for broadband sources with (a) fixed-phase relation, and (b) no fixed-phase relation.

broader the source (i.e. the more wavelengths) the shorter the coherence length. For simplicity, the effective waveform from a broadband source will always be represented as a pulse as opposed to the more realistic varying waveform.

TD-OCT, which was the original implementation of OCT, is based on interferometry with a broadband source instead of a monochromatic source. The light from the sample and reference arms can be represented as the pulses of light previously described (Figure 16.10a). If the pulses do not overlap at the beam splitter, then the time-averaged intensity measured by the detector is constant. However, if the pulses overlap (i.e. the path length difference between the two arms is less than twice the coherence length), then the time-averaged intensity will vary as a function of the path length difference (Figure 16.10b). Detecting the envelope of the signal and locating the maximum point can determine the position at which the path lengths match. This process is shown in Figure 16.11 where the reference mirror is mechanically moved and the intensity for each position

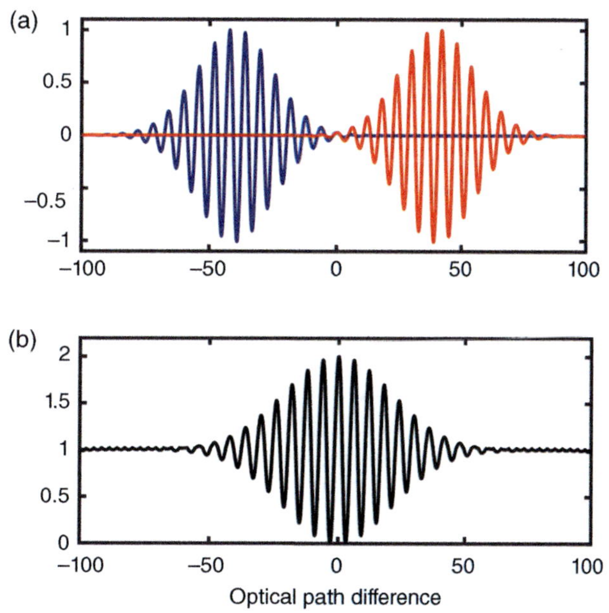

Figure 16.10 Principle of interferometry with a broadband source. (a) Wave pulses from sample and reference arms, (b) Time-averaged intensity of interfered wave as a function of the offset between pulses.

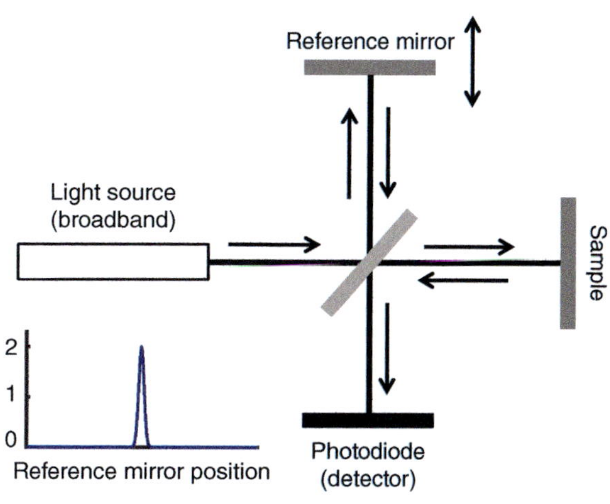

Figure 16.11 TD-OCT system with the sample represented by a single mirror. Envelope of detected signal is shown, which gives the depth location of the mirror.

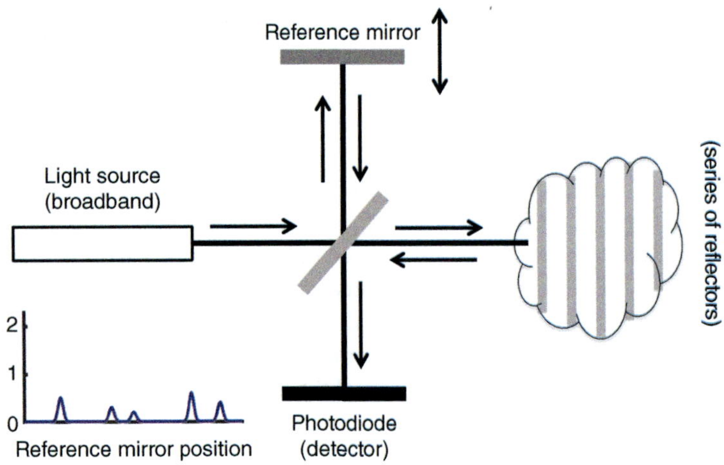

Figure 16.12 TD-OCT system with the sample represented by a series of semitransparent mirrors. Envelopes of the detected signal are shown, which give depth and reflection coefficient information.

is measured. The graph shows the envelope of the signal and the distance that corresponds to the peak is equal to the distance to the sample mirror. Most importantly, the ambiguity that was present in the interferometer with a monochromatic source is eliminated.

If the single sample mirror is replaced with a more realistic model of a series of semi-reflective mirrors, then the detector signal will be a series of interference signals (each of which corresponds to one of the sample mirrors). Once again the envelopes are determined (as shown in Figure 16.12); the locations and heights give the depth and reflection coefficient of each sample mirror, respectively. In total, the detected signal provides a depth-resolved profile of the sample (i.e. an A-scan). Note that the coherence length of the source dictates the width of the envelope. Therefore, the coherence length limits the axial (depth) resolution of the system (i.e. the axial resolution is improved with the use of a broader source). Recall that the beam can then be scanned in a single direction along the sample to create a cross sectional image (a B-scan). The resolution in this direction (i.e. the lateral resolution) is limited by the spot size of the light source, which is a function of the source's center wavelength and the NA of the objective lens.

16.1.5 Spectral-Domain OCT (SD-OCT)

TD-OCT relies on mechanically moving the reference mirror and is therefore relatively slow. Recall that the photodiode measures the intensity of the sum of all wavelengths, meaning that information about the intensity of individual wavelengths is lost. However, encoded in this data is all the depth information. By measuring the signal of the individual wavelengths, all the depth information can be retrieved using only a single position of the reference mirror; this is the operating principle of SD-OCT.

A diffraction grating is used to separate light into its various wavelength components and a CCD can be used to measure the intensity of each (Figure 16.13). The setup for SD-OCT, shown in Figure 16.14, uses the same source as TD-OCT but the reference mirror remains stationary and the photodiode is replaced with a diffraction grating coupled to a CCD.

The CCD signal as a function of wave number (k), which is inversely proportional to the wavelength, is related to the distance between the reference mirror and sample mirrors as follows:

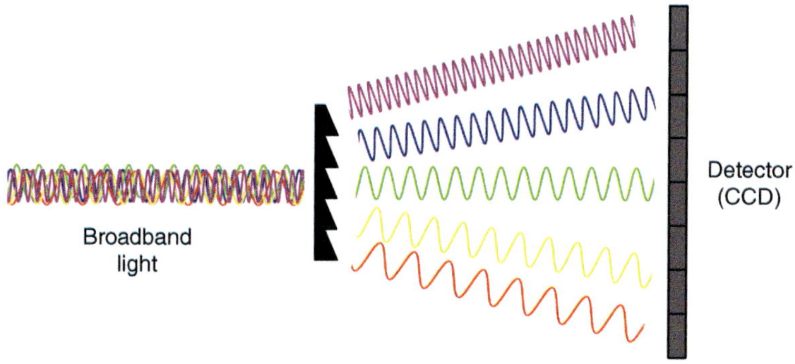

Figure 16.13 Schematic of a diffraction grating coupled to a CCD for measuring intensities of various wavelength components of a broadband source.

Figure 16.14 Schematic of SD-OCT system.

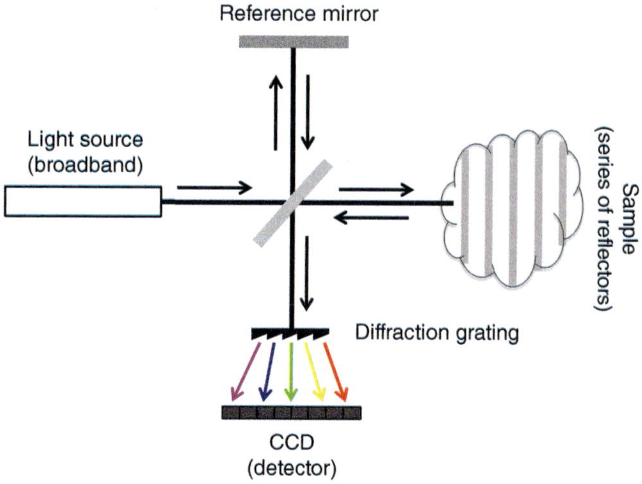

$$I_D(k) \propto S(k)\cos\left(2k\left(z_R - z_{S_n}\right)\right),$$

where I_D is the intensity on the CCD, S is the source spectrum, z_R is the distance to the reference mirror, and z_{S_n} is the distance to the nth sample mirror. The signal is a sum of cosines whose frequencies are dependent on the path length difference between the reference mirror and each sample mirror. Therefore, to determine the depth locations of each mirror, the frequencies of each cosine term need to be determined. This is achieved with a Fourier Transform. Recall that the Fourier Transform of a cosine is a sum of delta functions at the positive and negative values of the frequency. The signal in k is a product of the cosines with the source spectrum; therefore, the Fourier Transform is a set of delta function convolved with the source spectrum as shown in Figure 16.15. Similar to TD-OCT, the depth and reflection coefficient of each sample mirror can be calculated from the location and height of the peaks, respectively. Note that because the Fourier Transform gives signal at the positive and negative frequency values, half of the signal is cut off to obtain the depth profile of the sample. In summary, by acquiring the interferometry signal as a function of wavelength, the entire depth profile of a sample is obtained using only a single reference mirror position.

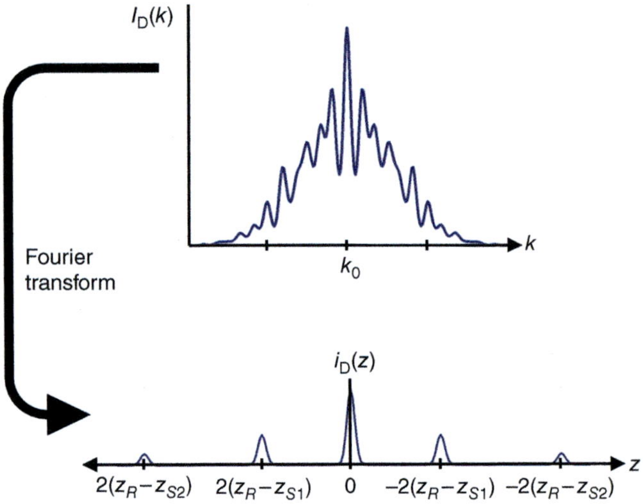

Figure 16.15 Intensity signal on the CCD from an SD-OCT system (top) and the Fourier Transform of this signal (bottom). The Fourier Transform gives depth locations and reflection coefficients of each sample mirror.

16.1.6 TD-OCT versus SD-OCT

As previously discussed, the data acquisition speed of SD-OCT is superior to that of TD-OCT since it requires only a single position of the reference mirror. In both SD-OCT and TD-OCT, axial and lateral resolutions are dictated by the same parameters; therefore, neither implementation has an advantage over the other. The coherence length of the source determines the axial resolution. The center wavelength and NA of the objective lens determine the lateral resolution. The penetration depth of light fundamentally limits the maximum imaging depth in both TD-OCT and SD-OCT, but in SD-OCT, it is also limited by the resolution of the spectrometer. The finite sampling of the spectrometer leads to aliasing in the spatial image. Poor spectrometer resolution causes aliasing at a shallow depth, which corrupts data from deep in the sample. Since TD-OCT samples in the spatial domain, it does not suffer from aliasing issues. Finally, the signal-to-noise ratio (SNR) in SD-OCT is typically higher compared to TD-OCT due to the longer exposure time. In TD-OCT, for a given scan time, the exposure time is split amongst all the reference arm positions. In SD-OCT, the exposure time is equivalent to the scan time. The faster acquisition and enhanced SNR make SD-OCT the implementation of choice for the majority OCT applications.

16.2 Applications of OCT

Applications of OCT are dictated by the limited imaging depth capabilities. For an application to be viable, it must be possible to place a light source and light collection mechanism close to the sample. As stated earlier, ophthalmology is the most advanced application of OCT, but many others are targets currently being explored including the esophagus, arteries, skin, and bladder.

16.2.1 Retina

OCT machines are becoming ubiquitous in ophthalmology and optometry clinics, where they are mainly used to image the retina (located at the back of the eye). However, machines capable of

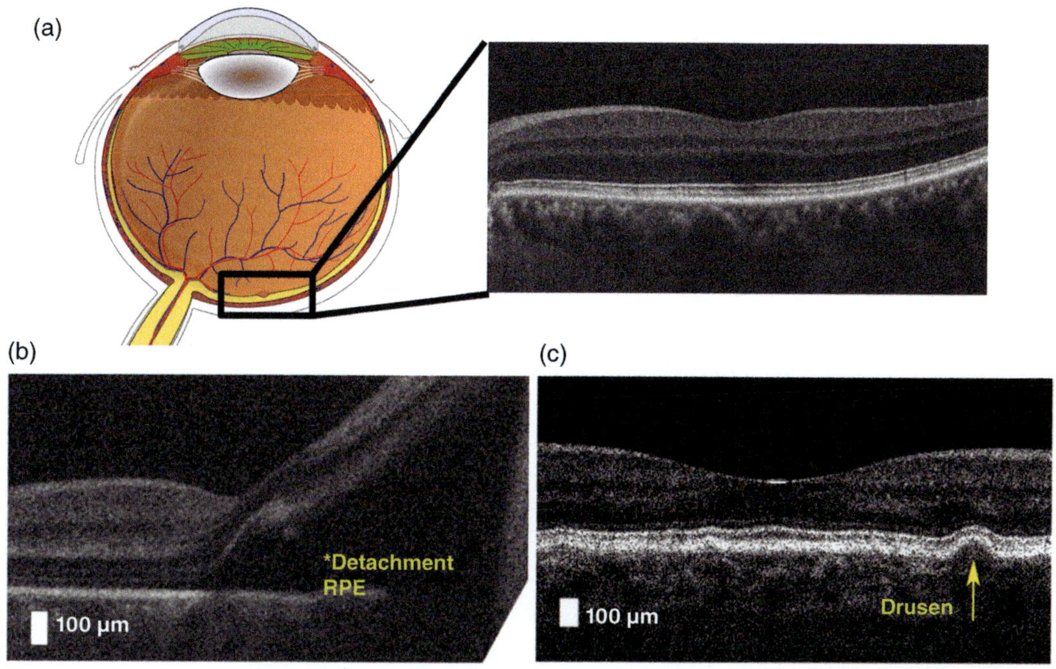

Figure 16.16 (a) Location of retina/foveal pit and an OCT image from a healthy patient. *Source:* Jmarchn [1]. Used under CC-BY-SA 3.0 https://creativecommons.org/licenses/by-sa/3.0/ (b) OCT image of a retinal detachment. (c) OCT image of a patient with age-related macular degeneration. *Source:* Lee et al. [2].

imaging the cornea are also becoming popular. Light is sent and collected outside of the eye, which requires the optics of the eye be taken into account when designing the system. Figure 16.6a shows a cross sectional OCT image of a retina. The indentation in the retina is the foveal pit, which is responsible for central sharp vision. The OCT image reveals that the retina is made up of several layers of different types of tissue, which are characterized by their attenuation coefficient (discussed in Chapter 15) and thickness. Since OCT operates in the near-IR window, the absorption of light is minimal compared to scattering. Therefore, the attenuation coefficient is dominated by the scattering coefficient and the two are often used interchangeably in reference to OCT. In OCT images, tissue with a higher attenuation coefficient appears brighter. Many ocular diseases can be diagnosed and tracked using OCT. A few examples include assessing the degree of retinal detachment (Figure 16.16b), diagnosing macular degeneration by identifying lipid deposits (drusen) under the retina (Figure 16.16c), and tracking the progression of glaucoma by quantifying the attenuation coefficient (Table 16.1). For example, it has been found that the attenuation coefficient of one of the layers in the retina (the retinal nerve fiber layer) decreases as glaucoma progresses.

16.2.2 Skin

Skin is an easily accessible tissue and is therefore a prime target for OCT. While not nearly as advanced as ophthalmic systems, clinical OCT machines for dermal applications are available. In dermal applications, OCT is used for tasks ranging from skin cancer diagnosis/staging to the assessment of burn tissue. Figure 16.17a shows an example of healthy skin imaged with OCT. Skin, like the retina, is made up of several distinct layers, which are clearly discernible in healthy skin. The thick arrow shows the surface of the skin, while the thin arrow shows the junction

Table 16.1 Average attenuation coefficient of the retinal nerve fiber layer in patients with varying severities of glaucoma.

Disease status	Average attn. coeff.
Healthy	4.78 ± 0.46
Mild glaucoma	4.09 ± 0.34
Moderate glaucoma	3.14 ± 0.22
Advanced glaucoma	2.93 ± 0.33

Source: Schoot et al. [3]. Republished with permission of Association for Research in Vision and Ophthalmology: Investigative Ophthalmology; permission conveyed through Copyright Clearance Center, Inc.

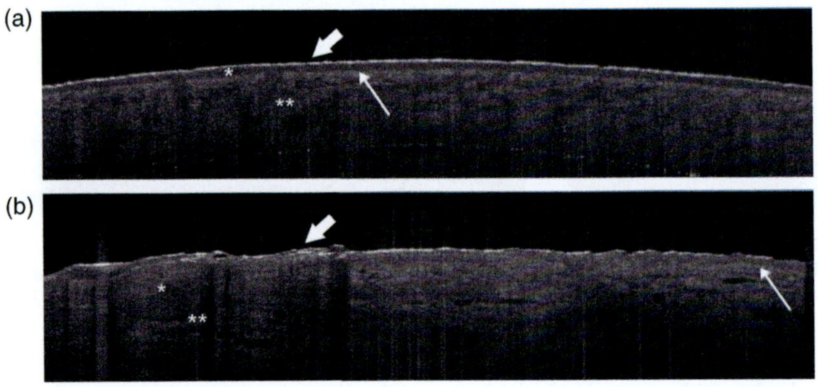

Figure 16.17 OCT images of (a) healthy skin and (b) an area of basal cell carcinoma. (*Source:* Olsen et al. [4]. Reprinted from Elsevier, Copyright © 2016, with permission from Elsevier.)

between the top two layers of the skin – the epidermis (*) and dermis (**). Many diseases, including skin conditions, initially manifest as changes in the tissue structure beneath the surface. The left side of Figure 16.17b shows an area of basal cell carcinoma (a type of skin cancer). The surface has become more irregular (thick arrow) and the junction between the epidermis and dermis is no longer clearly discernible (the thin arrow shows an area with a clear junction). Finally, there is a faint ovoid structure present between * and **. OCT is not only useful as a cancer diagnostic but also as a tool for staging tumors. Traditionally, a suspicious lesion is biopsied, sliced thinly, stained, and then imaged with a standard microscope. This information allows clinicians to determine the presence and stage of cancer. OCT provides the same information without the need for the physical removal of any tissue. OCT can provide an optical biopsy which not only reduces the procedure cost but also reduces patient risk.

16.2.3 Esophagus

Thanks to the miniaturization of optical components, OCT systems can be deployed to image surfaces deep within the body. One example is a tethered capsule that is swallowed and then used to image the stomach and esophagus as it is pulled back out (Figure 16.18a). Inside the capsule is an optical fiber, which is responsible for both delivering the light and collecting the reflections. To

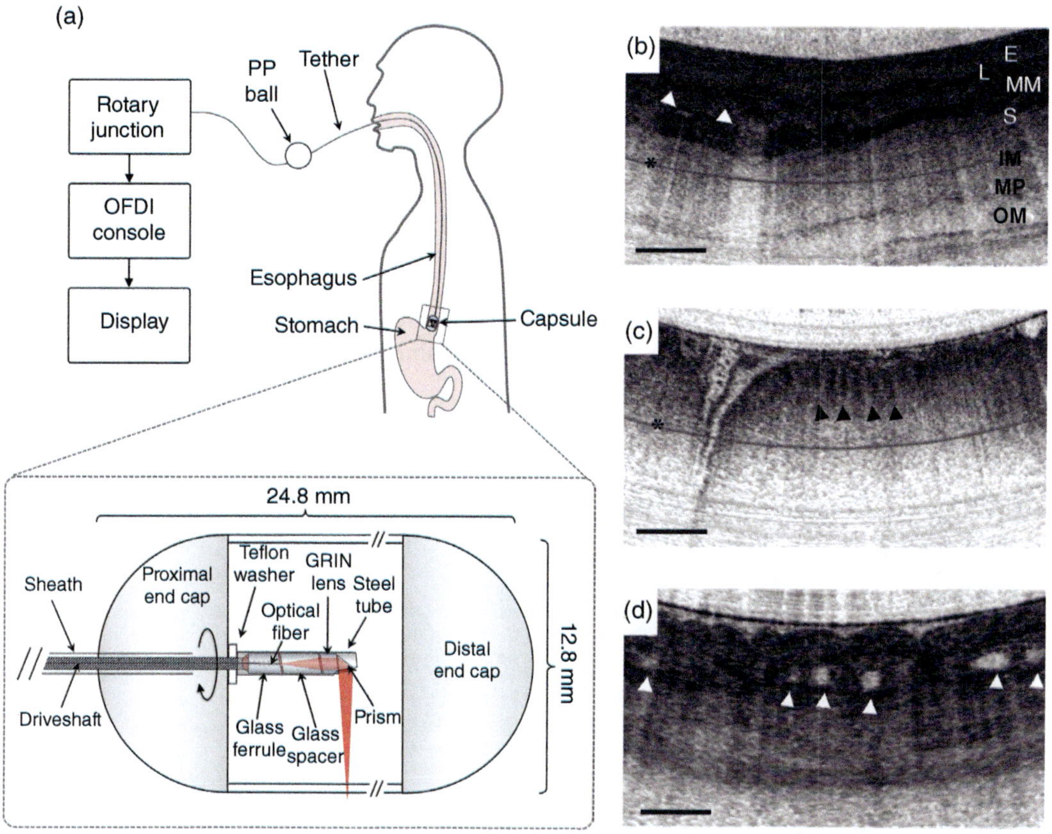

Figure 16.18 (a) Schematic showing the operation and components of a tethered OCT capsule. (b) OCT image of healthy esophagus tissue. (c) OCT image of healthy stomach tissue. (d) OCT image from a patient with Barrett's Esophagus. *Source:* Gora et al. [5]. Reprinted by permission from Springer Nature: Nature Medicine. Copyright © 2013 by Springer Nature.

collect data from all parts of the esophagus, the capsule also contains a driveshaft that rotates the optical components as images are collected. Figure 16.18b is an image of a healthy esophagus, which is made up of many layers: epidermis (E), muscularis mucosa (MM), lamina propria (L), submucosa (S), inner muscularis (IM), myenteric plexus (MP), and outer muscularis (OM). Blood vessels located in the submucosa are identified with arrows. Figure 16.18b is an image of healthy stomach tissue, which contains characteristic glandular pits (black arrows). Finally, Figure 16.18c is an image of tissue afflicted with Barrett's esophagus, which is diagnosed by the presence of submucosal glands (white arrows).

16.2.4 Artery

Similar to the tethered capsule, optical components can be inserted into cardiac catheters, which are commonly used for angioplasty procedures and stent placements (see Chapter 5). Similar to esophagus imaging, OCT images of the entire artery are obtained as the catheter is rotated and slowly pulled back through the artery. Intravascular OCT is used to assess the composition of plaques to determine whether or not they are vulnerable (that is, whether the plaque has a high chance of dislodging, which can lead to a stroke). Similar to previously described tissues, healthy arteries are regularly layered as shown in the top portion of Figure 16.19a. A fibrous plaque appears as an area of homogeneous and rich signal, as seen in the bottom part of Figure 16.19a. As plaques age, they become increasingly calcified; calcification within the plaque appears as signal poor regions that are well-delineated (Figure 16.19b). Lipid pools, which are a precursor to plaque formation, can also be identified using OCT; they appear as signal poor regions with diffuse boundaries (Figure 16.19c). Finally, an irregular protrusion from the surface indicates the presence of a thrombus (i.e. a blot clot), which can dislodge and then block blood flow to various organs (Figure 16.19d). The thrombus can also grow within the artery, which can eventually lead to a heart attack or stroke. Clinical intravascular OCT systems are currently in use, but such systems are currently not as advanced or widely available as ophthalmic systems.

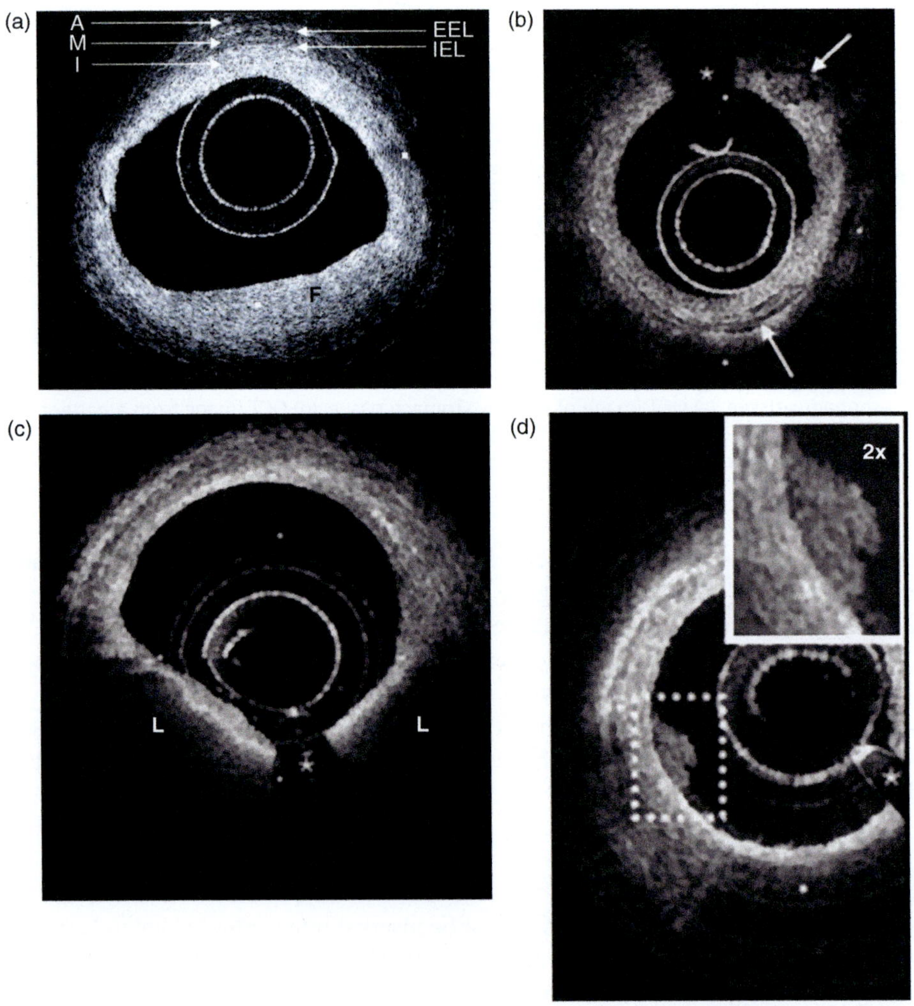

Figure 16.19 Intravascular OCT scans of (a) healthy tissue and fibrous plaque. (b) calcification within a plaque. (c) Lipid pools and (d) thrombus (blood clot). *Source:* Yabushita et al. [6].

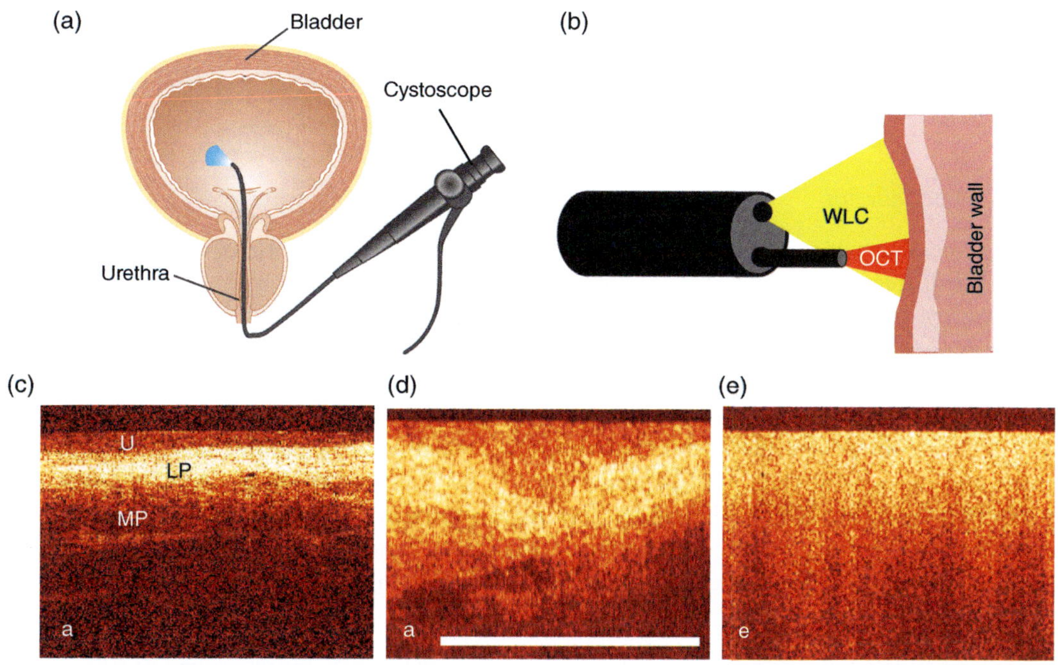

Figure 16.20 (a) Schematic of traditional white light cystoscope (WLC). (b) Schematic showing the integration of an OCT probe into a WLC. OCT images of (c) healthy bladder tissue. (d) Dysplasia and (e) urothelial cell carcinoma tumor. *Source:* Schmidbauer et al. [7], Reprinted from Elsevier: European Urology Copyright © 2009, with permission from Elsevier.

16.2.5 Bladder

Bladder imaging is another application of OCT. Typical bladder exams involve white light cystoscopy (WLC) in which a long tube is outfitted with a white light source and a camera (Figure 16.20a). With this tool, physicians are limited to observing the surface of the bladder. As stated earlier, many diseases initially manifest below the surface. For example, some cancerous tumors will grow into the bladder wall instead of protruding from the surface. These tumors appear flat when viewed from the surface, making them very difficult to identify with WLC alone. To overcome this challenge, an OCT probe can be inserted into the working channel of the cystoscope to obtain subsurface images of the bladder wall (Figure 16.20b). All cystoscopes are already equipped with a working channel; it is normally used for inserting additional tools into the bladder, such as forceps. Figure 16.20c shows an image of a healthy bladder, which is composed of well-defined layers; the top three layers are visible with OCT (U = urothelium, LP = lamina propria, and MP = muscularis propria). Figure 16.20d shows dysplasia (a precancerous lesion), which is characterized as a thickened urothelium. Finally, Figure 16.20e shows an advanced flat tumor. The tumor is characterized by a complete loss of layered structure; it has grown down into the muscle layer and has displaced the healthy layered tissue.

16.3 Contrast Enhancement

Various strategies have been employed to increase the power of OCT, ranging from image processing of traditional OCT images to using nanoparticles to add multiplexing capabilities. Contrast enhancement can be broken down into two categories: exogenous and endogenous. Exogenous refers to externally added contrast agents; fluorophores and SERS particles are examples of exogenous contrast agents. Endogenous enhancement does not alter the sample in any way; enhancement is achieved either through software or hardware changes to the system. Examples of each type follow.

16.3.1 Endogenous

Image processing, which could include de-noising or quantitation, is a form of contrast enhancement. Recall that the contrast in OCT images is due to differences in attenuation coefficient. However, the image intensity is complicated by the Gaussian nature of light beams and the fact that areas deep in the sample appear darker because less light is able to penetrate that far. To overcome this complication and allow clinicians to more accurately assess OCT images, the attenuation coefficient of each pixel in an image can be estimated. Figure 16.21a and b shows the original OCT intensity image and the attenuation image of a phantom, respectively. In the attenuation image, the intensity of each pixel is proportional to the attenuation coefficient of the sample. Notice that the fourth layer of the sample appears very dark in the intensity image, which could lead one to believe that it has a low attenuation coefficient. As shown in the attenuation image, this layer actually has a very high attenuation coefficient. The layer appears dark in the intensity image

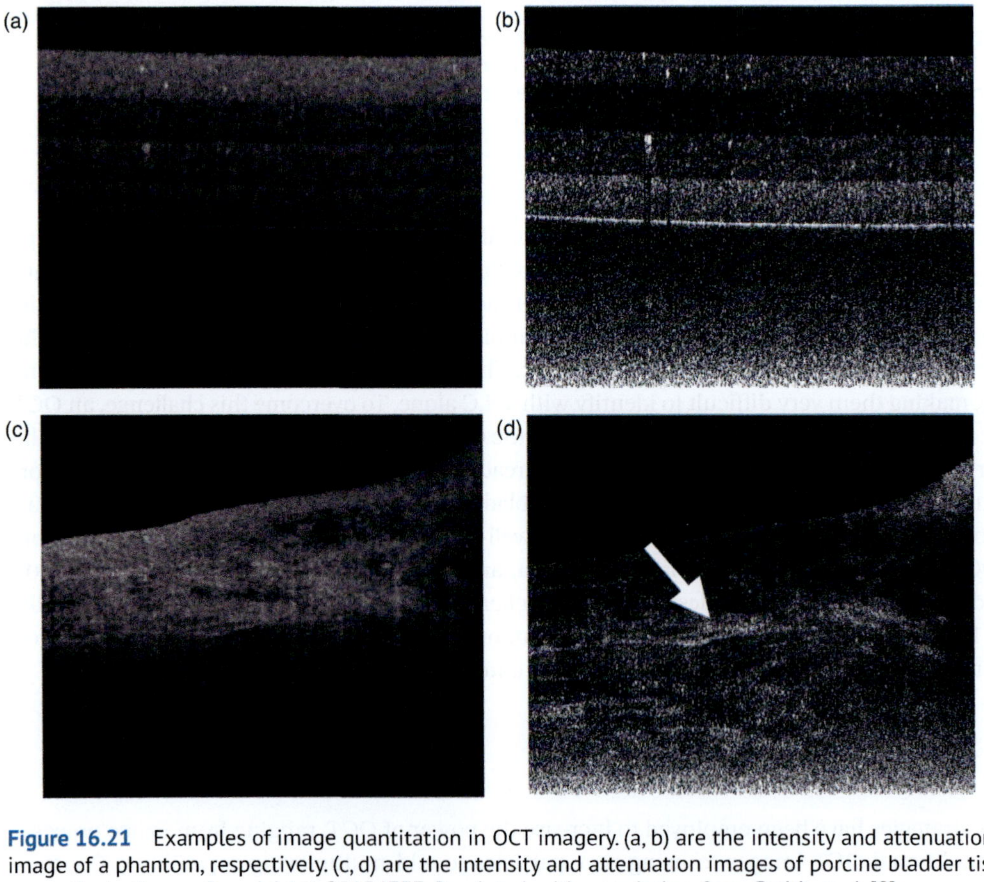

Figure 16.21 Examples of image quantitation in OCT imagery. (a, b) are the intensity and attenuation image of a phantom, respectively. (c, d) are the intensity and attenuation images of porcine bladder tissue, respectively. *Source:* Copyright © 2015 IEEE. Reprinted, with permission, from Smith et al. [8].

simply because it is deep within the sample. Figure 16.21c and d shows an additional example of contrast enhancement through image quantitation. The highly scattering muscle fibers (indicated by the arrow) in the porcine bladder tissue are difficult to discern in the intensity image (Figure 16.21c), but they become very clear in the attenuation image (Figure 16.21d). In addition to increased contrast, image quantitation is relevant for diagnostic, classification, and surveillance applications. Recall that the attenuation of the retinal nerve fiber layer is used to track the progression of glaucoma. Attenuation coefficient measurements have also been implicated in atherosclerotic plaque characterization, renal cancer diagnosis, bladder cancer tumor staging, burn scar assessment, and cerebral edema detection.

Another technique for endogenous contrast enhancement relies on measuring physical parameters of tissue other than attenuation coefficients. Two examples are polarization-sensitive OCT (PS-OCT) and Doppler OCT. Polarization is a characteristic of a light wave and it refers to the orientation of the oscillations of the electric field (recall that light is an electromagnetic wave). The polarization can be linear, circular, or elliptical. In traditional OCT, an unpolarized source (i.e. one that contains a mixture of polarization states) is used. In PS-OCT, the source is replaced with a polarized light source and the detector is replaced with a pair of CCDs, which can be used to assess the polarization state of the resultant wave. Dermal imaging is one application where PS-OCT has proven useful. When light propagates through healthy skin, the polarization state of the light is maintained due to highly ordered collagen particles. When light propagates through a tumor, the polarization state gets scrambled because the collagen in a tumor is very disorganized. This difference can be measured using PS-OCT. Figure 16.22 shows an example of dermal imaging with PS-OCT. The three rows are images from different mouse tissue samples. The left column shows the

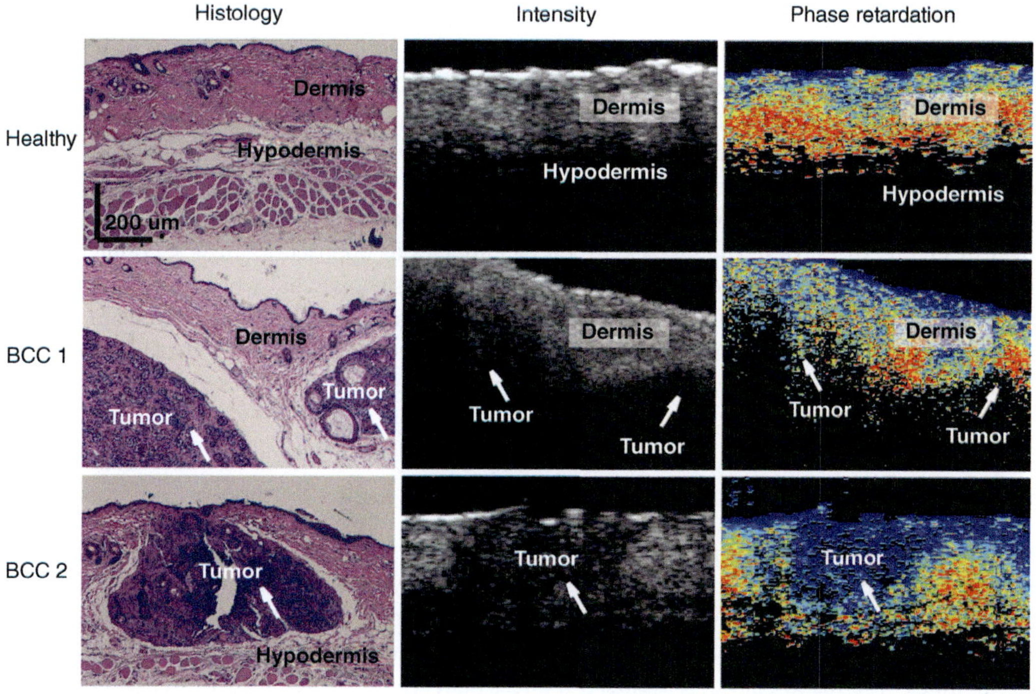

Figure 16.22 Histology (left column), traditional OCT scans (middle column), and PS-OCT images (right column) of both healthy tissue and basal cell carcinoma tumors in a mouse. *Source:* Duan et al. [9].

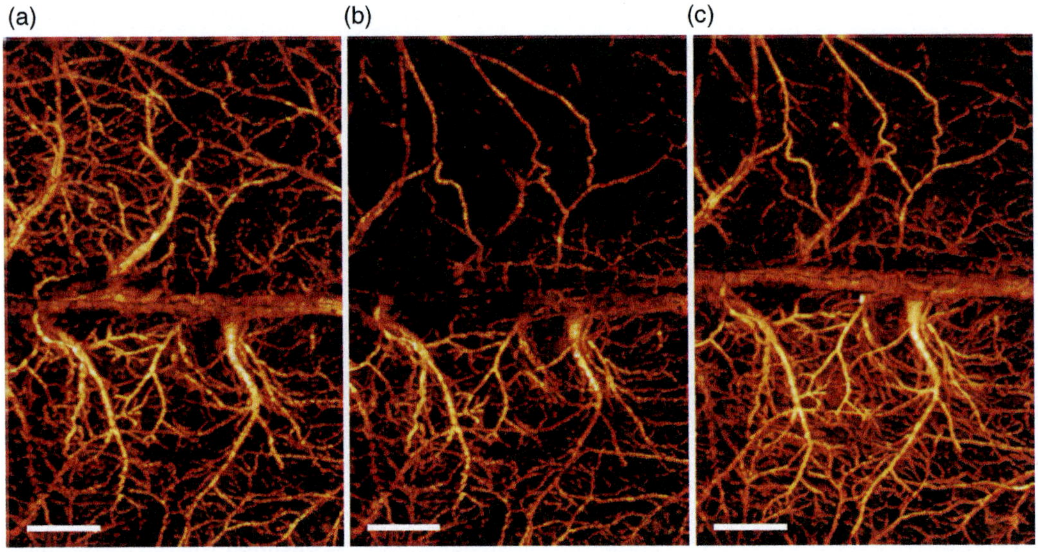

Figure 16.23 En face Doppler OCT scans of a mouse brain (a) before an induced stroke, (b) after an induced stroke, and (c) after reperfusion of the vasculature. *Source:* Jia and Wang [10].

histology images, the middle column shows traditional OCT intensity images, and the right column shows PS-OCT images. In the healthy tissue (top row), the PS-OCT has a characteristic banded nature. The middle row and bottom row are tissues that contain basal cell carcinoma (BCC) tumors. Notice the disruption to the banded nature in the PS-OCT images in both cases, and the low contrast between normal and tumor tissue in the intensity image of the first BCC tumor. The additional contrast from the PS-OCT images can be useful for both tumor detection and boundary definition for tumor removal surgery.

Doppler OCT is sensitive to flow within a sample. For example, it can be used to image blood flow within arteries and enhance the contrast of small vasculature. Doppler OCT measures flow by tracking the phase of the interference signal (the specifics of which are beyond the scope of this book). Doppler OCT has been used to study the effects of stroke on the vasculature of the brain, as shown in Figure 16.23. Here the images are en face images as opposed to cross sectional slices. While cross sectional images show a side view, en face images show what would be seen if a portion of the sample was removed from the top and the remaining sample was imaged from above. Figure 16.23a, b, and c shows a mouse brain before an induced stroke, after the stroke (notice the lack of blood flow to the top part of the image), and after reperfusion of the vasculature (i.e. reintroduction of flow), respectively.

16.3.2 Exogenous

Research around exogenous contrast agents for OCT is still an emerging area, but two will be described here: glycerol and nanoparticle-based contrast. Glycerol is a common type of alcohol that is often used as a laxative; when applied topically to skin, it both increases contrast and the imaging depth of OCT. When glycerol is applied topically, it displaces the interstitial fluid. Because it has an index of refraction closer to tissue, it reduces light scattering; reduced scattering results in a larger imaging depth. Glycerol also dehydrates the sample by pulling water out of the cellular structures, which reduces the volume of the scattering centers. The reduction in volume results in

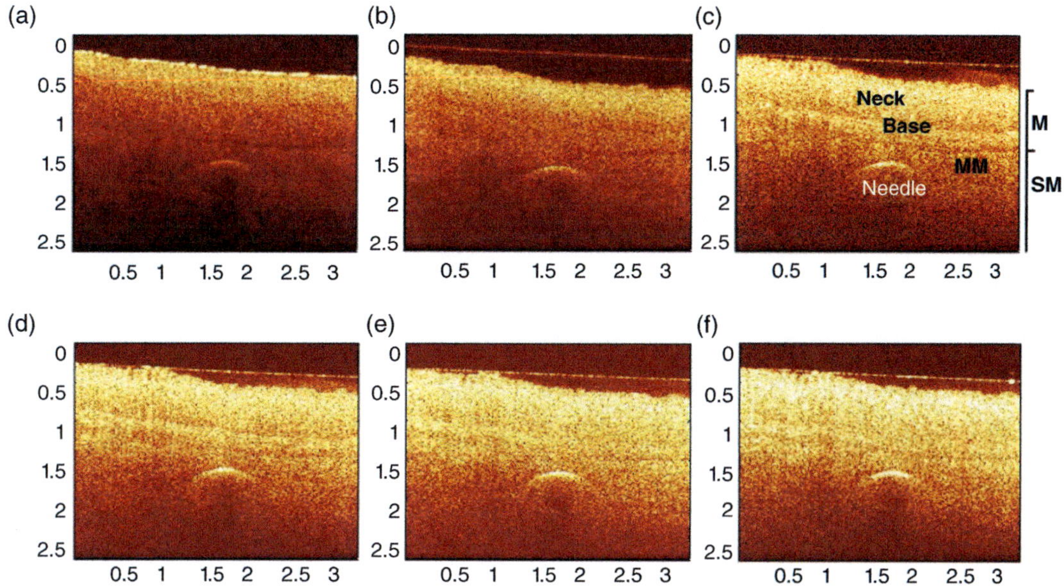

Figure 16.24 OCT images from 50-minute time progression of a needle embedded in porcine tissue after topical application of a 50% glycerol solution. *Source:* He and Wang [11].

an increase of the local back reflection and thus increases contrast. Figure 16.24 shows images of a needle embedded in porcine stomach tissue at various time points after topical application of a 50% glycerol solution. Notably, the imaging depth increased over time, as evidenced by higher signal from deep in the sample. In Figure 16.24c and d, the needle surface appears sharper which demonstrates increased contrast. Glycerol works over a limited time period as the tissue clears the chemical, which is evidenced by the decreased effects in Figure 16.24f.

Gold nanocages and large gold nanorods (LGNRs) are also examples of exogenous contrast agents. Both structures exhibit optical resonance at wavelengths typically used in OCT, giving them extremely large absorption and scattering coefficients at those wavelengths. For both nanocages and LGNRs, this wavelength can be adjusted by altering their size. The large absorption coefficient of the nanocages allows them to be easily distinguished in an OCT image, as demonstrated in Figure 16.25. The area on the right was injected with gold nanocages, which caused the signal to die very quickly. Other absorptive dyes have been tested as contrast agents, but gold nanocages have absorption coefficients approximately five orders of magnitude larger than typical absorptive dyes. On the other hand, LGNRs exhibit large scattering coefficients and can be detected directly by their scattering instead of relying on light attenuation because of absorption. Figure 16.26a shows a single LGNR as observed in high-resolution transmission electron microscopy (TEM). Figure 16.26b is a scanning electron microscope (SEM) image that shows that LGNRs exhibit a high degree of uniformity in terms of shape and size. This uniformity is important because it ensures that the particles all exhibit a well-defined, narrow spectral peak that makes them easily detectable with OCT. Figure 16.26c shows LGNRs prepared in glass capillary tubes at different particle concentrations in water. LGNRs produce such a strong OCT signal that single particles can be seen at very low concentrations. In other words, LGNRs are very high-sensitivity OCT agents. While the image in Figure 16.26c shows that LGNRs can be detected by their scattering intensity, one of their biggest advantages is that they have very unique spectral scattering peaks. This

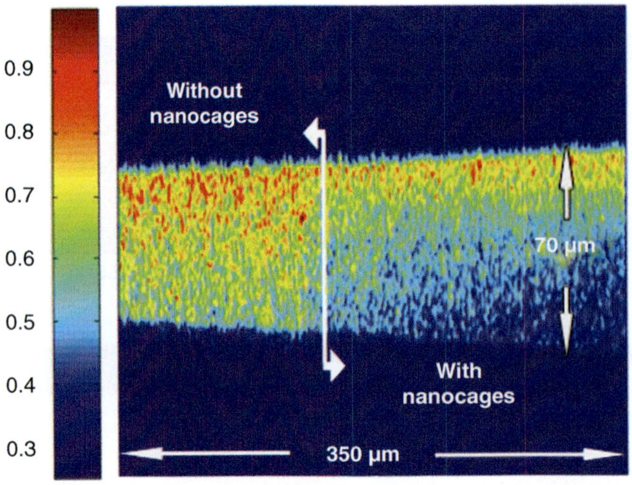

Figure 16.25 OCT image of a phantom with embedded gold nanocages in the right portion. *Source:* Chen et al. [12]. Reprinted with permission from Nano Letters: American Chemical Society, Copyright © 2005, American Chemical Society.

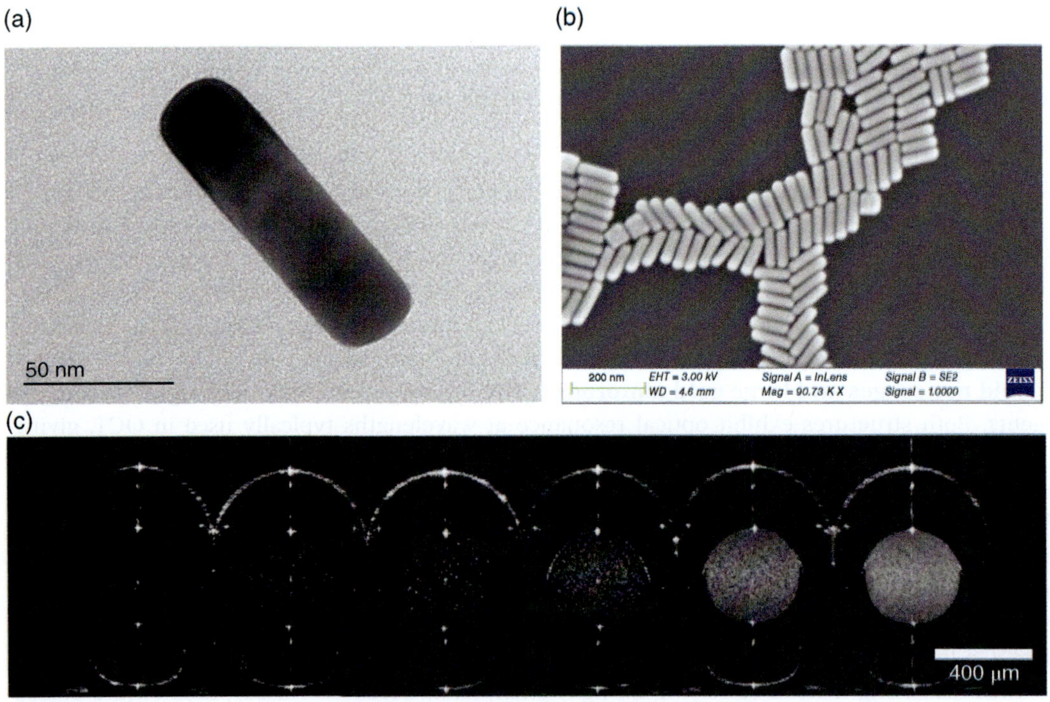

Figure 16.26 (a) TEM image of a single LGNR, (b) SEM image of a population of LGNRs, and (c) OCT intensity image of various concentrations of LGNRs in water within glass capillary tubes. The tube on the far left is water only. The highest concentration, on the far right, is ~50 pM.

property means that LGNRs can be detected and distinguished from tissue scattering with the help of spectral processing algorithms. Detecting LGNRs by their unique spectral signatures can be used to enhance the detection of tumor blood vessels in live animal models of cancer. Figure 16.27a depicts an OCT intensity image of a human glioblastoma xenograft (U87MG tumor cells) implanted within the ear of a live mouse. Spectral processing algorithms reveal the locations of several major

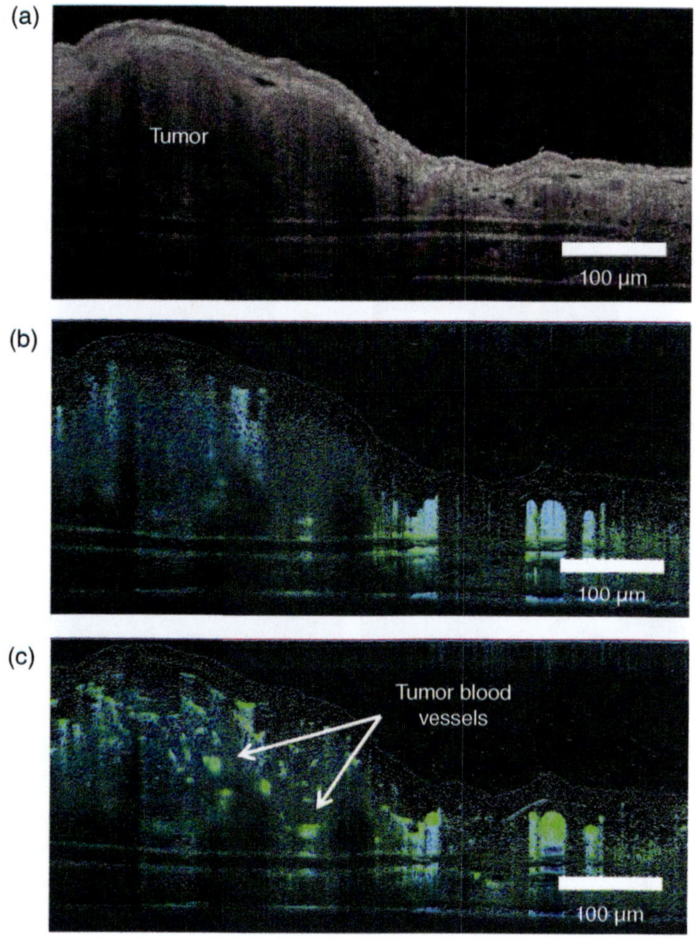

Figure 16.27 (a) OCT intensity image of a mouse ear with a tumor (glioblastoma), (b) Spectral contrast OCT image of the region before the injection of LGNRs. Blood vessels can be seen in cyan, and (b) The same region after injection of LGNRs. LGNRs appear in green and reveal numerous small blood vessels in the tumor.

blood vessels within the ear (Figure 16.27b), but almost no blood vessels can be seen within the tumor itself. In order to observe the vast network of blood vessels within the tumor, LGNRs were injected into blood circulation through the mouse's tail vein. After the injection, LGNRs (green signal) within a dense network of small blood vessels can be seen in the tumor (Figure 16.27c). LGNRs can be used for more than tumor imaging alone – they can also be used to image the lymphatic vessels within living subjects. Lymph vessels serve important immune functions in mammals that help preserve health. To image different networks of lymph vessels, LGNRs can be made with different spectral properties to enable multicolor and multiplexed contrast enhancement with OCT. Figure 16.28 demonstrates these multiplexing capabilities possible with LGNRs. Figure 16.28a is an en face view of blood vessels in a healthy mouse ear with no LGNRs. Figure 16.28b was taken after the subcutaneous injection of LGNRs, which drain from the injection site into the lymphatic system. The LGNRs filled the lymph vessels and drained from the injection site at the edge of the ear (top of image) to the base of the ear (bottom of image). LGNRs with a different scattering peak were then injected into a different site within the ear and the drainage of those LGNRs was also observed (Figure 16.28c). Because the two LGNR populations have different spectral peaks, they can be distinguished by looking at different bands of wavelengths in the raw OCT signal. In addition to multiplexing capabilities, LGNRs are a promising contrast agent because they can be

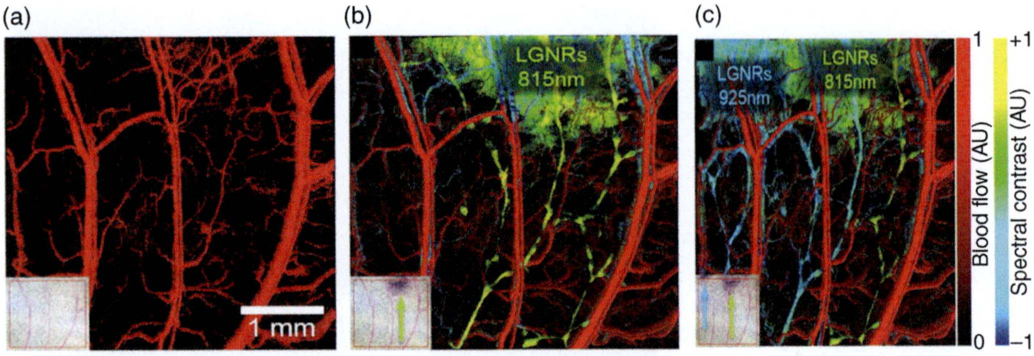

Figure 16.28 En face OCT scans of a mouse ear. (a) Blood vessels in the ear. (b) OCT scan after the injection of LGNRs (absorption peak at 815 nm) into the lymphatic system. (c) OCT scan after the injection of an additional set of LGNRs (absorption peak at 925 nm) into a different site in the ear. *Source:* Liba et al. [13].

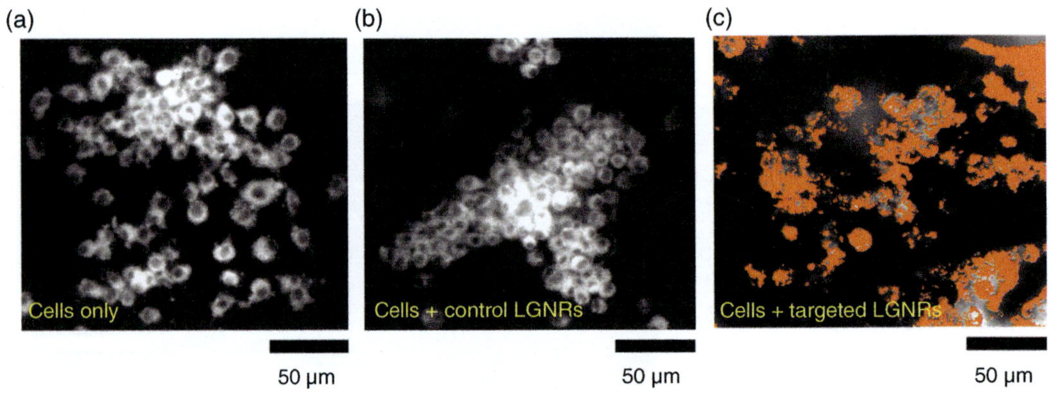

Figure 16.29 *In vitro* study of targeted LGNR cell uptake. (a) U87MG cells only (no LGNRs), (b) cells incubated with nonspecific LGNRs (control), and (c) cells incubated with LGNRs targeted to specific proteins on the cell surface.

functionalized with bio-specific tags to target areas of interest (e.g. anti-EGFR antibodies for targeting cancerous tumors). It is possible to characterize the specific binding of functionalized LGNRs to cell receptors of interest in labeled cell culture experiments. Figure 16.29 shows several cultures of tumor cells (U87MG) that were exposed to LGNRs with different surface coatings. The presence of LGNRs within each cell population was determined using different spectral detection methods. For all images in Figure 16.29, the presence of LGNRs is shown as an orange mask on top of a grayscale image. Figure 16.29a shows a high-resolution dark-field microscope image of tumor cells (40× magnification). As expected, no LGNRs are detected within the cells-only sample. Figure 16.29b shows a similar image of cells incubated with LGNRs that are not functionalized to bind a specific cell surface protein expressed by the tumor cells (e.g. "Control LGNRs"). This sample also shows a lack of LGNRs bound to the tumor cells. By comparison, Figure 16.29c shows cells that were incubated with LGNRs conjugated to antibodies that are specific for proteins expressed on the U87MG cell surface. These cells are densely covered with the targeted LGNRs (depicted in orange). These results suggest that functionalized LGNRs could be used as targeted contrast agents in OCT molecular imaging studies in the future.

While the optical scattering of nanoparticles holds great promise, they have the caveat of limited contrast over highly scattering tissue background. Two contrast mechanisms that aim to overcome this downfall are photothermal OCT (PTOCT) and magnetomotive OCT (MMOCT). In PTOCT, the strong optical absorption of small metal nanoparticles is exploited; the strong absorption causes a change in temperature around the particle (via the photothermal effect, which is discussed further in the next chapter). This change in temperature results in a variation of the index of refraction and therefore the optical path length. Using an amplitude-modulated laser in the sample arm of an OCT system creates photothermal oscillations in the sample, which can be imaged directly via the phase info of the measured light (there is a linear relationship between the phase and optical path length). Simulations and experiments have shown that there is a linear relationship between the photothermal signal and both the pump power of the amplitude-modulated laser and the nanoparticle concentration. PTOCT shows a sensitivity as low as 14 parts per million and has been used to measure EGFR expression levels from live cells in 3D tissue constructs.

MMOCT relies on tiny displacements of magnetic nanoparticles induced by an external magnetic field. The nanometer-scale displacements, which induce changes in local scattering, are measured using phase-sensitive OCT (similar to PTOCT). Phase-sensitive OCT can achieve a sensitivity of a few tens of nanometers, which is equivalent to approximately a 2nM concentration of magnetic nanoparticles. MMOCT is particularly attractive because the magnetic nanoparticles are already FDA-approved as a contrast agent for MRI. The contrast achievable with MMOCT is significant due to the low magnetic susceptibility of tissue (i.e. the external magnetic field has a negligible effect on tissue). Magnetic nanoparticles have been conjugated to antibodies for evaluation of EGFR expression levels; they have also been inserted in platelets to identify areas of endothelial damage. MMOCT can also be used to enhance the Doppler OCT signal as red blood cells contain iron and therefore exhibit magnetomotion in an external magnetic field. Finally, by observing the relaxation time of the nanoparticles (i.e. the time required for the particles to return to their original location after the magnetic field has been turned off) enables characterization of tissue properties such as stiffness.

16.4 Conclusion

OCT is an optical imaging technique. Similar to fluorescence and Raman spectroscopy, it has a high resolution, relatively low scan time, and (with the help of contrast agents) multiplexing capabilities. OCT uses interferometry with a broadband source to probe the subsurface structure of a sample. While OCT can only image a few millimeters below the surface, the miniaturization of optical components has made access to internal surfaces (e.g. bladder, artery) possible and thus greatly expanded the applications for OCT. Clinically, OCT is widely accepted in the ophthalmology community and is becoming more common in other areas, such as cardiology and dermatology.

Acknowledgment

The authors would like to thank Gennifer Smith for contributing this chapter.

Problems

16.1 Draw the measured output signal from an interferometer with the following parameters: a 1300 nm laser as the source, a moveable reference mirror, and a series of sample mirrors at distances of 4980, 5005, and 5025 μm from the beam splitter and with reflection coefficients of 0.3, 0.5, and 0.8, respectively. Refer to Figure 16.8 for the interferometer setup. Assume the following: the position of zero path length difference occurs when the reference mirror is positioned 5000 μm from the beam splitter, all mirrors are placed in air, and the reference mirror has a reflection coefficient of 1.

16.2 Discuss the advantages and disadvantages of OCT compared to imaging modalities discussed in previous chapters (e.g. MRI, PET, fluorescence, Raman).

16.3 Another scheme of OCT not discussed in the chapter is full-field OCT (FF-OCT). Rather than point scanning, which requires scanning the beam in two directions to acquire 3D volumes (in addition to depth scanning for TD-OCT), FF-OCT utilizes full-field sample imaging onto an array detector such as a CCD or CMOS camera. That is, an entire en face image is collected using an array detector; so only a depth scanning needs to be performed to acquire 3D volumes. Many FF-OCT systems use filtered lamps to obtain a source spectrum of about 600–900 nm. Given this info, what are the advantages and disadvantages of FF-OCT compared to SD-OCT?

References

1 Jmarchn, https://commons.wikimedia.org/wiki/File:Simple_diagram_of_human_eye_multilingual.svg

2 Lee, G.C.F., Smith, G.T., Agrawal, M. et al. (2015). Fabrication of healthy and disease-mimicking retinal phantoms with tapered foveal pits for optical coherence tomography. *Journal of Biomedical Optics* 20 (8): 085004.

3 van der Schoot, J., Vermeer, K.A., de Boer, J.F., and Lemij, H.G. (2012). The effect of glaucoma on the optical attenuation coeffiecient of the retinal nerve fiber layer in spectral domain optical coherence tomography images. *Investigative Ophthalmology* 53: 2424–2430.

4 Olsen, J., Themstrup, L., De Carvalho, N. et al. Diagnostic accuracy of optical coherence tomography in actinic keratosis and basal cell carcinoma. *Photodiagnosis and Photodynamic Therapy* 16: 44–49.

5 Gora, M.J., Sauk, J.S., Carruth, R.W. et al. (2013). Tethered capsule endomicroscopy enables less invasive imaging of gastrointestinal tract microstructure. *Nature Medicine* 19: 238–240.

6 Yabushita, H., Bouma, B.E., Houser, S.L. et al. Characterization of human atherosclerosis by optical coherence tomography. *Circulation* 106 (13): 1640–1645. http://circ.ahajournals.org/content/106/13/1640.

7 Schmidbauer, J., Remzi, M., Klatte, T. et al. Fluorescence cytoscopy with high-resolution optical coherence tomography imaging as an adjunct reduces false-positive findings in the diagnosis of urothelial carcinoma of the bladder. *European Urology* 56 (6): 914–919.

8 Smith, G.T. et al. (Dec. 2015). Automated, depth-resolved estimation of the attenuation coefficient from optical coherence tomography data. *IEEE Transactions on Medical Imaging* 24 (12): 2592–2602.

9 Duan, L., Marvdashti, T., Lee, A. et al. (2014). Automated identification of basal cell carcinoma by polarization-sensitive optical coherence tomography. *Biomedical Optics Express* 5 (3717–3729).

10 Jia, Y. and Wang, R. K. (2011), Optical micro-angiography images structural and functional cerebral blood perfusion in mice with cranium left intact. *Journal of Biophotonics*, 4: 57-63. doi:https://doi.org/10.1002/jbio.201000001

11 He, Y.H. and Wang, R.K. (2004). Dynamic optical clearing effect of tissue impregnated with hyperosmotic agents and studied with optical coherence tomogoraphy. *Journal of Biomedical Optics* 9 (1).

12 Chen, J., Saeki, F., Wiley, B.J. et al. Gold nanocages: bioconjunction and their potential use as optical imaging contrast agents. *American Chemical Society* 5 (3): 473–477.

13 Liba, O., SoRelle, E., Sen, D. *et al*. Contrast-enhanced optical coherence tomography with picomolar sensitivity for functional *in vivo* imaging. *Scientific Reports* **6,** 23337 (2016) doi:https://doi.org/10.1038/srep23337

Further Reading

https://www.thorlabs.com/images/TabImages/OCT_PW11.pdf

https://www.healthcheckup.com/blog/general/cystoscopy-test-for-bladder-cancer/

Boas, D.A., Pitris, C., and Ramanujam, N. (2011). *Handbook of Biomedical Optics*. CRC Press.

Dwork, Nicholas, et al. (2016). "Automated estimation of OCT confocal function parameters from two B-scans." Lasers and Electro-Optics (CLEO), 2016 Conference on IEEE, 2016.

Marvdashti, T. et al. (2016). Classification of basal cell carcinoma in human skin using machine learning and quantitative features captured by polarization sensitive optical coherence tomography. *Biomedical Optics Express* 7 (9): 3721–3735.

Skala, M.C. et al. (2008). Photothermal optical coherence tomography of epidermal growth factor receptor in live cells using immunotargeted gold nanospheres. *Nano Letters* 8 (10): 3461–3467.

Smith, G.T., Dwork, N., O'Connor, D. et al. (2015). Automated, depth-resolved estimation of the attenuation coefficient from optical coherence tomography Data. *IEEE Transactions on Medical Imaging* 34 (12): 2592–2602.

SoRelle, E. et al. (2015). Biofunctionalization of large gold nanorods realizes ultrahigh-sensitivity optical imaging agents. *Langmuir* 31 (45): 12339–12347.

Vo-Dinh, T. (ed.) (2014). *Biomedical Photonics Handbook: Therapeutics and Advanced Biophotonics*. CRC Press.

17

Photoacoustic Imaging

17.1 Photoacoustic Effect

The **photoacoustic effect** describes a process by which energy from photons gets converted to acoustic waves (i.e. sound waves). It occurs when absorption of photons from a pulse of light produces heat, which then causes localized thermal expansion, and therefore, acoustic waves due to pressure variation in the surrounding medium. Alexander Graham Bell discovered the photoacoustic effect and used it as the basis for the first phone system. Bell found that sound waves could modulate a ray of light. This modulation can be achieved by speaking to a thin mirror-like membrane. Vocally produced acoustic vibrations in the membrane caused the light hitting the membrane to be reflected in different directions based on the specific sound waves. As a modulated ray of light was received on the other end of Bell's photoacoustic device, the ray was absorbed by a thin metal, which produced sound waves according to the photoacoustic effect, reconstructing the original voice. A drawing of Bell's original photoacoustic device is shown in Figure 17.1.

If both the thermal and the stress confinement conditions are satisfied (see detailed discussion of the confinements below), the photoacoustic effect can be seen in an object illuminated with light, which will thermally expand and produce a pressure wave with an initial pressure p_0 propagating outward from the object at velocity c as an ultrasound wave:

$$p_0 = \left(\frac{\beta c^2}{C_\mathrm{p}}\right)\mu_\mathrm{a} F = \Gamma A,$$

where β is the isobaric volume expansion coefficient (units of K^{-1}) due to photon absorption, C_p is the specific heat (the energy required to raise the temperature of 1 kg of the material by 1 K, units of $\mathrm{J\,K^{-1}\,kg^{-1}}$), μ_a is the absorption coefficient (units of cm^{-1}), F is the light fluence (energy per unit area of light illumination, units of $\mathrm{J\,cm^{-2}}$), p_0 is the initial photoacoustic pressure (units of Pascal = Pa = $\mathrm{N\,m^{-2}}$), $A = \mu_\mathrm{a}\,F$ is the local energy deposition density (units of $\mathrm{J\,cm^{-3}}$), and $\Gamma = \beta c^2/C_\mathrm{p}$ is the Grüneisen coefficient (with typical values of 0.1–1 for different tissues; unitless). Thus, the exact pressure wave response from illuminating a certain type of tissue can be predicted. By measuring the time required for the pressure wave to arrive at a detector, an object's depth can be determined. Note that in the context of photoacoustic imaging, the following terms are all synonymous and interchangeably used in literature: pressure wave, sound wave, ultrasound wave, photoacoustic wave, and optoacoustic wave.

Biochips and Medical Imaging, First Edition. Adam de la Zerda and Shan Xiang Wang.

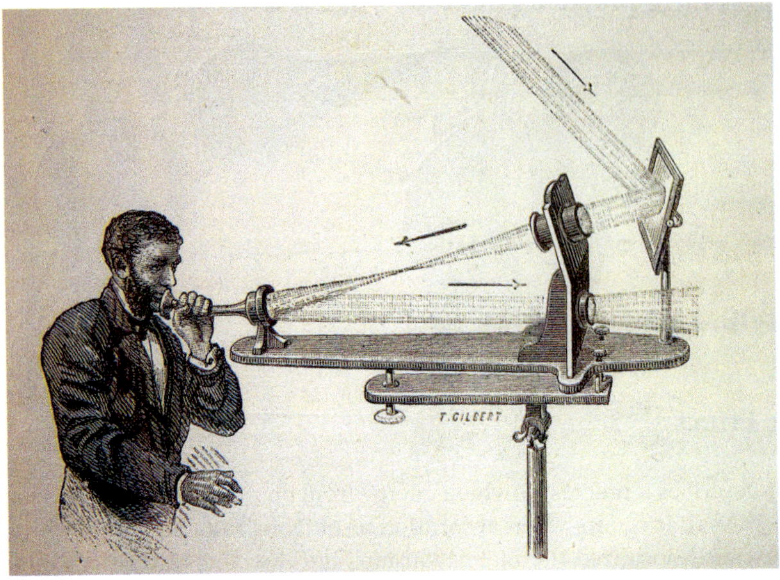

Figure 17.1 Bell's original photoacoustic setup. *Source:* Harryzilber [1]. CC0–1.0 public domain https://creativecommons.org/publicdomain/zero/1.0.

17.2 The Thermal and Stress Confinements

17.2.1 Thermal Confinement Condition

The **thermal confinement condition** states that over the course of the excitation pulse of light, the heat produced by the object should not diffuse a length greater than the size of the object (Figure 17.2). The distance that heat diffuses is given by the **thermal diffusion length**:

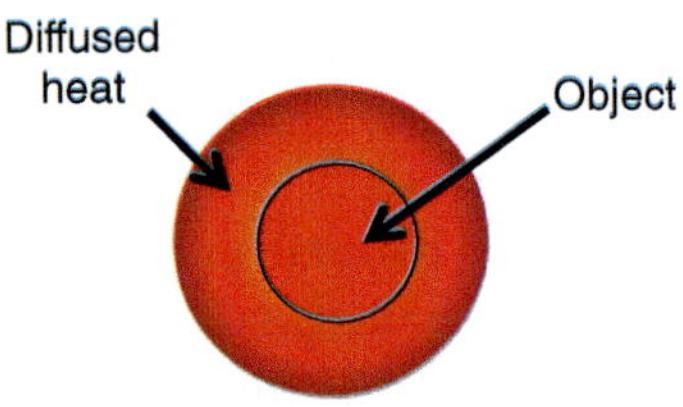

Figure 17.2 Thermal confinement.

$$\delta_T = 2\sqrt{D_T \tau_p},$$

where D_T is the thermal diffusivity (a constant depending on the type of tissue, with a typical value for most tissues of ~1.4×10^{-3} cm^2 s^{-1}), and τ_p is the laser pulse duration (units of seconds). Thermal confinement is then given by:

$$L_p > \delta_T$$

where L_p is the characteristic length of the smallest absorbing structure in the tissue. For example, for a laser pulse duration of $\tau_p = 0.5$ μs (a relatively long optical pulse), the thermal confinement condition requires that $\delta_T = 0.5$ μm, be smaller than L_p. This can easily be achieved, as the spatial resolution of photoacoustic imaging systems is typically at least 10 μm.

17.2.2 Stress Confinement Condition

The **stress confinement condition** requires that over the course of the light excitation pulse, acoustic waves produced by the object should not travel longer than the size of the object (Figure 17.3). Since acoustic waves travel over a distance of $\tau_p c$ in a time of τ_p (where $c = 1.54$ mm μs^{-1}

in soft tissues), this means that the stress confinement condition is $\tau_p c < L_p$. For example, for a laser pulse duration of $\tau_p = 0.5$ μs, the acoustic waves must travel no farther than $\tau_p c = 770$ μm (a relatively poor resolution). To allow a spatial resolution of 150 μm (i.e. $L_p = 150$ μm), the laser pulse duration τ_p must be no more than 97 ns. It is much harder to satisfy the stress confinement condition than the thermal confinement condition.

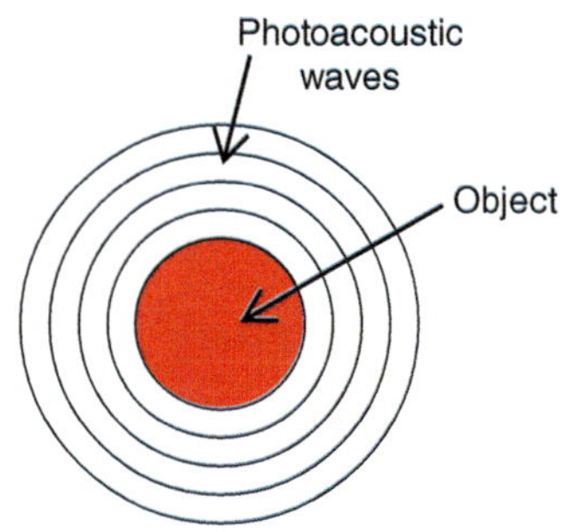

Figure 17.3 Stress confinement.

17.3 Photoacoustic Imaging

17.3.1 Imaging Steps

Photoacoustic imaging is performed according to the steps given in Figure 17.4a. First, an imaging agent is administered to the subject; single-walled nanotubes (SWNTs) are an example of an imaging agent (Figure 17.4b). Next, a pulsed laser (typically on the order of tens of nanoseconds in duration) is applied to the subject. The light is distributed instantaneously within the tissue (compared to the time scale of the laser pulse duration, τ_p). As the tissues absorb the light (especially in areas where the contrast agent has accumulated), the temperature of the tissue rises and rapid thermal expansion of tissue produces pressure waves. The pressure waves propagate radially outward, reach the surface of the object, and get detected by ultrasound detectors (a.k.a. transducers). The sound wave intensity and time of arrival provide information on the concentration and depth of the imaging agent in the body, respectively.

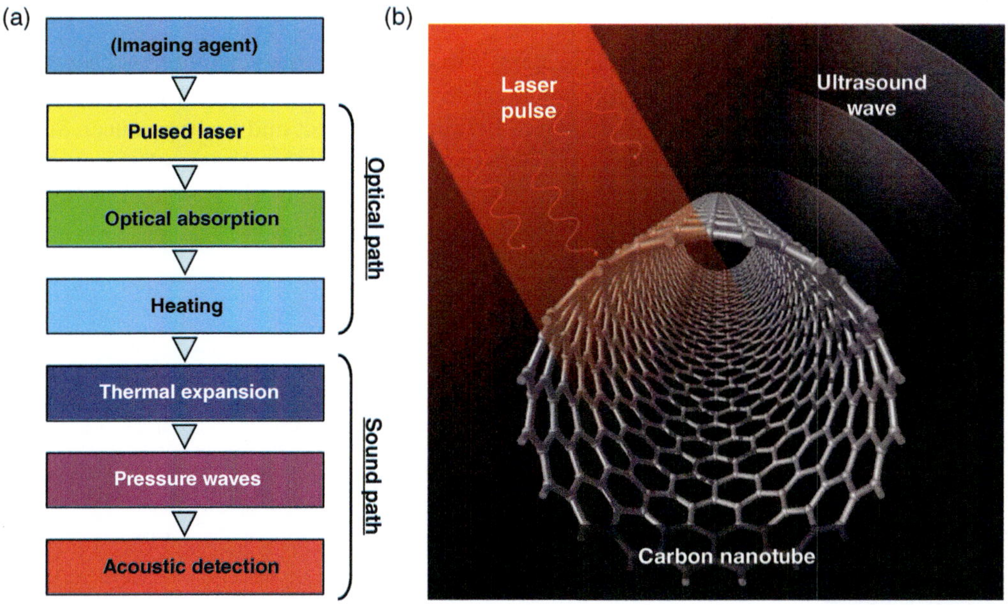

Figure 17.4 (a) Photoacoustic imaging steps, (b) photoacoustic effect on SWNT. *Source:* Courtesy of Jim Strommer.

17.3.2 Detection

An **ultrasound detector (transducer)** measures the ultrasound signal *p*(*t*) over time. Since the received signal is a function of time, it is possible to differentiate the signals from shallower versus deeper objects (e.g. signals from deeper objects arrive later in time). The signal intensity is given by:

$$I(t) = |p(x = ct)|^2,$$

which provides information on depth in the time domain. The transducer may be focused, allowing the transducer to be most sensitive to waves originating in front of it (Figure 17.5). The photoacoustic waves frequency bandwidth is $[0, 1/\tau_p]$; for $\tau_p = 10$ ns, frequencies up to 100 MHz will emerge. Transducers have a limited frequency bandwidth, e.g. a transducer of 5 ± 2 MHz (FWHM) is said to have 80% bandwidth (where the percent bandwidth is the bandwidth divided by the central frequency). The higher the frequency and bandwidth, the better the spatial resolution is; hence, high ultrasound frequencies are desirable. However, a higher frequency also results in higher tissue absorption of ultrasound. Thus, the typical range of ultrasonic frequencies used in clinical settings is 1.5–40 MHz, depending on the required depth of penetration and spatial resolution.

17.3.3 Advantages and Disadvantages

The main advantage of photoacoustic imaging over other optical techniques is its high depth of penetration and spatial resolution. As light propagates only once through the tissue (compared to twice for typical optical imaging), depth of penetration increases markedly and can reach several centimeters (about an order of magnitude higher than fluorescence imaging). Also, acoustic waves are not scattered or absorbed much by tissues, resulting in improved spatial resolution in the submillimeter range (as compared to fluorescence imaging which loses resolution exponentially as the depth increases). In addition, depth is encoded in the time domain ultrasound signal, which allows for reconstruction of 3D images.

One major disadvantage of photoacoustic imaging is that acoustic waves cannot travel between different media easily due to acoustic impedance mismatches. Hence, only soft tissues can be imaged and no bones or air structures are allowed between the object and the transducer. Since ultrasound waves cannot move easily from the soft tissue to air structures, the transducer must be in contact with the skin (or object surface). Impedance matching with the skin is typically achieved by using a water bath or simple ultrasound gel.

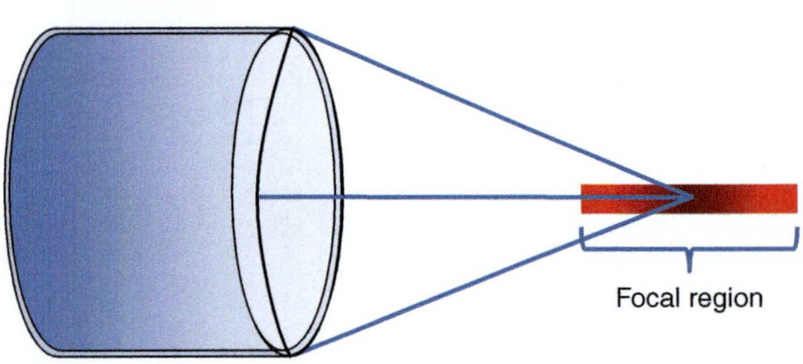

Figure 17.5 Ultrasound transducer (detector). *Source:* Rakruger [2]. Used under CC-BY-SA 3.0 https://creativecommons.org/licenses/by-sa/3.0.

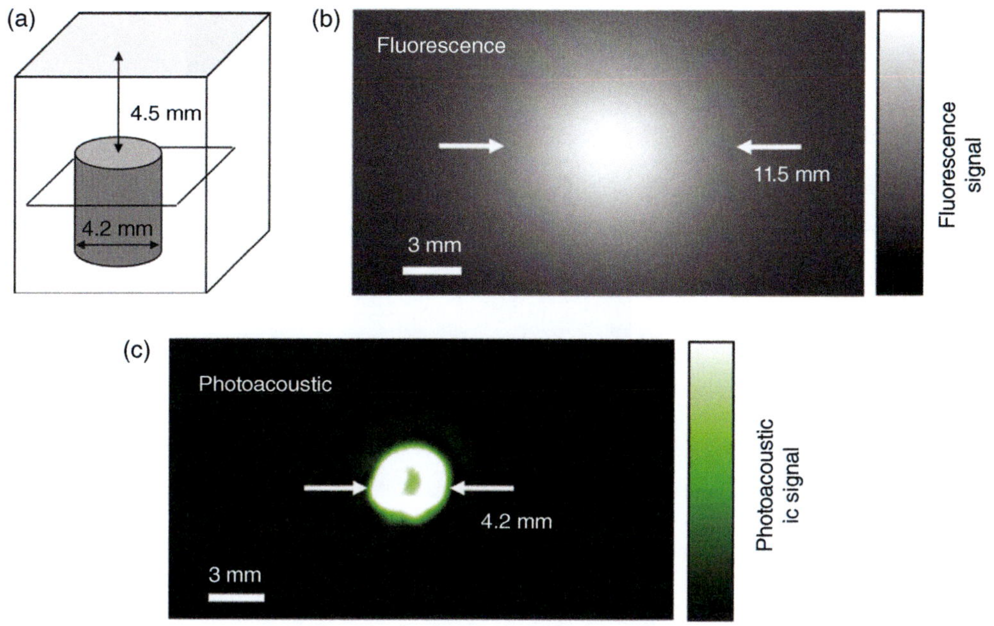

Figure 17.6 (a) Tissue-mimicking phantom with an inclusion filled of fluorescent quantum dots at 800 nm and single walled carbon nanotubes (black). (b) Epifluorescence of the phantom showing a full half-width max FWHM = 11.5 mm for the 4.2 mm wide inclusion. (c) A horizontal slice through the photoacoustic image of the phantom showing the accurate inclusion width. *Source:* de la Zerda et al. [3]. Reprinted by permission from Springer Nature. Copyright © 2008 by Springer Nature.

17.3.4 Photoacoustic Versus Fluorescence Imaging

To compare the resolution of photoacoustic and fluorescence imaging, consider a tissue-mimicking phantom that contains an inclusion filled with fluorescent quantum dots (QDs) emitting at 800 nm and single-walled carbon nanotubes (SWNTs). Recall that the fluorescence signal was 11.5 mm wide (FWHM) for a 4.2 mm wide inclusion. Photoacoustic imaging of this same phantom shows the accurate inclusion width of 4.2 mm (Figure 17.6). This demonstrates the greater depth of penetration and improved spatial resolution of photoacoustic imaging as compared with fluorescence imaging. The reason for high resolution in photoacoustic imaging is the fact that the ultrasound waves scatter very little compared to the optical waves as they travel to the surface.

17.4 Contrast Agents

17.4.1 Endogenous Contrast Agents

Endogenous contrast agents for photoacoustic imaging include molecules naturally found in the body that absorb light, such as melanin (skin pigment) and hemoglobin, which comes in deoxygenated and oxygenated forms (Hb and HbO_2, respectively). For example, a 3D photoacoustic image of hemoglobin in a mouse brain was taken with the skull and skin intact, allowing for visualization of the vasculature, as shown in Figure 17.7 (A is the superior sagittal sinus, B is the transverse sinus, and C is the inferior cerebral vein).

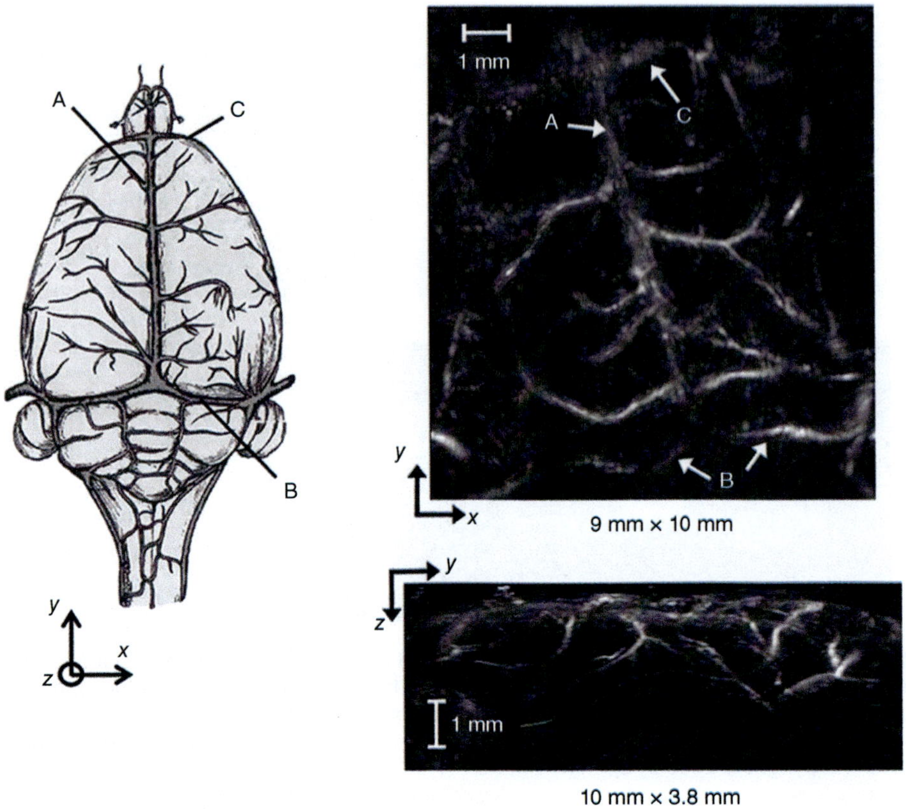

Figure 17.7 Photoacoustic image of mouse brain vasculature. *Source:* Laufer et al. [4].

Photoacoustic imaging can also be used for blood oxygenation measurements (Figure 17.8). By acquiring photoacoustic images at different excitation wavelengths, each voxel in space will be associated with multiple photoacoustic intensities (i.e. spectrum). Therefore, using a simple least squares technique, the spectral components in this voxel, such as Hb and HbO_2, can be separated and oxygen levels can be calculated as:

$$\mathrm{Oxy}(\%) = \frac{\mathrm{HbO_2}}{\mathrm{Hb} + \mathrm{HbO_2}}$$

Photoacoustics can also be applied in other ways to image-living subjects. For example, healthy tissue and scar tissue generate different levels of contrast in photoacoustic images and can therefore be distinguished from each other (Figure 17.9a). Like hemoglobin, melanin can also be used as an endogenous contrast agent. Using melanin as a photoacoustic contrast agent can be very useful for acquiring high-resolution images of melanomas. The image in Figure 17.9b shows one such image in which the location of a melanoma relative to the surrounding blood vessels can be observed.

17.4.2 Exogenous Contrast Agents

Exogenous contrast agents for photoacoustic imaging include any substance that absorbs light and does not emit all of it as fluorescence, including various small molecules and nanoparticles. Small molecule contrast agents include non-perfect fluorophores (e.g. Indocyanine Green – ICG)

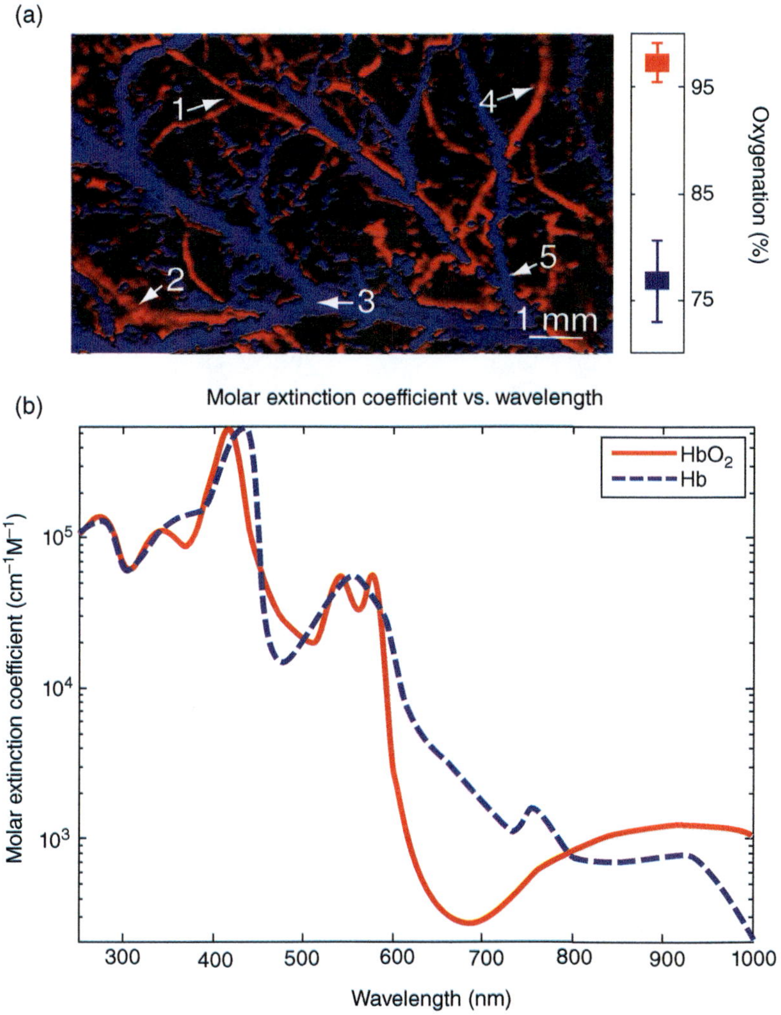

Figure 17.8 (a) In-vivo oxygenation measurement in a rat. Arteries, which have a higher oxygen level, are shown in red (arrows 1, 2, and 4). Vessels, which have a lower oxygen level, are shown in blue (arrows 3 and 5). *Source:* Zhang et al. [5]. Reprinted by permission from Springer Nature. Copyright © 2006 by Springer Nature. (b) Absorption spectrum of Hb and HbO_2. *Source:* German [6]. Used under CC-BY-SA 3.0 https://creativecommons.org/licenses/by-sa/3.0.

and nonfluorescent optical dyes (e.g. methylene blue). For example, only 15% of the photons absorbed by ICG are converted into fluorescent photons and the rest are converted to heat. Small molecule contrast agents have the disadvantage of low absorption coefficient, resulting in relatively low signal. However, their clearance from the body through the urinary system is much preferred over that of nanoparticles, which are secreted by the reticuloendothelial system (RES) (e.g. liver and spleen).

Nanoparticles can also be used as contrast agents. Commonly used nanoparticles in photoacoustic imaging include: single-walled carbon nanotubes (SWNTs), gold-based nanoparticles, liposomes, and hybrid particles (Figure 17.10). Nanoparticle agents have the advantage of high absorption coefficient (and hence high photoacoustic signal), and absorption in the near-infrared spectrum to minimize background signal and maximize signal-to-background ratio (SBR).

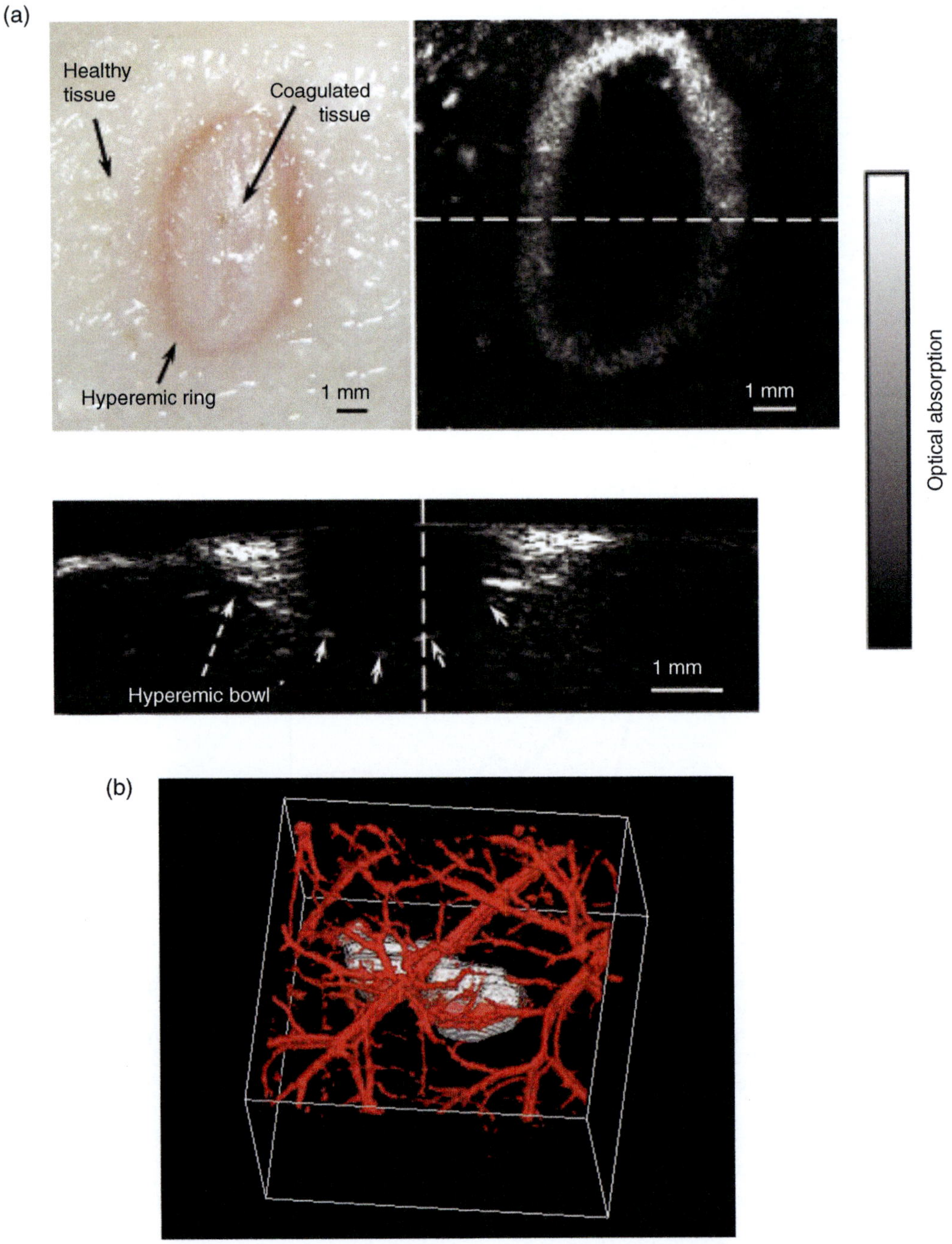

Figure 17.9 (a) Determining the depth of skin burns. *Source:* Zhang et al. [7]. (b) Imaging skin cancer (gray = Melanin, red = blood). *Source:* Zhang et al. [5]. Reprinted by permission from Springer Nature. Copyright © 2006 by Springer Nature.

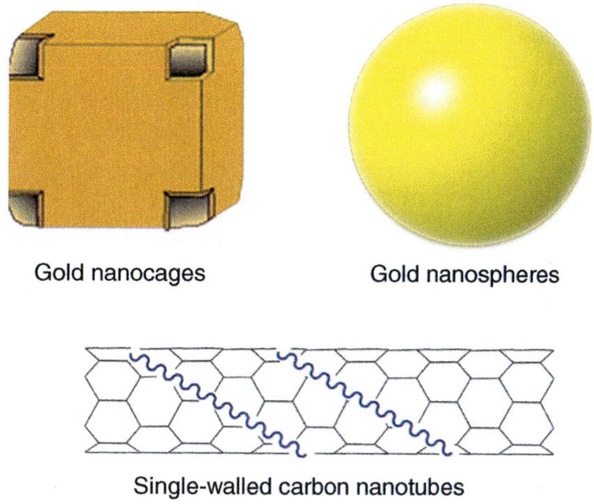

Figure 17.10 Different types of nanoparticle contrast agents. *Source:* Cobley et al. [8]. Reprinted by permission of Taylor & Francis Ltd.

One interesting fact about the gold nanoparticles is that their shape affects the absorption spectrum of the particle. For example, the gold nanosphere shown in Figure 17.10 has a peak absorption around 530 nm (green). However, if you create a rod-shaped gold particle, the peak absorption can red-shift significantly – up to 1000 nm and beyond. These elongated gold nanoparticles are called gold nanorods. The absorption of red light is highly desirable in many optical imaging systems because that is where the body's optical window is (i.e. red light is absorbed less by the tissues, which leads to higher depth of penetration of the incident source light).

17.4.2.1 SWNT Targeted to $\alpha_v\beta_3$ Integrin

The photoacoustic images shown in Figure 17.11 were taken using an SWNT imaging agent targeted to $\alpha_v\beta_3$ integrin, which is a receptor that is overexpressed in areas of active angiogenesis. The imaging agent is targeted through a peptide (small protein fragment), RGD, which is known to have binding affinity for $\alpha_v\beta_3$ integrin. Control SWNTs do not have the RGD peptide, in order to test the ability of the imaging agents to truly bind to the $\alpha_v\beta_3$ integrin. Finally, since photoacoustic images always have some background signal due to blood vessels and other endogenous contrasts, a subtraction image between the postinjection and preinjection images is calculated to produce the final image. Unlike fluorescence imaging, photoacoustic images can determine, with high resolution, where angiogenesis is occurring (i.e. the "hot spots" in the tumor where high activity is likely occurring).

17.4.2.2 Hybrid Imaging Agents

While nanoparticles such as SWNTs have high absorbance, small molecules are much more "efficient" absorbers than nanoparticles on a per-weight basis. For example, even though an SWNT (of ~2 nm in diameter and ~200 nm in length) exhibits an absorbance 30 times higher than an individual ICG molecule, it is also 220 times heavier. Therefore, on a per-weight basis, ICG is seven times more "efficient" in absorbing light than an SWNT (Figure 17.12). Hence, hybrid imaging agents, where an SWNT is coated with many ICG molecules to obtain a much stronger absorbance peak, show significant improvement in signal (Figure 17.13). Such new imaging agents will have the characteristic spectrum of SWNT and ICG combined and will therefore peak at ~780 nm. Such imaging agents were synthesized and showed a significant 20-fold improvement

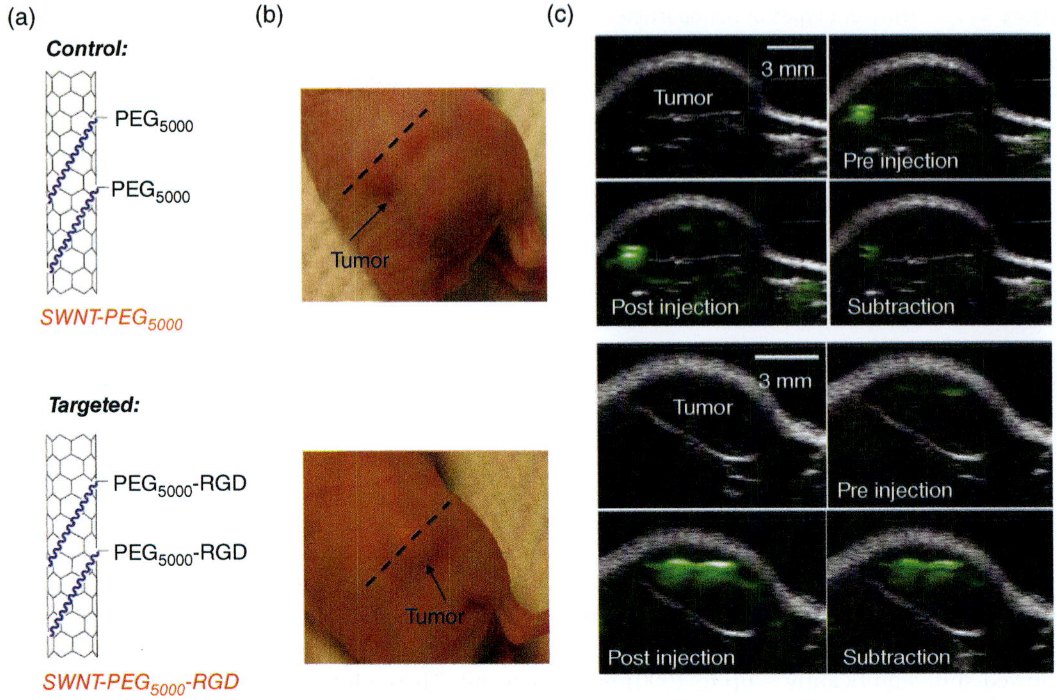

Figure 17.11 (a) Control and targeted contrast agents. *Source:* de la Zerda [9]. Reprinted with permission from ACS Nano. Copyright © 2012, American Chemical Society. (b) Mice with human glioblastoma. The dotted line corresponds to the slice being imaged. *Source:* de la Zerda et al. [3]. Reprinted by permission from Springer Nature. Copyright © 2008 by Springer Nature. (c) Control images (top 4) and targeted images (bottom 4). The photoacoustic signal is shown in green and overlaid on regular ultrasound images. *Source:* de la Zerda et al. [3]. Reprinted by permission from Springer Nature. Copyright © 2008 by Springer Nature.

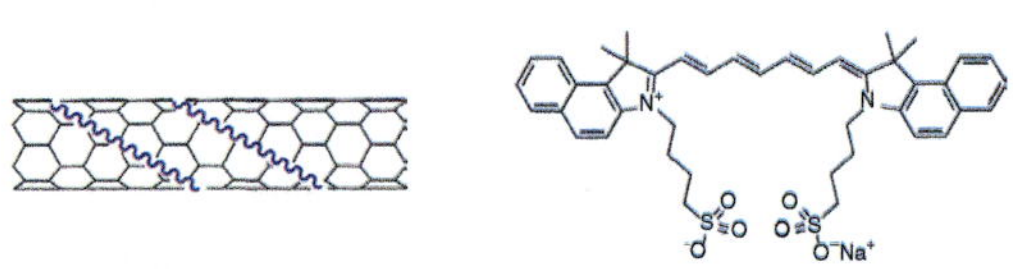

	Nanotube		ICG
Absorbance ($cm^{-1}M^{-1}$)	30	:	1
Weight (Da)	220	:	1
Absorbance/weight	**1**	**:**	**7**

Figure 17.12 Comparison of SWNT and ICG. *Source:* Edgar181 [10]. CC0–1.0 public domain https://http://creativecommons.org/publicdomain/zero/1.0.

in optical absorption compared to plain SWNTs. These agents improve the sensitivity of photoacoustic imaging to ~200 pM in living subjects.

17.4.2.3 Multiplexing with Photoacoustics

The surface of SWNTs can be coated with other optical dyes, rendering different absorption spectra (Figure 17.14). By acquiring multiple photoacoustic images at different wavelengths, a photoacoustic spectrum can be calculated and the spectral components can be isolated using least-squares.

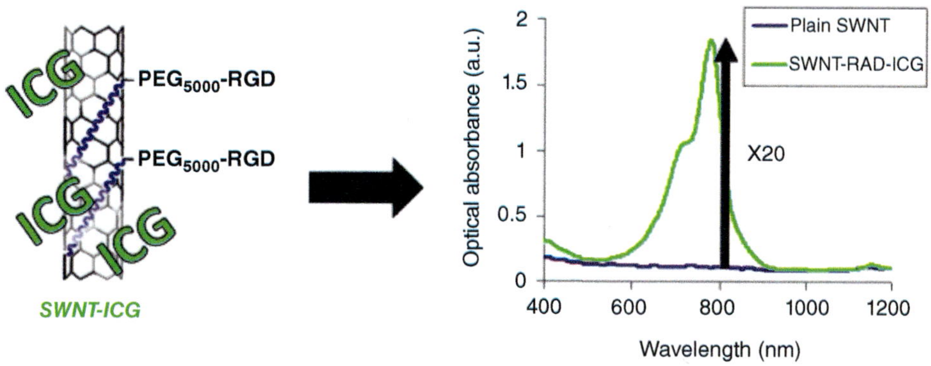

Figure 17.13 Hybrid SWNT-ICG contrast agent and the increase in absorption peak at 800 nm. *Source:* de la Zerda [9]. Reprinted with permission from ACS Nano. Copyright © 2012, American Chemical Society.

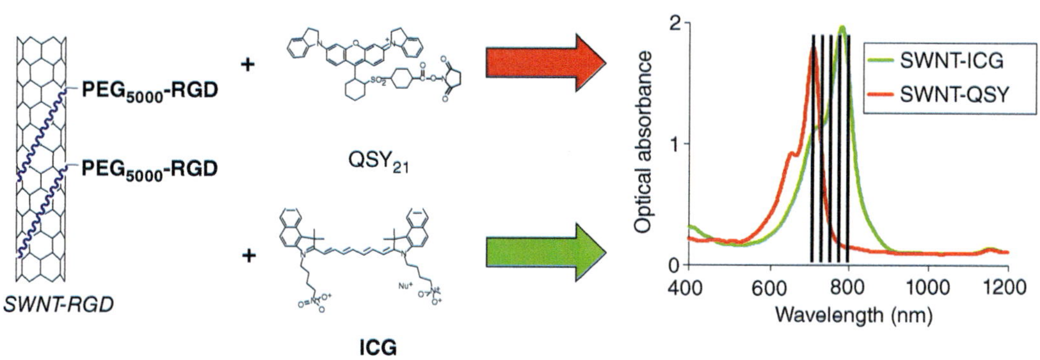

Figure 17.14 Photoacoustic multiplexing schematic. *Source:* de la Zerda [9]. Reprinted with permission from ACS Nano. Copyright © 2012, American Chemical Society.

17.5 Conclusion

Photoacoustic imaging is based on the photoacoustic effect, which refers to the conversion of photons to acoustic waves (i.e. sound waves) that occurs when absorption of photons from a pulse of light causes localized thermal expansion, producing acoustic waves due to pressure variation in the surrounding medium. Photoacoustic imaging is advantageous because it offers increased depth of penetration, on the order of several centimeters (about an order of magnitude higher than fluorescence imaging), and acoustic waves are not scattered or absorbed much by tissues, giving improved spatial resolution in the submillimeter range. One major disadvantage of photoacoustic imaging is that acoustic waves cannot pass through certain tissue boundaries due to acoustic impedance mismatches; hence, only soft tissues can be imaged with no bones or air in the way. Many possible contrast agents may be designed for photoacoustic imaging; whether based on small molecules or nanoparticles, the primary characteristic that contributes to the production of the photoacoustic signal is the contrast agent's light absorption. Table 17.1 provides a comparison between photoacoustic, fluorescence, and Raman spectroscopy imaging.

Table 17.1 Comparison of fluorescence, Raman, and photoacoustic imaging.

Differences	Fluorescence imaging	Raman spectroscopy imaging	Photoacoustic imaging
Spatial resolution	2–10 mm	2–10 mm	10–500 μm
Temporal resolution	< 1 s	Minutes	Seconds – minutes
Sensitivity	1 nM	10 pM	100 pM
Depth of penetration	< 5 mm	< 5 mm	< 5 cm (!)
Background level	High	Low	High
Cost/system complexity	Low	High	Low
Multiplexing ability	Low	High	Low
Intrinsic signal	Autofluorescence	Very low	Hb, HbO_2, Melanin
Contrast agents	Small molecules and nanoparticles	Nanoparticles	Small molecules and nanoparticles

Problems

17.1 Local fractional volume expansion dV/V of the heated tissue at position r can be expressed as:

$$\frac{dV}{V} = -\kappa p(r) + \beta T(r),$$

where p is the change in pressure [Pa], T is the change in temperature [K], κ is the isothermal compressibility [Pa^{-1}], and β is the isobaric volume expansion coefficient [K^{-1}].

A What is the desirable work confinement for the laser pulse duration to confine acoustic waves near the object or tissue of interest?
Hint: This is not related to the equation above.

B With the work confinement found in part (a), the fractional volume expansion is negligible. What is the relationship between the pressure and temperature of the tissue?

C If we assume that all absorbed optical energy is completely converted into heat in the tissue, the light fluence is F [J m^{-2}], and the absorption coefficient of the tissue is μ_a [m^{-1}], what is the temperature rise in the tissue generated by the laser pulse with the same work confinement found in part (a)?
Hint: Specific heat capacity is the required heat energy to change the temperature by 1 K per unit mass of a material. C_p and C_v are the specific heat capacities at constant pressure and volume, respectively [J K^{-1} kg^{-1}].

D If the isothermal compressibility is defined as $\kappa = \frac{C_p}{\rho c^2 C_v}$ (ρ is the density of the material, and c is the speed of sound), what is the pressure generated by the laser pulse with the same work confinement found in part (a)?

17.2 Explain the following in your own words:

A What are the advantages and disadvantages of photoacoustic imaging compared to fluorescence imaging?

B What kinds of contrast agents can be used in photoacoustic imaging? List at least two examples and discuss their advantages or disadvantages.

References

1 Harryzilber, https://commons.wikimedia.org/wiki/File:Photophone_transmitter_4074931746_9f996df841_b.jpg
2 Rakruger, https://commons.wikimedia.org/wiki/File:Focused_Transducer.jpg
3 de la Zerda, A., Zavaleta, C., Keren, S. et al. (2008). Carbon nanotubes as photoacoustic molecular imaging agents in living mice. *Nature Nanotechnology* 3: 557–562.
4 Laufer, J., Zhang, E., Raivich, G., and Beard, P. (2009). Three-dimensional noninvasive imaging of the vasculature in the mouse brain using a high resolution photoacoustic scanner. *Appl. Opt.* 48: D299–D306.
5 Zhang, H.F., Maslov, K., Stoica, G., and Wang, L.V. (2006). Functional photoacoustic microscopy for high-resolution and noninvasive in vivo imaging. *Nature Biotechnology* 24: 848–851.
6 German, https://commons.wikimedia.org/wiki/File:HbAbs_v3.png
7 Zhang, H.F., Maslov, K., Stoica, G., and Wang, L.V. (1 September 2006). Imaging acute thermal burns by photoacoustic microscopy. *Journal of Biomedical Optics* 11 (5): 054033.
8 Cobley, C.M., Au, L., Chen, J., and Xia, Y. Targeting gold nanocages to cancer cells for photothermal destruction and drug delivery. *Expert Opinion on Drug Delivery* 7: 577–587.
9 de la Zerda, A., Bodapati, S., Teed, R. et al. (2012). Family of enhanced Photoacoustic imaging agents for high-sensitivity and multiplexing studies in living mice. *American Chemical Society* 6 (6): 4694–4701.
10 Edgar181, https://commons.wikimedia.org/wiki/File:Indocyanine_green.png

Further Reading

Mgrdichian, L. (2006). Superconductivity in entirely end-bonded multiwalled carbon nanotubes. *Physical Review Letters* 96: 057001.

de la Zerda, A., Liu, Z., Bodapati, S. et al. (2010). Ultrahigh sensitivity carbon nanotube agents for photoacoustic molecular imaging in living mice. *Nano Letters* 10 (6): 2168.

18

Imaging Controls and Concepts

18.1 Controls

Control experiments are very important for any scientific observation in biology (biochips, imaging, nanomedicine, and beyond). They are necessary in every scientific study to prove a hypothesis. Since biology is a "black box" with very complex mechanisms, many processes beyond our control may occur, leading us to get the same results we would have otherwise expected from our hypothesis. Those processes may be at multiple levels: cellular (intra- or extracellular), tissue, organ, or system.

To find out which control experiments are needed to truly support a certain hypothesis, the following questions must be asked:

- What is the hypothesis?
- What could have gone wrong?
- What other circumstances might lead to the same observation?

Example 1: Photoacoustic imaging of $\alpha_V\beta_3$ integrin using SWNT-RGD. Suppose an experiment is performed where a photoacoustic image is taken using SWNT-RGD-targeted imaging agents and signal is in the tumor. One potential conclusion is that the imaging agents indeed targeted the tumors intended. However, this experiment and observations mean nothing without the use of a proper control. For example, what if the signal from the tumor postinjection is actually due to blood vessels (which have hemoglobin that produces photoacoustic signal) and not SWNTs? A control of a *preinjection* photoacoustic image of the same animal before the injection is needed to observe the difference between the preinjection and postinjection images (Figure 18.1). Now with a control image, conclusions that the signal in the tumor is truly due to the SWNT-RGD can be made.

Example 2: Photoacoustic imaging of $\alpha_V\beta_3$ integrin using SWNT-RGD. What if the SWNT-RGD leaked out nonspecifically from the tumor's leaky blood vessels? In other words, how do we really know that the signal is coming from particles that successfully bound $\alpha_V\beta_3$ integrin? A control with non-targeted SWNTs must be performed, e.g. with a mutated peptide that does not bind to $\alpha_V\beta_3$ (like RAD instead of RGD), or simply no attached RGD. If under identical conditions, the non-targeted particles produce a lower or no signal from the tumor, then the conclusion that the signal

Biochips and Medical Imaging, First Edition. Adam de la Zerda and Shan Xiang Wang.

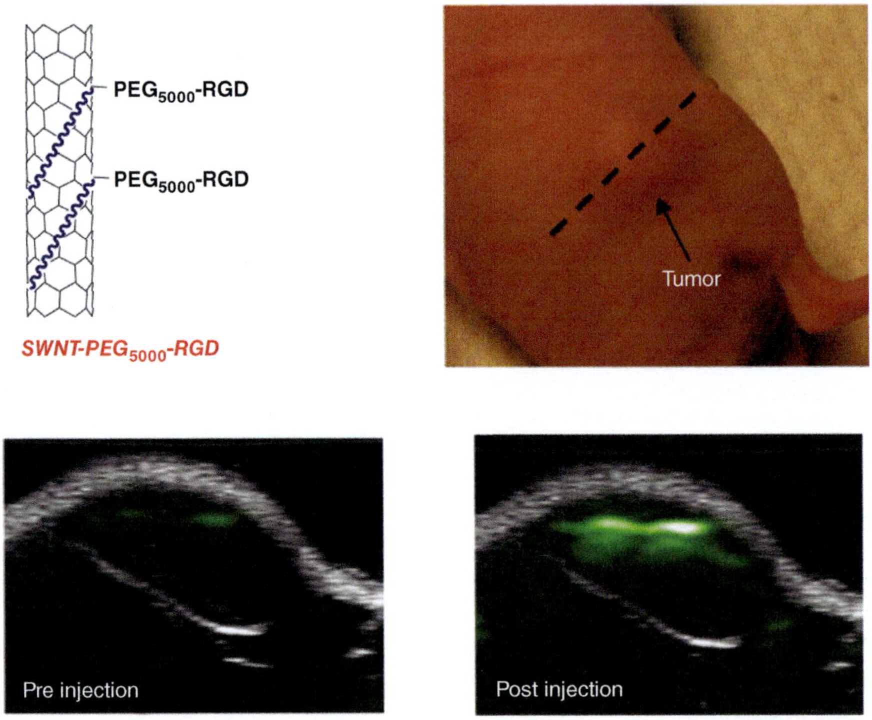

Figure 18.1 SWNT-RGD with subtracted image (post-minus preinjection images). *Source:* Zerda et al. [1]. Reprinted by permission from Springer Nature: Nature Nanotechnology. Copyright © 2008 by Springer Nature.

we observed with SWNT-RGD was indeed specific to $\alpha_V\beta_3$ can be made. As seen in the control experiment in Figure 18.2, not all of the signal was specific to $\alpha_V\beta_3$ as some low amount of SWNTs are either still circulating in the blood vessels or have leaked out of the tumor vasculature. Fortunately, this does not appear to be a major effect and only mildly contributes to the overall tumor signal.

Example 3: Photoacoustic imaging of $\alpha_V\beta_3$ integrin using SWNT-RGD. What if the one measurement was a fluke? For example, what if the specific control animal has clogged blood vessels, less leaky blood vessels than the experimental animal (that was injected with SWNT-RGD), or simply had thicker skin that allowed less light to go through. To control for these unforeseen circumstances, it is important to run the same experiment multiple times (e.g. $n = 4$ animals per group), measure the signal at multiple time points, and use statistics to calculate the p-value (i.e. the probability that the measurement from the two groups does not support our hypothesis), which should typically be below 0.05. Measurement of the signal over time helps remove time-dependent artifacts (Figure 18.3).

Example 4: Photoacoustic imaging of $\alpha_V\beta_3$ integrin using SWNT-RGD. What if the photoacoustic measurement is unreliable, or what if the SWNT-RGD caused a reaction by the body (e.g. immune system) that led to hemorrhage at the tumor, and hence the signal that is measured from the tumor is not from SWNT-RGD? To control for that, an independent method to measure the existence of the SWNTs in the tumor is necessary, e.g. Raman spectroscopy on tumors ex vivo (Figure 18.4).

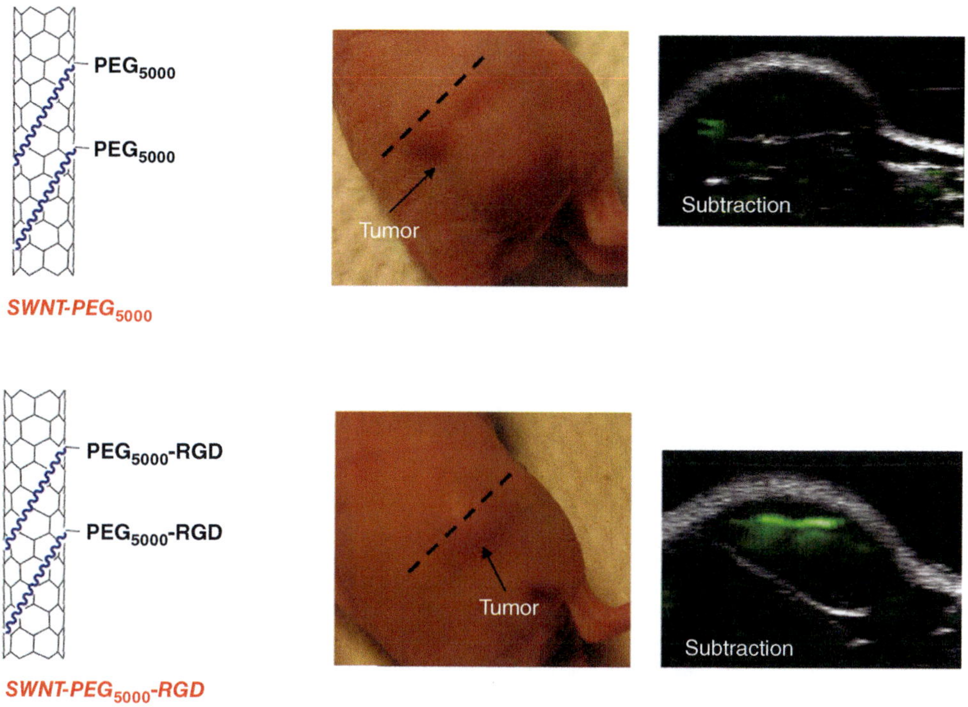

Figure 18.2 SWNT-RGD with subtracted image (postminus preinjection images). *Source:* Zerda et al. [1]. Reprinted by permission from Springer Nature: Nature Nanotechnology. Copyright © 2008 by Springer Nature.

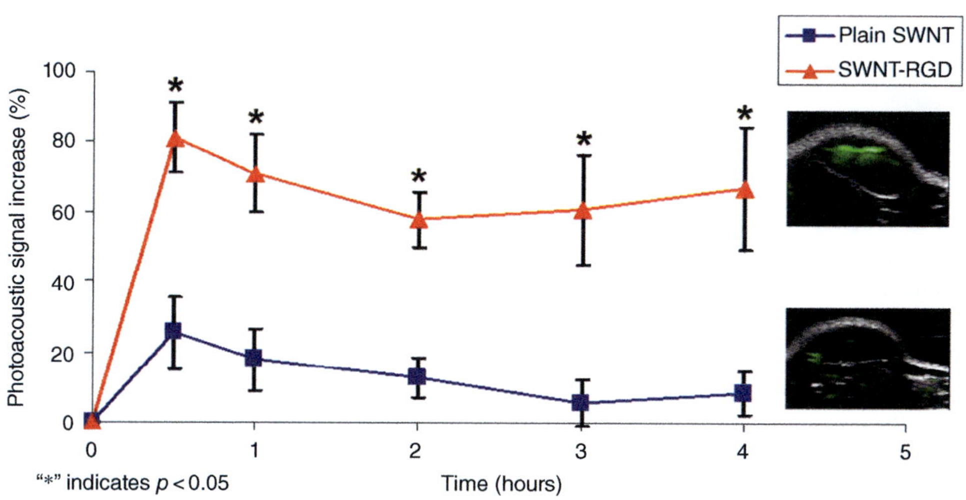

Figure 18.3 Photoacoustic signal from the experimental and control groups as a function of time. *Source:* Zerda et al. [1]. Reprinted by permission from Springer Nature: Nature Nanotechnology. Copyright © 2008 by Springer Nature.

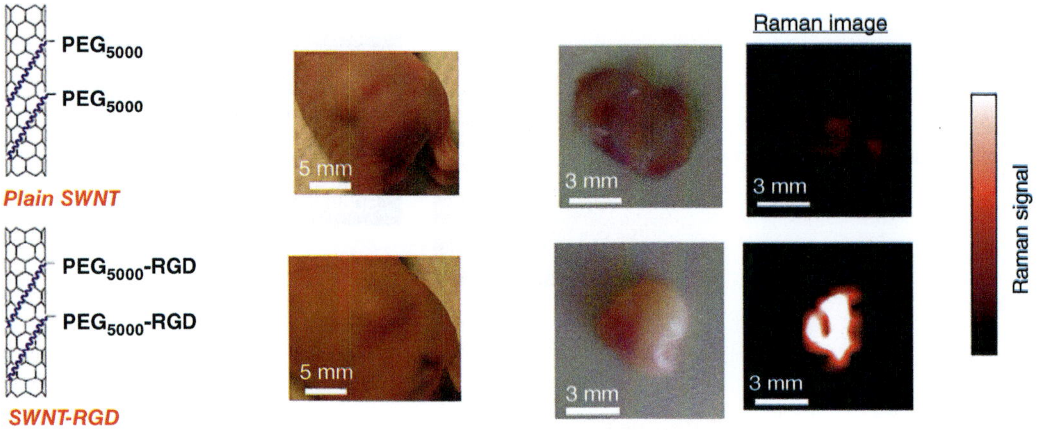

Figure 18.4 Raman imaging of SWNTs in tumor. *Source:* Zerda et al. [1]. Reprinted by permission from Springer Nature: Nature Nanotechnology. Copyright © 2008 by Springer Nature.

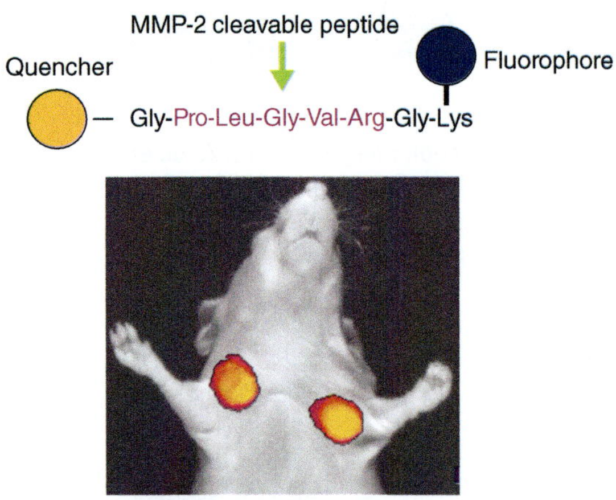

Figure 18.5 MMP-2 smart imaging agent design. *Source:* Bremer et al. [2]. Reprinted by permission from Springer Nature: Nature Medicine. Copyright © 2001 by Springer Nature.

Example 5: Suppose a research group claims to have developed a smart agent against MMP-2 enzyme, which plays a role in metastasis. The smart agent is activatable and uses FRET to produce a signal by the MMP-2 enzyme cleaving the sequence of amino acids between the fluorophore and the quencher (Figure 18.5). However, what if a different enzyme in the tumor was instead cleaving the peptide regardless of MMP-2 existence in the tumor, or if the pH environment in the tumor was responsible for the peptide cleavage? Hence, an important control would be the insertion of a mutation into the peptide sequence. By inserting such a mutation, a new peptide would result and the mutate peptide will likely not be cleaved by MMP-2 nor by any other peptide-specific enzyme. If administering this control agent to an animal results in a signal, then the original imaging agent was *not* specific to MMP-2.

In summary, multiple controls are needed to truly demonstrate that a proposed imaging modality or imaging agent is effective. Controls are necessary to make accurate conclusions from the observed phenomenon.

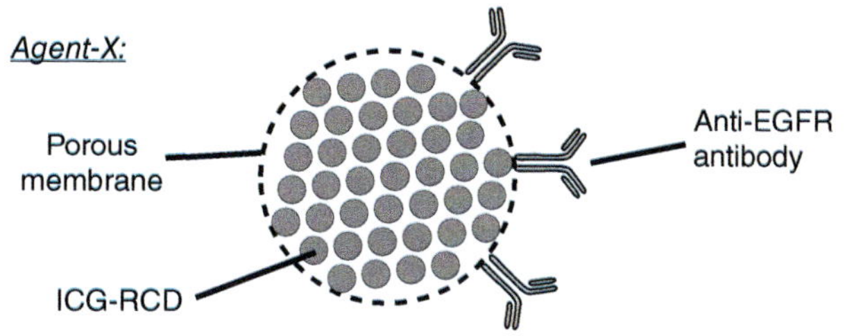

Figure 18.6 Agent-X schematic.

18.1.1 Example

Agent-X, shown in Figure 18.6, is a new fluorescent imaging agent. This imaging agent is made of a nanoparticle that is coated with anti-EGFR antibodies (i.e. antibodies against epidermal growth factor receptor). EGFR is a common receptor on cancer cells, that assists the cancer cells in self-growth. Each nanoparticle is loaded with 1000 ICG-RGD molecules (ICG = Indocyanine Green – a fluorescent dye; RGD = a peptide against $\alpha_v\beta_3$ integrin – a protein that assists tumors in angiogenesis). The nanoparticle is made of a porous material that releases its content (i.e. ICG-RGD molecules) over a course of 60 minutes from the time of injection. The particle is injected into mice that carry a human tumor that expresses EGFR and $\alpha_v\beta_3$ integrin. You can also assume the anti-EGFR antibody causes Agent-X to fully bind to EGFR in the tumor within 10 minutes after injection. Fluorescent images of the mouse are taken 1.5 hours after the injection and a bright signal emerges from the tumor.

a) What does this imaging agent aim to image? What is the likely targeting mechanism?

b) Explain some control experiments that would help prove the specificity of Agent-X to $\alpha_v\beta_3$ integrin and EGFR. Your answer should include:
   1) The possible scenario the control experiment is testing (the "what if?").
   2) The possible outcomes of each control experiment.
   3) How each of the possible outcomes will reflect on the specificity of the original Agent-X.

c) Agent-X was injected intravenously to mice carrying three different tumor types, as listed below. Draw hypothetical curves representing the fluorescence intensity versus time for each of the tumors. Assume Agent-X successfully binds and images its target(s).
   1) Tumor expressing EGFR and $\alpha_v\beta_3$ integrin.
   2) Tumor expressing EGFR but *no* $\alpha_v\beta_3$ integrin.
   3) Tumor not expressing EGFR and not expressing $\alpha_v\beta_3$ integrin.

18.1.2 Example – Answers

a) The imaging agent is imaging tumors that express *both* $\alpha_v\beta_3$ integrin as well as EGFR, and hence are actively proliferating as well as undergoing angiogenesis. The mechanism of targeting: upon injection to the bloodstream, Agent-X travels through the body and targets the EGF receptors on the tumor. Then ICG-RGD is slowly leaking and hence locally deposited in the tumor region. This allows ICG-RGD to target tumor cells expressing $\alpha_v\beta_3$ integrin. If either one of the targets is missing, no sustained binding will occur. This process allows imaging at 1.5 hours postinjection as required.

b)

Control experiment #1: Agent-X with ICG instead of ICG-RGD:

1) Tests for *what if* upon binding to EGFR, the ICG-RGD is simply staying in the tumor area nonspecifically regardless of the existence of $\alpha_v\beta_3$ integrin.
2) Upon injection of this control agent, either we see signal from the tumor or not.
3) If we do, it means that Agent-X is probably not specific to $\alpha_v\beta_3$ integrin, and if we do not, then it likely is.

Control experiment #2: Agent-X without the anti-EGFR antibody:

1) Tests for *what if* the initial attachment of the particle to the tumor occurred regardless of the expression of EGFR by the tumor.
2) Upon injection of this control agent, either we see signal from the tumor or not.
3) If we do, it means that Agent-X is likely not specific to EGFR, and if we do not, then it likely is.

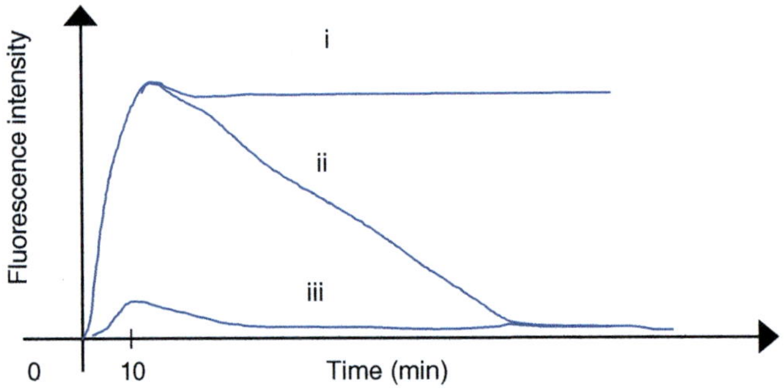

c)

1) The tumor is expressing EGFR and $\alpha v\beta 3$ integrin. The imaging agent arrives at the tumor within 10 minutes. ICG-RGD then diffuses and attaches to the tumor (local deposition), while some ICG-RGD leaks out.
2) The tumor is expressing EGFR but no $\alpha v\beta 3$ integrin. The imaging agent arrives at the tumor within 10 minutes. ICG-RGD then diffuses out of the tumor, while some ICG-RGD stays in the tumor creating a background signal.
3) The tumor is not expressing EGFR and not expressing $\alpha v\beta 3$ integrin. Hence, no tumor binding occurs. Probe circulates in the blood stream until cleared.

18.2 Imaging Concepts

18.2.1 Imaging Parameters (Sensitivity, Specificity, and Amplification)

Sensitivity and specificity are two important figures of merit for a given imaging modality. **Sensitivity** measures the minimal concentration of imaging agent that can be detected in a living tissue, and depends on the signal per imaging agent molecule (which should be maximized), the signal-to-background ratio (SBR) (e.g. autofluorescence in fluorescence imaging or blood vessel signal in photoacoustic imaging), and the signal-to-noise ratio (SNR). For some imaging modalities, SNR limits the sensitivity because the background signal is very low, e.g. PET/SPECT (since the body has almost zero natural radioactivity) and Raman imaging. For other imaging modalities, SBR limits the sensitivity because of endogenous contrasts, e.g. MRI (most tissues), fluorescence imaging (autofluorescence in skin and food), and photoacoustic imaging (melanin and hemoglobin).

Table 18.1 Sensitivity and specificity of mammography, MRI, and ultrasound.

	Mammography	MRI	Ultrasound
Sensitivity	33–40%	77–91%	33–40%
Specificity	93–99%	81–97%	91–96%

Source: Saslow et al. [3].

The **specificity** of an imaging modality describes how much of the signal obtained was caused by imaging agents that arrived to the target tissue. In contrast, the nonspecific signal is the signal not caused by true imaging agents that arrived to the target tissue and bound to their target. This signal can be caused by imaging agents with long circulation times that are still in circulation, imaging agents that localized where they should not have (e.g. imaging agents that accumulated in tumors due to the EPR effect of tumor vasculature, i.e. leaky vessels), or imaging agents that accumulate in the kidney, liver, bladder, or other organs as they are cleared from the body.

In contrast, **clinical sensitivity** and **clinical specificity** refer to a disease diagnosis based on the image, as defined in the biochips chapter. Hence, the definitions are: Sensitivity = TP/(TP + FN) and Specificity = TN/(TN + FP). Sometimes sensitivity and specificity can be improved by using multiple imaging modalities. For example, mammography and ultrasound may both have a sensitivity of 33–40% for screening breast cancer. However, combining the two screening methods may result in a sensitivity that exceeds either method alone. The sensitivity and specificity for mammography, MRI, and ultrasound are shown in Table 18.1.

Finally, **amplification** is a critical aspect of molecular imaging that aims to improve the sensitivity. Two common methods to improve the sensitivity of an imaging modality (by increasing its signal) are: (a) increase the signal per imaging agent, or (b) increase the imaging agent per target molecule through accumulation. For example, an imaging agent made of a liposome with 90 000 Gd-DPTA molecules coated onto its surface (Figure 18.7) provides a significant amplification over the alternative of targeting one Gd-DPTA per one molecular target on the cell. Another example is the use of hybrid imaging agents consisting of thousands of small ICG molecules on a single SWNT

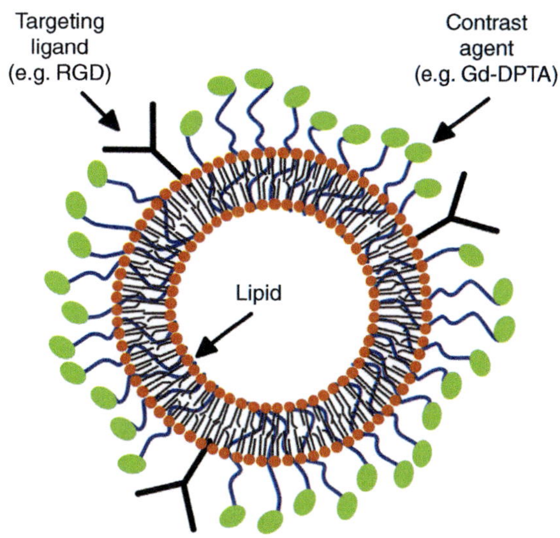

Figure 18.7 Gd-DPTA liposome-targeted contrast agent.

for Raman imaging, giving a 20-fold increase in absorption (Figure 18.8). A third example is the photomultiplier tube (PMT) in PET/SPECT imaging that increases the number of photons contributing to signal.

Finally, FDG and FLT are examples of methods to increase accumulation in targeted areas (Figure 18.9). For every one hexokinase enzyme (or thymidine kinase enzyme), many thousands of FDG (or FLT) are trapped in the cell due to their phosphorylation.

18.2.2 Multimodality Imaging

Multimodality Imaging is the use of a combination of multiple imaging modalities. This can produce synergistic benefits, e.g. a PET/CT system can combine a PET image that provides information about metabolism (e.g. FDG-PET with glucose metabolism) with a CT image that provides

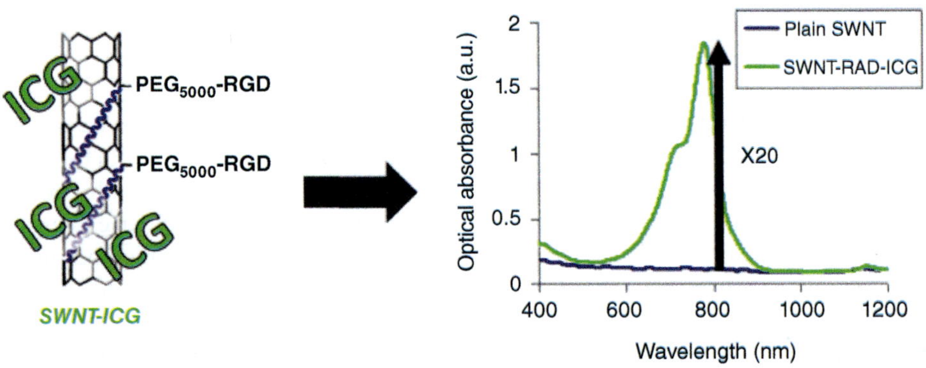

Figure 18.8 Hybrid SWNT-ICG contrast agent and increase in absorption peak at 800 nm. *Source:* Zerda et al. [4]. Reprinted with permission from ACS Nano: American Chemical Society. Copyright © 2012, American Chemical Society; Zerda et al. [5]. Reprinted with permission from Nano Letters: American Chemical Society. Copyright © 2010, American Chemical Society.

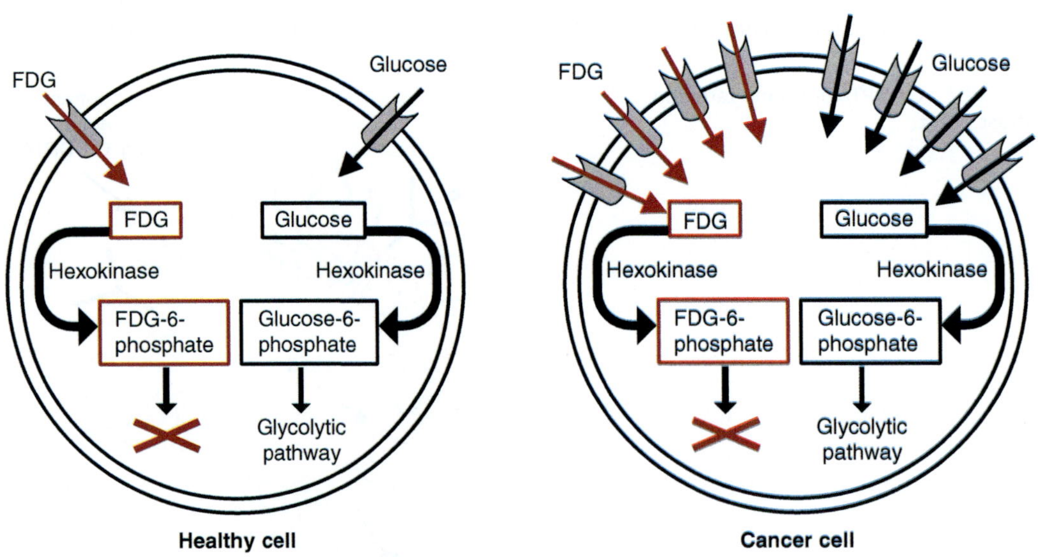

Figure 18.9 FDG accumulation in cancer cell compared to normal cell.

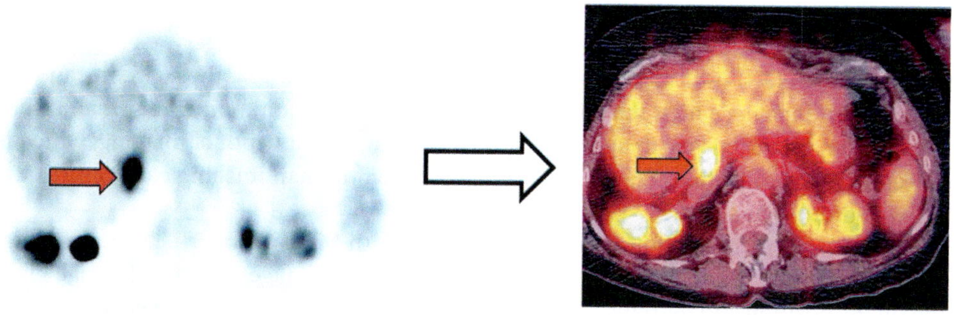

Figure 18.10 PET and PET/CT imaging. *Source:* Cohade et al. [6]. This research was originally published in JNM. Figure 1. © by the Society of Nuclear Medicine and Molecular Imaging, Inc.

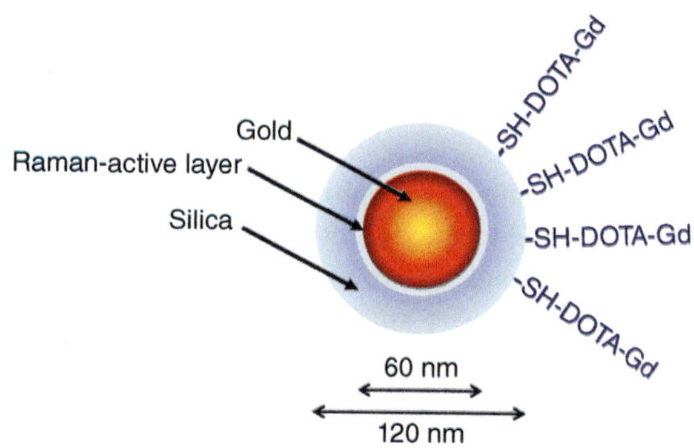

Figure 18.11 Structure of MPR nanoparticles. *Source:* Kircher et al. [7]. Reprinted by permission from Springer Nature: Nature Medicine. Copyright © 2012 by Springer Nature.

anatomical context to the molecular information (Figure 18.10). Multimodality imaging can also complement the advantages and disadvantages of each imaging modality, e.g. MPR nanoparticles can be used to produce contrast on three imaging modalities: MRI (T_1-weighted), photoacoustic, and Raman imaging.

MPR (MRI, Photoacoustic, and Raman) **Nanoparticles** have the structure depicted in Figure 18.11. The nanoparticle is composed of an inner core of gold surrounded by a layer of Raman-active material and silica. About 80 000 DOTA-Gd molecules can be conjugated to this Raman-active particle (recall that Gd must be kept chelated by DOTA to surround the Gd and prevent toxic exposure). By plotting $1/T_1$ versus concentration of MPR nanoparticles, we can find the relaxivity of the MPR nanoparticle by calculating a linear fit to the data, which gives a relaxivity of about 3 million $(\text{mM s})^{-1}$ (compared to 4 $(\text{mM s})^{-1}$ for each individual Gd-DTPA molecule). The Gd relaxivity is enhanced due to the heavier weight of the nanoparticle, which moves slower and allows more interaction time with water. This MPR nanoparticle structure also produces a photoacoustic signal because it has strong characteristic absorption, and the Raman dye layer between the gold core and the silica shell give the particle a strong Raman signature.

The MPR nanoparticles described above can be used during surgical planning steps, deep tumor localization, and fine margin resection of a tumor in a mouse model. The ability to image tumor margins with high resolution is critical because tumor cells may be extravasating out of the surrounding leaky blood vessels, especially in the case of glioblastoma – an aggressive form of brain tumor. We want the contrast agents to go only into the tumor and not into the healthy brain tissue so that we can image the entire outline of the tumor for surgery and remove only tumor and not healthy brain tissue. During surgery, imaging is important to guide the surgery, e.g. to indicate when a tumor portion is left over after cutting. As shown in Figure 18.12a, the surgeon can take advantage of Raman imaging's high sensitivity for fine margin resection to find any small tumor that may be left over. Photoacoustic imaging provides the advantage of depth of imaging, which is useful for deep tumor localization. Finally, postsurgery ex vivo Raman imaging can confirm the clean margins of the resected tissue.

Figure 18.12b illustrates three different images obtained with MPR nanoparticles. Each imaging modality was scanned twice for preinjection and postinjection images. The MRI image gives information on the position and margins of the brain tumor, which is useful for surgical planning. The photoacoustic images taken before and after injection have more green signal after injection, which indicates the accumulation of nanoparticles in the tumor. This is useful for deep tumor localization intraoperatively. The Raman signal (red) does not have background signal in the body; thus the preinjection image is free of Raman signal, while the postinjection image shows a specific signal from the tumor area. Due to Raman's ultrahigh sensitivity, it can be used for identifying the fine margins of the tumor intraoperatively. All images were taken with the mouse's skin and skull intact.

MPR nanoparticles can be used in Raman imaging during tumor resection surgery (intraoperative imaging). A series of photographs and Raman images of a tumor-bearing mouse with its skull removed are shown in Figure 18.13. As the tumor was resected out, Raman images were taken. After all of the visible tumor was removed, (second image from the right), a Raman image indicated the existence of two small focal regions from which signal was still observed (boxed region). Resecting this tissue and further analysis under a microscope (in which the tumor cells were stained with and visualized green), revealed that the two focal regions were indeed part of the tumor not visible with the naked eye. In real surgical scenarios, surgeons often remove a few extra millimeters of healthy brain around the tumor (margins) to make sure no tumor was left behind. However, removal of healthy brain tissue is very intrusive and harmful and therefore such imaging techniques to visualize tumor margins are highly desirable. Specifically, with brain tumors, the tumors do not typically grow radially as a sphere, but rather in finger-like protrusions (Figure 18.14).

18.3 Clinical Translation

There are 11 steps in clinical translation to develop a clinical imaging agent (Figure 18.15). First, pathology (the study of diseases) determines the characteristics of a disease and a molecular target is identified for imaging (e.g. $\alpha_V\beta_3$ integrin). Next, an imaging modality is chosen for the specific clinical application. Then, the chemistry of the imaging agent is developed, e.g. optimized preparation of imaging agents for radionuclide imaging (due to radioactive decay), along with labeling methods for the imaging agent. An in vitro test is then performed using molecular and cell biology methods followed by experiments on small and large animal models. Mice are, in most cases, the ideal small animal model due to the relatively low cost and ease of experiments. Next, the imaging setup and parameters are designed and computer modeling measures the biodistribution of imaging agents in the body. Finally, the clinical imaging technique is fully developed and tested on humans. Bringing a new molecular imaging agent to the clinic can cost several hundreds of millions of dollars and last 5–10 years, similar to the drug development process.

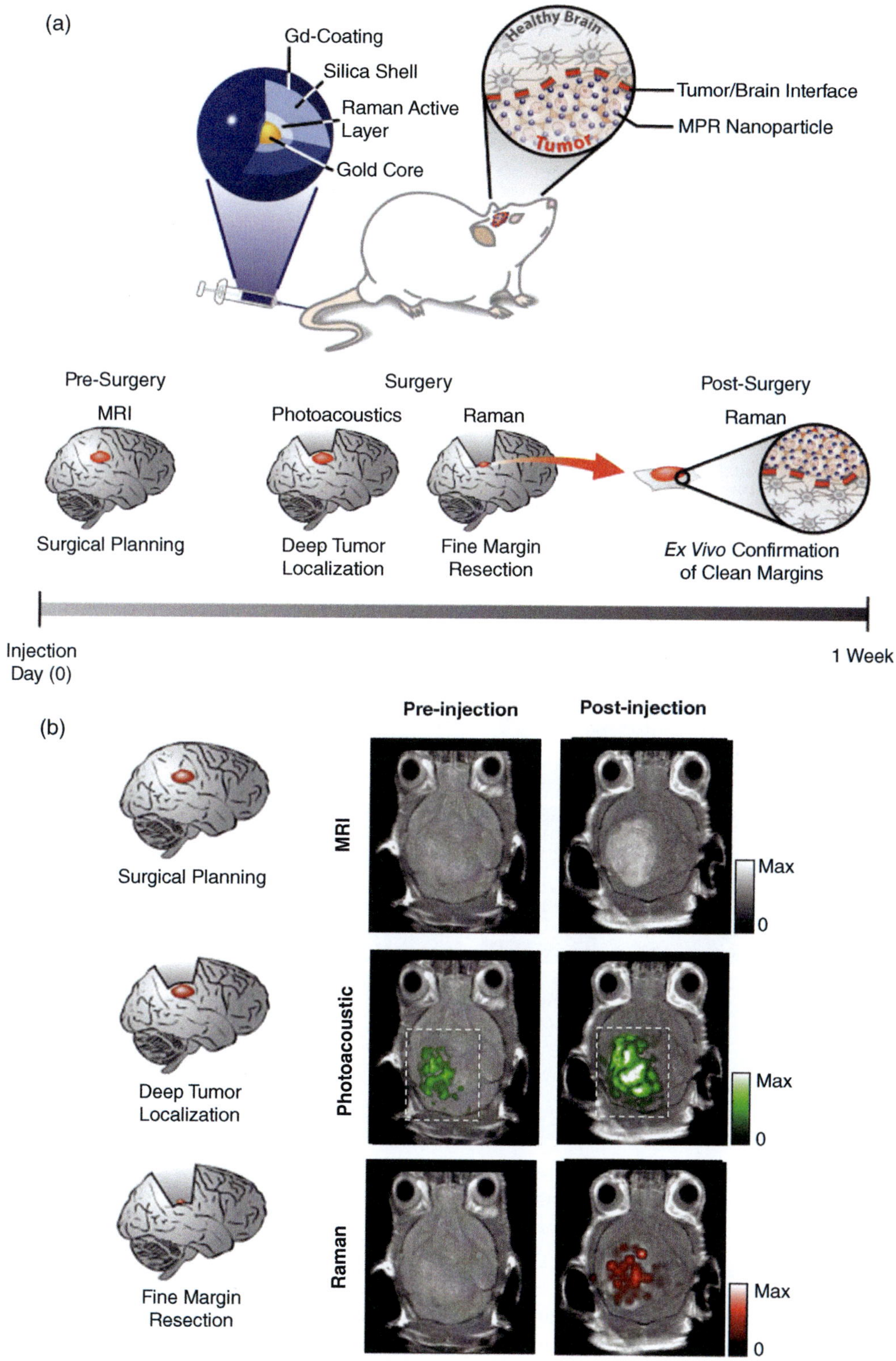

Figure 18.12 (a) Applications of MPR nanoparticle in mouse model. (b) Preinjection and postinjection images of MPR nanoparticles. *Source:* Kircher et al. [7]. Reprinted by permission from Springer Nature: Nature Medicine. Copyright © 2012 by Springer Nature.

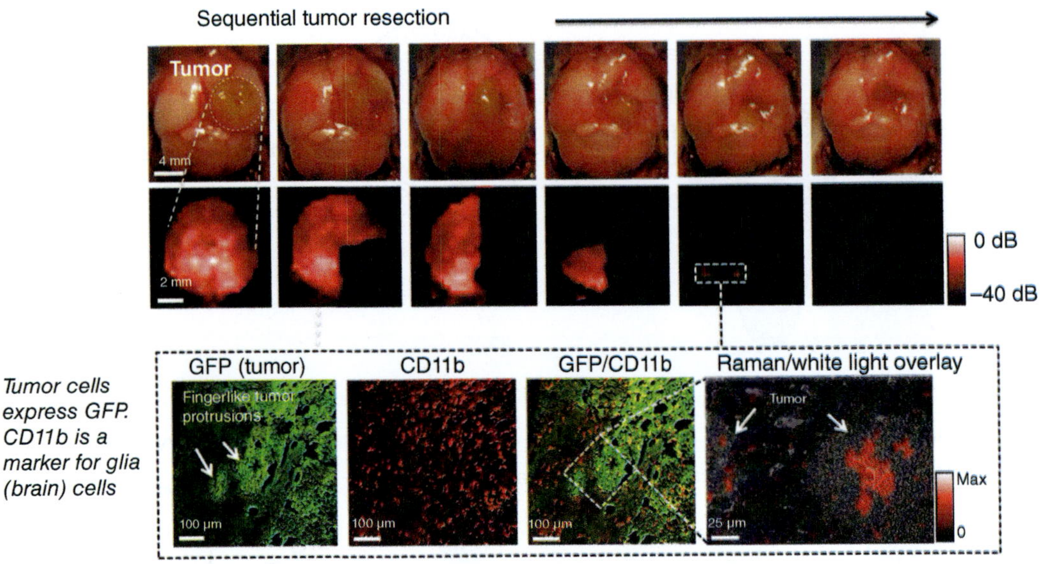

Figure 18.13 Sequential tumor resection and intraoperative Raman imaging. *Source:* Kircher et al. [7]. Reprinted by permission from Springer Nature: Nature Medicine. Copyright © 2012 by Springer Nature.

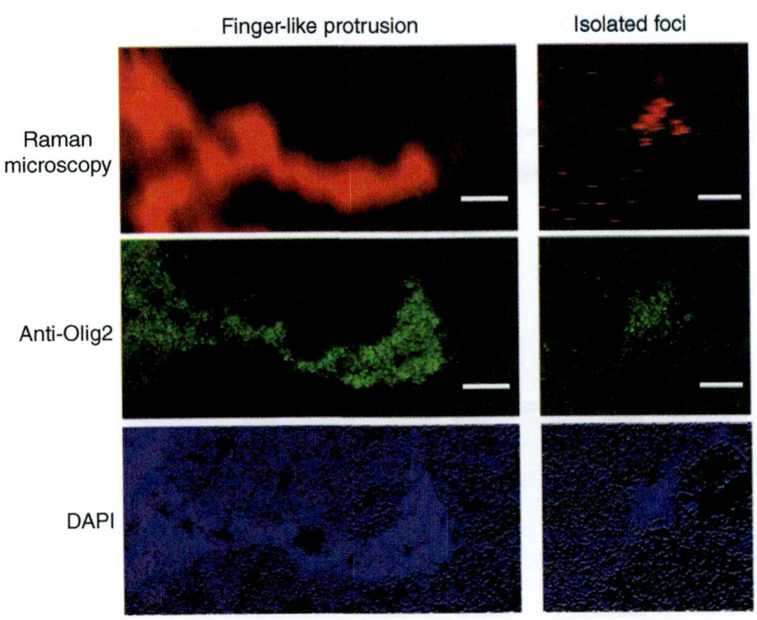

Figure 18.14 Imaging invasive tumor extensions. *Source:* Kircher et al. [7]. Reprinted by permission from Springer Nature: Nature Medicine. Copyright © 2012 by Springer Nature.

18.3.1 Clinical Needs for Imaging

There are many clinical needs for imaging. Early detection of diseases, such as mammography (breast X-ray image) for detection of breast cancer, is an important clinical goal. Imaging can also help in the development of personalized medicine, which can predict the most beneficial treatment for a patient, e.g. breast cancer patients who have an overexpression of Her2/neu, as well as

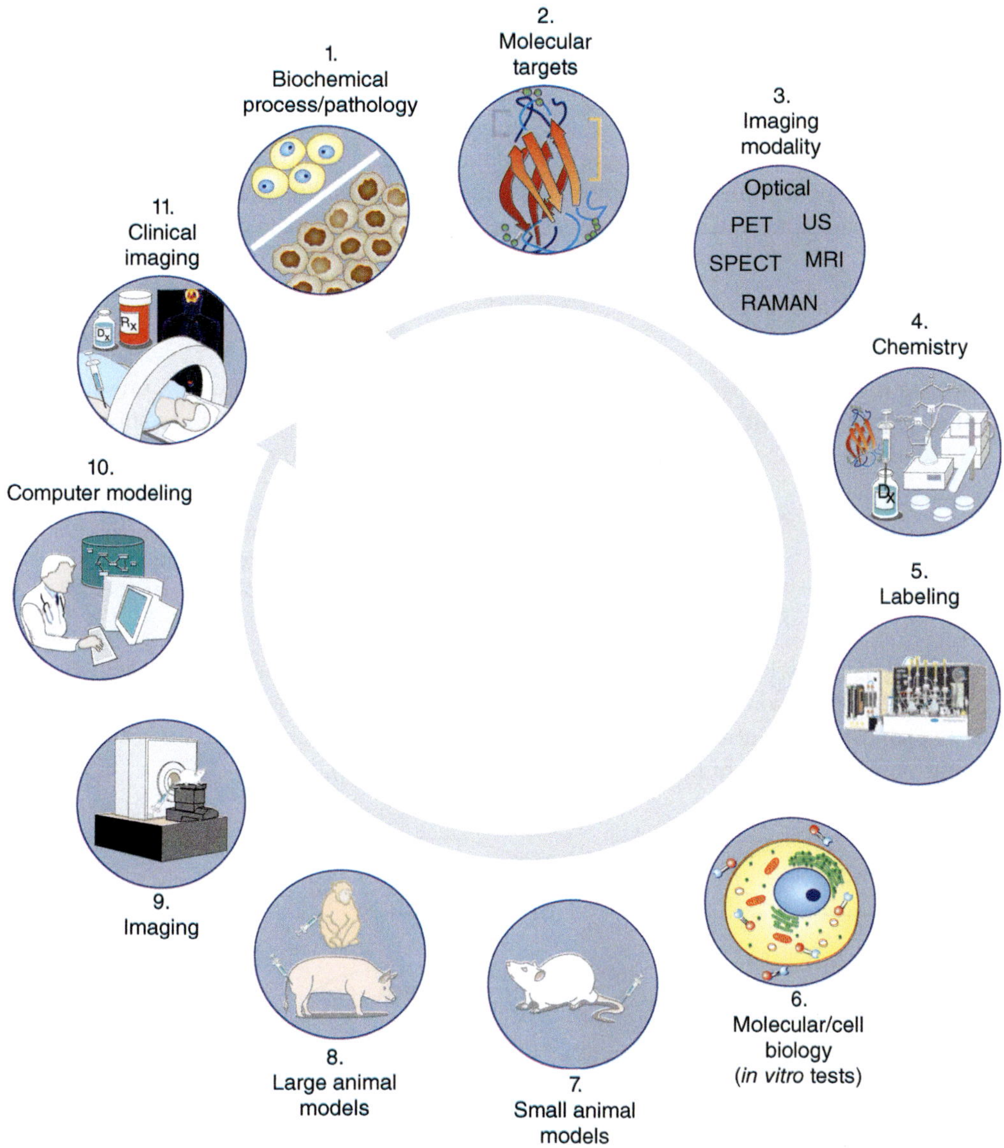

Figure 18.15 11 steps of clinical translation. *Source:* James and Gambhir [8]. Reprinted by permission from The American Physiological Society: Physiological Reviews. Copyright © 2012 by The American Physiological Society.

provide early assessment of treatment efficacy. For example, imaging in personalized medicine could significantly decrease the three-month time period that is currently necessary to evaluate if a proposed chemotherapy treatment is effective, which increases the flexibility of selecting different treatments. In addition, imaging can enable early detection of disease relapse, in which cancer can come back, but to do so, relapse markers must be identified and imaged. This is difficult because patients at risk for relapse may have residual markers that would confound early detection methods. Intraoperative imaging can be used for surgical guidance, e.g. for brain tumor resection guidance. Finally, imaging can help assess new drug efficacy, such as the monitoring of an MMP-2 inhibitor drug.

18.4 Conclusion

This course has presented some of the commonly used medical imaging technologies and some of the upcoming molecular imaging technologies. The underlying physical basis of these imaging instruments and the physical mechanisms that produce imaging contrast were covered. Some powerful real-world applications of imaging technologies, as well as illustrations of why there are several very important clinical needs where imaging is necessary have been presented.

Problems

18.1 We constructed the imaging agent shown in Figure 18.16, where molecule X prevents the entire agent from going into the cell, and the MMP-2 cleavable sequence is a short amino acid sequence that is recognized and cut by the matrix metalloproteinase-2 (MMP-2).

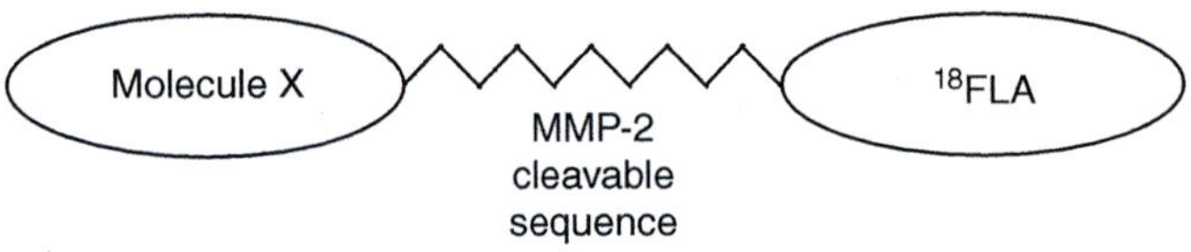

Figure 18.16 Schematic of a new imaging agent, which contains two molecules held together by a cleavable sequence.

A From your knowledge of MMP-2 action and ^{18}FLA, what does this imaging agent aim to image? Explain your answer and refer to the likely targeting mechanism.

B Explain how each of the following control imaging agents helps prove the specificity of the new imaging agent to the targets you mentioned in (a).

i.

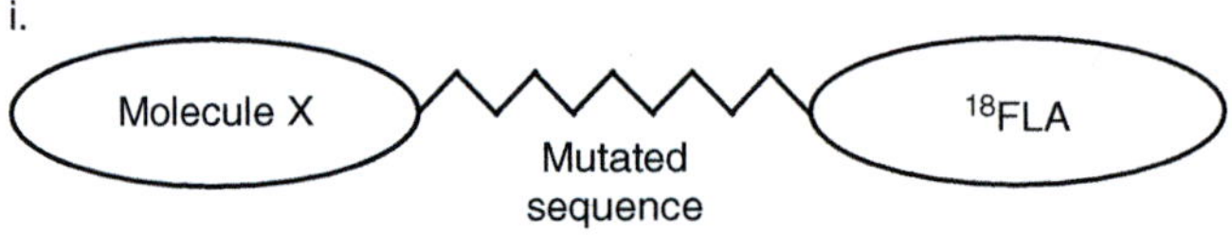

ii.

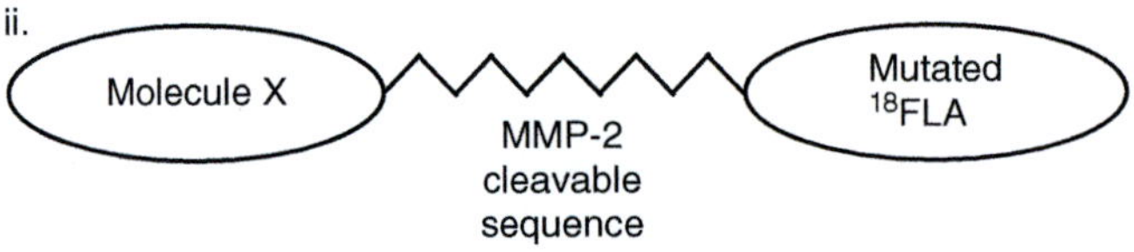

18.2 After finding that CA-1891 is upregulated in the bloodstream of stomach cancer patients, your research team observed this protein is also expressed on the surface of the stomach cancer cells. To detect the tumor, anti-CA-1891 antibody has been generated, and tested with photoacoustic imaging techniques. Single-walled carbon nanotubes (SWNT) were conjugated with anti-CA-1891 antibodies, and injected into immunodeficient mice bearing human stomach tumors. A clear photoacoustic signal was observed four hours post injection to the mice. What kinds of control experiments can you do to confirm that these observed signals are real? List at least 4 "what ifs" for this experiment, and describe corresponding control experiments to address the question. Also, outline what are the possible outcomes of the control experiments and the meaning of them.

18.3 A group of researchers have developed a novel imaging method for fluorescence imaging. Instead of one imaging agent that contains both a targeting moiety and a signaling moiety,

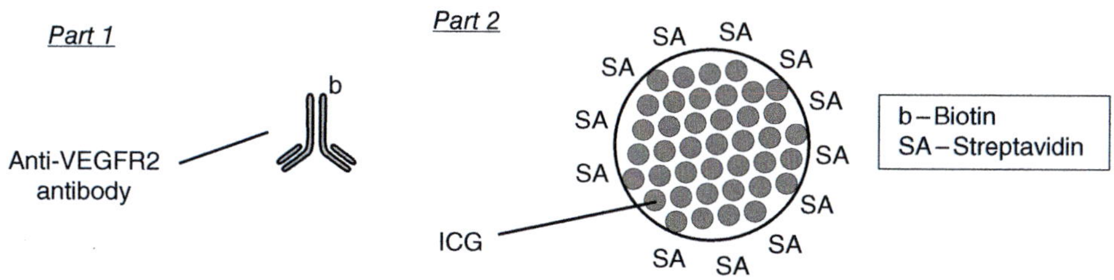

Figure 18.17 Schematic of a new two-part imaging agent against VEGFR2.

they have separated the two functionalities into two parts (Figure 18.17). The first part is an **antibody** against VEGFR2 (vascular endothelial growth factor receptor 2 – a receptor that is commonly over-expressed on the blood vessels of tumors undergoing angiogenesis). However, the anti-VEGFR2 antibody has been modified with a biotin molecule. The second part of the agent is a micron-sized bead (a.k.a. **microbead**) filled with millions of ICG molecules (see illustration) and covered on its surface with streptavidin. This microbead is so bright that a single such bead can be detected with a fluorescence imaging signal when implanted superficially in a mouse. Streptavidin and biotin bind with each other very strongly. However, the researchers are a little concerned that since the microbead is so large, a single biotin-streptavidin bond will not suffice to keep it attached to a target, especially when targeting a protein like VEGFR2 that is expressed on the blood vessels, where there is a constant flow of blood that may knock off the microbead.

The researchers have tested their imaging agent in mice that were administered with breast cancer tumors. First the researchers have intravenously injected the antibodies (part 1 of the imaging agent), and five hours later, they intravenously injected the microbeads (part 2 of the imaging agent). The microbeads circulate in the blood for 20 minutes after which they were cleared from the blood and the researchers took a fluorescence image of the tumor area and the surrounding healthy tissue. Much to their excitement, they saw the tumor lighting up with bright fluorescence signal while the healthy tissue surrounding the tumor was completely dark.

A Describe what is the mechanism of targeting that allows visualizing overexpression of VEGFR2 in the tumor but does not show *any* signal in healthy tissues. You may use Figure 18.18 to explain.

Figure 18.18 Drawing for explaining the targeting mechanism of a new imaging agent.

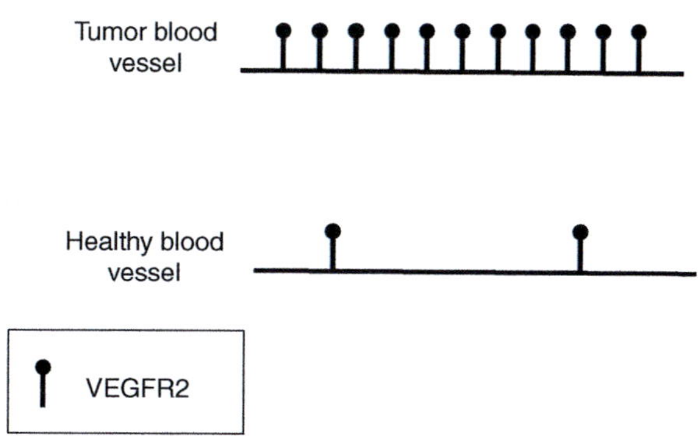

B Control experiments:

vi) Clearly based on this experiment alone, one cannot fully prove the hypothesis that this agent is able to image the overexpression of VEGFR2 in the tumors. Still, based on this experiment, what can you say about the imaging agent and its ability to target?

vii) The researchers were also a little concerned that this experiment did not fully proof their hypothesis about the imaging agent being able to image overexpression of VEGFR2 in tumors. For the following control experiments, *find a reasonable "what if" statement, explain the rationale behind this control design, describe what are the possible outcomes* and *their meaning regarding the hypothesis of the researchers.*

a) Replace part 1 with antibodies against VEGFR2 but without biotin.

b) Replace part 2 with microbeads without streptavidin on their surface.

viii) A new anticancer drug just entered the market by storm as it is able to reduce the levels of VEGFR2 in the tumor's blood vessels back to their normal level in healthy tissues. However, it only works well in 50% of breast cancer patients, and does not affect the VEGFR2 levels in the other 50% of patients. You would like to use the imaging agent in this question to help patients undergoing treatment by this drug know if they respond to the drug or not. Your hypothesis is that three days after the treatment by this drug started, the imaging agent should be able to indicate whether the drug is effective or not. Design a lead experiment and one control experiment to prove this hypothesis (notice you are asked to design two experiments!). For the control experiment, explain what was the rationale for this control experiment and which "what if" statement it tackles.

18.4 A group of researchers developed a new chemotherapy drug against breast cancer. Now, they would like to develop a photoacoustic imaging agent that will be used on every patient receiving this drug to help identify, as early as possible, which patients respond to the drug and which do not. To achieve that, the researchers took a gold nanorod and attached it to Annexin-V. Annexin-V is known to bind to PS, a protein that is expressed on the surface of cells that undergo apoptosis (programmed cell death). They called their new photoacoustic imaging agent Agent-X.

To prove Agent-X works well, the researchers took mice implanted with human breast tumors, gave the mice the chemotherapy drug, waited 24 hours, injected agent-X intravenously (i.e. into the mouse blood vessels), and 4 hours later, acquired a photoacoustic image of the tumor and its surroundings. Much to their excitement, the tumor lit up in the photoacoustic image, while the surrounding tissues seemed to have remained mostly dark in the photoacoustic image.

c) The researchers were a little concerned that perhaps this result isn't really proving their hypothesis and that perhaps something else led to these seemingly good results. For the following "what if" statements, *design a control experiment, explain the rationale behind this design, describe what are the possible outcomes* and *their meaning regarding the hypothesis of the researchers.*

i) What if some cells in the tumor are dying regardless of any chemotherapy?

ii) What if Agent-X gets trapped by the tumor nonspecifically through the EPR effect?

d) After running the control experiments, the researchers discovered that while Agent-X bound to all cells that undergo apoptosis (by binding to the PS on their surface), Agent-X *also* got into all areas of the tumor nonspecifically through the EPR effect. However, a cancer researcher from the lab next door, who is studying MMP-2, told them that he tested their new chemotherapy drug and that it has an effect of reducing MMP-2 activity.

Hence, areas of the tumor that respond to the chemotherapy will exhibit low MMP-2 activity, while areas that do not respond will exhibit high MMP-2 activity.

Based on this new information, help the researchers design a *photoacoustic* imaging agent that can measure MMP-2 activity in the tumor. Describe in detail *what your imaging agent looks like and the mechanism of action that allows it to image MMP-2.*

Hint: You can assume that your new imaging agent will also experience the same EPR effect as Agent-X. You may also find fluorophore F useful, as it is very small but has 100% quantum yield (i.e. 100% of the photons it absorbs are converted into emitted fluorescent photons). As a reminder, MMP-2 cuts the following amino acid sequence in the middle: GPLGVRGK.

e) List 2 "what if" statements that will prevent the imaging agent you created in (b) from working properly. Explain why they are truly a concern.

18.5 Particle X is a new dual-modality imaging agent (Figure 18.19). It is composed of a gold nanorod (which produces strong photoacoustic signal) conjugated with Anti-EGFR antibodies. The nanorod is also linked to two fluorescent dyes that make up a FRET pair. These two dyes are linked together by a peptide sequence that is recognized and cleaved by the enzyme MMP-2. Recall that for FRET probes, if the two dyes stay coupled together, they will emit red fluorescence. However, if the two dyes become physically separated from each other, the observed fluorescent signal will be green.

Biology Notes: EGFR is a protein commonly expressed by human tumor cells. MMP-2 is an enzyme that is present within the margin of actively growing tumors.

Particle X is injected into mice that carry human tumors. You can assume that the anti-EGFR antibody causes Particle X to fully bind to EGFR on the tumor within 10 minutes after injection. You can also assume that MMP-2 cleaves the peptide it recognizes within one hour. Photoacoustic images and fluorescence images are acquired two hours after the injection, and bright photoacoustic signal and green fluorescence are observed within the tumor. No such signals are observed within the surrounding healthy tissue.

f) What does Particle X aim to image? Explain and refer to the likely mechanism that results in (1) the observed photoacoustic signal and (2) the observed fluorescent signal.

g) Suppose that you switch the positions of the dyes within the FRET pair. In other words, the nanorod would now be linked to the red fluorophore instead of the green fluoro-

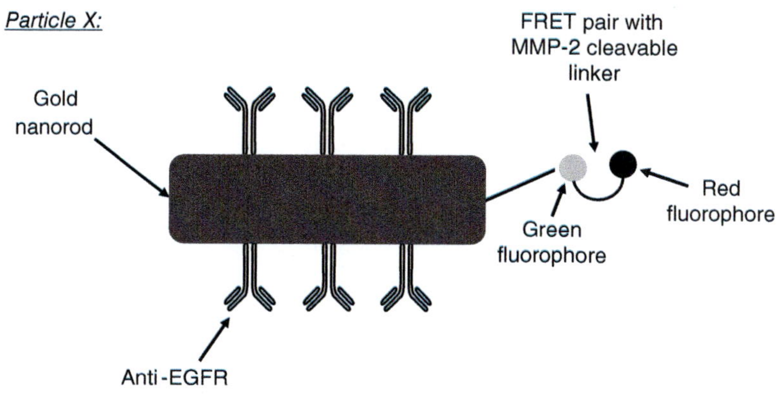

Figure 18.19 Schematic of a new imaging agent consisting of a gold nanorod and FRET pair.

phore. The peptide linker between the two dyes is still recognized by MMP-2. Assuming that you do not change the fluorescent excitation wavelength, do you expect to see red, green, or no fluorescence in EGFR-positive tumors with active MMP-2 at two hours? Explain the rationale for this result, and plot the expected photoacoustic and fluorescent signals (both green and red fluorescence levels) over the two-hour time period.

References

1 de la Zerda, A., Zavaleta, C., Keren, S. et al. (2008). Carbon nanotubes as photoacoustic molecular imaging agents in living mice. *Nature Nanotechnology* 3: 557–562.
2 Bremer, C., Tung, C.-H., and Weissleder, R. (2001). in vivo molecular target assessment of matrix metalloproteinase. *Nature Medicine* 7: 743–748.
3 Saslow, D., Boetes, C., Burke, W., Harms, S., Leach, M. O., Lehman, C. D., Morris, E., Pisano, E., Schnall, M., Sener, S., Smith, R. A., Warner, E., Yaffe, M., Andrews, K. S., Russell, C. A. and (2007), American Cancer Society guidelines for breast screening with MRI as an adjunct to mammography. *CA: A Cancer Journal for Clinicians*, 57: 75-89. doi:https://doi.org/10.3322/canjclin.57.2.75
4 de la Zerda, A., Bodapati, S., Teed, R. et al. (2012). Family of enhanced photoacoustic imaging agents for high-sensitivity and multiplexing studies in living mice. *American Chemical Society* 6 (6): 4694–4701.
5 de la Zerda, A., Liu, Z., Bodapati, S. et al. (2010). Ultrahigh sensitivity carbon nanotube agents for photoacoustic molecular imaging in living mice. *American Chemical Society* 10 (6): 2168–2172.
6 Cohade, C., Osman, M., Leal, J., and Wahl, R.L. (2003). Direct comparison of 18F-FDG PET and PET/CT in patients with colorectal carcinoma. *Journal of Nuclear Medicine* 44 (11): 1797–1803.
7 Kircher, M.F., de la Zerda, A., Jokerst, J.V. et al. (2012). A brain tumor molecular imaging strategy using a new triple-modality MRI-photoacoustic-Raman nanoparticle. *Nature Medicine* 18: 829–834.
8 James, M.L. and Gambhir, S.S. (2012). A molecular imaging primer: modalities, imaging agents, and applications. *Physiological Reviews* 92 (2): 897–965.

Further Reading

Burnside, E.S., Trentham-Dietz, A., Kelcz, F. et al. (2006). J. An example of breast cancer regression on imaging. *Radiology Case Reports. [Online]* 1: 4.
Thibodeau, G.A. (2008). *Structure & Function of the Body*, 13ee. Mosby.
Adam de la Zerda, unpublished results
Zhang et al. (2006). *Nature Biotechnology* .

Index

Biochips and Medical Imaging, First Edition. Adam de la Zerda and Shan Xiang Wang.

b

c

m

n

o

p

q

r

Printed and bound by CPI Group (UK) Ltd, Croydon, CR0 4YY

16/09/2026

14963428-0001